Little, Brown's Paperback Book Series

Basic Medical Sciences

Boyd & Hoer	Basic Medical Microbiology
Colton	Statistics in Medicine
Hine and Pfeiffer	Behavioral Science
Kent	General Pathology: A Programmed Text
Levine	Pharmacology
Peery & Miller	Pathology
Richardson	Basic Circulatory Physiology
Roland et al.	Atlas of Cell Biology
Selkurt	Physiology
Sidman & Sidman	Neuroanatomy: A Programmed Text
Siegel, Albers, et al.	Basic Neurochemistry
Snell	Clinical Anatomy for Medical Students
Snell	Clinical Embryology for Medical Students
Streilein & Hughes	Immunology: A Programmed Text
Valtin	Renal Function
Watson	Basic Human Neuroanatomy

Clinical Medical Sciences

Clark & MacMahon	Preventive Medicine
Daube et al.	Medical Neurosciences
Eckert	Emergency-Room Care
Grabb & Smith	Plastic Surgery
Green	Gynecology
Gregory & Smeltzer	Psychiatry
Judge & Zuidema	Methods of Clinical Examination
MacAusland & Mayo	Orthopedics
Nardi & Zuidema	Surgery
Niswander	Obstetrics
Thompson	Primer of Clinical Radiology
Wilkins & Levinsky	Medicine
Ziai	Pediatrics

Manuals and Handbooks

Alpert & Francis	Manual of Coronary Care
Arndt	Manual of Dermatologic Therapeutics
Berk et al.	Handbook of Critical Care
Bochner et al.	Handbook of Clinical Pharmacology
Children's Hospital Medical Center, Boston	Manual of Pediatric Therapeutics
Condon & Nyhus	Manual of Surgical Therapeutics
Friedman & Papper	Problem-Oriented Medical Diagnosis
Gardner & Provine	Manual of Acute Bacterial Infections
Iversen & Clawson	Manual of Acute Orthopaedic Therapeutics
Massachusetts General Hospital	Clinical Anesthesia Procedures
Massachusetts General Hospital	Diet Manual
Massachusetts General Hospital	Manual of Nursing Procedures
Neelon & Ellis	A Syllabus of Problem-Oriented Patient Care
Papper	Manual of Medical Care of the Surgical Patient
Shader	Manual of Psychiatric Therapeutics
Snow	Manual of Anesthesia
Spivak & Barnes	Manual of Clinical Problems in Internal Medicine: Annotated with Key References
Wallach	Interpretation of Diagnostic Tests
Washington University Department of Medicine	Manual of Medical Therapeutics
Zimmerman	Techniques of Patient Care

Little, Brown and Company
34 Beacon Street
Boston, Massachusetts 02106

Pharmacology: Drug Actions and Reactions

Pharmacology:
Drug Actions and Reactions

Second Edition

Ruth R. Levine, Ph.D.
Professor of Pharmacology and
Chairman, Division of Medical and
Dental Sciences, Boston University
School of Medicine, Boston

Foreword by Byron B. Clark, Ph.D.
Director, Pharmacology-Toxicology Program,
National Institute of General Medical Sciences,
National Institutes of Health, Bethesda

Little, Brown and Company   Boston

To Martin

The second edition of this book is dedicated to
the memory of a beloved friend and
respected colleague

Aldo P. Truant
1920–1973

FOREWORD

The mode of action of drugs is not generally understood by people outside certain health professions. However, public awareness and concern about the intermittent or daily exposure of large segments of the population to drugs and other chemicals is greater today than ever before. Interest in drugs now extends far beyond their therapeutic use in the treatment of disease. For the first time, a large population of normal people receive drugs over long periods, as illustrated by the oral contraceptives. Recently, the dramatic increase in the use of street drugs and drugs of abuse in all age groups has greatly expanded public awareness of drugs. In addition, increasing numbers of chemicals appear in our environment as food additives, economic insecticides, and fertilizers and as industrial pollutants in air, water and food. It is abundantly clear that the science of pharmacology has relevance to a growing number in our society.

There is an obvious need for an authoritative book covering the general aspects of pharmacology and addressed to individuals of diverse backgrounds and occupations who wish to acquire an understanding of how chemical agents affect living processes. Such a book should be useful not just to students in the health professions but to biologists, chemists, public health officials, lawyers, legislators, administrators, science instructors and intelligent laymen as well.

Pharmacology: Drug Actions and Reactions is the consummate result of an earnest, scholarly and pioneering effort to present an explanation of the science of pharmacology in terms of general concepts and principles governing chemical-biologic interactions. This is a logical approach to cover the multitude of chemical agents and the diversified interests of the intended reader; the principles will endure even though today's drugs may change. With the background provided by this book, one will be prepared to understand the actions of most individual drugs. In addition, a sufficient number of important, specific examples are included to illustrate the application of the principles.

Much of the material presented in the book is oriented toward therapeutic agents, but the concepts and principles apply equally to most nontherapeutic and toxic chemicals; furthermore, specific attention is given to toxicology. Great effort has been expended in making the text self-contained and understandable. The style is straightforward and lucid. The carefully selected illustrations and examples are simple and clear.

The author of this book is well known for her many research contributions in pharmacology over the years and for her thorough understanding of the subject. She has been a dedicated scholar and teacher of students in the health professions and in recent years has been a lecturer to nonprofessional groups as well. It was my pleasure to have guided her doctoral studies and to have collaborated in research with her during my tenure as chairman of the Department of Pharmacology at Tufts University School of Medicine.

The above was written as the foreword to the first edition. It is still relevant in its entirety, since the present edition incorporates additional and new material without changing the approach that has proved to be so successful in presenting the general aspects of pharmacology. The new chapter on drug actions affecting the fundamental properties of all cells and those influencing the autonomic nervous system, as well as the appended details of the pharmacology of various important classes of drugs, will, moreover, greatly enhance the reader's understanding of the mode of action of drugs. The thought-provoking questions newly provided at the end of each chapter will guide the serious student in mastering the fundamental principles of the interaction of drugs and living organisms.

Byron B. Clark

PREFACE TO THE SECOND EDITION

The philosophy guiding the writing of this textbook, as stated in the preface to the first edition, was to present a comprehensive and coherent explanation of the science of pharmacology in terms of its basic concepts and principles. The text's wide acceptance by college students majoring in diverse fields as well as by students in medicine, nursing and veterinary medicine affirms that this was a logical approach to use. I am most grateful for this favorable reception. That the guiding concept was also realistic is evident from the fact that, despite rapid advances in the medical sciences, no revisions have been needed in these aspects of the original text. The text and references have been updated, however, to reflect advances in our understanding of receptors, of kidney function and of various other processes, and to indicate the changes in environmental and occupational toxicology and in new drug development brought about by recent legislation. Since students have indicated the usefulness of the Glossary, this portion of the book has also been amended to include additional terms in current usage. But it is the wholly new sections which have been added that clearly distinguish the present edition from its predecessor.

The textbook has been enlarged by addition of a new chapter and study guide questions at the end of each chapter, and by new appendixes prepared to meet the needs of students who wish to supplement their knowledge of the basic principles of drug action with more specific information about some of the therapeutic agents currently in widespread use. These sections were developed originally as teaching aids in my own undergraduate course in pharmacology. Their proved usefulness to several hundred students and the favorable comments of many colleagues have encouraged the incorporation of these teaching materials into the textbook itself.

The new Chapter 13, How Drugs Alter Physiologic Function: A Recapitulation, is a summary of the various mechanisms by which drugs may influence and alter physiologic functions and biochemical processes. The major portion of this chapter is concerned with the general aspects of the anatomy, physiology and biochemistry of the autonomic nervous system and with the ways in which drugs affect autonomic nervous system activity.

The approach used in the presentation of Appendixes 1-6 is both descriptive and operational. The material presented is, however, only introductory; comprehensive sources such as those listed in Chapter 2 should be consulted for more detailed information about the drugs discussed as well as those that are not included. Appendix 1 deals with two groups of nonprescription drugs widely used by the laity — the antacids and laxative-cathartics. Appendix 2 is a synopsis of drugs that influence kidney function, a topic chosen primarily because the action of these drugs can be so well identified and characterized in terms of known physiologic functions and processes. Appendix 3 summarizes some important aspects of the use of chemotherapeutic agents in the treatment of parasitic and neoplastic diseases. Appendix 4 discusses the nature of pain and the principal classes of drugs used to treat pain: local anesthetics, nonnarcotic analgesics, narcotic analgesics, and general anesthetics as exemplified by alcohol. Appendix 5 continues the discussion of central nervous system depressants by summarizing the actions of drugs used as sedatives and hypnotics. Finally, Appendix 6 deals briefly with drugs used in the treatment of mental disorders.

I want to express my gratitude to my publishers, Little, Brown and Company, whose careful editing and sound judgment added immeasurably to the success this text has enjoyed. In addition to acknowledging again my debt to all those who helped launch the first edition of this book, my thanks are due to the many students and readers whose enthusiastic reception of the first edition encouraged and promoted the preparation of this new one.

R. R. L.

Boston

PREFACE TO THE FIRST EDITION

Pharmacology is the unified study of the properties of chemical agents (drugs) and living organisms and all aspects of their interactions. So defined, it is an expansive science encompassing areas of interest germane to many other disciplines. The specific pharmacologic knowledge needed by the physician, who uses chemicals as therapeutic agents, differs from that of the biochemist or physiologist, who uses chemicals as tools in research. Likewise, this knowledge is different for the ecologist or legislator, who is sensitive to the consequences or responsibilities inherent in the widespread use of chemical agents. There is, however, a body of information dealing with the basic concepts and principles that is fundamental to understanding the actions of drugs in every aspect of this science, theoretical or applied, and at any level of complexity.

The purpose of this book is to provide a concise source of that core of pharmacologic knowledge that can be shared by all wishing to acquire an understanding of how chemical agents affect living processes. The emphasis is placed, therefore, on fundamental concepts as they apply to the actions of most drugs. In order to illustrate the underlying principles, some agents that are in general use or are subjects of public concern are singled out for fuller discussion. Certain therapeutic conditions are also discussed in order to provide an understanding of the basis of drug therapy. The nontherapeutic or toxicologic aspects of drug action are given special attention since the widespread exposure of living organisms to a multitude of chemicals is of grave public significance.

This book is written for individuals of diverse backgrounds who have in common a working knowledge of general chemistry and biology. The biochemical and physiologic principles needed to understand pharmacologic principles form an integral part of the text. In order to provide more coherence and greater ease in reading, individual statements have not been scientifically documented with references to the pertinent literature. At the end of each chapter, however, some specific as well as some general references are listed for those who desire more extensive information. And in the body of the text certain words or phrases are printed in boldface type to indicate that a fuller explanation of the term is contained in the Glossary. The Glossary of more than one hundred entries also provides a handy reference for most terms defined throughout the text.

I have tried to prepare a text that alone will provide the nonprofessional with a basic understanding of pharmacology but that may also serve as an introduction for those who will be professionally concerned with the interactions of drugs and living organisms. I hope, too, that this book will serve the further purpose of implementing the presentation of pharmacology in nonprofessional schools so that students in biology, chemistry, psychology, physical education, and premedical programs as well as those in other fields will have the opportunity to acquire some training in one of the youngest of the experimental medical sciences — pharmacology.

R. R. L.

Boston

CONTENTS

Foreword by Byron B. Clark   vii
Preface to the Second Edition   ix
Preface to the First Edition   xi

1. **THE HERITAGE OF PHARMACOLOGY**   1
   The Beginnings   1
   The Rise of Pharmacology   8
   Synopsis   14

2. **THE SCOPE OF PHARMACOLOGY – DEFINITIONS**   17
   Drug Nomenclature   19
   Sources of Information about Drugs   21

3. **HOW DRUGS ACT ON THE LIVING ORGANISM**   27
   Site of Action   31
   Mechanism of Action   34
   Synopsis   46

4. **HOW DRUGS REACH THEIR SITE OF ACTION: I. GENERAL PRINCIPLES OF PASSAGE OF DRUGS ACROSS BIOLOGIC BARRIERS**   49
   Passive Diffusion   51
   Specialized Transport Processes   63
   Filtration   68
   Synopsis   69

xiii

5. HOW DRUGS REACH THEIR SITE OF ACTION: II. ABSORPTION
   AND DISTRIBUTION   73
   Absorption   74
   Distribution   99

6. HOW THE ACTIONS OF DRUGS ARE TERMINATED   117
   Excretion   118
   Biotransformation   139
   Synopsis   165

7. GENERAL PRINCIPLES OF THE QUANTITATIVE ASPECTS OF
   DRUG ACTION: I. DOSE-RESPONSE RELATIONSHIPS   169
   Quantitative Aspects of Drug-Receptor Interactions   170
   The Quantal Dose-Response Relationship   184
   The Selectivity of Drug Action   195
   Synopsis   197

8. GENERAL PRINCIPLES OF THE QUANTITATIVE ASPECTS OF
   DRUG ACTION: II. TIME-RESPONSE RELATIONSHIPS   205
   Rate of Drug Absorption   209
   Rate of Drug Elimination   211
   The Time Course of Drug Action after Single Doses   224
   The Kinetics of Drug Accumulation following Multiple Doses   228
   Synopsis   236

9. FACTORS MODIFYING THE EFFECTS OF DRUGS IN
   INDIVIDUALS: VARIABILITY IN RESPONSE ATTRIBUTABLE
   TO THE BIOLOGIC SYSTEM   241
   Body Weight and Size   242
   Age   243
   Sex   247
   Genetic Factors   247
   General Conditions of Health   261
   Psychologic Factors: The Placebo Effect   262

10. FACTORS MODIFYING THE EFFECTS OF DRUGS IN
    INDIVIDUALS: VARIABILITY IN RESPONSE ATTRIBUTABLE
    TO THE CONDITIONS OF ADMINISTRATION   267
    Modified Drug Effects after Repeated Administration of a Single Drug   267
    Drug Interactions   283
    Synopsis   293

11. **DRUG TOXICITY** — 301
Classifications of Toxic Reactions — 303
Evaluation of Drug Toxicity — 310
Incidence of Poisoning — 319
Treatment of Toxicity — 326
Synopsis — 336

12. **THE PHARMACOLOGIC ASPECTS OF DRUG ABUSE AND DRUG DEPENDENCE** — 341
The Functional Organization of the Central Nervous System — 342
General Characteristics of Drug Dependence — 348
General Depressants of the Central Nervous System — 352
Narcotic Analgesics — 355
Stimulants of the Central Nervous System — 359
Psychedelics (Hallucinogens) — 361
Synopsis — 366

13. **HOW DRUGS ALTER PHYSIOLOGIC FUNCTION: A RECAPITULATION** — 371
Drug Actions Influencing the Fundamental Properties Common to all Cells — 372
Drug Actions Influencing the Autonomic Nervous System — 373

14. **THE DEVELOPMENT AND EVALUATION OF NEW DRUGS** — 391
Development and Evaluation in the Laboratory — 391
Clinical Studies — 400
The New Drug Application (NDA) — 407
Concluding Remarks — 409

GLOSSARY — 413

APPENDIXES — 431
1. Locally Acting Drugs Affecting the Gastrointestinal Tract — 433
2. Drugs Influencing Renal Function — 438
3. Chemotherapy — 444
4. Drugs Used to Alter the Perception of and Response to Pain — 454
5. Sedatives and Hypnotics — 469
6. Drugs Used in the Treatment of Mental Disorders — 475
7. Weights and Measures — 482

Index — 485

Pharmacology: Drug Actions and Reactions

1. THE HERITAGE OF PHARMACOLOGY

An acquaintance with the history of a subject frequently reveals the true nature
of the subject. Tracing the growth of pharmacology, then, from its earliest beginnings
will give us a sharper perspective of the scope of the field and a clearer understanding
of what distinguishes pharmacology today as an orderly science in its own right. In
the words of the Nobel laureate Albert Szent-Györgyi, "If we want to see ahead we
must look back."

THE BEGINNINGS

Man's use of medicinals is as old as man himself, since his need to find measures to
combat sickness has always been as important to his survival as his need for food and
shelter. Early man's efforts in dealing with disease, colored as they were by his superstitious concepts of the causes of illness, led him to search for animate and inanimate objects in his environment with which to drive away the evil spirits. But the
successes of science frequently have their roots in the absurdities of magic, and some
of our important drugs were discovered through primitive man's experiments with
the plants that grew around him. The use of alcohol and opium to ease pain, of
cinchona bark (the source of quinine) to treat malaria and of ipecac for amebic dysentery can be cited as examples of early man's therapeutic successes despite his ignorance of the causes of these ailments. Some of his failures can also be called
valuable discoveries, since drugs like curare, veratrine and ouabain, known only as
fatal poisons by primitive cultures in various regions of the world, have now become
valuable therapeutic agents when used in proper amounts. Thus the accumulation
of this primitive medical lore and its dissemination and use by midwives, priests,
witch doctors and other practitioners were the beginnings of **materia medica,**[1]medi-
cine and toxicology.

Egypt and Babylonia

The Egyptians are to be credited with handing down to us the oldest known records
of medicine, even though the medical systems of Sumaria, Babylonia and India are

[1]Terms appearing in **boldface type** are defined in the Glossary.

probably of equal antiquity. The most ancient of the records devoted entirely to medicine is the Medical Papyrus of Smith (ca. 1600 B.C.E.).[2] It clearly indicates that the Egyptians had developed a codified and conventionalized form of therapy for a great variety of diseases and had differentiated between those clinical conditions that could be treated successfully and those that could not. The Ebers' Papyrus (1550 B.C.E.), the largest of the Egyptian medical papyri, lists more than seven hundred remedies and describes in detail the procedures for their preparation and administration for specific ailments. Many of these prescriptions plainly show their magical origins in the inclusion of incantations together with ingredients such as lizard's blood, an old book boiled in oil, the thigh bone of a hanged man and excreta or organs of various domestic animals. But there is also reference to liver as a remedy for anemia and to modern drugs, such as castor oil, squill and opium. This close alliance of medicine and religious beliefs was to continue for many, many centuries and even today has not been completely broken.

As Egyptian medicine developed, it gave rise to great physicians and surgeons whose knowledge was unsurpassed even by the famous Greek physicians who came later. The Egyptians not only advocated professional standards of conduct that were to influence the Hippocratic code of medical ethics but also developed medical specialization. For example, some physicians limited their practice to obstetrics, gynecology or gastric disorders. For the first time the patient was given the choice of witch doctor or which doctor. The Egyptians can also take credit for some of the earliest concerns about public health in their promotion of public sanitation through a system of copper pipes for the collection of rainwater and the disposal of sewage.

The known contributions of the Babylonians to medicine appear to be fewer and of lesser consequence than those of the Egyptians. This may be related to the differences in their religious philosophies. The Egyptian had a comforting mythology that made him feel secure in his world; he believed that the supernatural powers were concerned with promoting his welfare. The Babylonian, on the other hand, lived in a hostile world in which demons were everywhere and were always ready to descend upon a victim in the form of sickness. Although the code of Hammurabi (2123–2081 B.C.E.) established the profession of physician as separate from that of clergy, with doctors' fees set by law, the highly superstitious populace demanded the irrational treatment purveyed by the sorcerers. Yet despite this contrast in medical culture between the Egyptians and the Babylonians, it was the latter who transmitted the foundations of medicine to India and Greece and even supplied the names of many Greek drugs.

Greece and India
In both the Greek and Indian cultures, the earliest records disclose that secular medicine was practiced but still had to compete with that of the priesthood. For even though disease was treated by both medicinals and charms, the most common

---

[2]B.C.E.: before the common (Christian) era; C.E.: common era.

place for treatment was the temple. In Greece, with its luxuriant mythology and its plethora of deities, separate temples were built to Asclepius, the God of Healing, and these became virtually sanatoriums or hospitals for the sick. The greatest of these temples was built atop a high mountain peak at Epidaurus, to which people flocked from all parts of the Mediterranean area. Near the present-day ruins of this temple-sanatorium is an almost perfectly preserved theater built in the fourth century B.C.E. and paid for by the fees and largess of the temple's patients.

Secular medicine was fostered by and developed around the celebrated centers of learning. In India, the universities at Taxila (present-day Pakistan) and Benares, famous for their medical schools, and in Greece the four prestigious schools at Cos and Cnidus (in Asia Minor), Crotona (in Italy) and Acragas (in Sicily) produced some of the most illustrious men associated with the medical sciences of antiquity.

Sushruta (ca. 500 B.C.E.), one of the renowned names of Hindu science, was professor of medicine at the University of Benares. He described and laid down elaborate rules for many surgical procedures and was also probably the first to graft skin from one portion of the body to another and to attempt aseptic surgery by sterilization of wounds. Sushruta also recommended diagnosis by inspection, palpation and auscultation for the detection of the 1,120 diseases he described.

In the sixth century B.C.E., vaccination for smallpox was known and probably practiced in India. Evidence for this appears in writings attributed to one of the earliest Hindu physicians, Dhanwantari (550 B.C.E.): "Take the fluid of a pock on the udder of the cow . . . upon the point of a lancet, and lance with it the arms between the shoulders and the elbows until the blood appears; then, mixing the fluid with the blood, the fever of the small-pox will be produced." Yet vaccination for smallpox and the aseptic surgery practiced by Sushruta were unknown in Europe for another two thousand years. It may well be that there were still other advances that the Hindus could have contributed to Europeans, if the latter had had wider acquaintance with the culture of India and if there had been better transmission and acceptance of Indian knowledge.

The impact of the Indians on the advancement of medicine depends on whether one speaks about their contributions to European medicine or about the practice of medicine in India itself. In contrast, the preeminent Greek physicians of this period had a far-reaching effect on medicine and pharmacy; their influence was to pervade the ensuing years.

Development of Medical Ethics
It was the great teacher Hippocrates (460–377 B.C.E.) and his successors who really freed medicine from mysticism and philosophy and made it reliant upon rational therapy. Hippocrates taught the doctrine that disease stems from natural causes and that knowledge is gained only through study of the natural laws; he sought to explain Nature in Nature's terms. Since Hippocrates believed that the body has ample natural resources for recuperation and that the role of the physician was to remove or reduce the impediments to this natural defense, he made little use of drugs. He relied mainly upon fresh air, good food, purgatives and enemas, blood-letting,

massage and hydrotherapy, and used sparingly only a few of the four hundred drugs mentioned in his writings. However, Hippocrates is known as the Father of Medicine not just for his rational doctrine but mainly for his emphasis on medical ethics. The famous oath attributed to him did much to ennoble the medical profession by setting a standard of professional conduct to which subsequent generations of physicians have sworn fealty.

The emancipation from religious beliefs and the setting of high standards of ethics were the two most important contributions that the Greeks made directly to medicine; the art itself was not advanced to any degree beyond that achieved by the Egyptians of a millenium earlier. The Age of Greece did contribute to some important progress, however, in pharmacy, anatomy and physiology.

Development of Pharmacy

Theophrastus (372–287 B.C.E.), in his classic treatise *The History of Plants,* provided a summary of all that was known about the medicinal properties of plants. This work was later used by Dioscorides (57 C.E.), Nero's surgeon, in the preparation of a materia medica which scientifically described six hundred plants, classified for the first time by substance rather than by disease. It remained the chief source of pharmaceutic knowledge until the sixteenth century, and Dioscorides is honored as the Father of Materia Medica.

Development of Anatomy and Physiology

Herophilus, perhaps the greatest anatomist of antiquity, and Erasistratus, probably the most outstanding physiologist of ancient times, were contemporaries of Theophrastus. They developed their respective disciplines to heights which would be attained only once again before the Renaissance. Herophilus carried out remarkable dissections, named various parts of the human body and even understood the role of nerves, differentiating for the first time between sensory and motor nerves. He understood so completely the function of the artery that he might well be credited with the discovery of the circulation of blood nineteen centuries before Harvey.

Erasistratus also made noteworthy advances in dissection and in understanding the function of arteries, veins and nerves as well as some of their interrelationships. Although Hippocratic medicine developed the rational approach to therapy, it was Erasistratus who rejected the final ties of medicine to mystical entities. Hippocratic medicine was bound to the doctrine of so-called humors, the composition of the body being blood, phlegm, yellow bile and black bile, and illness or pain being brought about by a change in the proportion of these humors. Erasistratus abandoned this humoral theory and tried to account for all physiologic phenomena on the basis of natural causes. Unfortunately, it was the Hippocratic theory which became the heritage of medicine, being ultimately discarded only in the nineteenth century.

The Roman Era

After the conquest of Greece, the heritage of Greek medicine migrated to Rome. With their great sense of order, the Romans organized medicine, trained physicians in state schools, built military and private hospitals and provided for public sanitation. But their most useful contribution was the compilation of encyclopedic summaries of knowledge which prepared the way for future advances. In medicine, the foremost was that of Aurelius Celsus (first century B.C.E.); when rediscovered in the fifteenth century, his *De Medicina* played a major role in fostering the reconstruction of medicine.

Although the Romans formulated and applied their borrowed medicine in able fashion, they contributed little of real significance to the development of Western medical science. Even the one outstanding original scientist of this period — Galen (131–201 C.E.) — was a Greek physician.

Galen was one of the first true experimental physiologists. For example, in neurology he performed experiments by which, in serial sectioning of the spinal cord, he was able to distinguish the sensory and motor functions of each segment of the cord. Galen also made many contributions to the field of pharmacy; most noteworthy are his extensions of the work of Dioscorides, introduction of a complicated polypharmacy and origination of the use of **tincture** of opium and preparations of vegetable drugs, still known as "**galenicals**."

Galen missed anticipating the science of pharmacology, however, since he did not carry over the experimental approach to the study of the drugs he used. He further tarnished his record as an experimentalist by ignoring the work of Erasistratus and adopting and enlarging the Hippocratic doctrine of the origin of human illness. Galen added the four elements — earth, air, fire and water — to the four humors — blood, phlegm, yellow bile and black bile — and ascribed the cause of all diseases to derangement of these elements and humors. In Galen's voluminous writings (of the five hundred books reputed to him, one hundred eighteen have survived), he set forth his ideas and his system of medicine and pharmacy with such authority and conviction in his own invincibility that he profoundly affected medicine for fifteen hundred years. Unfortunately, to the detriment of medieval medicine, it was the serious errors embodied in Galen's system of the cause of disease which went uncriticized; these far outweighed in influence his valuable contributions as an accurate observer and experimentalist.

The Middle Ages

In the long span of years between the distinguished Greek physicians and Paracelsus (1493–1541) there were no significant new advances in medical science. This is not to say, however, that progress was not made during the Dark Ages. While the medical sciences were marking time in Europe, the wealth of knowledge that had been accumulated and preserved in the Roman manuscripts passed to the East. Sustained and enriched in turn by the Arab and Jewish physicians, this medical knowledge came back to Europe with the Western movement of the Arabs and the travels of the Crusaders. The diligence of the Christian religious orders in copying manuscripts and in making their monasteries the repositories of all the learning of the past also helped in preserving this knowledge. Notable among those responsible for maintaining the continuum of medicine during the Dark Ages were the Moslem physicians

Abu Bekr Muhammad Al-Razi (844–926), famous in Europe as Rhazes, and Abu Ali al-Husein ibn Sina (980–1037), known as Avicenna, and the Jewish physicians Isaac Israeli (ca. 855–ca. 955) and Moses Maimonides (1135–1204). The medical writings of these men left their mark on European medicine for hundreds of years, being used as authoritative texts as late as the seventeenth century. In addition, Avicenna and his successors preserved the pharmaceutic art of the sixth to sixteenth centuries by compiling and condensing the detailed directions for concocting hundreds of drugs.

The Arab Influence

Although the synthesis of accumulated knowledge, rather than original findings or scientific research, was characteristic of all medieval science, the Arabs between the seventh and eleventh centuries made certain contributions that would prove to be of great consequence to the future development of pharmacology. In chemistry and alchemy, the Saracens, by introducing precision in observation, control in experimentation and meticulous record-keeping, developed the experimental method that was to stimulate the growth of European chemistry five hundred years later. Second, the Moslems, by establishing the first apothecary shops and dispensaries and by founding the first medieval school of pharmacy, dissociated the practice of pharmacy from the profession of medicine. Third, the Arabs, by subjecting pharmacists to state regulations and inspections and by producing the first pharmaceutical formulary, developed standards for preparing and storing drugs. Since druggists who violated these standards by selling deceptive or deteriorated drugs were subject to punishment by law, the medieval Moslems can also be credited with one of the earliest efforts at consumer protection.

Pharmacies as separate establishments for the compounding and dispensing of medicinals began to appear and spread throughout Europe only after the thirteenth century. An illustration contained in a book published just forty-seven years after the invention of printing permits us to visualize one of these medieval apothecary shops (Fig. 1-1). What this early drawing does not show, however, is the close resemblance between the fifteenth century drugstore and that of the present day. Even in medieval times, the druggist sold stationery, confections, jewelry and miscellany along with his pills and drugs in order to augment his income. But the kind of pharmacy practiced in Europe at the end of the Middle Ages was really an art that required a special training. This is perhaps best exemplified by the most popular of all drugs, triaca or theriaca, a weird mixture which in the lifetime of Dioscorides had 57 components and by the fifteenth century had grown to 110 constituents.

As the alchemy of the Arabs swept over Europe in the fifteenth century, it brought, together with its search for the elixir of life and the philosopher's stone, new chemical methods and simpler, relatively pure substances (sulfur, iron and arsenic) which were diverted to medical use. In this period, too, the awakening of medicine and its reliance on ancient therapy, the introduction of new drugs from the East and the proliferation of formularies for the preparation of a vast arsenal of medicinals all pointed toward the necessity of having official regulations and standards. The city

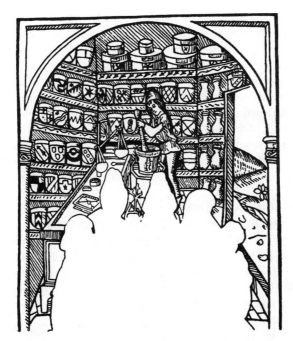

FIGURE 1-1. A medieval apothecary shop. (From P. Schöffer, Gart der Gesundheit, Mainz, 1485, as modified in H. Peters, Pictorial History of Ancient Pharmacy and Medicine. Chicago: Netter, 1889.)

of Florence, Italy, is credited with issuing the first European book endowed with legal sanction for standardization and uniformity in drug preparation. This *Nuovo Receptario,* published in 1498, was distinguished not only as the first official European pharmacopeia, but also as the first *printed* compilation of medicinal preparations. The sixteenth century saw pharmacy come into its own in the Western world, and it will not serve our purpose here to trace further the varied endeavors to standardize drugs which have culminated in national and international pharmacopeias, formularies and other publications in current use.

The Influence of Paracelsus

Aureolus Paracelsus (1493–1541), whose real name was Phillipus Theophrastus Bombastus von Hohenheim, has been called the Grandfather of Pharmacology. As such, he deserves special attention.

Paracelsus was one of the angry young men of his day. He possessed a brillant mind, but his restlessness, arrogance and defiance – his bombast – frequently brought him into conflict with the law as well as with the medical profession. He studied medicine but never obtained a degree, giving it up to experiment with chemistry and alchemy. Even though he never completely separated science from magic, he nevertheless revolutionized therapy by boldly advancing the application of chemistry to medicine. Paracelsus believed that man's body is composed of chemicals; he discarded Galen's theory of humors and advocated the theory that illness is a disturbance of the chemical constituents of the body. He popularized the use of chemical tinctures and extracts and compounded laudanum, the tincture of opium which remains in use today. He spoke out against the indiscriminate use of drug mixtures derived from the plant and animal world, recognizing that any useful substance which they contained was probably diluted to ineffective concentrations by their inert ingredients. He stressed the curative powers of single agents, particularly inorganic materials, such as the use of mercury to treat syphilis. He recognized the relationship between the amount of a drug administered and the beneficial or harmful effects produced, for he wrote: "All things are poisons, for there is nothing without poisonous qualities. It is only the dose which makes a thing a poison."

THE RISE OF PHARMACOLOGY

The advances made by a few men like Paracelsus frequently are too far ahead of most people, and contemporary society as a whole remains almost completely indifferent to their value. Perhaps a maverick like Paracelsus is too hostile, too intolerant and impatient to be able to infuse his influence into his own time. The experimental methods and work of Paracelsus certainly forecast the modern approach to pharmacology, but a century was to elapse before another significant milestone appeared

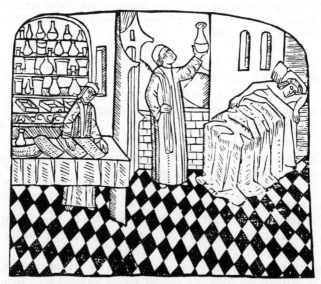

FIGURE 1-2. A pharmacist at work, while a physician examines a urine sample from the patient. It may be the earliest depiction of the concept of the "triad of medical care" to appear in an English book. (The illustration introduces Book 7 of the encyclopedia On the Properties of Things by Bartholomew [13th century], Westminster, 1495.) (From G. Sonnedecker [Ed.], History of Pharmacy, by Kremers and Urdang [4th ed.]. Philadelphia: Lippincott, 1976. P. 34.)

along the road of progress. This noteworthy event followed close on the heels of William Harvey's (1578–1657) explanation of the circulation of the blood.

The Forecasters of Experimental Pharmacology

The publication of Harvey's *Exercitatio anatomica de motu cordis et sanguinis in animalibus* in 1628 not only was the most momentous event in medicine to occur in the fifteen centuries since Galen, but also signaled the beginning of the scientific study of drug action. It opened the way for administering drugs in a new manner — by the intravenous route — and thus made it possible to demonstrate temporal connections between biologic effects produced and the administration of a drug. It is interesting to note that it was not a physiologist but a great chemist and physicist, Robert Boyle, who apparently was among the first to use this new route to investigate drug action in animals. About the year 1660, Boyle and an associate, Timothy Clarke, showed by well-controlled pharmacologic experiments that drugs are active when administered by vein. They also indirectly proved that these drugs, when taken by mouth, could produce the same effects only after being absorbed into the circulation.

There are only a few other events in the science of the seventeenth and eighteenth centuries that can be singled out as meaningful to the development of pharmacology. Those that are notable herald the great advances of the nineteenth century. The work of the Swiss physician John Jacob Wepfer (1620–1695) was the first critical publication of careful and large-scale pharmacologic experiments designed and carried out to determine the toxicity of drugs and poisons in animals. Felix Fontana (1720–1805), following the example set by Wepfer, also performed thousands of experiments on the toxicity of various crude drugs. His results suggested to him that a crude drug contains an *active principle* which preferentially acts upon one or more discrete parts of the organism to produce a characteristic effect. Thus Fontana's premise was preamble to the pioneering demonstrations of François Magendie (1783–1855) and Claude Bernard (1813–1878) that the site of action of a drug could be located in specific structures of the body.

The work of a young pharmacist's apprentice, Peter John Andrew Daries, in the late eighteenth century, was of equal or perhaps greater importance to pharmacology than that of Fontana. The results of Daries' carefully controlled studies were published as his doctoral dissertation in 1776. Through his astute deductions, he anticipated by many years the establishment of one of the fundamental pharmacologic principles, namely, that there is a relationship between the amount of a drug administered and the magnitude of the biologic response evoked.

The Influence of Advances in Physiology and Chemistry

The aforementioned pharmacologists of the seventeenth and eighteenth centuries recognized the need and value of animals as experimental tools and used them in their studies. They were hampered in their investigations, however, by a lack of refined physiologic techniques and methods with which to pinpoint where and how drugs interact with living tissue. In the early nineteenth century this impediment to the development of pharmacology as a science was removed by the achievements of the illustrious French vivisectionists. To pioneers like Magendie and Bernard, modern pharmacology owes a debt equal to that owed by modern physiology. The methods of physiologic experimentation which they established and employed were as fundamental and essential to understanding normal physiologic processes as they were to understanding the dynamic actions of chemicals on biologic processes and materials. They provided the means for discovering just what drugs do in the living organism.

The revolutionizing changes that occurred in chemistry almost simultaneously with those in physiology were of equal import to the subsequent rapid rise of pharmacology. Until this time, most of the drugs in medical or experimental use were impure, crude preparations or extracts of plants; the chemical methods needed to separate active ingredients were unknown. The German apothecary Frederick W. A. Sertürner (1783–1841) altered all this in 1806 when he isolated a white crystalline substance, morphine, from opium. This *first isolation* of an active principle of a medicinal plant stimulated so much enthusiastic research on other vegetable drugs that Magendie was able to publish a medical formulary in 1821 which contained only pure chemical agents.

After the momentous discovery of Sertürner, pharmaceutical chemistry rapidly took its place as an important branch of chemistry. With new isolation procedures, many natural drugs became available for investigation and use, and with the invention of chemical syntheses, many derivatives of natural products were made. The advances in organic chemistry also resulted in the production of totally synthetic drugs, many of which had chemical structures entirely different from compounds of plant origin.

Pharmacology as a Separate Discipline

Now that chemistry had provided the pure chemicals, and physiology the experimental methods with which to determine their biologic activity, pharmacologists had the implements they needed to advance their science to a discipline in its own right. From this time on, no lapses occurred between significant findings; new developments in all aspects of pharmacology followed one another in quick succession.

Localization of Site of Drug Action

The investigations of the pioneering physiologist Magendie ushered in this new era in pharmacology. He not only studied the action of a number of the newly purified drugs, but, more importantly, by using his new methods of experimentation, he was able to show that their effects were the results of actions within specific organs of the body. Thus, fifty years after Fontana had made the suggestion that each active component of a crude drug exerts its own characteristic effect at one or more specific sites in the body, Magendie concluded the experiments which established this as fact.

Magendie's work was continued and extended by his brilliant pupil Claude Bernard, one of the most outstanding physiologists of all time. Among the many valuable contributions Bernard made to our understanding of the sites and modes of action of various drugs, his studies of the arrow poison curare are perhaps the most remarkable. In a series of prodigious experiments culminating around 1856, he clearly demonstrated that curare exerts its muscle-paralyzing effect by acting at the junction between the muscle and the nerve stimulating the muscle. He further showed that the drug does not affect the nerve or the muscle itself. Therefore, by pharmacologic means, Bernard proved that there is a specialized area between the nerve and the muscle which is directly concerned with muscular activity. From this time on, the determination of the locus of action of a drug became an essential part of the study of the drug.

Cellular Mechanisms of Drug Action

Claude Bernard stated that drugs are the means of "dealing with the elementary parts of organisms where the elementary properties of vital phenomena have their seat." He therefore inferred that to understand the action of a given drug, it is essential both to know which tissues are primarily involved and to explain how the drug interacts with the biologic system to produce its effect. Rudolf Buchheim (1820–1879), in his masterly experiments with various drugs, advanced the thesis that drug activity could be explained on the basis of physicochemical reactions between cell constituents and the particular drug. The work of Buchheim foreshadowed the great conceptual contributions made at the turn of the present century by J. N. Langley (1852–1926) and Paul Ehrlich (1854–1915) concerning the nature of the cellular combining sites for drugs, and by A. J. Clark (1885–1941) on the quantitative aspects of this interaction between drug and cell. The work of these men is discussed in more detail in later chapters.

Chemical Structure and Biologic Activity

In 1841 James Blake (1815–1893), an English physician who emigrated to the United States in 1847, employed a novel methodologic approach that was to be profitably exploited by the future developers of synthetic drugs. By using a systematic series of chemically related inorganic salts, Blake established the principle that *the chemical structure of drugs determines their effect on the body.* The first steps toward disclosing the relationship between the chemical structure of organic compounds and their pharmacologic activity were made by the English physician T. R. Fraser (1841–1920) in collaboration with the chemist A. Crum Brown (1838–1923). Paul Ehrlich's work in the preparation of more than nine hundred compounds in the course of his search for a drug effective in the treatment of syphilis is a classic example of the structure-activity approach to the development of new and effective agents. The use of structure-activity relationships was also to become a powerful tool in the twentieth century in helping to bring to light the ultimate mechanisms by which drugs interact with biologic materials to produce their characteristic effects.

Fate of Drugs in the Body

James Blake, in the studies already referred to, also established the fact that drugs are effective only if, after administration, they are able to reach a responsive tissue. Oswald Schmiedeberg (1838–1921), a pupil of Buchheim, enlarged upon this and added the concept that drug activity is the consequence of a dynamic equilibrium, i.e., that the activity of a given drug is related to its ability to reach its site of action and to be removed from it. The means by which the body is able to eliminate drugs and terminate their action therefore became of primary concern.

That the body eliminates many chemical substances, particularly in the urine, had been known for centuries. But clear-cut proof that the living organism can also turn off the activity of a drug by carrying out chemical reactions which change the drug was obtained for the first time in 1842 by W. Keller. Schmiedeberg and his co-workers discovered a number of additional chemical reactions carried out by the body on various groups of drugs and strengthened the concept that drug activity can be terminated by chemical conversion within the body.

Pharmacology as a Profession

Buchheim and Schmiedeberg are important figures in pharmacology not only for their contributions to its substantive matter but also for the stature to which they raised the discipline. Buchheim was the first professor of pharmacology as well as the founder of the first laboratory devoted exclusively to experimental pharmacology as an independent part of physiology. The excellent textbook of pharmacology that he authored grouped drugs according to their chemical and pharmacologic actions rather than by their therapeutic effects.

Oswald Schmiedeberg, as professor of pharmacology at Strassburg, Germany, continued this transformation of the traditional materia medica into the modern science of pharmacology. He defined the purpose of pharmacology — to study the reactions brought about in living organisms by chemically acting substances (except foods) whether used for therapeutic purposes or not. Schmiedeberg, with Naunyn and Klebs, also founded *Archiv für experimentelle Pathologie und Pharmakologie,* the first modern journal devoted to reports of pharmacologic experimentation. But it was Schmiedeberg's renown as a teacher that drew students to him from all over the world. Through these students, many of whom attained eminence in their own right, he influenced the worldwide development of professional pharmacology. Noteworthy among Schmiedeberg's pupils were John Jacob Abel (1857–1938) and Arthur Robertson Cushney (1866–1926).

Abel officially founded pharmacology in the United States and became the Father of American Pharmacology. He occupied the first full-time professorship of pharmacology at the University of Michigan in 1891 and started the American Society for Pharmacology and Experimental Therapeutics in 1908 and the *Journal of Pharmacology* thereafter. When Abel left Ann Arbor in 1893 to chair the Department of Pharmacology at The Johns Hopkins University, Cushney took Abel's place at the University of Michigan and established an outstanding laboratory of pharmacologic research.

The Modern Era

Together with the tremendous achievements in the advancement of pharmacology to the status of a science, the nineteenth and early part of the twentieth centuries

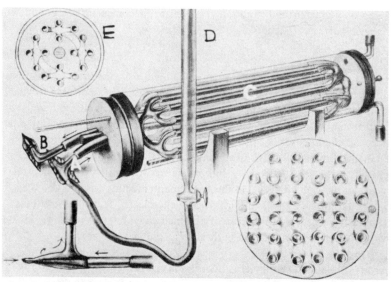

FIGURE 1-3. "Artificial kidney" as envisioned by John Jacob Abel years before one was finally developed that would work on human patients. The view, reproduced from an old drawing, shows the artificial kidney used by Dr. Abel on animals in 1913. A cannula (tube) was inserted in the animal's artery (A) to lead blood into the device's apparatus (C), a series of collodion tubes through which the blood flowed and from which substances in the blood were diffused into a fluid introduced from outside. A cross-section of these tubes is shown in the circle at the upper left (E). Anticoagulant was introduced through the burette in the center of the drawing (D). Blood was returned to the animal's vein through the upper cannula at left (B). (From J. J. Abel, L. G. Rowntree and B. B. Turner, Trans. Assoc. Am. Physicians, p. 28, 1913.)

witnessed dramatic discoveries of new pharmacologic agents. The character of surgery and obstetrics was changed by Morton (1819–1868) with the introduction of ether and by Lister (1827–1912) and Semmelweis (1818–1865) with the use of antiseptics to prevent infection. Ehrlich's work showing that drugs can be developed which are capable of destroying invading organisms without disabling the host ushered in the era of chemotherapy. The discovery of insulin by Banting and Best in 1921 led to dramatic success in the treatment of diabetes; it also focused attention on the therapeutic use of normally occurring substances as replacement for what the body is unable to provide in adequate quantities to maintain health. All these events and more formed the basis for the rational therapy of disease. And the growth of the pharmaceutical industry, with its extensive programs of research and development, assured the continued availability of an ever-increasing number of new drugs for the treatment and prevention of more and more diseases.

We shall cease our narration of the history of pharmacology at this point, for as Albert Szent-Györgyi has stated: "The future is the continuum of the past, the present being the dividing line between the two." The progress made in the recent past, probably greater than in all the years before, becomes our present and forms the subject matter of this book.

SYNOPSIS

Primitive man used drugs with about as much logic as he used magic, charms and incantations to drive away the evil spirits that he thought responsible for his illness. The rational use of drugs began only in the more recent past with the understanding of the real causes of disease. The emergence of pharmacology from a purely empiric part of medicine to a science in its own right was dependent on the development of sound medical therapy. But the real impetus for the growth of pharmacology was supplied by advances in chemistry and physiology. Chemistry provided pure compounds, and physiology provided the experimental techniques and knowledge essential in evaluating the biologic effects of pure chemicals. Many able scientists contributed significantly to the rise of pharmacology, but certain ones may be singled out as the innovators and pathfinders. Among these are:

Paracelsus (Phillipus Theophrastus Bombastus von Hohenheim) (1493–1541), who united chemistry with medicine; he discarded the ancient theories of the causes of disease and advocated the belief that illness is a derangement of body chemistry to be treated by simple chemical therapeutic agents

William Harvey (1578–1657), who explained the circulation of the blood; this momentous discovery signaled the beginning of the scientific study of the medical sciences

François Magendie (1783–1855), who pioneered the experimental approach to the study of pharmacology as well as physiology

Frederick W. A. Sertürner (1783–1841), who isolated morphine from opium in 1806, the first isolation of an active ingredient of a natural drug

Claude Bernard (1813–1878), the first to demonstrate and explain how a drug produces its action in the body

James Blake (1815–1893), who first set forth the principles that drugs are effective only after reaching a responsive tissue and that there is a relationship between the structure of drugs and the effects that they produce

Rudolf Buchheim (1820–1879), the first professor of pharmacology as well as founder of the first laboratory devoted exclusively to experimental pharmacology; he raised pharmacology to a position of equal importance with other branches of medicine

Oswald Schmiedeberg (1838–1921), the first great teacher of pharmacology; his textbook, techniques and students set the pattern for the worldwide development of pharmacology

Paul Ehrlich (1854–1915), who ushered in the era of chemotherapy by showing that chemicals can be made which are capable of destroying particular invading organisms; he also formulated the concept of receptors, i.e., that part of a chemical component of living tissue with which a drug combines to produce its biologic effect

John Jacob Abel (1857–1938), the Father of American Pharmacology, who occupied the first full-time professorship of pharmacology in the United States and founded the American Society for Pharmacology and Experimental Therapeutics and its journal

GUIDES FOR STUDY AND REVIEW

What great physiologist was the first to demonstrate and explain how a drug produces its action in the body?

Who ushered in the era of chemotherapy and formulated the concept of receptors?

Who is known as the Father of American Pharmacology? What were some of his major contributions to pharmacology as a profession?

SUGGESTED READING

Black, W. G. *Folk-Medicine: A Chapter in the History of Culture.* London: Eliot Stock, 1883.

Bryan, C. P. *The Ebers' Papyrus.* London: Geoffrey Bales, 1930.

Castiglioni, A. *A History of Medicine.* (Translated and edited by E. B. Krumbhaar.) New York: Knopf, 1947.

Chatard, J. A. Avicenna and Arabian medicine. *Johns Hopkins Hosp. Bull.* 19:157, 1908.

Garrison, F. *History of Medicine,* 4th ed. Philadelphia: Saunders, 1929.

Holmstedt, B., and Liljestrand, G. (eds.). *Readings in Pharmacology.* Oxford, Eng.: Pergamon, 1963.

Jarvis, D. C. *Folk Medicine.* New York: Holt, 1958.

Krantz, J. C., Jr. *Historical Medical Classics Involving New Drugs.* Baltimore: Williams and Wilkins, 1974.

La Wall, C. H. *Four Thousand Years of Pharmacy.* Philadelphia: Lippincott, 1927.

Meek, W. J. *Medico-Historical Papers: The Gentle Art of Poisoning.* Madison: University of Wisconsin Press, 1954.

Paracelsus. *Four Treatises of Theophrastus von Hohenheim Called Paracelsus.* (Edited by H. E. Sigerist.) Baltimore: Johns Hopkins University Press, 1941.

Shuster, L. (ed.). *Readings in Pharmacology.* Boston: Little, Brown, 1962.

Withering, W. An account of the foxglove, and some of its medical uses; with practical remarks on dropsy, and other diseases. *Med. Classics* 2:305, 1937.

2. THE SCOPE OF PHARMACOLOGY – DEFINITIONS

The word *pharmacology* comes from the Greek *pharmakon,* equivalent to "drug," "medicine" or "poison," and *logia,* meaning "study." But the question "What is pharmacology?" is only partially answered by the derivation of the term. We have seen that it is a branch of biology, since it is concerned with living organisms, and as such it borrows heavily from kindred subjects like physiology and biochemistry for much of its substantive matter and experimental techniques. Pharmacology is equally related to chemistry, since it deals with chemical agents and is dependent upon knowledge of their sources and properties. Also, pharmacology is an essential part of medicine. For although a *drug,* in broad terms, is any chemical agent other than food that affects living organisms, in its medicinal sense, a drug is any chemical agent used in the treatment, cure, prevention or diagnosis of disease. Pharmacology makes use of mathematics to express its principles in quantitative terms and of behavioral sciences, such as psychology, to understand the actions of drugs that lead to changes in mood or emotion. Thus *pharmacology is the unified study of the properties of chemicals and living organisms and all aspects of their interactions;* it is an *integrative* rather than an autonomous science, drawing on the techniques and knowledge of many allied scientific disciplines.

The broad science of pharmacology may be divided into four main categories: pharmacodynamics, toxicology, pharmacotherapeutics and pharmacy. In each of these subdivisions the emphasis is on those aspects of pharmacology that meet the specific requirements and objectives of the professional engaged in the particular field of specialized study.

Pharmacodynamics may be defined as *the study of the actions and effects of chemicals at all levels of organization of living material and of the handling of chemicals by the organism.* The similarity of the definition of pharmacodynamics to that of pharmacology itself is indicative of the fundamental nature of this aspect of pharmacology and of its place as the foundation on which the study of all other facets of pharmacology must be based. Indeed, pharmacodynamics is frequently referred to simply as pharmacology. Pharmacodynamics may also be used in a narrower sense to mean the science and study of how chemicals produce their biologic effects; this definition distinguishes pharmacodynamics from *pharma-cokinetics,* the science and study of the factors which determine the amount of drug at sites of biologic effect at various times after application of an agent to a biologic system. The professional pharmacologist, whether physician or nonphysician, depends on his knowledge of pharmacodynamics for a productive career.

Pharmacodynamics includes the study of (1) the effects produced by chemicals; (2) the site(s) at which and mechanism(s) by which the biologic effects are produced; (3) the fate of a chemical agent in the body: its absorption, distribution and elimination; and (4) the factors which influence the safety and effectiveness of an agent, i.e., the factors attributable to the physicochemical properties of the agent and those attributable to the biologic system.

General pharmacodynamics includes the fundamental principles or properties involved in the actions of all drugs, and *special pharmacodynamics,* the additional factors necessary to understand the action of individual drugs or drugs of similar action. In this book we are concerned primarily with the study of general pharmacodynamics. We shall deal with certain aspects of the specific pharmacology of some common drugs only to help in elucidating the general principles applicable to most drugs. We shall use the term *drug* in its broad sense to apply to *any chemical agent that affects living organisms.*

Toxicology is *the study of the toxic or harmful effects of chemicals as well as of the mechanisms and conditions of occurrence of these harmful effects.* It is also concerned with the symptoms and treatment of poisoning as well as the identification of the poison.

As Paracelsus pointed out, all drugs are toxic in overdosage. But what may constitute an overdose of insecticide for a particular insect may be entirely harmless to animals and human beings. Thus toxicity, while always indicating a harmful effect on some biologic system, is a relative term and requires definition of the system on which the toxic effect is produced. Although the toxic effects of therapeutic agents are part of their pharmacodynamics, the study of toxicology has developed into a separate discipline because large masses of people are exposed to a great variety of other potentially toxic substances. The toxicologist, in addition to training in pharmacodynamics, requires special training in drug identification and poison control.

The field of toxicology has developed into three principal subdivisions:

1. *Environmental toxicology* is concerned with the toxic effects of chemicals that become incidental or occupational hazards as contaminants of the atmosphere, water or food.

2. *Economic toxicology* deals with the toxic effects of those chemicals that are intentionally administered to a living organism in order to achieve a specific purpose. Thus economic toxicology deals with (a) all the therapeutic agents for human and veterinary use;.(b) the chemicals used as food additives and cosmetics; and (c) the chemical agents used by humans to selectively eliminate another species. In the last case, the human is considered the *economic* species, and the undesirable species, e.g., an insect, is considered the *uneconomic* species.

3. *Forensic toxicology* refers to the medical aspects of the diagnosis and treatment of poisoning and the legal aspects of the relationships between exposure to and harmful effects of the chemical. It involves both intentional and accidental exposure to chemicals.

Pharmacotherapeutics is *the application of drugs in the prevention, treatment or diagnosis of disease and their use in purposeful alteration of normal functions,* such as in the prevention of pregnancy or in the use of anesthetics for surgical procedures. Pharmacotherapeutics is of primary concern to those individuals engaged in the healing professions. It is that division of pharmacology which correlates pharmacodynamics with the pathologic physiology or microbiologic or biochemical aspects of disease.

Pharmacy is concerned with *the preparing, compounding and dispensing of chemical agents for therapeutic use.* It includes (1) *pharmacognosy,* the identification of the botanical source of drugs; (2) *pharmaceutical chemistry,* the synthesis of new drugs either as modifications of older or natural drugs or as entirely new chemical entities; and (3) *biopharmaceutics,* the science and study of the ways in which the pharmaceutic formulation of administered agents can influence their pharmacodynamic and pharmacokinetic behavior.

We have seen that pharmacy was the first branch of pharmacology to achieve professional status in its own right. But the pharmacist today bears little resemblance to his predecessor. He is no longer called upon to prepare or package drugs, since this is done for him by the pharmaceutical manufacturing companies. The role he is now called upon to play, and which will become progressively more important as the complexity of therapeutics increases, is that of an essential assistant to the physician, since the pharmacist has specific knowledge of the properties of drugs and drug preparations.

DRUG NOMENCLATURE

Drugs used as therapeutic agents may be conveniently divided into two main groups: (1) nonprescription drugs, which may be sold "over the counter" since they are judged safe for use without medical supervision; and (2) prescription drugs, which are considered to be unsafe for use except under supervision and which are, therefore, dispensed only by the order of practitioners licensed by law to administer them, i.e., physicians, dentists and veterinarians. In the United States, the Food and Drug Administration (FDA), under the provisions of the Durham-Humphrey Act of 1952, is empowered to make decisions on which drugs require prescription and which may be sold over the counter.

Drugs may also be classified *generically* to designate a chemical or pharmacologic relationship among a group of drugs, such as sulfanomides, local anesthetics, sedatives and so forth. This is a particularly useful categorization, since it focuses attention on the pharmacologic similarities among the members of a class as a whole. Usually, attention is directed within the group to one or two drugs chosen as representatives, or prototypes, of the entire class. Procaine, for example, is commonly used as the prototype of the drugs classified as local anesthetics. The use of prototypes also permits easy recognition of the member of a group that displays different or unique properties. In this text we shall use this prototype device to characterize a generic class of drugs.

The problems in drug nomenclature arise in naming individual therapeutic agents. Not only is an overwhelming number of agents available for use, but each of these agents has at least three names. Every drug has a *chemical* name, a *nonproprietary* name and a *proprietary,* or *trade,* name. Many of the older drugs, in addition, have an *official* name, whereas the official name of newer drugs is usually synonymous with their nonproprietary name. The nonproprietary name is frequently referred to as the *generic* name of the drug. The latter by strict definition is inappropriate, however, and should be reserved to designate a family relationship among drugs, as already indicated.

The chemical name of a drug – its first name – is a precise description of its chemical constitution and indicates the arrangement of atoms or atomic groups. For example, one of the most popular drugs in the treatment of anxiety is 7-chloro-2-methylamino-5-phenyl-3H-1, 4-benzodiazepine-4-oxide. Although meaningful to a chemist, this name obviously is too complex and unwieldy for most persons to use. Consequently, chemical names are rarely employed to designate drugs except for the simplest compounds, such as sodium bicarbonate.

The nonproprietary name of a drug is the name assigned to it when it is found to be of demonstrated or potential therapeutic usefulness. New drugs are now given nonproprietary names by the United States Adopted Name (USAN) Council, an enterprise jointly sponsored by the United States Pharmacopeial (U.S.P.) Convention Inc., the American Pharmaceutical Association and the American Medical Association (A.M.A.), and with representation from the FDA. The USAN Council replaces the older A.M.A.-U.S.P. Nomenclature Committee. The nonproprietary name usually becomes the *official* name of the drug as well when the drug is finally admitted to official compendia, *The United States Pharmacopeia* or *The National Formulary* (see pp. 20-21). The names selected by the USAN Council for newer drugs may also be adopted for use on a worldwide basis through the mediation of the World Health Organization. Such uniformity of nomenclature is very desirable in view of the rapid proliferation of new agents and the rate at which people travel from one country to another.

The nonproprietary names selected for many drugs, however, frequently defeat the purpose for which they were originally established. These assigned names are, for the most part, too long, too difficult to pronounce or spell and, consequently, too hard to remember. For example, chlordiazepoxide is the nonproprietary name given to the previously mentioned agent widely used for the treatment of anxiety. The *trade* name selected by the pharmaceutical company for the same drug is *Librium.* And it is the rule rather than the exception that the proprietary name is shorter, more euphonious and easier to recall than the nonproprietary name. As a result, it is the trade name that is most frequently remembered and used.

Confusion about proprietary names arises from the fact that a single drug may have many different trade names. Unlike the nonproprietary or official name, which is public property, the trade name is registered and its use restricted to the owner of the copyright. Even when a drug is new and is protected by a patent, it may be licensed for use by a number of companies, and it then appears under a variety of trade names. The patent which covers the drug as a chemical entity, or protects its method of manufacture or use, expires at the end of seventeen years. After that time a single agent may be marketed under ten or twenty different trade names. For example, the names by which a local anesthetic — known in the United States by the nonproprietary name procaine — is designated in various parts of the world include the following:

Novocain	Atoxicocaine
Ethocaine	Bernacaine
Neocaine	Chlorocaine
Syncaine	Irocaine
Scurocaine	Juvocaine
Allocaine	Kerocaine
Anesthesol	Paracain
Cetain	Planocaine
Isocaine-Asid	Aminocaine
Isocaine-Heisler	Eugerase
Naucaine	Sevicaine
Alocaine	Topokain
Anestil	Westocaine

The nonproprietary name should be used, however, to designate a particular therapeutic agent in order to minimize confusion and ensure accurate recognition. This is the nomenclature that we shall use throughout this book.

SOURCES OF INFORMATION ABOUT DRUGS

In this text we will focus on the principles and mechanisms that are fundamental to understanding all the aspects of pharmacology and discuss specific drugs only to illustrate and exemplify. In the standard textbooks the emphasis is on drugs and their application to therapeutics, with only a relatively small section being devoted to basic principles. For those who desire supplemental information about drugs per se, these systematic textbooks provide a concise catalogue and detailed descriptions of prototypes that serve as standards of reference for the various classes of therapeutically useful agents. Certain periodically published monographs and journals which feature comprehensive reviews of selected subjects or fields are also excellent sources of pharmacologic information. The data which eventually find their way into review articles and textbooks are collected and synthesized from the numerous regular journals of pharmacology and related medical sciences. These journals publish the wealth of experiments and rechecked observations on which our present generalizations are founded.

Although textbooks and reviews provide information about established drugs and furnish the bases for understanding new ones, they obviously cannot include details on many older agents or keep abreast of those most recently introduced. This type of encyclopedic information is the province of the numerous compendia, only two of which, *The United States Pharmacopeia* and *The National Formulary,* are recognized as official in the United States.

A number of the compendia are revised annually. But even this frequency is often insufficient and too slow to keep up with the constant advances in the field of pharmacology. So to meet the need for current and critical sources of information, there are also several publications which furnish prompt and pointed assessment of new drugs and of recent developments in drug therapy and toxicity.

Some of these sources of general and current drug information are listed below. Although the sources are representative of those considered pertinent, the list is by no means complete.

Current Textbooks (Published Within the Last Five Years)
Goodman, L. S., and Gilman, A. (eds). *The Pharmacological Basis of Therapeutics,* 5th ed. New York: Macmillan, 1975. A multiauthored textbook of pharmacology, toxicology and therapeutics that has become a classic since the first edition was published in 1941.

Goth, A. *Medical Pharmacology,* 8th ed. St. Louis: Mosby, 1976. An excellent modest-sized textbook that deals with those aspects of pharmacology which are relevant to the practice of medicine.

Goldstein, A., Aronow, L., and Kalman, S. M. *Principles of Drug Action,* 2d ed. New York: Wiley, 1974. An advanced text emphasizing the principles of pharmacology, designed for investigators and students of the natural sciences.

Reviews
Elliot, H. W., George, R., Okun, R., and Dreisbach, R. H. (eds.). *Annual Review of Pharmacology.* Palo Alto, Calif.: Annual Reviews, Inc. Annual.

Garattini, S., Goldin, A., Hawking, F., and Kopin, I. J. (eds.). *Advances in Pharmacology and Chemotherapy.* New York: Academic. Annual.

Harper, N. J., and Simmonds, A. B. (eds.). *Advances in Drug Research.* New York: Academic. Annual.

Jucker, E. (ed.). *Progress in Drug Research.* Basel, Switzerland: Birkhauser. Annual.

Munson, P. (ed.). *Pharmacological Reviews.* Baltimore: Williams & Wilkins. Quarterly (The American Society for Pharmacology and Experimental Therapeutics).

Journals of Pharmacology
Some of the journals containing original articles dealing with the effects of drugs in animals and humans also regularly feature reviews on selected topics. These journals are identified by an asterisk.

Publications of the American Society for Pharmacology and Experimental Therapeutics:

Journal of Pharmacology and Experimental Therapeutics
*Clinical Pharmacology and Therapeutics
Molecular Pharmacology
Drug Metabolism and Disposition

Other Journals:

Archives Internationales de Pharmacodynamie et de Thérapie
Biochemical Pharmacology
British Journal of Pharmacology and Chemotherapy (British Pharmacological Society)
European Journal of Pharmacology
*Journal of Pharmacy and Pharmacology (Pharmaceutical Society of Great Britain)
*Journal of Pharmaceutical Sciences (American Pharmaceutical Society)
Naunyn Schmiedebergs Archiv für Pharmakologie
Toxicology and Applied Pharmacology (Society of Toxicology)

Compendia

Official Compendia
The Pharmacopeia of the United States of America, 19th revision. *(The United States Pharmacopeia; U.S.P.)* New York, 1974.

The first pharmacopeia was published in the United States in 1820 but was only given official status in 1906 by the Federal Food, Drug and Cosmetic Act. It is now revised every five years by outstanding pharmacologists, physicians and pharmacists who donate their services to the U.S.P. Convention.

The drugs included in the *U.S.P.* are selected on the basis of their proved therapeutic value and low toxicity. Trademarked or patented drugs of therapeutic usefulness may be included as long as their content and method of preparation are not secret; they are listed under their official names. Drugs may be deleted from the *U.S.P.* when they have been supplanted by newer or better drugs, or when there is a high incidence of toxic reactions after extensive use.

The official drugs in the *U.S.P.* are defined according to source; physical and chemical properties; standards for identity, quality, strength and purity; method of storage; and dosage range for therapeutic use. However, the *U.S.P.* does not provide information about the pharmacologic actions or therapeutic uses of the drugs. The *U.S.P.* is, therefore, more useful to individuals concerned with the preparation of drugs than to those concerned with the study of the actions of drugs.

The National Formulary (N.F.), XIV ed. Washington, D.C.: American Pharmaceutical Association, 1975.

The *N.F.* was also given official status in 1906 and is now similar in purpose, format and content to the *U.S.P.* When it was originally published in 1888 under the name *National Formulary of Unofficial Preparations,* it contained only formulas for drug mixtures. This changed slowly over the years to include single drugs, but the *N.F.,* unlike the *U.S.P.,* still lists drug mixtures along with a variety of materials of plant origin. With the present edition, the *N.F.* has changed its criteria for the inclusion of drugs. Previously, drugs had been admitted on the basis of demand as well as therapeutic merit; now only the latter criterion is used.

The *British Pharmacopoeia (B.P.),* published by the British Pharmacopoeia Commission under the direction of the General Medical Council, and the *British Pharmaceutical Codex (B.P.C.),* published by the Pharmaceutical Society of Great Britain, are counterparts of the *U.S.P.* and *N.F.,* respectively. Other countries also have their official compendia. Recently, a committee of the World Health Organization published *The Pharmacopoeia Internationalis (Ph.I.).* This compendium is not intended to convey official status, but to encourage the development of international standards and unification of national pharmacopeias.

Unofficial Compendia
Osol, A., and Pratt, R. *The United States Dispensatory.* Philadelphia: Lippincott, 1973.

The *Dispensatory* is an encyclopedia of all the official drugs in the *U.S.P., N.F., B.P.* and *Ph.I.,* a very large number of drugs not listed in these compendia, and drugs used in veterinary medicine. In addition to the types of information found in the official compendia, there are comprehensive monographs on the history, actions, uses and factual toxicology of individual agents, documented with references to the original literature. There are also general articles on pharmacologic classes of drugs.

Department of Drugs of American Medical Association. *AMA Drug Evaluations,* 3rd ed. Acton, Mass.: Publishing Sciences Group, Inc., 1977.

A useful reference book that evaluates information on virtually all therapeutic agents in the official compendia as well as new single-entity drugs and mixtures, arranged according to therapeutic category.

Hoover, J. (ed.). *Remington's Pharmaceutical Sciences,* XV ed. Easton, Pa.: Mack, 1976.

This is a comprehensive reference book containing almost all the drugs and chemicals used today in medicine and pharmacy, classified according to their therapeutic use as well as by chemical structure. There are also complete commentaries on the official drugs listed in the *U.S.P., N.F., B.P., Ph.I.* and other current reference sources. It is of particular value to students and practitioners of pharmacy.

Lewis, A.J. (ed.). *Modern Drug Encyclopedia.* New York: Donnelley. Annual.

This encyclopedia lists over five thousand prescription medications by trade names as well as by nonproprietary names. The information contained in monographs of individual drugs includes the drug's manufacture; its chemical name with structural formula when possible; the forms in which the drug is supplied; its actions, uses and methods of administration; and the principal cautions to be observed in its use.

Billups, N. F. *American Drug Index*. Philadelphia: Lippincott. Annual.

Essentially a dictionary providing a useful cross-indexed source of drug products and dosage forms, listed by both nonproprietary and trade names.

The Merck Index: An Encyclopedia of Chemicals and Drugs, 9th ed. Rahway, N.J.: Merck, 1976.

Contains the structural formulas and chemical and physical properties of a large number of chemical compounds, including many therapeutic agents. The *Index* is also an excellent source for the many synonyms by which an individual drug is known.

Physicians' Desk Reference. Oradell, N.J.: Medical Economics. Annual.

The *P.D.R.,* as it is best known, lists the products of all the major drug manufacturers. Although a convenient source of information about available products, dosage forms, composition and untoward reactions of the listed preparations, it is not useful as a critical guide to the pharmacologic actions or uses of drugs.

Legally, all the information contained in the *P.D.R.* must conform to that supplied in the small leaflets that are required by law to accompany each package of a drug. These package inserts are, in themselves, useful sources of information about the particular drug; they furnish a concise description of the product, its pharmacology, indications and contraindications for use, known adverse reactions and recommended doses. The contents of these brochures must be reviewed and approved by the FDA.

Current and Critical Sources of Information

The Medical Letter on Drugs and Therapeutics. New York: Drug and Therapeutic Information, Inc. Biweekly.

Contains concise, informative and critical comments on newly promoted drugs and those being currently evaluated. The comments are written by a board of distinguished, competent physicians affiliated with teaching hospitals and medical schools. The *Medical Letter* compares new drugs with older agents, critically analyzes the claims made for new drugs and also alerts physicians to reports of adverse drug reactions.

Modell, W. (ed.). *Pharmacology for Physicians.* Philadelphia: Saunders. Monthly.

A publication of the American Society for Pharmacology and Experimental Therapeutics, in which experts discuss the basic pharmacology of a particular group of drugs in order to provide the rationale for their proper therapeutic use.

Unlisted Drugs. New York: Special Libraries Association. Monthly.

Lists new drugs found in the literature or advertising which have not as yet appeared in *Modern Drug Encyclopedia, New Drugs,* or other standard sources.

GUIDES FOR STUDY AND REVIEW

What distinguishes "pharmacodynamics" from "pharmacokinetics"? How are toxicology, pharmacotherapeutics and pharmacy related to pharmacology?

What do we mean by the chemical name of a drug? the nonproprietary name? the proprietary name? the official name? Why is the term "generic name" an inappropriate synonym for "nonproprietary name"?

What are the names of the compendia that have official status in the United States? How are drugs selected for inclusion in these official compendia? What are some of the other compendia that furnish encyclopedic information about established and new drugs?

3. HOW DRUGS ACT ON THE LIVING ORGANISM

The eminent Canadian physician Sir William Osler made the witty comment that, "The desire to take medicine is perhaps the greatest feature which distinguishes man from the animals." Whatever truth there be to this quip, it is certainly true that from the dawn of history man has exercised his desire to assuage his suffering and combat illness by concocting thousands of medicinals and avidly partaking of them. But of this legion, only a handful continually enjoyed popularity through the ages and made their way to our own time. Why did the juice of the poppy seed, the beverages made from fermented fruits and vegetables, the infusion of the autumn crocus, the extract of willow bark or the seeds of the castor oil plant survive as useful remedies? These and similar nostrums (Fig. 3-1) survived not because they actually contain *effective* drugs, but because to both physician and patient the *effects they produced were immediately evident and unmistakable.* Opium and alcohol quickly relieved the patient's pain and suffering; within a few hours colchicine terminated the agony of an acute attack of gout; salicin (an ancestor of our aspirin) rapidly reduced fever; and castor oil was equally conspicuous in its activity. The effects of these agents were easily recognizable and readily measured as significant changes in the recipient's physiologic state. Physician and patient alike could answer the question "What does the drug do?"

The effect produced by a drug can be recognized only as an alteration in a function or process that maintains the existence of the living organism, since all drugs act by producing changes in some known physiologic function or process. Drugs may increase or decrease the normal function of tissues or organs, but they do not confer any *new* functions on them; effects of drugs are quantitative, never qualitative. As in the examples previously cited, the effects produced by a drug can be identified as an *increase* in the normal rate of evacuation of the bowels, a *reduction* in an elevated body temperature or the *lessening* of pain and return to the normal painless state. Thus the particular effect of a drug is always expressed in relative terms — relative to the physiologic condition that exists at the time of drug administration. The primary factor in the facility with which the effect of any drug can be

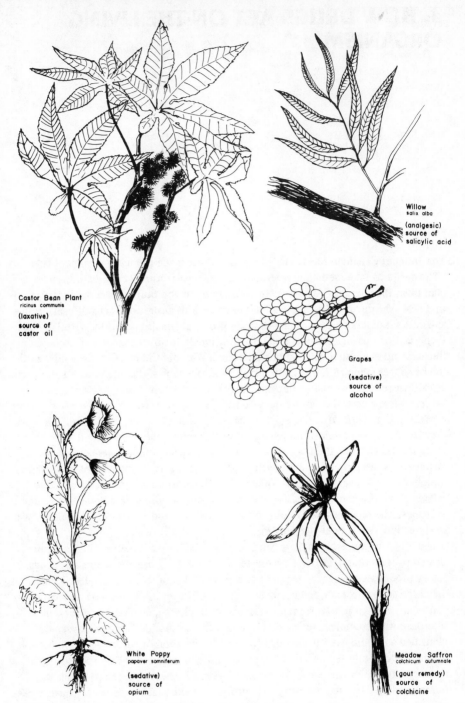

FIGURE 3-1. Sources of ancient remedies and modern drugs.

evaluated is that there are yardsticks or standards by which the presence or absence of an effect can be measured.

The importance of having an appropriate yardstick to measure the changes produced by drugs is well illustrated by an analysis of quinine's effectiveness under diverse physiologic conditions. Quinine was introduced into Europe in the middle of the seventeenth century as the powdered bark of cinchona, a tree indigenous to South America. The powder was found to have a striking effect in reducing the high fever of patients with malaria. This discovery led to its widespread use in all kinds of febrile illnesses. The cinchona preparations proved to be much less effective, however, in fevers of nonmalarial origin. On normal body temperature, the effect of cinchona was found to be negligible. The effect of quinine, easily measured as a change in body temperature, answers only the question of what quinine does. Evaluating quinine's effect in malaria, in other febrile disorders and in healthy individuals provides the answer to the additional question "When does the drug act?" It also tells us that normal body temperature is an inappropriate standard to choose for measuring quinine's effect.

Many other drugs resemble quinine in this respect, i.e., the changes they produce in a physiologic process can be detected only in the presence of a disease in which the process is functioning at an abnormal level. For most drugs, however, it is only necessary to know the conditions at the time of administration; their effects on a physiologic process can be measured using either normal or abnormal levels as the appropriate standard. For example, certain drugs that lower blood pressure produce this effect in patients with high, low or normal pressure; the yardstick in each condition is the blood pressure present before drug administration, and the lowering is measured relative to the initial state.

Why is quinine so much more effective in the treatment of malaria than in fevers associated with other disorders? Now we are really asking "How does quinine produce its effect?" The answer to this had to await the identification of the cause of malaria as well as the disclosure of the physiologic processes involved in maintaining normal body temperature. Following A. Laveran's famous discovery in 1880 that malaria is caused by the infecting parasite *Plasmodium,* it became relatively simple to show that quinine suppresses this organism. Quinine's significant effect on malarial fevers can now be attributed to its *specific action* on the agent responsible for the disease. On the other hand, quinine's effect on nonmalarial fevers can be explained not as an action on a causative agent, but in terms of what we now know about the regulatory processes of the body (Fig. 3-2). Certain distinct areas in the brain act as the "thermostat" of the body and maintain normal temperature by balancing heat production against loss of body heat. Fever results when the thermostat is "set at a higher level." The action of quinine is to readjust the controls to normal levels.

The answers to the question of how does quinine produce its effect on body temperature incorporate several points which are fundamental in answering this same question about any drug. First, they tell us that a particular effect measured as a change in a definite physiologic process may be brought about in several ways.

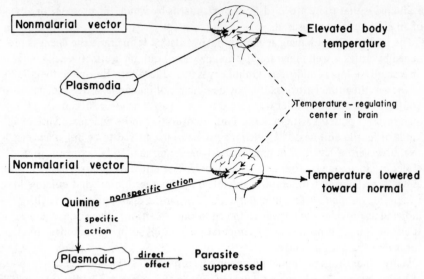

FIGURE 3-2. *Site of action of quinine in fevers of malarial and nonmalarial origin.
(A) Both the nonmalarial vector and the plasmodia act directly or indirectly on the
temperature-regulating center in the brain to produce an elevation in body
temperature. (B) In fevers of nonmalarial origin, quinine produces a lowering of
body temperature by acting on the temperature-regulating center to alter its
response to the nonmalarial vector. In malaria, quinine acts directly on the
plasmodia, thereby eliminating the cause of the elevation in body temperature.*

The action of the drug may be *specific,* i.e., aimed directly at the agent responsible
for the disease, or *nonspecific,* i.e., ameliorating a symptom of the disease, such as
fever, without getting to the basis of the disorder. Clearly, the distinction between
what is produced by an agent — its *effect* — and where and how the effect is produced — its *action* — becomes of consequence in determining the use to which the
drug may be put. But the most salient point is that, while the effects of many
drugs are amenable to measurement, their actions can be identified and characterized
only in terms of what we know about physiologic functions and processes. New
actions of drugs can be found only after a new physiologic or biochemical process is
uncovered on which the drugs may act. And what effect or action a drug has in a
particular disease depends on a basic knowledge of the disease — its cause and the
changes in normal body function brought about by the illness. For example, not
until the thyroid gland was revealed to be an organ with a definite physiologic role
was it possible to relate certain clinical symptoms to disturbances in the functioning
of this gland. Only then was it feasible to develop, test and find agents capable of
counteracting these disorders.

In arriving at an understanding of how drugs interact with a living organism, we
must address ourselves to some specific questions: "What is the action of the drug?,"
which includes "Where does it act?" and "By what means does it act?," "When does

it act?" "What does the drug do?" "What are its effects?" In discussing general phar-macodynamics we will be concerned only with answers common to most or all drugs. In this chapter we will consider the general answer to "What is the action of the drug?" by considering, first, where it acts, and then the means by which it acts.

SITE OF ACTION

The part of the body — organ, tissue or cell — where a drug acts to initiate the chain of events leading to an effect is known as *the site of action of the drug.* For quinine, the site of action in malaria is the plasmodium, the cell invading the host; in nonmalarial fever it is the discrete areas of the brain involved in the regulation of body temperature.

It should be obvious that different experimental approaches were required in order to arrive at these two conclusions about quinine's sites of action. For malaria, once the cause of the disease had been discovered and the fever shown to be one of its accompanying symptoms, it was only necessary to determine the effect of quinine on isolated plasmodia. For other fevers, various surgical procedures had to be carried out in febrile experimental animals in order to demonstrate that quinine could lower temperature only when the areas within the brain involved in temperature regulation were left intact. Although the two experimental approaches were markedly different, the "system" used in each case was identical. Each system included both the effector tissue, organ or cell — that entity in which the change in function could be observed or measured as an effect — and the site of action of the drug — that entity in which the drug acted to produce the response.

We saw earlier that an appropriate physiologic state had to be chosen as a standard in order to measure the effect of quinine on body temperature. In an entirely analogous fashion, it is essential to choose a suitable "intact living system," not only to disclose the site of action of the drug but also to determine its effect. The site of action and the effect of a drug are mutually dependent — one cannot be demonstrated in the absence of the other.

Let us consider the effects of drugs on the pupil of the eye as another example of the need for relevance in choosing the system on which these effects are to be measured. The muscles of the iris control the size of the pupillary opening in response to light; in bright light the opening is made smaller, in dim light, larger. Some drugs, like atropine, when applied to the *external* surface of the eyeball cause the pupil to become larger than it would be normally under the same light conditions (Fig. 3-3). The ophthalmologist frequently uses atropine or similar agents in just this way to aid him in eye examinations. Other drugs analogous to the organic phosphorus insecticides, when applied externally, cause the pupil to constrict. Application of drug solutions to the external surface of the eye can be used in these cases as a simple test system, since the system includes both the site of action — the muscles of the iris — and the target — the pupil, where the effect may be perceived as a change in diameter.

In contrast, if solutions of morphine are applied externally to the eyeball, no change in the size of the pupil is observed. Yet when morphine is administered

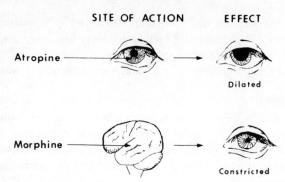

FIGURE 3-3. Sites of action of atropine and morphine in producing effects on pupillary diameter.

internally it produces marked pupillary constriction, and this effect is so characteristic that the presence of "pinpoint pupils" always leads to the presumption that an individual has taken morphine. This tells us that morphine cannot act *directly* on the muscles of the iris to produce its effect. Since the simple test system includes only half of what is essential — it does not include the site where morphine acts — no effect can be produced or seen. The site of action of morphine is not definitely known, but it is within the brain, probably in certain areas which influence the response of the pupil to light (Fig. 3-3). Thus, when morphine is taken internally, it has an opportunity to reach this site of action within the central nervous system.[1]

From the examples cited, we can see that a particular effect may be produced by a drug acting at a site close to the structure that ultimately responds, or by a drug acting at a site distant from the target organ. The more complex the physiologic process, the more sites at which drugs may act to produce the same alteration in function. For instance, blood pressure is regulated in the normal individual by the diameter of blood vessels, the rate of beating of the heart and the amount of blood forced out of the chambers of the heart at each beat, as well as by influences coming to the heart or blood vessels from several areas of the brain. A substance may lower blood pressure by acting at any one of these sites involved in its regulation: directly on the muscle of the blood vessel walls; indirectly through action on the heart muscle; or within the brain. Knowing only the effect of the drug tells us little about its site of action.

All that is necessary to determine the effect of a drug is to choose an appropriate standard and method of measurement and a relevant system that includes the effector organ and the site of action. Although determination of the effect of a drug is not always straightforward, determining the site at which a drug acts to produce a specific effect necessarily requires more experimental finesse. For example, it took little work to show that the iris of the eye was not the site at which morphine acts to constrict the pupil. But despite extensive investigation, the site at which morphine does

[1]The central nervous system includes the brain and spinal cord.

act is still not clearly defined. We need more knowledge of the manner in which individual areas of the brain influence physiologic function before we can determine exactly where and how drugs act in the brain.

Even when we can localize the site of action of a drug to a certain tissue or organ, this knowledge in itself may be insufficient, since different drugs producing the same or different effects may have different sites of action within the same tissue or organ. For example, caffeine, histamine and nitrites, such as nitroglycerin, all act on the muscle of blood vessels to increase their diameter, whereas cocaine produces constriction. It is then necessary to consider the separate components of the tissue or organ and to determine which of them is the specialized, functional element on which the drug acts. Ultimately it may be possible to show that the site of action is a particular kind of cell within an organ and that the drug acts either at the surface of this cell or within the cell itself. Alternatively, the site of action may be identified as extracellular, i.e., the site of action may be a component not contained within a cell. One of the fundamental objectives of pharmacodynamics is to be able to identify the site of action of each drug with this kind of precision. Although there are many drugs for which this has been possible, for many other important drugs we still do not have sufficient information to achieve this objective.

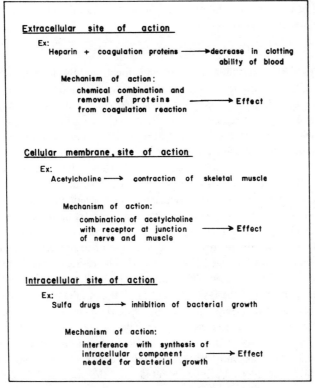

FIGURE 3-4. The different sites at which drugs may produce their effects.

MECHANISM OF ACTION

When the site of action of a drug has been identified to be either at the surface
of the cell, intracellular or extracellular, we are still at least one step away from
understanding *how* the drug acts. We know where the drug acts. Now knowledge is
needed of the *mechanism of action* — the means by which the presence of the drug
produces an alteration in function at the site and initiates the series of events that
we measure or observe as the effect (Fig. 3-4). The mechanism of action of some
agents, particularly those that act extracellularly, is relatively uncomplicated and
easy to understand. Other mechanisms, especially those of drugs that act intracellularly, are complex, and our understanding of them is usually not explicit. For still
other agents we have only a superficial explanation of how they act, since too little
is known of the cellular biochemical or physiologic functions involved in the effects
they produce.

Actions at Extracellular Sites

Let us consider first some of the drug reactions which occur extracellularly and
which are aimed at noncellular constituents of the body. One of the simplest
examples is that of the neutralization of excessive gastric acid by antacid drugs.
In this reaction a base, such as sodium bicarbonate, reacts chemically with the hydrochloric acid of the stomach and removes the acid by formation of new products,
salt, water and carbon dioxide:

$$NaHCO_3 + HCl \longrightarrow NaCl + H_2O + CO_2$$

Another type of extracellular mechanism is illustrated by the action of heparin
in preventing the coagulation of blood. Heparin is a high-molecular-weight **polymer**
in which the repeating units contain sulfuric acid. Such a structure makes heparin
a highly acidic organic substance with a negative charge. The strong electronegativity
allows heparin to react with substances of opposite charge. **Proteins**, also macromolecular substances, contain a number of groups in their structure which are
positively charged. Through the attraction of opposites, the electronegative heparin
combines with the electropositive groups of a variety of proteins to form new compounds. The anticoagulant effect of heparin is the consequence of its combining
with a protein in blood plasma which is essential for coagulation. The new compound formed by this combination, although containing heparin and the essential
protein, no longer has the properties of the uncombined protein and, thus, cannot
enter into the reactions involved in coagulation. The result is that clotting is inhibited.

The specific antidote, calcium disodium edetate, used to treat lead poisoning provides another example of the type of reaction that can take place extracellularly. The
drug removes lead that is free in blood and tissue fluids by a reaction in which the
calcium of the drug is displaced by the lead. The attractive force between the drug
and lead — its affinity for lead — is many orders of magnitude greater than that
between the drug and calcium. Thus the antidote renders the lead inert by complexing it so tightly that the lead can be excreted from the body as the soluble lead-
edetate complex.

In each of these examples, the action of the drug was the result of a chemical reaction. And this chemical reaction was easily definable since, in addition to the drugs involved, the other reactants could also be specifically identified. Thus, whenever a drug can be shown to interact with a distinct biologic entity and when the identified material is also a functionally important molecule in a living system, the mechanism of action of the drug can be readily explained.

Actions at Cellular Sites

Most functions of the living organism, however, do not take place extracellularly but are cellular in origin. Therefore, the vast majority of drugs produce their effects by interactions with cells, either with components of the interior of the cell or with those on the surface of the cell comprising the cellular membrane. Many of the constituents of the cell interior have been obtained as separate entities by complicated methods of isolation following careful disruption of the intact cell. Using the sophisticated techniques and instrumentation now available, it has also been possible to chemically identify or characterize many of these cellular substances and to determine their function. These efforts have been particularly fruitful in identification of the various molecules functioning to maintain the life of the *individual cell* — those involved in the processes of cellular respiration, energy production and reproduction.

When a drug is shown to act intracellularly, it may be possible to determine whether it affects one of these vital processes, since its effects can be measured in terms of the change in the function, e.g., a change in the utilization of oxygen or of a sugar. Just as with heparin, it then becomes feasible to determine the mechanism of drug action, since most of the reactants as well as the chemical reactions of a particular process have been identified. The mechanisms of action of many drugs used to treat infectious diseases have been elucidated, since they produce their effects on single-celled organisms. However, with a tissue like muscle or an organ like the heart, the specialized function of the tissue or organ is not dependent solely on the vital processes going on in the individual cells; it is also determined by the way in which the cells are integrated to form the organized structure. Breaking the heart up into its chemical components and showing that one or more of them can react chemically with a particular drug will not necessarily tell us how the drug acts to produce a slowing of the rate of the beating, intact heart. But even when our understanding of the mechanism of action is incomplete, the general concepts of the ways in which drugs act are valuable in analyzing specific drug effects. These concepts are based on the proposition that a drug can produce an effect on a living organism only through *interaction* with a *functionally important molecule,* whether that molecule exists as a free entity or as part of an organized structure.

The Concept of Receptors

The overwhelming majority of drugs show a remarkable amount of *selectivity* and *specificity* in their actions. That is to say, they act at some sites to produce their characteristic biologic effects, whereas their presence at other cells, tissues or organs leads to no measurable biologic response. This suggests that (1) there is something exceptional in the physicochemical properties of the biologic molecule at the sites where the responses are produced by drug interaction, and (2) this uniqueness is absent at other sites. There is also a definite relationship between the chemical structure of a drug and the biologic effect it produces at a particular site. Sometimes a very slight modification in the chemical structure of the drug molecule yields a compound that no longer produces the same effect at the site as did the parent compound. In other instances a variety of substitutions or additions can be made in some parts of the molecule without producing a qualitative change in the characteristic pharmacologic effects, provided that certain fundamental structural features are not altered. In still other cases, changes in the effect produced at a site can be shown to occur when there are no changes in the chemical formula of the agent, but only changes in the way a few atoms are arranged in the three dimensions of space — when the compounds are **stereoisomers.**

Even from these few brief statements about the relationship of the chemical structure of drugs to their activity at a particular site, it is possible to infer (1) that there is something unique in the physicochemical properties of the tissue constituent at the site of action, and (2) that the three-dimensional aspect of the site — its shape or configuration — also plays a role in determining whether an interaction with a drug will lead to a biologic effect. The macromolecules of tissue — substances such as proteins or **nucleic acids** — have physicochemical and spatial characteristics well suited to permit certain drugs, but not others, to interact with them. When this interaction initiates the events that lead to a biologic effect, these macromolecules are considered to be *the* functionally important tissue components at a site of drug action. These tissue elements with which drugs interact to produce their characteristic biologic effects are called *receptors.*

The concept of receptors originated with the work of Paul Ehrlich (1845—1915) and J. N. Langley (1852-1926). Ehrlich coined the word *receptor* to help explain the high degree of specificity which he first noted in his early work on the interaction between **antibodies** and the **antigens** which stimulated their production, and later in his pioneering investigations on the reactions between synthetic organic materials and microorganisms. He postulated that all cells have "side-chains" and that side-chains of different cells have different chemical compositions as well as a definite three-dimensional arrangement of their chemically reactive groups. He believed that drugs can be active only when bound to these side-chains, or receptors as he called them, and that chemicals can be attached only when they fit the receptors, as a key fits a lock.

Langley coined the term *receptive substance* to describe the specialized material in muscle on which drugs act. Much earlier, Claude Bernard had established that the site of action of curare, when it prevents the contraction of a muscle in response to stimulation of its motor nerve, is at the junction between the end of the nerve and the muscle. Langley showed that nicotine acts at this same site to elicit a muscular contraction and that curare can prevent this contractile response to nicotine. He then postulated that both nicotine and curare could bind to the same receptive substance, which was neither muscle nor nerve, but that only the combination of nicotine with the receptive substance triggers the contraction of the muscle. When curare combines with the receptive substance, no muscle action is elicited and, furthermore, the presence of curare prevents the binding of nicotine. Thus Langley used the concept of receptors to explain how drugs act to initiate a biologic effect as well as to inhibit one.

Binding Forces in the Drug-Receptor Interaction — Types of Bonds

According to the receptor theory of drug action, the drug must interact by *combining* or *binding* with the macromolecular tissue element at the site of action in order to produce its characteristic biologic effect. Therefore, there must be some forces that not only attract the drug to its receptor, but also hold it in combination with the receptor long enough to initiate the chain of events leading to the effect. These forces are the chemical bonds which hold two atoms, groups of atoms or molecules together with sufficient stability that the combination may be considered an independent molecular species. Since these forces underlie all interactions between drugs and the tissue elements of a living system, we shall briefly consider each of the four types of bonds that may be formed.

Let us first recall some features of the structure of the atom. The internal structure of the atom consists of a nucleus that has a positive electric charge and which can account for most of the mass of the atom. The nucleus is surrounded by electrons in sufficient number that their total negative charge is equal to the positive charge of the nucleus. This makes the atom electrically neutral. The simplest atom is hydrogen, which contains a single positively charged proton in its nucleus and a single negatively charged electron moving about the nucleus. Atoms larger than hydrogen also contain neutrons in their nucleus, and these, as the name implies, carry no charge. For example, carbon has six protons and six neutrons in its nucleus and six surrounding electrons; oxygen has eight protons and eight neutrons with eight surrounding electrons. The extranuclear electrons are the seat of chemical reactivity, and this reactivity is dependent on the configuration of the external electrons.

The external electrons move about the nucleus in groups and subgroups, referred to respectively as shells and subshells, each shell and subshell having a definite number of electrons that may be situated in it. The number of shells and subshells is determined by the total number of external electrons of the atom. The simplest atoms, hydrogen and helium, have only one external shell; two is the maximum number of electrons that can be accommodated in this shell. Successive shells may contain eight or more electrons, but there can be no more than eight electrons in the outermost shell of an atom *before* the next shell is started. In other words, in shells that can contain more than eight electrons, only eight enter initially, then a new shell is started and the incomplete shell is left to be filled in later. This electronic configuration of eight electrons in the outermost shell (two in the case of helium) corresponds to the structure of the inert, rare gases. The chemical inactivity of these gases indicates that their configuration must be a highly stable arrangement of electrons.

All atoms try to reach chemical stability and to attain the configuration of a rare gas. They do this by giving up or taking on electrons. For example, the sodium atom, with eleven external electrons, has two closed shells, the first with two electrons corresponding to helium, the second with eight electrons corresponding to neon and the remaining electron in the third outermost shell. When the sodium atom gives up this electron to reach the configuration of neon, the resulting particle is positively charged because it now has one more proton in its nucleus than it has electrons in its surrounding shells. Chlorine, with seventeen electrons, has seven of these in its outermost shell. When chlorine accepts an electron to attain the configuration of the inert gas argon, it also loses it neutrality and becomes negatively charged. Charged particles are called *ions*. Thus, chemical reactivity is associated primarily with the electrons in the outermost shell.

THE IONIC BOND.   The atoms of metallic elements, such as sodium, tend to give up their electrons easily, whereas the nonmetallic atoms, such as chlorine, tend to add electrons. These natural tendencies come into play when a metallic atom and a nonmetallic atom approach one another to form a stable molecule or crystal. In the electronic formulation of the interaction, the symbol of the element, i.e., Na for sodium, Cl for chlorine, represents the kernel of the atom, standing for the nucleus and the *closed* shells of electrons. The electrons of the outermost shell, the **valence** shell, are shown by dots. Thus,

$$Na \cdot \; + \; :\overset{..}{\underset{..}{Cl}} \cdot \; \longrightarrow \; Na^+ \; + \; \left[:\overset{..}{\underset{..}{Cl}} : \right]^-$$

An electron is transferred from the $Na \cdot$ to the $:\overset{..}{\underset{..}{Cl}} \cdot$ to yield a positively charged sodium *cation* and a negatively charged chloride *anion,* each with the configuration of a rare gas. These ions are stable and retain their electronic configuration essentially independently of each other in solution and even in the solid, crystalline form. However, they are held together to form a *molecule* by the electrostatic attraction between them. The bond formed between atoms involving the *outright transfer* of one or more electrons from one atom to the other is called the *ionic bond.* The ionic bond is defined, then, as the electrostatic attraction between oppositely charged ions. The strength of this bond depends on the distance between the two ions and diminishes as the square of the distance between them.

THE COVALENT BOND.   Whereas electrostatic attraction can explain the binding found in a simple salt like sodium chloride, or in a more complicated molecule such as that formed by heparin with a protein of the coagulation process, this type of binding can hardly account for the formation of molecules such as the gases hydrogen, H_2, or methane, CH_4, in which no ions can be detected. To explain this latter type of binding, G. N. Lewis proposed in 1916 that not only can a bond between atoms arise from outright transfer of electrons, but a rare gas configuration can also be attained from the *sharing* of a pair of electrons by the two bonded atoms. Thus we can write electronic structures such as:

$$H \cdot + H \cdot \longrightarrow H:H \quad \text{or} \quad \cdot \overset{\cdot}{\underset{\cdot}{C}} \cdot + 4H \cdot \longrightarrow H:\overset{H}{\underset{H}{C}}:H$$

in which a pair of electrons held jointly by two atoms is doing double duty and is effective in completing a stable electronic configuration for each atom. Each hydrogen can claim the shared pair and thereby attain the structure of helium. And the carbon, by being able to share in its own as well as in the four acquired electrons of hydrogen, has the configuration of the rare gas neon. The bond formed when two atoms share a pair of electrons is known as a *covalent bond.* It is about twenty times stronger than the ionic bond and is responsible for the chemical stability of organic molecules.

Covalent bonding resulting from electron sharing also accounts for the formation of double and triple bonds in molecules. Moreover, a covalent bond can result from the sharing of electrons supplied by one atom only, the resulting bond being called a *coordinate covalent bond.* The atom contributing the electron pair is called the donor atom and in biologic systems is usually nitrogen, oxygen or sulfur. Consider the formation of ammonium ion (NH_4^+) from ammonia (NH_3) and hydrogen ion:

$$H : \overset{..}{\underset{..}{N}} : + H^+ \longrightarrow \left[H : \overset{..}{\underset{H}{\underset{..}{N}}} : H \right]^+$$

The ammonia molecule has four electron pairs, of which only three are shared; thus each hydrogen has attained a stable helium configuration, and the nitrogen atom with five electrons in its outermost shell has attained its complete octet. When a hydrogen ion approaches the ammonia, the nitrogen allows the hydrogen proton to share with it the free pair of electrons. But the positive charge associated with the hydrogen ion is retained by the ammonium ion complex, since there has been no net gain or loss of electrons. We shall see that this coordinate covalent bond formation is important in the ionization of drugs and in certain interactions with receptors.

THE HYDROGEN BOND. The hydrogen atom, with only a single electon, can form only one covalent or one ionic bond with another atom. The hydrogen nucleus, however, being a bare proton, is strongly electropositive. When hydrogen is bound by an ionic or covalent bond to a strongly electronegative atom, the hydrogen may further coordinate two more electrons donated by another strongly electronegative atom, such as oxygen (O), nitrogen (N) or fluorine (F). This second bond of hydrogen is referred to as the *hydrogen bond,* and it forms a bridge between two strongly electronegative groups. Hydrogen bonding may form this bridge between different molecules or may lead to the association between like molecules, as in acetic acid:

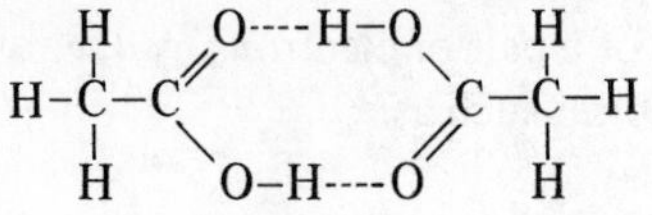

$$
\begin{array}{c}
\overset{\displaystyle H}{\underset{\displaystyle H}{H-C-C}} \quad \overset{\displaystyle O\text{----}H-O}{\underset{\displaystyle O-H\text{----}O}{}} \quad \overset{\displaystyle H}{\underset{\displaystyle H}{C-C-H}}
\end{array}
$$

The dotted lines represent hydrogen bonds, the solid lines, covalent bonds.

Although the hydrogen bond is ionic in character, its strength is less than that of a true ionic bond. A single hydrogen bond confers little stability on the association of two molecules, but *several* such hydrogen bonds can stabilize an interaction significantly. For example, in a compound like water, which can form hydrogen bonds readily, the hydrogen bonding does not stop at two molecules but may extend throughout the entire mass:

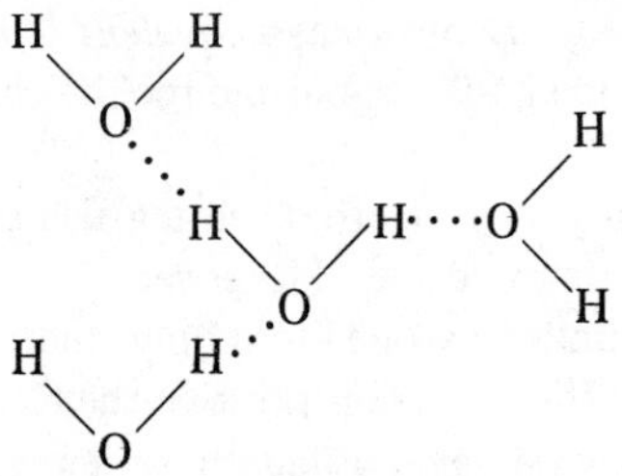

This association between molecules of water in the liquid state makes it more resistant to disruption by heat. This is why water has a higher boiling point than organic solvents such as chloroform, $CHCl_3$, which do not exist as associated liquids. Chloroform cannot form hydrogen bonds since the hydrogen is attached by a covalent bond to carbon, which is not a strongly electronegative atom.

VAN DER WAALS FORCES.   These are very weak attractive forces between any two neutral atoms or atomic groupings; they operate only at close range. Since the force of attraction is inversely proportional to the seventh power of the distance between the atoms, these forces decrease rapidly with a slight increase in interatomic distance.

Drug-binding at Receptors

We have stated that a drug can produce an effect on a living organism only through interaction with a functionally important molecule of that organism, and that for most drugs this means combining with a macromolecular tissue element, the hypothetical receptor. We have' also said that most drugs are selective in their action, combining only with certain receptors and not with others, and that receptors also show specificity by binding with some agents and not with others. Still another important characteristic of the drug-receptor interaction is that it is of sufficient stability to permit the initiation of the action-effect sequence. However, what is equally true, but which was not previously stated, is that for most drugs the binding to receptors is not so stable that it cannot be readily broken. In other words, the binding of most drugs to receptors is a reversible reaction. It is obvious that this selectivity, specificity and reversibility of drug-receptor interaction cannot be brought about by a single force but requires the synchronous operation of numerous bonds of the several types mentioned to achieve all these conditions.

Factors and processes involved in getting a drug to its site of action are discussed in the next chapter. Let us consider now only what may happen once the drug is present in the immediate vicinity of its receptor. As the drug molecule approaches, the first force to be exerted must be one that can overcome the random thermal agitation of the drug molecule and draw it to its receptor. What is needed, then, is a bond that can form rapidly, is of sufficient strength to hold the molecule to the receptor and, most importantly, can exert its influence when the drug molecule is still distant from its receptor. The ionic bond formed by electrostatic attraction is best suited to this purpose. The ionic bond acts at high velocity and is stronger than the hydrogen bond and the bond formed by Van der Waals forces. Also, whereas the force of the latter diminishes as the seventh power of the interatomic distance, the force of the ionic bond diminishes only as the square of the distance. The strength of the covalent bond is many times that of the ionic bond; so strong, in fact, that unlike the other three bonds, it is essentially irreversible at ordinary body temperature. Since the drug-receptor combination of most drugs can dissociate at body temperature, covalent bond formation in their interaction is rather improbable; covalent binding to receptors is characteristic of long-lasting drug actions.

Of course, what is needed for ionic bond formation is the presence of oppositely charged groups on a drug and on its receptor. This condition is readily satisfied for most drugs: the macromolecules of the receptors contain charged groups that are available for interaction, and most drugs have one or more groups that can act as either negatively or positively charged centers of attraction. Thus, even though only one or two ionic bonds may be formed, it is probably this electrostatic attraction that first ties a drug to its receptor.

Whereas the formation of one or two ionic bonds may be sufficient to initiate drug-receptor combinations, the strength of these bonds by themselves would be insufficient to hold the drug molecule in combination long enough to promote the action-effect sequence. The ionic bond must be reinforced by other bond formation in order to overcome the energy of thermal agitation, which is great enough at 37°C to break a single ionic bond. Thus the additional attractions of hydrogen bonds and Van der Waals forces must be called upon to give the drug-receptor combination the stability essential for drug action.

The formation of one or even two ionic bonds would also be insufficient to confer much specificity or selectivity on the drug-receptor interaction. The inference was made earlier, from brief statements about the relationship between the structure of a drug molecule and its activity, that the receptor requires not only unique physicochemical properties, such as charge, but also a definite shape in order to account for specificity. To use Ehrlich's analogy, a drug can produce an effect only when it fits its receptor as a special key fits a well-designed lock. The ionic bonds can be visualized, then, as the first major notches made in the blank key which permit it to approach the lock, to penetrate, as it were, the exterior of the lock — the keyhole.

The electrostatic attraction of hydrogen bonds, weaker than that of ionic bonds but still felt at a distance from the receptor, may be analogous to smaller notches in the key which bring it in still closer contact with the lock mechanism by allowing it to turn part way in the keyhole. The Van der Waals attraction, the weakest of all the binding forces, nevertheless is the force most critically dependent on the interatomic distance between reacting molecules. The Van der Waals forces may be considered, then, as special small notches in the key whose spatial arrangement is such as to fit the lock perfectly and permit it to turn the mechanism once the key is in position to do so. The Van der Waals forces may well be the major contributing forces in determining the specificity of drug-receptor interactions. A slight misfit, one tiny notch out of place, may hinder the perfect association of the drug molecule with the complementary aspects of the receptor and, despite the other bond formations, may prevent the drug action, i.e., the turning of the lock. Thus the concerted operation of ionic bonds, hydrogen bonds, Van der Waals forces and, in some cases, covalent bonds is needed to initiate the action of most drugs and to confer specificity on this action.

Figures 3-5 and 3-6 are schematic representations of the ways in which drugs are postulated to interact with hypothetical receptors. The hypothetical combination of naturally occurring acetylcholine with a receptor is shown in Figure 3-5. In acetylcholine, the nitrogen group has a strong positive charge which it acquired by donating its unshared pair of electrons to carbon to form a coordinate covalent bond. This is like the situation previously described for the formation of the ammonium ion, NH_4^+, in which the nitrogen atom of ammonia donated its unshared pair of electrons to the hydrogen proton. When a nitrogen atom donates this unshared pair to an atom other than hydrogen, the resulting compound is called a *quaternary ammonium compound.* The positive charge of the quaternized nitrogen in acetylcholine is thought to be ionically bonded to a negatively charged group of the receptor. This electrostatic attraction may be sufficient to draw acetylcholine close to the receptor. But the stability of the bond is conceived of as being increased by Van der Waals forces,

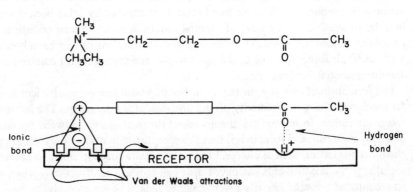

FIGURE 3-5. The hypothetical receptor for acetylcholine (see text for explanation).

produced by the close fit of two of the CH_3, or methyl, groups into the cavity in which the charged site of the receptor is embedded. Van der Waals attractions may contribute additional stability to the overall binding, since the chain of carbons between the nitrogen and oxygen is pictured as lying close to and fitting a flat part of the surface of the receptor. Finally, the formation of a hydrogen bond with oxygen may draw the other end of the molecule close to the receptor and thus further increase the stability as well as specificity of the entire acetylcholine-receptor combination.

Although this concept of a receptor is almost entirely hypothetical, the inferences concerning individual points of binding are based on the results of studies of structure-activity relationships. That is, the structure of acetylcholine was systematically altered, for example, by changing the groups attached to the nitrogen or by changing the length of the middle chain of carbons. The ability of the new compound to produce a specific biologic effect of acetylcholine, such as contraction of muscle, was then determined. A model of the receptor for acetylcholine was subsequently arrived at which would be consistent with all the data obtained.

The three-dimensional aspects of the drug-receptor combination may be seen more clearly, perhaps, by the interaction diagrammed in Figure 3-6. L-Epinephrine and D-epinephrine are identical molecules with respect to the number and kinds of atoms and the distances between atoms in their structures. They differ only in the arrangement in space of the groups attached to one carbon atom. The two structures cannot be superimposed but are mirror images of each other and are, therefore, optical stereoisomers. Since the biologic effect of these two isomers differs, the inference may be drawn that the receptor surface can distinguish between these two optical isomers. Both L-epinephrine and D-epinephrine could be bound to the receptor by hydrogen bonding of the two hydroxyl (OH) groups at one end of the molecule and by ionic bond formation at the other end, where nitrogen has become positively charged by coordinate covalent bonding with a hydrogen ion. But only the entire spatial arrangement of all the atoms in L-epinephrine permits a three-point attachment to the receptor, a condition which appears to be consistent with maximum biologic effect.

Evidence that receptors do exist appears to be incontrovertible, even though their properties are still largely presumptive since most receptors have not been isolated or purified. Recent attempts to isolate, purify and determine the molecular structure of receptors for acetylcholine, however, have met with significant success. Using highly specialized and sophisticated new techniques, a membrane-bound receptor for acetylcholine has been isolated from various sources and shown to be a high molecular weight **proteolipid**. The putative receptor displayed binding patterns and functional properties consistent with the known pharmacologic activities of acetylcholine. Promising results have also been obtained in the isolation and identification of the putative insulin receptor and in the detection of highly specific binding sites for morphine (cf. Chapter 12).

Recent advances in establishing the complete three-dimensional structures for

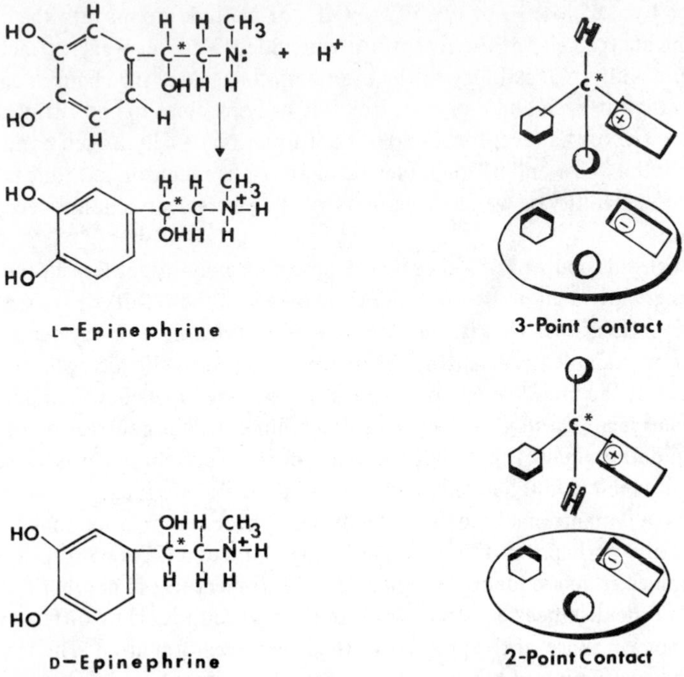

FIGURE 3-6. Combination of epinephrine with its hypothetical receptor, illustrating the influence of the three-dimensional structure of the receptor surface. In L-epinephrine, the spatial arrangements of the hydrogen atom and the three radicals bound to the asymmetric (*) carbon atom permit a three-point attachment to the complementary receptor. This perfect fit cannot be achieved with the D isomer. The symbol ⬡, written with or without double bonds, is the diagrammatic representation of benzene and indicates a ring structure of six carbons, each with one hydrogen atom, and alternating double and single bonds between the carbon atoms of the ring. (Modified from T. Z. Csaky, Introduction to General Pharmacology. New York: Appleton-Century-Crofts, 1969. P. 29.)

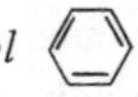

nucleic acids and many proteins also indicate the feasibility and potential validity of many inferences made concerning the binding of drugs to receptors that may not yet have been isolated. These recent advances also provide some insight into how this binding may lead to drug action. For example, the elucidation of the three-dimensional configuration of the red blood cell protein, hemoglobin, has shown us how and where the reversible attachment of oxygen occurs in the structure. Moreover, the discovery that the *shape* of hemoglobin changes when oxygen combines with it suggests that perhaps a drug can also change the spatial configuration of a receptor upon combining with it. This drug-induced change in the shape of the macromolecular receptor may be the trigger for the biologic effect seen, for example, as muscular contraction or increased secretion.

Actions Not Involving Receptors

We have already noted that certain drugs which act extracellularly produce their characteristic effects without combining directly with a receptor. The neutralization of gastric acid by antacid drugs and the interaction of a small molecule like lead with an antidotal drug are true chemical reactions that produce biologic effects. However, they are not considered *receptor* interactions by the definition of a receptor, since no macromolecular tissue elements are involved. Still other mechanisms of drug action are not mediated directly by receptors. These actions may occur at cellular sites and may involve macromolecular tissue components, but the biologic effects produced are nonspecific consequences of the physical or chemical properties of the drugs.

Drugs that are used primarily to destroy living tissue, such as germicides to kill bacteria, are obvious examples of agents with a nonspecific, and thus nonreceptor, mechanism of action. Detergents, alcohol, oxidizing agents such as hydrogen peroxide and phenol derivatives like lysol all act by irreversibly destroying the functional integrity of the living cell through disruption of cellular membranes or cellular constituents, such as nucleic acids or proteins.

Another group of agents whose mechanism of action does not involve direct combination with specific receptors, as they are defined, are the volatile general **anesthetics.** Their action on the living organism, however, is entirely different from that of the antiseptic agents, in that the action of the former is completely reversible and appears to involve no discernible chemical reactions. The inert gas xenon, the inorganic gas nitrous oxide and organic gases like cyclopropane, along with volatile substances like ether and chloroform, all produce similar effects on the brain. Such a diversity of chemical structure, indeed the remarkable lack of any obvious common molecular feature, makes it untenable that these agents produce a common pharmacologic effect by acting at a receptor with structural specificity. These agents do have some physicochemical properties — such as their solubilities in various solvents — which may be partially correlated with their pharmacologic activity. A number of theories on their mechanism of action have been built around these correlations. Until now, however, no theory has been advanced which can be considered entirely valid.

On the other hand, the mechanism of action of certain other types of drugs can be adequately explained on the basis of their physicochemical properties. Certain water-soluble cathartics, such as magnesium sulfate (Epsom salt), are almost completely retained within the alimentary canal after oral administration, since both the magnesium and the sulfate of the salt are only slightly absorbed. This excess of a salt within the intestinal lumen creates a solution that is much more concentrated than normal body fluids. The body tends to compensate for this high concentration by adding water, from the blood carried in vessels within the wall of the bowel, to the intestinal contents to bring them back to a normal level, i.e., to **isotonicity.** Thus magnesium sulfate acts as a cathartic by exerting an **osmotic effect** within the lumen of the intestine to bring fluid into the intestine, to retain fluid therein and to increase the total fluid bulk of the feces. The macromolecular blood plasma substitutes used in acute blood loss act by the same principle. These substances are administered directly into blood vessels and remain within them. By exerting an osmotic effect, they help to restore and maintain an adequate volume of blood.

SYNOPSIS

The action of a drug is the process by which the drug brings about a change in some preexisting physiologic function or biochemical process of the living organism. The effects produced by a drug can be measured and expressed only in terms of an alteration of some known function or process that maintains the existence of the organism. The alteration brought about by the action of a drug may be one that either returns a function or process to normal operating levels or changes a function or process in a direction away from normal levels. Drugs may also act to prevent changes by other factors, such as disease or other drugs. Although drugs do not confer any new function on the living cell or organism, they may be precise tools to disclose and analyze, as Claude Bernard said, "the most delicate phenomena of the living machine."

The part of the body in which the drug acts to initiate the chain of events leading to the response — the effect — is the site of action. It may be close to the effector organ or distant from the tissue or organ that ultimately responds. It may be at the surface of the cell, inside the cell or extracellular.

The means by which a drug in the immediate vicinity of its site of action initiates the series of events measured or observed as an effect is known as its mechanism of action. The mechanism of action of most drugs is believed to involve a chemical interaction between the drug and a functionally important component of the living system. When this component is identifiable as a distinct entity, the mechanism of action can be readily explained. This is frequently the case for drugs that act at extracellular sites. However, the majority of drugs do not act extracellularly, and to help understand their mechanisms of action the concept of receptors was formulated.

The hypothetical receptor is regarded as a macromolecular tissue constituent of functional significance at the site of drug action. Drugs are postulated to combine reversibly with receptors by means of ionic bonds, hydrogen bonds and Van der Waals forces. The concomitant formation of a number of these different types of bonds gives the drug-receptor complex sufficient stability to initiate the events that ultimately lead to the pharmacologic effect. For the most part, these interactions are readily reversible. The specificity and selectivity of drug-receptor interactions arise not just from the number and types of bonds formed, but also from the spatial configuration of the sites for bond formation at the surface of the receptor.

Whereas the majority of drugs produce effects by mechanisms involving a drug-receptor interaction, certain drugs produce their characteristic effects without combining directly with a receptor. The most notable among those drugs whose actions do not involve receptors are the volatile general anesthetic agents.

GUIDES FOR STUDY AND REVIEW

How do you distinguish between the effect of a drug and the action of a drug?

What are the only terms in which the effects of any drug can be expressed or measured? Do drugs produce quantitative or qualitative changes in bodily functions?

What is the site of action of a drug? What parts of the body can serve as sites of drug action? What is the relationship between the site of action of a drug and the tissue or organ of the body that ultimately responds to the drug?

The mechanism of action of most drugs involves what type of interaction? For most drugs, where does this interaction take place with respect to the cell?

What is a drug receptor? How do drugs interact with receptors? What are the forces responsible for this interaction? What force is best suited to initiate a drug-receptor interaction? What forces largely determine the specificity of drug-receptor interactions? How can the receptor concept explain the difference in the pharmacologic effect of two isomers?

May some drugs produce effects by chemical interactions other than drug-receptor interactions? Are these actions relatively specific or nonspecific? What are some examples of such interactions?

Does the mechanism of action of drugs such as the volatile general anesthetics involve discernible chemical reactions? How have the pharmacologic effects of such agents been explained? Are there classes of drugs other than the general anesthetics whose mechanism of action does not involve a chemical reaction? Examples?

SUGGESTED READING

Ariens, E. J. *Molecular Pharmacology: The Mode of Action of Biologically Active Compounds.* New York: Academic, 1964. Vol. 1, p. 197.

Barlow, R. B. *Introduction to Chemical Pharmacology,* 2d ed. London: Methuen, 1964.

Burgen, A. S. V. Receptor mechanisms. *Annu. Rev. Pharmacol.* 10:7, 1970.

Burger, A., and Parulkar, A. P. Relationship between chemical structure and biological activity. *Annu. Rev. Pharmacol.* 6:19, 1966.

Clark, A. J. *The Mode of Action of Drugs on Cells.* London: Arnold, 1933.

Ehrlich, P. *Collected Papers.* (Edited by F. Himmelweit.) London: Pergamon, 1957.

Furchgott, R. F. Receptor mechanisms. *Annu. Rev. Pharmacol.* 4:21, 1964.

Koshland, D. E., Jr. Conformation changes at the active site during enzyme action. *Fed. Proc.* 23:719, 1964.

Mautner, H. G. The molecular basis of drug action. *Pharmacol. Rev.* 19:107, 1967.

Pauling, L. *The Nature of the Chemical Bond,* 3rd ed. Ithaca, N.Y.: Cornell University Press, 1960.

Pauling, L. The hydrate microcrystal theory of general anesthesia. *Anesth. Analg. Curr. Res.* 43:1, 1964.

Porter, C. C., and Stone, C. A. Biochemical mechanisms of drug action. *Annu. Rev. Pharmacol.* 7:15, 1967.

Porter, R., and O'Connor, M. (eds.). *Molecular Properties of Drug Receptors.* Ciba Foundation Symposium. London: J. & A. Churchill, Ltd., 1970.

Rang, H. P. Receptor mechanisms. *Br. J. Pharmacol.* 48:475, 1973.

Van Rossum, J. M. The relation between chemical structure and biologic activity. *J. Pharm. Pharmacol.* 15:285, 1963.

4. HOW DRUGS REACH THEIR SITE OF ACTION
I. General Principles of Passage of Drugs Across Biologic Barriers

We have seen that a drug can produce an effect only when it is in the immediate vicinity of its site of action. With the obvious exceptions of chemicals that act like the cathartic magnesium sulfate or the plasma substitutes, drugs do not make their initial contact with the body at, or even near, their locus of action. In almost all cases, drugs must move from where they are administered to the tissues or cells where they will act. For example, when aspirin is swallowed for the relief of a headache or a barbiturate is taken to produce sleep, these agents must go from the gastrointestinal tract to their respective sites of action in the brain to exert their characteristic effects. (One would hardly consider rubbing an aspirin on the forehead to relieve the headache!) To do this, they must pass through various cells and tissues which act as barriers to their movement. Just as receptors show specificity with regard to the drugs with which they combine, so too do barriers show a certain degree of selectivity in the ease with which they permit drugs to pass through them. Thus the anatomic structures which act as barriers to the migration of materials are called *semipermeable,* allowing certain chemicals to pass freely, others to pass with difficulty and still others to be almost entirely excluded from passage. We have seen that the specificity of a drug-receptor combination is the consequence of the physiocochemical properties and structural configuration of the receptor at the site of action as well as of the physicochemical properties and structure of the drug molecule. In an analogous way, the selectivity of migration through the anatomic barrier is the consequence of the physicochemical properties and structural configuration of the barrier as well as of the migrating molecule. We have also noted that the forces responsible for a particular drug-receptor combination are not unique to that combination but underlie all the reactions between drugs and tissue elements of a living system. In a parallel fashion, the mechanisms that serve to move a drug across a particular barrier are those which move any substance across any biologic barrier. This movement is called *biotransport,* and the mechanisms underlying the transfer of chemicals across biologic barriers are called *transport processes* or *transport mechanisms.*

Biotransport is a specific case of the general phenomenon of transport, and *transport* is defined as the translocation of a *solute* from one *phase* to another, the solute appearing in the same form in both phases. A *phase* is a homogeneous, physically distinct part of a system which is separated from other parts of the system by definite bounding surfaces. In the physicochemical sense, the boundary may be any surface we choose to designate as separating two phases, but in the biologic sense we usually mean an anatomic structure which may be the membrane separating the outside from the interior of a cell, or may even be the whole structure, such as the epidermal layer of the skin. In the biologic sense, then, the phases are the environmental conditions on either side of the anatomic barrier. The material that is transferred from one phase to another is a solute, and implicit in any discussion of biologic transport is the fact that we are talking about *chemicals in solution in biologic media.* The explicit statement that the transferred solute must be in the same form in both phases also helps to distinguish biologic transport processes from other biologic processes. For example,

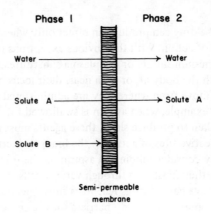

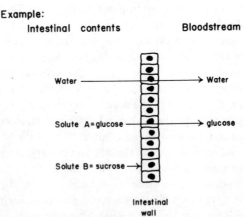

FIGURE 4-1. Translocation from one phase to another. The semipermeable membrane permits the passage of water and solute A (glucose), but not solute B (sucrose) from Phase 1, the side of higher concentration, to Phase 2, the side of lower concentration. Sucrose may disappear from Phase 1 since it is digested by intestinal enzymes and converted to glocuse and fructose, which are absorbed.

when the sugar sucrose is ingested, it quickly disappears from the intestine. However, its disappearance cannot be considered transport across the intestinal wall, since the substances leaving the intestine are glucose and fructose, the end products of a digestive process, and not the original sucrose (Fig. 4-1). Thus *biotransport* may be defined as *the translocation of a solute from one side of a biologic barrier to the other, the transferred solute appearing in the same form on both sides of the biologic barrier.*

The principal transport mechanisms underlying movement across biologic barriers are *passive diffusion, facilitated diffusion, active transport* and *pinocytosis.* Each of these will be discussed in terms of the forces responsible for the movement of solute and of the requirements of the process for energy derived from the cells or tissues of the biologic barrier.

PASSIVE DIFFUSION

Definitions

The term *diffusion* denotes the natural phenomenon by which molecules or other particles intermingle as a result of their ceaseless, chaotic motion — their inherent kinetic energy — during which they collide with each other and with the surface of any enclosure. The progression of the diffusion process can be readily observed with the naked eye if distilled water is carefully layered onto the surface of a water solution of a dye. Both water and dye molecules wander across the boundary, so that in the course of time the whole body of liquid attains nearly uniform color, i.e., uniform concentration (Fig. 4-2). If a barrier or membrane permeable to the dye molecule is placed between the two layers, the same phenomenon occurs. When the dye molecules collide with the surface of the membrane, some may pass through it from one side to the other. Obviously, the greater the number of molecules, the greater the number of collisions with the membrane and the greater the probability of transfer through the membrane. When equal numbers of molecules are present on both sides of the mem-

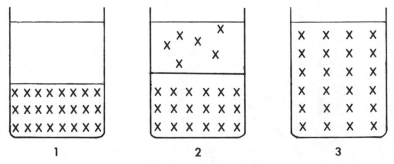

FIGURE 4-2. Diffusion. In the first beaker, distilled water is carefully layered over an aqueous solution of dye. Due to thermal agitation (Brownian movement) of both water and dye molecules, the dye molecules (X) migrate into the distilled water layer and water migrates into the solution of dye (beaker 2). Equilibrium is reached with time, and the dye molecules are equally distributed throughout the entire system (beaker 3).

brane, there will still be an exchange of dye molecules between the two sides, but there will be no *net* change in numbers. The diffusion of dye molecules through the membrane will continue from the side where there are more dye molecules — the side of higher concentration — to the side where there are fewer molecules — the side of lower concentration — until there are equal numbers on both sides, i.e., equal concentrations. Thus the transfer of solutes across a membrane by the process of diffusion, analogous to the movement of water "downhill" from a higher to a lower level, is the consequence of *the tendency of all naturally occurring processes to change spontaneously in a direction which will lead to equilibrium.*

The force which directs the movement of solute is the difference between concentrations of the solute on the two sides of the membrane — the *gradient* between the two phases. No energy has to be supplied to the system since no work is done to make the molecules move from a higher to a lower concentration. Thus the process is said to be a *passive* process. We may define *passive diffusion,* then, as *the directed movement of a solute through a biologic barrier from the phase of higher concentration to the phase of lower concentration, the process requiring no direct expenditure of energy by the biologic system.*

In diffusion, any increase in concentration leads to a proportional increase in the amount of solute transferred in a unit of time. Thus the rate of migration or diffusion of the solute is proportional to the gradient between the two phases. This is illustrated in Figure 4-3 for the transfer of ethyl alcohol from the lumen of the intestine to the blood. As the ethanol crosses the intestinal wall and diffuses into the blood vessels in the tissue, it is rapidly carried away from the intestine by the circulation. Therefore the concentration of the alcohol on the nonluminal side of the intestinal barrier tends to be negligible compared to that on the luminal side. And as a result,

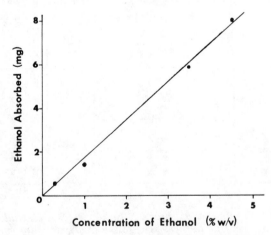

FIGURE 4-3. *Relationship between the amount of ethanol absorbed from the small intestine of the rat and the concentration of ethanol in the intestine (concentration of ethanol expressed as per cent, weight/volume X 100). (After T. Z. Csaky,* First International Pharmacological Meeting Symposia, *1963. Vol. 3, p. 230.)*

the amount of alcohol that leaves the intestine in one hour is directly proportional to the concentration of alcohol in the intestine.

Although a concentration gradient is indispensable for the passive diffusion of a solute, it does not follow that a solute will be able to diffuse across a biologic barrier just because it is in higher concentration on one side of the barrier. The concentration gradient is merely the force responsible for movement. But the facility with which a solute diffuses depends on the nature of the biologic barrier itself — on those factors determining the barrier's selective permeability: the physicochemical properties of its individual constituents and the way in which these constituents are organized within the barrier structure. One would anticipate, then, that the rate of diffusion of a particular solute across the wall of the intestine might be different from that across the wall of a blood capillary even if the concentration were the same at both barriers. This is indeed true. But even though the *absolute* rates of diffusion of given solutes vary according to the characteristics of the particular barrier, the *relative* rates of diffusion of given solutes appear to be much the same regardless of the barrier involved. In other words, if we rank a group of compounds according to the rate at which they diffuse across the intestinal wall, we find that they arrange themselves in much the same order with regard to rate of diffusion across most other biologic barriers. This implies that the diverse anatomic structures that serve as barriers to the free migration of solutes must have certain similarities in their properties and organization which are noteworthy with respect to the diffusion of solutes. Knowing the characteristics which biologic barriers have in common, we should be able to formulate some general principles of passive diffusion that would be applicable to all barriers.

Membrane Structure
Regardless of whether we designate the biologic barrier as a complete tissue or organ, e.g., the wall of a capillary or of the intestine, or as particular cells which make up the tissue or organ, the organizational architecture of the tissue is such that in most cases the migration of solutes occurs through cells and not between them. In order for a solute to pass through a cell, it must, of course, first penetrate the enclosure of the cell, the *cell membrane*. The membrane, then, becomes the ultimate barrier to the migration of solutes through any biologic structure. Moreover, studies have shown that the membranes of all types of cells are remarkably alike in their overall chemical composition and in the spatial arrangement of their chemical components. Therefore the characteristics which biologic barriers share in common and which make for similarities in solute diffusion at diverse sites reduce to *the characteristics common to cell membranes*. What is this generalized view of the cell membrane and how do its structure and properties regulate the diffusibility of chemicals?

Chemical analyses of various cell membranes show that, despite differences in specific details, all cell membranes are composed chiefly of proteins and lipids. The lipids of the membrane consist mainly of cholesterol and **phospholipids**. These compounds, like proteins, have groups that can form ionic or hydrogen bonds with other appropriate groups. We have seen that water can form hydrogen bonds within itself or with other molecules having suitable atomic groupings. Compounds with groups like —OH or —NH acquire solubility in water through this tendency toward hydrogen bond formation. Accordingly, the groups which can readily form hydrogen bonds are called *hydrophilic groups,* from the Greek *hydro,* for "water," and *philos,* meaning "loving" or "a tendency toward." The membrane lipids also have numerous groups which cannot form hydrogen bonds, such as the —CH_2— groups of the long hydrocarbon chains of the fatty acid esters in the phospholipids. They are called *hydrophobic groups,* from the Greek *phobos,* meaning "to fear." The hydrophobic groups of molecules tend to make the compounds insoluble in water but soluble in organic solvents. Since lipids are characterized by relative insolubility in water and by solubility in organic solvents (or fat solvents), substances which acquire fat-like solubility through their hydrophobic groups are said to be *lipid-soluble* compounds.

It is this dual nature of the membrane lipids, possessing both hydrophilic and hydrophobic groups, that causes them to orient themselves into an orderly configuration within the membrane core. The tendency of the hydrophobic portions of the molecule is to withdraw from the aqueous phase, whereas the tendency of the hydrophilic portions is to be surrounded by water. Both these tendencies must be satisfied

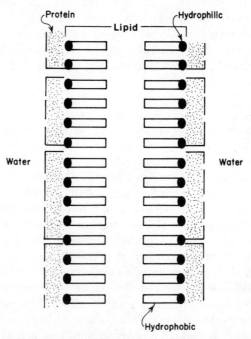

FIGURE 4-4. *The Davson-Danielli diagram of the cell membrane showing a double layer of lipid molecules covered by a protein coat. The hydrophobic end of each molecule is directed inward, while its hydrophilic end faces outward toward the protein coat. (From H. Davson and J. F. Danielli,* The Permeability of Natural Membranes. *Cambridge, Eng.: Cambridge University Press, 1952. P. 64.)*

simultaneously. This can be achieved most economically when the lipid organizes itself into two layers in which all the hydrophobic chains face each other and are surrounded by other hydrophobic chains, and all hydrophilic portions are oriented toward the water phase — toward the outer and inner membrane surfaces. Up until a few years ago, it was thought that this bimolecular lipid layer was covered on both sides by sheets of protein (Fig. 4-4). Another, newer concept of the cell membrane, and one that much recent evidence supports, views the proteins as globular molecules dispersed throughout the lipid and, in some instances, extending from one side of the membrane to the other (Fig. 4-5). The hydrophilic groups of the protein protrude from the membrane surface and are in contact with an aqueous phase; the hydrophobic residues are buried in the interior of the membrane sequestered from contact with water. The surfaces of the membrane have the appearance of tightly packed hydrophilic groups of phospholipids interspersed with globular proteins. The interior of the membrane is more loosely ordered, since the embedded proteins produce discontinuities in the lipid bilayer that forms the matrix of the mosaic. Thus the characteristic feature of the cell membrane is a bimolecular lipid layer, oriented perpendicular to the plane of the membrane, and forming the matrix of a mosaic in which globular proteins are randomly embedded.

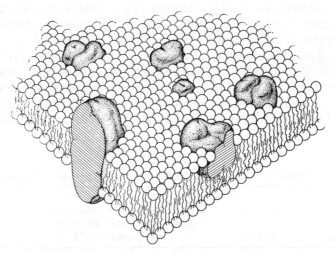

FIGURE 4-5. The lipid-globular protein mosaic model of the cell membrane with a lipid matrix. Schematic three-dimensional and cross-sectional views. The circles represent hydrophilic groups of the phospholipid molecules; wavy lines represent the hydrophobic fatty acid chains; solid bodies with stippled surfaces represent the globular integral proteins. (From S. J. Singer and G. L. Nicolson, The fluid mosaic model of the structure of cell membranes. Science 175:720, 1972. Copyright © 1972 by the American Association for the Advancement of Science, Washington, D.C.)

Diffusion Across Membranes

The barrier action of the membrane, its ability to restrict and sometimes prevent the passive penetration of many solutes, is believed to arise from the compact arrangement of the hydrocarbon chains of the lipids within it. Historically, the concept that the cell is surrounded by a lipid membrane which acts as a barrier to free diffusion arose indirectly from studies of the actual rates of penetration of various substances into cells; it did not come from morphologic evidence obtained by microscopic examination. We have stated earlier, in the discussion of the actions of drugs which do not involve a receptor-drug interaction, that there is great diversity of chemical structure among compounds which produce the common pharmacologic effect of general anesthesia. Ernest Overton and Hans H. Meyer, at the turn of this century, carried out independent investigations intended to explain the action of general anesthetics. In doing so, they found a systematic relationship between the solubility properties of the chemicals they used and the rates at which the chemicals entered cells.

These investigators used intact plants and animals to study the permeability characteristics of living cells. For example, Overton placed tadpoles in solutions of different alcohols and used disappearance of movement of the tadpoles as an indication of penetration of the agents into cells. He noted both the concentration at which the various alcohols produced this cessation of movement and the time required for the alcohols to act. Results typical of those obtained are shown in Table 4-1. The relative rates of penetration of these four alcohols are expressed in terms of the concentration of each agent that produced equivalent effects on tadpoles. The alcohols differ from each other by the length of their hydrocarbon chains. A series of compounds whose successive members possess, in addition to structural similarity, a regular difference in formula (in this case a $-CH_2-$group) is known as a *homologous* series. It can be seen that the concentration required to produce an equivalent disappearance of movement of the tadpoles becomes lower and lower as the length of the hydrocarbon chain of the alcohols increases. Thus the rate of penetration increases within the

Table 4-1.   Effect of Alcohols on the Movement of Tadpoles in Aqueous Medium

Alcohol	Formula	Concentration to Produce Equivalent Cessation of Movement (moles/liter[a])	Partition Coefficient (oil/water)
Methyl	CH_3OH	0.57	0.00966
Ethyl	C_2H_5OH	0.29	0.0357
Propyl	C_3H_7OH	0.11	0.156
Isobutyl	C_4H_9OH	0.045	0.588

[a] See Glossary for definition of **molarity.**

Data from E. Overton, *Studien über die Narkose zugleich ein Beitrag zur allgemeinen Pharmakologie.* Jena, Germany: Gustav Fischer, 1901. P. 101; and from K. H. Meyer and H. Hemmi, Beiträge zur Theorie der Narkose: III. *Biochem. Z.* 277:39, 1935. P. 45.

homologous series, since it takes less and less of a concentration gradient to move successive members of the series to the site of action.

As might be anticipated, the addition of a hydrophobic $-CH_2-$ group makes successive compounds less water soluble and more lipid soluble — it makes them less **polar** and more **nonpolar**. These changes in solubility cannot be measured, however, in terms of *absolute* solubility, i.e., how much of an agent will dissolve in water or in a lipid solvent. If absolute solubility alone were measured, we would see no differences among methyl, ethyl or propyl alcohols since they are all infinitely soluble in water and in a fat solvent such as ether. Only isobutyl alcohol would appear to be different since it has limited solubility in water. Differences in solubility characteristics can be demonstrated when *relative* solubilities are determined, i.e., when the tendency of an agent to *distribute* itself between water and lipid is measured in the presence of both an aqueous and a lipid phase. The tendency of an agent to distribute itself between these two phases can be expressed as the *ratio* of its concentration in the lipid phase to its concentration in the aqueous phase after the agent has come to equilibrium in the two-phase system. This ratio is known as the *lipid/water partition coefficient.* The lipid phase may be any fat solvent, such as ether, chloroform or a vegetable oil. Overton chose cottonseed oil as the lipid phase for his determination of the lipid/water partition coefficients of the alcohols in Table 4-1. He found that in this homologous series, the partition coefficient between the two solvents water and oil changed in favor of the latter as the chain length increased. It follows that the rate of cellular permeability of the alcohols also increased as the oil/water partition coefficient increased. Thus the lipid/water partition coefficient can be an external measure of the relative tendency of agents to leave the aqueous medium outside a cell and enter the lipid within the membrane.

Overton and Meyer summarized the results of their studies by suggesting that (1) the cell membrane is lipoid in nature; (2) the facility of substances to diffuse across the membrane is determined by their ability to dissolve in the membrane; and (3) this ability is proportional to their lipid/water partition coefficients. This view was later supported by the classic experiment of Collander and Bärlund. These investigators found a very good correlation between olive oil/water partition coefficients of an extensive series of organic substances and their rates of penetration into plant cells (Fig. 4-6). Many other studies since then, using various two-phase solvent systems to determine lipid/water partition coefficients, have shown that these early findings are generally applicable to the permeability of many other types of cells. Thus one of the general principles governing the passive diffusion of substances across membranes may now be stated: *the rate of passive diffusion is dependent on the degree of lipid solubility, and compounds that are highly soluble in lipids diffuse rapidly, whereas those that are relatively lipid insoluble diffuse more slowly.*

As we have said, these first deductions about the lipoid nature of the cell membrane were based on its functional properties. Even the evidence which led Danielli and Davson in 1935 to visualize the structure of the membrane as depicted in Figure 4-4 was not obtained from direct morphologic examination. Only within the last decade or so, after the sophisticated tools of electron microscopy, polarized light microscopy

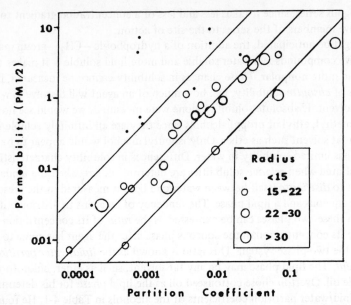

FIGURE 4-6. Permeability of cells of Chara certatophylla to organic nonelectrolyes of different lipid solubility and different molecular size. Abscissa: olive oil/water partition coefficient. Ordinate: permeability (PM ½); P is the permeability constant in centimeters per hour, and M is the molecular weight of the penetrating substance. Each circle represents a single compound; the radius of each circle symbolizes the molecular radius in angstroms, as indicated. (Modified from A. Collander, Physiol. Plant. 2:300, 1949.)

and x-ray diffraction analysis became available, has it been possible to obtain evidence of structure directly from observations of the cell membrane. The structure of the cell membrane that has emerged from these recent studies incorporates the earlier deductions concerning the bimolecular arrangement of its phospholipids. This newer model presents a different conceptual organization and role, however, for the membrane proteins.

Although Collander and Bärlund found good correlation between rates of penetration and lipid/water partition coefficients for the majority of the compounds they examined, they noticed that certain very small molecules penetrate more rapidly, and some very large molecules somewhat more slowly, than would be predicted on the basis of their partition coefficients. In Figure 4-5 the size of the symbol used for each compound indicates its relative molecular size, or molecular radius. It can be seen that many of the compounds of radius below 15 angstroms[1] are high above the line and some of those of larger size fall well below the line, indicating a deviation from the relatively good proportionality shown by the other compounds. The small

[1] An angstrom is a unit of length equal to one ten-thousandth of a micron or one hundred-millionth of a centimeter.

molecules that diffused faster than predicted were water-soluble particles like urea (NH_2CONH_2) and thiourea, and water itself was found to penetrate with extreme rapidity. These findings led Collander and Bärlund to propose that the surface of the cell membrane is not a continuum of lipid, but is interspersed with tiny holes through which certain molecules can leak in spite of their relative lipid insolubility.

As this "pore theory" developed, the assumption was made that water-filled channels extend through the membrane from one side to the other and that small molecules diffuse through these hydrophilic passageways. The presence of pores in the cell membrane has not yet been verified by direct observation because their postulated diameter is beyond the maximum resolving power of the electron microscope; the evidence of their existence is only inferential. Future research will tell whether the proteins that protrude from the outer membrane surface and traverse the entire breadth of the membrane can serve as watery channels for these small molecules; such aqueous passageways could open and close as the proteins are induced to aggregate or disaggregate. However, the fact remains that relatively small water-soluble molecules do passively diffuse across the cell membrane, whether through pores or otherwise, at rates which are inversely proportional to their molecular size (the smaller the molecule, the faster it penetrates).

The slower-than-predicted rate of diffusion for relatively large organic molecules may have a more factual explanation. When a substance traverses a membrane, not only does it have to diffuse through the interior lipid of the membrane but, in order to reach or to leave the lipid core, it has to diffuse through water-lipid interfaces on both sides of the membrane. Large organic molecules with a great number of hydrophobic groups are so water insoluble that they may encounter difficulty in passing through the water-lipid interface, and therefore their rate of passage across the cell membrane is slowed despite the high degree of lipid solubility. Thus some water solubility conferred on a molecule by the presence of hydrophilic groups is also essential for rapid diffusion across cell membranes. We can now modify our statement of the principles governing passive diffusion to include this factor of molecule size and say that *the rate of diffusion of a solute across a biologic barrier is dependent on its lipid solubility and on its molecular size.*

Weak Electrolytes

The early investigators, in arriving at the theory concerning the relationship of the rate of passive diffusion to lipid solubility, used organic compounds which do not form ions when dissolved in water, in other words, nonelectrolytes. But the majority of the agents of pharmacologic interest are organic compounds which do form ions in aqueous solutions and which are electrolytes. Their ability to ionize, however, is different from that of inorganic compounds like sodium chloride or hydrochloric acid. Whereas inorganic electrolytes exist in water almost completely as their respective ions, only a fraction of the molecules of most organic electrolytes dissociate into ions in aqueous solution. Since the conductance of electricity in solution is dependent on the number of ions present, substances like the inorganic salts are known as *strong electrolytes,* and the organic compounds, which ionize only partially, as *weak electro-*

lytes. The way in which these weak electrolytes diffuse across the cell membrane needs some additional clarification.

Some weak electrolytes form ions by giving up, or donating, a proton (hydrogen ion) and are called *weak acids.* Thus, for the weak electrolyte acetic acid:

$$CH_3COOH \rightleftharpoons CH_3COO^- + H^+$$

or for aspirin:

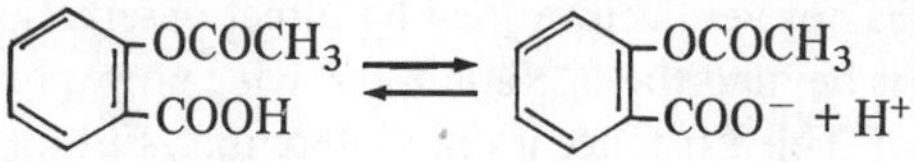

Other weak electrolytes are *bases,* which ionize by accepting a proton. In the discussion of bond formation we pointed out that certain atoms like oxygen, sulfur and nitrogen can donate an electron pair to the naked proton of the hydrogen ion to form a coordinate covalent bond and retain the positive charge associated with the hydrogen ion. Since so many drugs are organic compounds containing nitrogen, this type of coordinate covalent bond formation plays an important role in the ionization of drugs. Figure 4-7 shows this ionization for three different drugs. Norepinephrine, which has a nitrogen attached to only one carbon, is an example of a *primary amine;* epinephrine, with its nitrogen attached to two carbon atoms, is an example of a *secondary amine;* and cocaine, with three carbons attached to the nitrogen, is an example of a *tertiary amine.* All drugs which have one of these structures are *weak bases* and have the potential of becoming positively charged ions (cations) by the mechanism illustrated earlier for ammonia (p. 36).

The degree to which a weak electrolyte will ionize is an inherent property of the molecule and is determined by the electron-attracting and electron-repelling properties of its constituent atoms. This tendency to ionize is a constant for a given weak electrolyte when measured in pure water at a given temperature and is expressed as the *ionization constant.* Moreover, the fraction that is ionized is always in equilibrium with the fraction that is undissociated. Thus,

$$HA \rightleftharpoons H^+ + A^-$$

and

$$B + H^+ \rightleftharpoons BH^+$$

where *HA* symbolizes the undissociated acid and *B*, the nonionized base.

Since such equilibria exist for the ionization of weak electrolytes, the law of mass action should be applicable to them, and it should be possible to change the fraction of ionized or nonionized material present in solution by changing the hydrogen ion concentration. You will recall that the law of mass action states: when a chemical reaction reaches equilibrium at a constant temperature, *the product of the active masses on one side of a chemical equation, when divided by the product of the active*

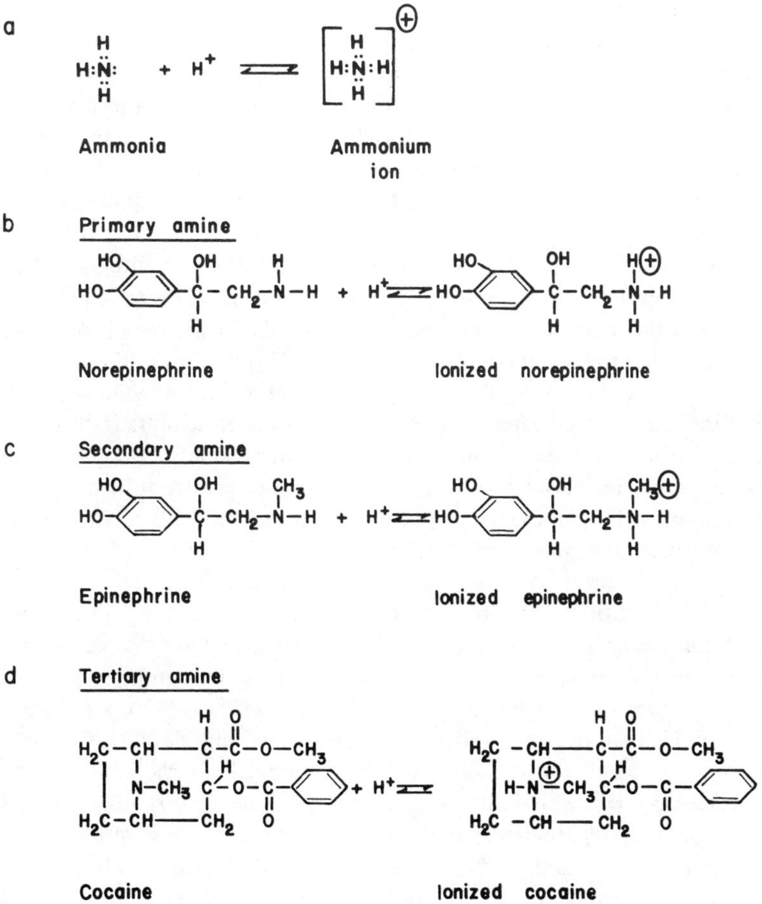

FIGURE 4-7. *Ionization of amines by coordinate covalent bond formation.*

masses on the other side of the equation, is a constant regardless of the amount of each substance present at the beginning of the action. Thus, for an acid:

$$\frac{[H^+] \times [A^-]}{[HA]} = \text{a constant}$$

where [ ] stands for concentration. For a base:

$$\frac{[BH^+]}{[B] \times [H^+]} = \text{a constant}$$

If we add hydrogen ions to a solution of a weak acid, the concentration of the ionized portion, $[A^-]$, in the numerator must decrease and the concentration of the undissociated acid, [HA], in the denominator must increase in order to keep the relationship constant. The converse would be true for the addition of hydrogen ions to a solution of a weak base. In both cases, an excess of hydrogen ions drives the ionization reaction of the weak electrolytes to the *side of the equation which does not have hydrogen ions.* Therefore, an excess of hydrogen ions in a solution of a weak acid tends to *decrease* the extent of ionization of the weak acid, and an excess of hydrogen ions in a solution of a weak base tends to *increase* the extent of ionization of the weak base.

It is much simpler to use the convention **pH** to express the hydrogen ion concentration of a solution, as long as we always remember that pH is an expression of the *reciprocal* of the hydrogen ion concentration; i.e., the higher the pH of a solution, the lower the hydrogen ion concentration, and vice versa. From the relationships between the ionization of weak electrolytes and pH, we can now draw the following generalizations: (1) the degree of ionization of a weak electrolyte is dependent on its ionization constant and on the pH of the aqueous medium in which it is dissolved; (2) the degree of ionization of a weak acid tends to be greater at higher pH's and lower at lower pH's; and (3) the degree of ionization of a weak base tends to be greater at lower pH's and lower at higher pH's.

The degree of ionization of weak acids and bases has a great deal of significance when we consider their diffusion across biologic barriers. At the pH's of biologic fluids, weak electrolytes are present partly in the dissociated or ionized form and partly in the undissociated or nonionized form. The ionized groups of the weak electrolytes interact strongly with water, which makes them more water soluble and less fat soluble than the undissociated molecule. If we consider diffusion only in terms of a solute's ability to dissolve in the membrane lipid, then the ionized form of a weak electrolyte would diffuse across the membrane much more slowly than the more lipid-soluble, undissociated form. However, in the case of ions, an additional barrier to passage through the membrane may arise from their interaction with negatively or positively charged groups at the protein surfaces. These two factors — the greater electrical resistance to passage and the much lower lipid solubility — combine to make the rate of penetration of the ionized form so slow that, for all practical purposes, the rate of diffusion of a weak acid or base may be entirely attributed to the concentration gradient of the undissociated fraction itself. For weak electrolytes, then, we must now add another factor to the general principles governing their passive diffusion across cell membranes: *The rate of passive diffusion of weak electrolytes is dependent on their degree of ionization: the greater the fraction that is nonionized, the greater the rate of diffusion, since the rate of diffusion is mainly determined by that of the undissociated portion.*

The stability of the pH of most fluids within the body is vigorously maintained at levels near neutrality by the body's regulatory mechanisms. But the fluids within the stomach are characteristically at a low pH, whereas those within the intestines vary from a relatively acid pH near the stomach to more neutral values farther from it, and the pH of the urine as it is formed in the kidney can be either lower or higher than 7

Table 4-2. Effect of pH on Rate of Absorption of Strychnine from the Stomach[a]

pH of Solution in Stomach	% Undissociated Strychnine	Interval to Death Following Injection (min.)
8.0	54.0	24
6.0	1.2	83
5.0	0.1	150
3.0	0.001	Survived

[a]Strychnine (5 mg) was injected into the stomach of anesthetized cats.
Source: Modified from J. Travell, *J. Pharmacol. Exp. Ther.* 69:21, 1940.

under various normal conditions. In certain abnormal states, even the pH of plasma or other body fluids may be above or below their normal range.

It can be readily appreciated, then, that the degree of ionization of a given compound may vary considerably at different biologic barriers or at a particular barrier under different conditions of pH. It follows from the relationship between rate of diffusion and degree of dissociation that the rate of penetration of a weak electrolyte across a particular barrier also depends on the pH of its solution at the barrier site. This is well illustrated by the results obtained in studies of the effect of pH on the absorption of the weak base strychnine from the stomach of animals (Table 4-2). At pH 8.0, more than half of strychnine exists in solution in the more lipid-soluble, undissociated form. Consequently, when strychnine was administered in alkaline medium, it rapidly crossed the stomach wall as measured by the fact that the animals died within a relatively short time. In contrast, when an equivalent amount of strychnine was administered in solution at pH 3.0, the concentration gradient of the undissociated form was markedly reduced. As a result, the quantity of poison absorbed from the stomach was insufficient to produce any deleterious effects.

In summary, then, passive diffusion may be defined as a transport process in which the driving force for movement across the cell membrane is the concentration gradient of the solute, the rate of diffusion being proportional to this gradient and dependent on the lipid solubility, degree of ionization and molecular size of the solute.

SPECIALIZED TRANSPORT PROCESSES
The concept of a membrane as a simple lipid barrier, interspersed perhaps with aqueous pores, provides the cell with little discriminatory power to move material into or out of its environment except by virtue of size, solubility and charge of the solutes. The cell must have greater latitude than this for acquiring the substances it needs as energy sources or building materials and for getting rid of its waste products. Indeed, we know that cell membranes are able to distinguish between optical isomers of sugars and amino acids as well as among a variety of other substances, irrespective of their lipid solubility, molecular size and charge. Also, many

substances of physiologic importance, such as glucose, do penetrate membranes at rates much faster than would be predicted merely on the basis of passive diffusion and the properties of an inert barrier. However, specialized transport processes in which the barrier theoretically plays an active role can account for these and many other experimental observations. These specialized transport processes give the cell membrane the flexibility and selectivity it requires to control the movement of specific substances into and out of the cell.

Facilitated Diffusion

Many molecules, especially those which are primarily hydrophilic, show peculiarities in their migration through the membrane even though their movement is *with* the concentration gradient and ceases when the gradient disappears. First, as already mentioned, the rate of penetration is greater for many substances than would be expected on the basis of either their lack of lipid solubility, as in the case of glucose, or the presence of a charge, as in the case of many ions such as sodium ion. Furthermore, optical isomers with the same lipid solubility and the same charge may have very different rates of penetration. What is also observed is that the rate of penetration is initially proportional to the concentration gradient. but as the gradient increases, the rate of migration stops increasing and, instead, reaches a limiting or maximal value (Fig. 4-8). This is also different from what happens in passive diffusion, in which the rate of migration always increases with a rise in the concentration

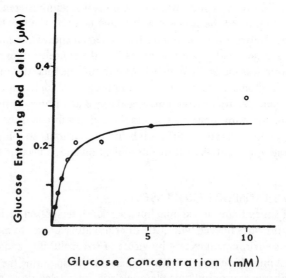

FIGURE 4-8. *Facilitated diffusion of glucose into human red blood cells. Abscissa: glucose concentration (mM) in the bathing medium. Ordinate: μM glucose entering intracellular water (1 ml) of red blood cells during 15-second incubation at 5° C. (Modified from W. D. Stein,* The Movement of Molecules Across Cell Membranes. *New York: Academic, 1967. P. 134.)*

gradient, provided that the cell membrane is not structurally damaged by high concentrations of solute. One may also frequently observe that the rate of migration of a particular compound is markedly reduced by the presence of another compound of similar chemical structure.

The transport processes with the characteristics just described are obviously diffusion processes since, by definition, the moving force is a concentration gradient. But how can we account for the other characteristics which are so different from those of simple passive diffusion? To explain the specificity and selectivity of drug action, the concept of a hypothetical receptor was developed. And to account for the same properties of specialized transport processes, a somewhat analogous concept has been formulated. The specificity and selectivity of solute transport are postulated as arising from temporary binding of solute to some site or component of the membrane. This hypothetical binding site has been given the name *carrier*, and since binding of carrier and solute facilitates the transmembrane movement of solute, the process has been termed *facilitated diffusion* (Fig. 4-9).

Carriers, as in the case of receptors, are viewed as having special groups or structural configurations which lead to their binding only with solutes that are complementary. Also, the interaction between the transferred molecules and the transfer system is reversible and does not modify the solute or the carrier. This implies that

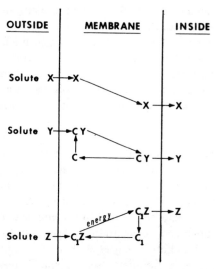

FIGURE 4-9. Passive diffusion, facilitated diffusion and active transport. X is a lipid-soluble drug, freely diffusible in the membrane. Y is a lipid-insoluble drug which combines with carrier, C, at the outside surface of the membrane to form a complex, CY, which moves across the lipid membrane. At the inner surface of the membrane, CY dissociates to release Y into the intracellular space. Both X and Y are transferred with the concentration gradient. Z is a drug, insoluble in the membrane, which combines with carrier C_1. Z is actively transported against a concentration gradient.

the temporary binding involves the same kind of bond formation that can occur between a drug and its receptor — hydrogen bonding, ionic bonding and Van der Waals attractive forces. Proteins have the properties necessary to impart the specificity characteristic of carrier transport systems, and there is much evidence to support the hypothesis that membrane proteins function as carriers.

The carrier concept also postulates that the complex of solute and carrier is able to cross from one side of the membrane to the other, but that solute can cross the membrane at only a negligible rate when not combined with carrier. Thus the presence of carrier can account for the greatly increased transport capacity of those substances which can combine with it. However, the availability of sites on a membrane which can act as carrier is necessarily limited; the rate of diffusion will be proportional to the concentration gradient only as long as there is sufficient carrier to accommodate all the solute. Thus the carrier hypothesis can also account for the limited rate of diffusion reached at higher concentration gradients, when the carrier ability is saturated.

Facilitated diffusion may be defined, then, as a transport process in which the driving force for movement across the cell is the concentration gradient of the solute, the rate of diffusion being dependent on the binding capacity of the solute and its hypothetical carrier and being limited by the availability of carrier. As in passive diffusion, no cellular energy is required beyond that needed to maintain the integrity of the cell and cell membrane. But in facilitated diffusion, the membrane can no longer be considered an inert barrier, as it is in passive diffusion, since it participates by making carrier available for the transfer of solute.

A number of physiologically important facilitated diffusion systems have been adequately characterized. Their presence at most cell membranes favors the cell's acquisition of essential substances, such as sugars, amino acids and various ions. For drugs, there is evidence, although inconclusive, to suggest that facilitated diffusion processes may exist for the transport of some water-soluble agents.

Active Transport

In some cases of carrier-mediated transport, the solute continues to move across the membrane even though there no longer is a concentration gradient in the direction of movement. Obviously, the driving force cannot be the concentration gradient, since the migration proceeds beyond the concentration equilibrium and, in fact, against a higher concentration. This movement across the membrane from the side of lower concentration to that of higher concentration is analogous to water being raised from a lower to a higher level. In both instances work has to be done, and this requires energy. The energy needed to transport a solute "uphill" must be supplied by the cell. Thus the cell is now actively involved in the transport process, and these processes are accordingly termed *active transport* (Fig. 4-9). With the exception of this requirement for expenditure of energy by the cell, the characteristics of active transport are the same as those for facilitated diffusion. Thus, *active transport* may be defined as a transport process requiring energy of cellular origin to move solute across a biologic barrier from a lower to a higher concentration gradient, the rate of transport being dependent on the binding capacity of the solute and its hypothetical carrier and being limited by the availability of carrier.

The physiologic need for transport systems that will allow a cell to accumulate substances essential for growth and maintenance and to eliminate waste products against concentration gradients is obvious. It is not surprising that active transport processes have been shown to exist for ions, sugars, amino acids, some vitamins and various other substances vital to the cell. And evidence for the active transport of drugs appears to be limited to those agents which bear close structural similarities to normal body constituents and to water-soluble compounds which share processes used for elimination of waste products.

Pinocytosis
The transfer process of pinocytosis almost defines itself in its derivation from the Greek *pino*, meaning "I drink," *kytos,* meaning "hollow vessel" (denoting a cell),

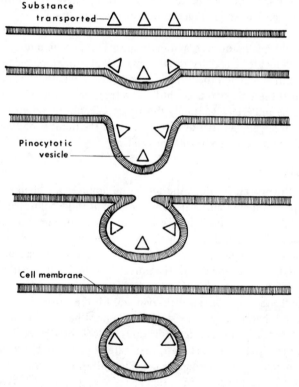

FIGURE 4-10. Stages of pinocytosis. Macromolecular solutes in contact with the membrane are trapped in microscopic cavities or cups – invaginations – formed on the surface of the membrane. The membrane fuses around and completely encloses the fluid to form a vesicle. The vesicle is pinched off, passing some fluid and solutes across the membrane into the interior of the cell.

and *osis,* "a process." Pinocytosis is just that: the engulfing of fluid by a cell. The mechanism involves the infolding of a microscopic part of the cell membrane, local invagination and the subsequent budding off within the cell interior of this small sac, or vesicle, which contains the solute (Fig. 4-10). In some cases, particulate matter can also be transferred by local invagination of the cell membrane; but then the process is more properly termed *phagocytosis,* from the Greek *phagein,* "to eat." These mechanisms also require the expenditure of cellular energy and, therefore, are appropriately classified as active transport processes. There is also a degree of specificity in some of the transfer processes believed to be pinocytotic.

The process of engulfing particles or dissolved materials by vesiculation is the most primitive mechanism for the ingestion of food. In the course of evolution the process was lost, but not completely, since the intestinal cells of newborn mammals still possess the ability to absorb certain substances by pinocytosis. In the newborn calf, for example, the capacity for absorbing soluble protein by pinocytosis is present at birth but disappears shortly thereafter. Poisoning by botulinus toxin and allergic reactions resulting from the ingestion of offending proteins (cf. **antigens** in the Glossary) are well-known phenomena in humans and certainly leave no doubt that the adult mammal can absorb intact macromolecules. The amount absorbed appears to be extremely small, however, and mechanisms other than pinocytosis may be responsible. Pinocytotic activity is rather marked at other biologic barriers, such as the alveoli of the lungs and the walls of blood vessels. Whether the numerous vesicles that are seen at these barriers account for the transfer of solute has not always been related as cause and effect. Certainly this process cannot represent the transfer mechanism for large quantities of materials, since the number of vesicles that would have to be formed would be beyond possibility.

FILTRATION

Filtration is the process in which the solids and liquid of a system are separated by means of a porous membrane that allows passage of fluid, solutes and some particulate materials, while retaining particles too large to pass through the pores. It is a purely physical process in which the driving force for movement is a *pressure gradient,* the rate of filtration being dependent on this gradient and on the size of the particle to be filtered in relation to the size of the pore. Thus filtration is markedly different from the transfer processes already described.

We have indicated that there is little evidence for the existence of pores in cell membranes and that, if they do exist, their size must be very small indeed. However, we know that intact proteins can pass various biologic barriers such as the capillary wall, and at the capillary level at least, their rate of movement is strongly dependent upon a pressure gradient. So when we consider filtration in terms of a biologic barrier, we are led to the conclusion that the process probably does not occur *across cell membranes* but *through spaces between cells.* Filtration may be extremely important for the movement of large macromolecules and is certainly an important process in the formation of urine and the ultimate elimination of substances from the body.

SYNOPSIS

Drugs or chemicals foreign to the body move across biologic barriers using the pre-existing processes which serve to transport substances required for the maintenance and growth of living organisms. This movement of solutes across complex barriers is determined by the general principles governing movement across the membrane of the cells which comprise the barrier. The membranes of all cells have functional similarity derived from their similar structural organization and chemical composition. The cell membrane is currently viewed as a structure containing a bimolecular layer of lipids with the hydrophobic groups of the lipid oriented toward each other and the hydrophilic groups aligned at both surfaces. This lipid bilayer forms the matrix of a mosaic in which proteins are embedded; the highly polar and ionic groups of the proteins protrude into the aqueous phase and the nonpolar residues are largely buried in the interior of the membrane. These membrane proteins are thought to perform many important functions, including (1) contributing to the strength of the membrane; (2) acting as enzymes (cf. p. 136) to promote chemical reactions; (3) acting as carrier protein for transport of substances through the membrane; and (4) providing discontinuities in the lipid bilayer which then serve as "pores" for passage of water-soluble materials through the membrane.

The mechanisms underlying biotransport can best be defined in terms of the forces responsible for movement of the solute and of the requirements of the process for cellular energy. Basic to all the mechanisms is the cellular energy needed to maintain the integrity and organization of the cell and its membrane. *Passive,* or *simple, diffusion* requires no additional expenditure of cellular energy, and movement occurs in the direction of the concentration gradient and in proportion to the physical force provided by the gradient. The rate of passive diffusion is also determined by the lipid solubility, the degree of ionization and the molecular size of the solute. *Facilitated diffusion,* like passive diffusion, requires no further expenditure of cellular energy, and movement occurs only with the concentration gradient. It differs from passive diffusion in that the physicochemical properties of the constituents of the membrane and those of the solute are insufficient to account for the rate of movement of the solutes. Therefore, the concept of temporary combination of solute with a hypothetical chemical structure or site —*carrier*— of the membrane must be invoked to explain the total phenomenon. *Active transport* also requires the concept of carrier-mediated passage across the membrane, but it is clearly distinguished from facilitated diffusion by the movement of the solute in a direction opposite to that of the concentration gradient. Thus active transport requires an energy source for the work to be done in moving the solute "uphill." *Pinocytosis* is a transport mechanism which also requires an expenditure of cellular energy. It differs from active transport in that the transfer of the solute is not mediated by combination with a carrier, but by the local invagination of the cell membrane and subsequent budding off of a vesicle containing the solute.

Nonelectrolytes, with the exception of very small or very large molecules, can diffuse passively across biologic barriers at rates proportional to their lipid/water partition coefficients. Very small molecules appear to move faster, and very large ones slower, than would be predicted on the basis of their lipid/water partition coefficients. Weak electrolytes, among them the majority of compounds of pharmacologic interest, diffuse passively across cell membranes at rates which are relatively proportional to their degree of ionization and to the lipid/water partition coefficient of their undissociated form. The foregoing general principles apply equally to substances of physiologic and pharmacologic importance. Many of the former are nonelectrolytes such as glucose, weak electrolytes such as amino acids or strong electrolytes such as inorganic ions. For these poorly lipid-soluble substances, the specialized transport processes of facilitated diffusion and active transport are available to assist their rapid ingress or egress from cells. Agents of pharmacologic interest may also use these specialized transport processes when their chemical structures are similar enough to those of the solutes normally transferred to permit temporary combination with the same specific carrier.

The question of whether the cell membrane is interspersed with tiny holes or pores through which small water-soluble molecules can readily diffuse awaits a definitive answer. It appears more likely, however, that the large protein molecules embedded in the lipid bilayer and traversing the entire thickness of the membrane provide direct watery passage through the interstices of the protein molecules. But at several biologic barriers the space *between* cells appears to provide a means of more ready passage for some substances. At these barriers, the process of filtration, proportional to a *pressure* gradient and related to the size of the transferred molecules, can account for the movement of these solutes.

GUIDES FOR STUDY AND REVIEW

What common characteristics do diverse biologic barriers have that account for similarities in solute movement at different sites? What is the general view of the cell membrane and how do its structure and properties regulate solute transport?

What are the mechanisms that account for the transfer of drugs (or other solutes) across biologic barriers? How do these mechanisms differ from one another?

In passive diffusion, what is the force responsible for solute movement and what are the requirements of the process for cellular energy? How do lipid solubility, degree of ionization and molecular size influence the rate of passive diffusion? How does an alteration in pH affect the diffusion of a weak acid? a weak base? Does a change in pH affect the diffusion of a strong acid? a strong base?

In facilitated diffusion what is the force responsible for solute movement and what are the requirements of the process for cellular energy? How does facilitated diffusion differ from passive diffusion? What factor determines and what factor limits the rate of facilitated diffusion?

What factor clearly distinguishes the process of active transport from the processes of passive and facilitated diffusion? Why is active transport essential for the life of the cell?

What is pinocytosis? What role, if any, does this process play in the movement of drugs across biologic barriers?

How does the process of filtration differ from other transport processes with respect to the pathway of solute movement across a barrier? with respect to the force responsible for transfer across a barrier? How does molecular size influence filtration? At what biologic barrier is filtration an important transport process?

SUGGESTED READING

Christensen, H.M. *Biological Transport.* New York: Benjamin, 1962.

Cohn, V.H. Transmembrane Movement of Drug Molecules. In B.N. La Du, H.G. Mandel, and E.L. Way (eds.), *Fundamentals of Drug Metabolism and Drug Disposition.* Baltimore: Williams & Wilkins, 1971.

Csaky, T.Z. Transport through biologic membranes. *Annu. Rev. Physiol.* 27:415, 1965.

Davson, H., and Danielli, J.F. *Permeability of Natural Membranes.* New York: Cambridge University Press, 1952.

Green, D.E. (ed.). Symposium: Membrane structure and its biological applications. *Ann. N.Y. Acad. Sci.* 226:1, 1973.

Stein, W.D. *The Movement of Molecules Across Cell Membranes.* New York: Academic, 1962.

Wilbrandt, W., and Rosenberg, T. The concept of carrier transport and its corollaries in pharmacology. *Pharmacol. Rev.* 13:109, 1961.

5. HOW DRUGS REACH THEIR SITE OF ACTION
II. Absorption and Distribution

In order for a drug to exert its characteristic effects, it must reach its site of action. This usually entails movement, since most drugs make their initial contact with the body some distance away from where they act. Although the transport processes described in Chapter 4 can adequately account for passage of drugs across any biologic membrane that impedes their progress, they can hardly explain movement over any great distance. The forces which drive passive or facilitated diffusion, or active transport and pinocytosis, are sufficient only to move solutes across the very short span of cellular membranes themselves. How, then, is the movement of drugs over greater distances accomplished? Just as oxygen from the lungs or food substances from the intestine gain access to every cell of the organism by way of the bloodstream, so too does the circulatory system serve as the *common pathway* for carrying drugs from the *inner side* of a biologic barrier to any tissue or organ. Hence, unless a drug is purposely administered to produce its effect locally, or is injected directly into the bloodstream, getting to its site of action involves two separate processes. The first of these is *absorption,* the movement of the solute into the bloodstream from the side of administration. The second process is *distribution,* the movement of solute from the blood into the tissue (Fig. 5-1).

The rate at which a drug reaches its site of action depends on both its rate of absorption and its rate of distribution. These rates, in turn, are determined by the rates of translocation across the specific barriers interposed between the sites of absorption and action. But we have already seen that there are notable similarities in the movement of materials across any biologic barrier. No matter how grossly different the barriers, the mechanisms responsible for solute movement are those which serve to transfer material across any cell membrane. In addition, the principles governing these transport mechanisms apply equally at all barriers. If no inequalities exist at diverse barriers with respect to the mechanisms available for biotransport, it follows that the explanation for the known and observed disparities in the overall movement of materials across the different biologic barriers must lie in the anatomic arrangement of the barriers themselves within their contiguous environment.

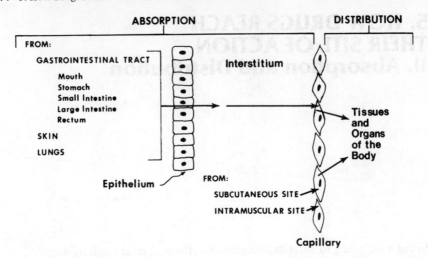

FIGURE 5-1. Absorption and distribution. Drugs entering the body by way of the gastrointestinal tract, skin or lungs must first traverse an epithelial barrier before entering the interstitium. Drugs given subcutaneously or intramuscularly bypass the epithelial barrier. Drugs given by any of the routes shown must traverse the capillary wall in order to enter the circulation.

From the physiologic viewpoint, the differences in the structure of biologic barriers subserve their particular function in relation to their normal external environment. For example, an alcohol sponge bath can be used to cool the body of a fevered child without the danger of producing any of the symptoms that would follow if the same quantity of alcohol were ingested by the child. The normal function of the skin is to protect the individual from material of the external environment, whereas that of the alimentary canal is to afford a more or less open gateway into the body for materials of exogenous origin. And the structure of each of these barriers is such that its main function can be realized.

Let us now examine some of these biologic barriers more closely to see how each structure with its normal physiologic function and its normal environmental conditions influences the absorption and distribution of drugs. In Chapter 6 we shall consider these same variables with respect to the barriers that a drug encounters on its way out of the body.

ABSORPTION

Routes of Administration

We defined absorption as the movement of solute from the site of administration across a biologic barrier into the bloodstream. To be more explicit this definition should also embrace the movement of solute into the *lymphatic system* — the tubular system which supplements the blood circulation. This second vascular system is like the blood vasculature, in that the smaller lymphatic tubules resemble capillaries and the large vessels, called lymphatic ducts, are comparable to veins. But the lymphatic system has no vessels corresponding to arteries; its fluid, lymph, does not flow in a circuit and is not self-contained. Lymph flow begins in the lymphatic capillaries, which collect fluid from the tissue spaces, and ends at the level of the neck where the chief vessels, the thoracic duct and the right lymphatic duct, empty into the large veins (Fig. 5-2). Thus the lymph functions only to deliver or carry back to the bloodstream substances, particularly water and macromolecules, that have entered the extracellular fluid from the cells or the blood capillaries. Indeed, in the intestinal tissue, the lymphatics serve as the chief route by which nutrients like fat and proteins make their way to the blood after leaving the intestine. Since the lymphatics can act as potentially important channels for absorption of materials that have gained access to interstitial fluid, we should amplify our statement of absorption: *only after a substance has entered the blood or lymph capillaries can it be said to be truly absorbed.*

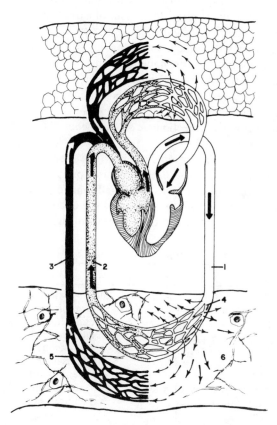

FIGURE 5-2. *Highly schematic diagram comparing blood and lymph circulation: artery* (1); *vein* (2); *lymphatic vessel* (3); *blood capillary* (4); *lymph capillary system* (5); *and interstitial space* (6).

It follows from the definition of absorption that a very important factor in determining the rate of entry of a solute into the circulation after its passage through the barrier is the vascularity at the site of absorption. The greater the vascularity, the greater the flow of blood and lymph within the tissue, and the greater the opportunity for removal of a drug from tissue into the circulation. Since the rate of blood flow is many hundred times that of lymph flow, the *amount of blood flowing* through the tissues on the inner side of the biologic barrier is really the determinant of the rate of absorption for most substances. Consequently, one of the environmental variables we shall have to consider with respect to the overall absorption at each site of administration is blood flow. This factor is equally important, as we shall see, in determining the rate of distribution of drugs to various organs and tissues.

In man and other terrestrial mammals, the lungs, the alimentary canal and the skin represent the most important sites of absorption of material from the external environment. When a drug or chemical is a *therapeutic agent* used in the treatment, prevention, cure or diagnosis of disease, the gastrointestinal tract is the most commonly used route of administration. Placement of a drug directly into any part of the gastrointestinal tract is called *enteral* (Gk. *enteron,* "an intestine") administration. This includes the usual mode of administration, i.e., swallowing the drug (oral, per os, p.o.), as well as placing the drug under the tongue (sublingual) and administration into the rectum. Other routes are called *parenteral* (Gk. *para,* "aside from"), since they bypass the gastrointestinal tract. Thus the administration of drugs by injection, by topical application to the skin or by inhalation through the lungs are all parenteral. The most common routes of injection are subcutaneous (S.C.), intramuscular (I.M.) and intravenous (I.V.).

From the standpoint of absorption, however, the various routes of administration can be more conveniently classified into those used primarily for *local effects* and those used for *systemic effects* (Table 5-1). The former do not require the intervention of the vascular system to get the drug to its site of action; agents may be regarded as acting locally when the manner of their placement ensures effects without the

Table 5-1.   Administration of Drugs

For Local Effect	For Systemic Effect
Application to skin	Sublingual administration
Application to mucous membranes	Oral administration
Nose	Rectal administration
Throat	Inhalation
Mouth	Subcutaneous administration
Eye	Intramuscular administration
Genitourinary tract	Intravenous administration
Oral administration (limited) — only	Intrathecal (injection into spinal sub-
for cathartics, antacids or drugs	arachnoid space)
used to treat parasitic or bacterial	
infections of gastrointestinal tract	
Various techniques for administering	
local anesthetics	

necessity of being distributed by the blood. As examples we can cite the application of calamine lotion to the skin for treatment of poison ivy, the use of nose drops to ease nasal congestion and the intradermal injection (placement into the upper layers of the skin) of various materials when testing for allergic reactions. The routes used for systemic effects require both absorption of the agents into the circulation and their distribution by the blood to the cells and tissues capable of responding to them. Only after intravascular administration is absorption completely bypassed; drugs are ready for immediate distribution to the various tissues of the body. We shall discuss only those routes which involve the more important sites from which chemicals or therapeutic agents enter the body.

Absorption from the Gastrointestinal Tract
The tissue covering the surface of the skin and lining every canal, tract and cavity which communicates with the external air is *epithelial* tissue. This tissue is made up of very closely associated cells with very little intercellular material, and the close approximation of each cell to its neighbor virtually precludes passage of material between cells. Thus, the barriers to absorption common to all parts of the alimentary canal as well as to the respiratory tract and skin are the epithelial cells themselves. After a substance passes through the epithelial barrier and reaches the inner side — the interstitial tissue containing vascular vessels — it comes in contact with internal environmental conditions which are nearly identical for each site, regardless of whether it is part of the gastrointestinal, respiratory or integumental epithelium. The fluids on the interior of these barriers are maintained at relatively constant composition, pH and temperature. On the inside of each of these barriers the resistance to movement of solutes into the blood or lymphatics is also nearly the same. However, the organization of the epithelium and the environmental conditions on its *external* surface are different for each site. Even in the alimentary canal, the epithelial lining and intraluminal environment vary from one part to another in accordance with the function of the particular segment. And it is these factors which account for differences in absorption in different parts of the gastrointestinal tract and at the different sites of entry into the body.

The Oral Cavity
The oral cavity is lined with a smooth-surfaced epithelium made up of several layers of cells. Its normal function is to secrete saliva into the mouth in order to moisten dry foodstuffs and start digestion. As a result of these secretions, the normal external environment of the epithelial cells has a slightly acidic pH and is composed mainly of water.

The thin epithelium, the rich vascularity and the external pH of the oral mucosa are highly conducive to rapid absorption. Many of those drugs which are weak electrolytes, even the weak bases, would be present in significant amounts as the undissociated molecule. But not much absorption occurs in the mouth, mainly because it is so difficult to keep solutions in contact with the oral mucosa for any length of time.

Placement of solid drugs under the tongue — sublingual administration — so that they may be retained for longer periods can prove a very effective method of administration if the drugs meet certain requirements. It was stated earlier that transport across biologic barriers is almost exclusively the prerogative of *solutes*. Hence, drugs given as solids by the sublingual route must be able to dissolve rapidly in the salivary secretions before they are ready for absorption. From the standpoint of patient comfort, the drug also must be able to produce its desired effects when given in small amounts. These two restrictions, combined with the need for the patient's cooperation in keeping the drug under the tongue until it has dissolved and is absorbed, limit the potential usefulness of this route of administration.

When the sublingual route *can* be used, it has certain advantages over the other enteral routes. Following absorption within the oral cavity, the drug gains access to the general circulation without first traversing the liver. All the blood leaving the stomach or small intestine passes first through the liver before entering the general circulation to be distributed to other tissues and organs. In the large intestine, only the blood coming from the lower part of the rectum circumvents the liver on its way to the heart. The liver is the principal locus for the chemical reactions (to be discussed in Chapter 6) which may inactivate a drug or transform it into a less effective substance. For any drug *on which the body acts,* more drug will be available to *act on the body* when it is administered in a region served by veins that bypass the liver and go directly to the heart.

The effectiveness of sublingual administration is well demonstrated by the rapidity with which nitroglycerin relieves the pain of *angina pectoris*.[1] A nitroglycerin tablet placed under the patient's tongue usually acts within two minutes to terminate the attack. The same quantity of nitroglycerin is totally ineffective if swallowed, since it must pass through the liver before reaching its site of action.

The Stomach

Beyond the oral cavity the alimentary canal becomes a hollow tube extending from the larynx to the anal sphincter. Throughout its length the tube is surrounded by four concentric layers of tissue: *mucosa, submucosa, muscularis* and *serosa*. The mucosa is made up of three components: a superficial epithelium composed of a single layer of cells; an underlying layer, the *lamina propria,* containing connective tissue, blood vessels and lymphatics; and, innermost, a relatively thin layer of muscle fibers.

The superficial epithelium of the gastric mucosa, in contrast to that of the oral cavity, is not a smooth surface but contains many folds. These folds increase the number of epithelial cells and, thereby, the total area available for absorption over that afforded by a flat, smooth lining.

The normal function of the stomach is to act as a storage depot for food and to assist in its digestion. It accomplishes the latter by secreting hydrochloric acid and

[1] Angina pectoris, a transient interference with the flow of blood, oxygen and nutrients to heart muscle, is associated with severe pain.

the enzyme pepsin, the catalytic protein which accelerates the initial digestion of food proteins. The secretions are usually sufficient to make the gastric contents very acidic (in man, about pH 2).

Although the stomach does not function primarily as an organ for absorption, its considerable blood supply combined with the potential for prolonged contact of an agent with a relatively large epithelial surface is conducive to the absorption of various drugs. The length of time a substance remains in the stomach, however, is the greatest variable determining the extent of gastric absorption. The rate at which the stomach empties its contents into the small intestine is influenced by the volume, viscosity and constituents of those same contents; by physical activity and the position of the body; by drugs themselves; and by many other factors. For example, lying on the left side decreases the rate of stomach emptying compared with lying on the right side; the presence of fat in the gastric contents also leads to a decreased rate of emptying compared with the effect of carbohydrate foods. The sum total of so many influences makes any prediction concerning the length of sojourn of an agent in the stomach highly unreliable. Only when a drug is taken with water on a relatively empty stomach is it possible to say that it will reach the small intestine fairly rapidly.

From our considerations of the principles governing transport across cell membranes, it follows that water, small molecules, lipid-soluble nonelectrolytes and weakly acidic drugs can pass through the gastric epithelium by passive diffusion. The low pH of the stomach contents discourages ionization of weak acids while promoting that of weak bases. Consequently, a larger fraction of weak acids than of weak bases is present in the undissociated form, and the former are more rapidly absorbed than the latter. For example, studies on drug absorption have shown that at normal gastric pH, weak acids such as aspirin and phenobarbital are absorbed from the stomach, whereas weak bases such as atropine and nicotine are not absorbed to any significant degree. We have already seen that the base strychnine was negligibly absorbed when the gastric pH was 3.0, but when the pH was made increasingly alkaline, increasingly greater amounts of strychnine reached the general circulation (cf. Table 4-2). The absorption of alcohol from the stomach is also in conformity with the concept that lipid-soluble, small nonelectrolytes diffuse relatively readily

Table 5-2. Influence of Lipid Solubility on Rate of Absorption

Drug	Partition Coefficient[a]	% Absorbed from Stomach in 1 Hour
Barbital	1	4
Secobarbital	52	30
Thiopental	580	46

[a]Concentration in organic solvent, methylene chloride, divided by concentration in water. Partition coefficient data from M. T. Bush, Sedatives and Hypnotics: 1. Absorption, Fate, and Excretion. In W. S. Root and F. G. Hofman (Eds.), *Physiological Pharmacology*. New York: Academic, 1963. Vol. I, pp. 185–218. Absorption data from L. S. Schanker, P. A. Shore, B. B. Brodie, and C. A. M. Hogben. *J. Pharmacol. Exp. Ther.* 120:528, 1957.

across biologic barriers. However, the influence of lipid solubility on transport is more strikingly illustrated by the observed rates of gastric absorption of three derivatives of barbituric acid (Table 5-2). Barbital, secobarbital and thiopental are each present in excess of 99.99 per cent as nonionized molecules when placed in the stomach at normal gastric pH. There is, however, considerable dissimilarity in lipid solubility among the undissociated forms of the three drugs, and this condition leads to marked differences in their rates of absorption.

Absorption of various drugs can and does occur in the stomach. Nevertheless, under the normal conditions of oral administration, the contribution of gastric absorption to total absorption is not only variable but, at best, exceedingly small compared with that of the small intestine.

The Small Intestine

The epithelial lining of the mucosal layer of the small intestine, like that of the stomach, is composed of a single layer of cells. But the unique arrangement of this lining makes the intestine exquisitely suited to its prime function of absorbing the end-products of digestion for utilization by the organism. These exceptional features provide the small intestine with the means for increasing the surface area of its absorbing epithelium out of all proportion to that of the area of its flat serosal surface. To the naked eye, the mucosal surface is heaped up into folds which, in man, are known as the folds of Kerckring. These folds are more numerous and deeper than the folds of the gastric epithelium; they alone increase the intestinal epithelial surface about three times relative to that of the serosal surface (Fig. 5-3). Using the light microscope, one sees that these folds give rise to slender, delicately ruffled projections called *villi*. These projections make an additional ten-fold relative increase in the luminal surface area. Individual villi are lined with the primary absorbing units — the epithelial cells — and with goblet cells, the mucus-secreting cells. The central portion of each villus contains the blood and lymph capillaries. Visualized with the electron microscope, the free surface of the epithelial cell at the luminal border is seen to bear an array of finger-like structures called *microvilli*. It has been estimated that there are about six hundred microvilli per cell, and this produces another twenty-fold increase in relative epithelial surface area. As Figure 5-4 illustrates, the small intestine of man, approximately 280 cm long and 4 cm in diameter, would have about 200 m^2 of available absorbing surface area!

The environmental conditions within the intestinal lumen change somewhat along its length. In the duodenum — the segment of the intestine closest to the stomach — the pH remains acidic, about 4 to 5, due to the gastric contents that have been emptied into it. However, the somewhat alkaline secretions of the pancreas and the secretions of bile and of the intestine itself quickly neutralize this acid. From about the first quarter of the small intestine to the end of the large intestine, the intraluminal pH changes only from slightly acidic to barely alkaline. Obviously, the ingestion of food and liquids markedly affects the composition of the contents of the entire alimentary canal and also stimulates gastrointestinal secretions.

For *any* substance which can penetrate the gastrointestinal epithelium in measurable

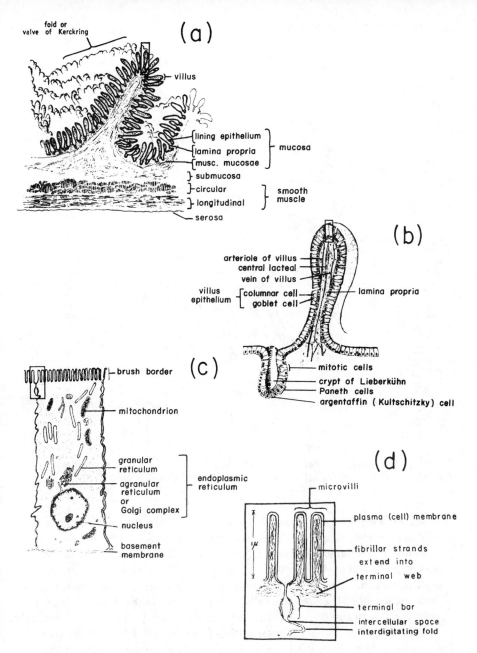

FIGURE 5-3. The small intestine. The boxed-in area of figure portions A to C is shown in greater magnification in the succeeding figure portion. (A) The several layers forming the wall of the small intestine; (B) the villi and the crypts of Lieberkühn; (C) highly schematic interpretation of the electron microscopic appearance of the columnar absorbing cell; (D) details of the brush border and the intercellular space. (Modified from L. Laster and F. J. Ingelfinger, N. Engl. J. Med. *264:1138, 1961.)*

81

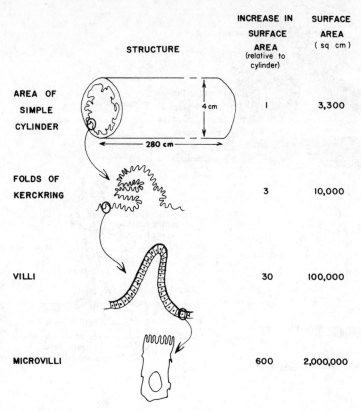

STRUCTURE	INCREASE IN SURFACE AREA (relative to cylinder)	SURFACE AREA (sq cm)
AREA OF SIMPLE CYLINDER	1	3,300
FOLDS OF KERCKRING	3	10,000
VILLI	30	100,000
MICROVILLI	600	2,000,000

FIGURE 5-4. Three mechanisms for increasing surface area of the small intestine. (From T. H. Wilson, Intestinal Absorption. *Philadelphia: Saunders, 1962. P. 2.)*

amounts, *the small intestine represents the area with the greatest capacity for absorption.* This is true whether the molecule is relatively lipid-soluble and nonionizable, like alcohol, or is a weak electrolyte, either base or acid. For example, in animal studies, when the rates of absorption were determined for various agents placed directly into the intestine or into the stomach and prevented by a ligature from emptying into the intestine, the following results were obtained (Table 5-3): alcohol was found to be at least *six times,* and weak acids such as phenobarbital *twelve times* more rapidly absorbed from the small intestine than from the stomach. A weakly basic, antihistaminic drug, promethazine, was insignificantly absorbed from the stomach but was absorbed relatively quickly from the intestine. These data may at first glance appear to be a partial contradiction of the stated general principles of biotransport. For although one would predict that a weak base would be more completely absorbed under the pH conditions of the intestine, one would hardly anticipate faster absorption from the intestine than from the stomach for drugs like alcohol, whose absorption is independent of pH, or for weak acids, which are more ionized at the higher intestinal pH. These are not, however, deviations from the general rules

Table 5-3. Comparison of Absorptive Capacity of Rat Stomach and Small Intestine[a]

Drug	% Absorbed from Stomach in 1 Hour[b]	% Absorbed from Small Intestine in 10 Minutes[c]
Phenobarbital	17.1 ± 4.7	52.4 ± 2.3
Pentobarbital	23.7 ± 3.8	54.6 ± 4.6
Promethazine	-0.2 ± 3.2	38.2 ± 6.1
Ethanol	37.7 ± 8.6	64.1 ± 7.5

[a]All values are means $\pm$ standard deviation of 6 to 22 determinations.
[b]Drugs dissolved in 0.01N HC1.
[c]Drugs dissolved in solution, pH 6.0, containing NaC1, KC1 and CaC1$_2$.
Data from M. P. Magnussen, *Acta Pharmacol. Toxicol.* (Kbh.) 26:130, 1968.

governing transport across biologic barriers. They are simply manifestations of the *qualitative difference* in the primary function of the stomach and intestine and of the enormous *quantitative difference* in the *area available for absorption* in these two regions of the gastrointestinal tract.

The great epithelial area of the intestine provided by the many villi and microvilli presents many more surfaces than the gastric mucosa for the absorption of neutral, lipid-soluble substances and more than compensates for the decrease in the relative proportion of the nonionized molecules of weak acids. It follows from this that the rate at which the stomach empties its contents into the intestine markedly affects the overall rate at which drugs reach the general circulation after oral administration. The absorption of weak bases, which constitute the majority of commonly used drugs, would be particularly dependent on the speed with which they arrive in the intestine. But for all drugs, it is essentially valid to say that slowing the rate at which the stomach empties will decrease the overall rate of gastrointestinal absorption, and vice versa. That is why so many agents are administered on an empty stomach with sufficient water to ensure their rapid passage into the intestine.

Under normal conditions, substances usually take several hours to pass from one end of the small intestine to the other. In contrast to the stomach, this slow transit through the intestine enhances absorption, since absorption can take place along the entire length. Only when intestinal motility is abnormally increased, as in marked diarrhea, is the residence time in the small intestine too short to ensure maximal absorption.

Passive diffusion and the laws governing it appear to be sufficient to account for the intestinal absorption of the majority of drugs which are either lipid-soluble or are weak electrolytes. Usually these drugs are completely absorbed. However, lipid-insoluble drugs and agents which are completely ionized at all physiologic pH's, such as the quaternary ammonium compounds referred to earlier (e.g., acetylcholine; cf. pp. 39–40), are also partially absorbed from the small intestine. This poor yet partial absorption was a demonstrated fact long ago. Although primitive man did not know that the active ingredient in his arrow poison curare was a quaternary ammonium compound, he was well aware that he could eat with impunity the flesh of animals killed with it. Man absorbed too little of the curare present in the meat to produce deleterious effects. On the other hand, the ingestion of certain species of mushroom has long been known to produce poisonous effects. It was not until Schmiedeberg isolated muscarine from *Amanita muscaria* that it was shown to be the culprit and subsequently identified chemically as a quaternary ammonium compound. The mushroom contains sufficient muscarine so that poisoning results even from partial absorption. Even large macromolecules like proteins may be absorbed, as such, to a very small degree. An excellent example of this is the poisoning by botulinus toxin, which occurs after eating canned foods contaminated with the causative microorganism. It is possible that mechanisms like facilitated diffusion and pinocytosis are responsible for the absorption of quaternary ammonium compounds and proteins, respectively. Active transport has been shown to account for the absorption of only those drugs that closely resemble the normal nutrients known to be actively absorbed.

The Large Intestine

The structure of the epithelial lining of the large intestine reflects the change in primary function of this part of the gastrointestinal tract compared with the small intestine. The epithelial cells of the colon do not possess microvilli, and their function is primarily that of secreting mucus rather than of absorption. However, the large intestine retains the ability to actively transport sodium ion and to reabsorb water.

Even though the function of the colon is not fundamentally that of absorption, drugs which escape absorption in the small intestine may continue to be absorbed during their passage out of the body. Moreover, the terminal segment of the large intestine — the rectum — can serve as a useful site for drug administration, particularly when the oral route is unsuitable. Rectal administration is advantageous in the unconscious patient, in patients unable to retain material given by mouth, and for drugs with objectionable taste or odor or those destroyed by digestive enzymes. This route protects susceptible drugs not only from alteration by the digestive processes of the mouth, stomach and small intestine, but also from the chemical reactions occurring in the liver. It should be recalled that the blood draining the lower part of the rectum bypasses the liver on its way to the heart.

Absorption of Drugs Administered as Solids

Under normal conditions, ingested material is transferred across the gastrointestinal epithelium as a *solute* in the fluid at the site of absorption. While there may be a few exceptions to this rule in the case of nutrients absorbed by pinocytosis, no such exceptions have been demonstrated for therapeutic agents. However, for convenience and for practical reasons of solubility, stability and consumer acceptance, most drugs are administered orally in some form of solid dosage. Therefore, drugs administered as solids must first go into solution in the gastrointestinal tract. And the rate at which dissolution takes place determines how much of the drug is made available for absorption and how quickly:

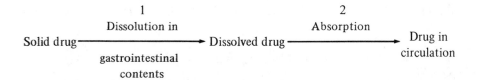

In this two-step process, if the rate of solution is slower than the rate of absorption, then the second step becomes initially dependent on the physicochemical principles which apply to the dissolution of substances in aqueous media. Only after dissolution would the rate of absorption be governed by the principles established for the passage of solutes across biologic barriers. If the rate of dissolution is faster than the rate of absorption, however, then the first step is no longer rate-limiting, and the rate of absorption will be governed entirely by the principles of passive diffusion.

Of course, the greater the inherent solubility of a drug, the greater its rate of dissolution from the solid-dosage form. The salts of acidic or basic drugs are usually more soluble than the parent compounds, which is why many acidic drugs are prepared as salts of sodium or other cations and basic drugs as salts of hydrochloric or other acids. But formation of salts is only one of many ways in which the pharmaceutical chemist has successfully manipulated the form or formulation of an agent to change its dissolution rate.

The size of the drug particle presented to the dissolving medium is one of the more important factors determining rate of dissolution. The smaller the particle size, the greater the rate of solution, since the proportion of surface area exposed to the solvent compared to the volume of the particles increases with decreasing particle diameter. For example, in human subjects, the administration of sulfadiazine as microcrystalline particles results in a more rapid and complete absorption than when the same drug is given in "ordinary" particle size with a surface area approximately one-seventh that of the micronized substance. However, reduction in particle size, while almost always increasing rate of solution, is potentially beneficial to absorption only for substances with dissolution rates slower than their rates of absorption. Equal amounts of the antibiotic tetracycline hydrochloride, for instance, administered to humans either as capsules containing small particles or as compressed pellets, were equally well absorbed despite the thirty-fold difference in surface area between the two dosage preparations. Tetracycline hydrochloride dissolves rapidly in the acidic gastric environment but is only poorly absorbed from the stomach, and even from the intestine its absorption is slow and incomplete.

Almost all solid dosage forms of drugs contain other ingredients besides the active agent. The excipients are considered pharmacologically inert but are included in the pharmaceutical preparation for a variety of reasons, e.g., to mask an unpleasant taste, to increase solubility or stability, or to add bulk to active agents used in extremely small quantities. But the inclusion of these inert constituents adds another dimension to be considered in the availability of a drug for absorption — the disintegration of the dosage form itself and the dispersion of the active ingredients within the gastro-intestinal tract. Thus:

Drug in solid dosage form

| Disintegration

Smaller particles and free solid drug

| Dissolution

Drug dissolved in gastrointestinal fluids

Hence, in the majority of instances of drug administration by the oral route, drug absorption is not only dependent on the rate of dissolution of the *therapeutic agent,* but also influenced by rates of disintegration of the solid dosage form.

These points are extremely well illustrated by the results of studies carried out with twelve brands of tablets of a single agent, phenylbutazone (Table 5-4). A fifteen-fold variation was found among the different brands with respect to the time required for tablet disintegration. The time necessary for 50 per cent of the phenylbutazone to dissolve showed a more than seventy-fold difference among the tablets tested. Additionally, there was no significant correlation between disintegration and dissolution times. From the clinical viewpoint, however, the most important finding was

Table 5-4.   Disintegration and Dissolution Data for 12 Brands of the Antiinflammatory Agent Phenylbutazone

Brand	Disintegration Time[a] (min)		Dissolution Data[b] (mg in solution)			
	Mean	Range	2 hr	4 hr	6 hr	$t_{1/2}$[c] (min)
A	17	11−22	80	94	99	54
B	12	8−16	60	83	93	86
Cq	4	3−4	99	99	99	9
D	20	19−21	78	98	104	57
E	41	18−83	21	56	76	210
G	43	30−45	98	100	100	31
H	35	20−48	75	96	99	80
L	41	28−52	80	94	99	54
Pq	42	28−55	86	87	88	36
Q	44	39−53	39	59	70	174
W	61	46−120	29	64	88	188
X	51	23−62	0	7	48	369
Pure drug	. . .	. . .	99	100	100	5

[a]Mean of six tablets from each brand.
[b]Average of two tablets from each brand, subjected separately to the dissolution test.
[c]$t_{1/2}$ is the time required for 50 per cent of the quantity of drug to be dissolved.
Data from R. O. Searl and M. Pernarowski, *Can. Med. Assoc. J.* 96:1513, 1967.

that there was such a wide variation in the rate and extent of absorption among the four brands chosen for study in human subjects, this despite the fact that equal amounts of phenylbutazone were administered (Fig. 5-5). Different brands of the same drug certainly produce quantitatively different therapeutic responses. The equality of the analytic content of a given agent in a particular preparation is obviously no guarantee that there will be equality of availability for absorption or for therapeutic effectiveness.

A comparison of the absorption rates of three different commercial aspirin tablets also documents the dependence of absorption on the pharmaceutical formulation (Fig. 5-6). This particular example also demonstrates the effect of another variable in oral administration — the quantity of water ingested along with the solid dosage form. The amount of each preparation absorbed by the subjects in Group B, who ingested a large quantity of water with the aspirin tablets, was greater than in Group A, even though the same relationship between absorption and dissolution rate was maintained.

Recognition of the fact that different formulations of the identical quantity of the same drug may not result in equal therapeutic response has led the Food and Drug Administration to set new standards for biologic availability. The Federal Food, Drug and Cosmetic Act as amended in 1977 requires sponsors of drugs to provide data of **bioequivalence** whenever there is evidence that drug products containing the same active drug are intended for the same therapeutic effect (cf. Chapter 14).

Special pharmaceutical formulations can also be employed to decrease the rate of disintegration and dissolution when this is desired. Tablets or capsules can be exter-

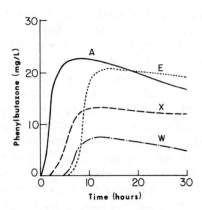

FIGURE 5-5. Concentration of phenylbutazone in serum of patients after the oral administration of four different products (A, E, X and W). Each product contained the same amount of phenylbutazone. Curves are composite curves of results obtained in 3 subjects per product, but the individual data points were sufficiently close to permit the construction of reasonably accurate composite curves. (Modified from R. O. Searl and M. Pernarowski, Can. Med. Assoc. J. 96:1513, 1967.)

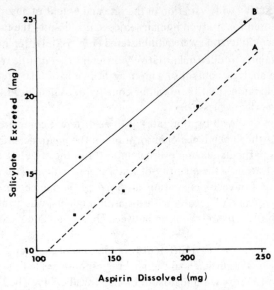

FIGURE 5-6. Mean amount of apparent salicylate excreted in one hour after administration of three different commercial aspirin tablets (2 tablets of 0.3 g each) as a function of in vitro dissolution rate. Lower line, group A: 14 subjects ingested aspirin with exactly 100 ml water. Upper line, group B: 10 subjects ingested aspirin with exactly 200 ml water. (Adapted from G. Levy, J. Pharm. Sci. 50:388, 1961. Reproduced with permission of the copyright owner.)

nally coated to prevent their disintegration within the stomach. When such *enteric* coatings are used, the drug is not presented to an absorbing surface until it reaches the small intestine, where the environment is conducive to destruction of the coating and release of the drug. This is a particularly useful procedure to protect drugs which are prone to alteration by the extremely acidic gastric medium.

Other types of oral preparations contain drugs coated in various ways so as to release only a limited amount of active agent at any one time and thus provide for sustained therapy by making additional small quantities of drug available for absorption over a relatively long period. However, if the *sustained-release medication* leaves the intestine before all the drug has been delivered for absorption, an unused portion will be excreted in the feces. Still other disadvantages, of a more serious nature, may be associated with the use of sustained-release preparations. Since the liberation of the drug depends upon certain reactions taking place in appropriate segments of the gastrointestinal tract, there is usually a great deal of variability in the rate of release among individuals, and even in the same individual at different times. A single sustained-release tablet or capsule contains a greater amount of drug than does a conventional form. If release is more rapid than is assumed, too much drug may be absorbed too quickly and thus lead to adverse effects. Conversely, if the rate of discharge is slower than expected, amounts of drug may be provided that are inadequate to produce the desired therapeutic effect. Sustained-release preparations are justified only when a drug is so rapidly absorbed — and, following absorption, so quickly eliminated — that a sufficient amount reaches the site of action for only a short period following administration. If continued action of such a drug is needed, it would require taking the drug more than three or four times a day. In such cases, sustained-release preparations provide the means to avoid fluctuations in the amount of drug delivered and to obviate the necessity of repeated ingestion of the more usual oral preparations.

Although sustained-release preparations for enteral administration do not appear to be the desired panacea for prolonged, uniform drug absorption, some promising results have been achieved using such preparations for parenteral administration. For example, pilocarpine, a drug useful in the treatment of glaucoma,[2] has been successfully incorporated into a thin membrane for placement by the patient in the conjunctival sac to provide slow release of the drug over a week's time. The permeable membrane is made from Silastic, a silicon rubber with most desirable properties — it is practically inert and does not irritate tissues. The rate of pilocarpine release is sufficient to maintain a constant reduction in intraocular pressure but the amount released is too small to produce significant systemic effects. A single weekly administration of the drug is obviously more convenient than periodic daily application of eye drops. Contraceptive agents incorporated into devices for placement intravaginally are other examples of sustained-release preparations using silicon rubber.

Absorption Through the Skin

The epidermis, the outer layer of the skin, is composed of epithelial cells. From a functional point of view, it is a two-ply structure consisting of the dead *stratum corneum,* or the *cornified* or *horny layer,* and an underlying layer of living cells, the *stratum germinativum* (Fig. 5-7). The stratum corneum is normally made up of many tiers of cells bound tightly together into a dense, coherent membrane whose intercellular spaces are submicroscopic. The function of the skin as a barrier to the movement of solutes resides almost entirely in its dead product. "The raison d'etre of the viable layer is to make the horny layer; this is its specific biologic mission. Its aim in life is to die usefully so that its horny shroud forms a continually renewable wrapping around the body."[3]

The integumental epithelium differs in still other ways from the rest of the epithelial barriers. With the possible exception of a portion of the mucous lining of the nose, the skin is the only tissue whose free surface is usually exposed to relatively

---

[2]Glaucoma is a disease of the eye marked by increased pressure within the eyeball. Untreated, there may be damage to the optic disk and gradual loss of vision. Drugs useful in the treatment of glaucoma reduce intraocular pressure by providing better drainage of the aqueous humor; contraction of muscles of the eye innervated by the parasympathetic system widens the passage through which fluid drains from the aqueous humor back to the blood.

[3]A. M. Kligman, The biology of the Stratum Corneum. In W. Montagna and W. C. Lobitz, Jr. (eds.), *The Epidermis.* New York: Academic, 1964.

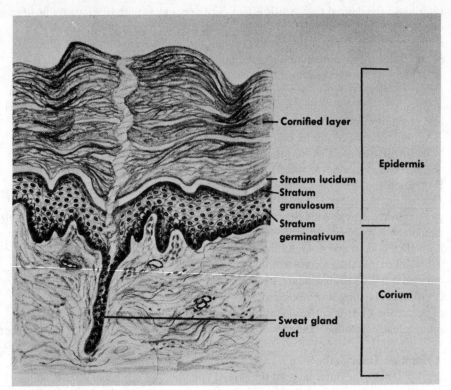

FIGURE 5-7. Structure and layers of the skin. A thick, cornified layer is charac-teristic of areas such as the fingertip. The cornified layer is made up of flat, dead, dry, keratinized cells. Cell division in the epidermis takes place in the stratum germinativum. The corium, or dermis, is a compact layer of connective tissue containing sweat glands and numerous collagenous and elastic fibers. (Modified from G. Bevelander, Outline of Histology *[6th ed.]. St. Louis: The C. V. Mosby Co., 1967.)*

dry air. This dry outer environment leads to a comparatively low water content of the several cell layers on the outside of the skin and, generally speaking, of the entire stratum corneum. In no other normal epithelium is there dry tissue on the environ-mental side. The cells of the horny layer also contain less phospholipid and lipid than those of other epithelia and are unique in being densely packed with the complex protein keratin. Thus this horny layer may derive its true barrier function from its lack of water and lipid and the presence of keratin, which together account for the density and packing of the cells.

The epidermis affords the body protection; this is really its exclusive function, and it is a two-way process. Its dead product, the horny layer, obstructs the passage of materials both to and from the environment. No multicellular membrane of biologic origin is as "waterproof" as the skin, and water loss from the body by diffusion and evaporation is equally retarded, except at the sweat glands. It is well to note that there is no evidence that sweat or sebaceous glands act as the entrance pathways for exogenous materials. It is not surprising, then, that absorption through the skin, when it does occur, is ordinarily extremely slow. Once a solute passes this barrier, it encounters no further significant obstacles to absorption. The underlying tissue, the dermis, is well supplied with lymph and blood capillaries.

Passage of chemicals through the skin, as determined by direct measurement, appears to be simply by passive diffusion. Although rates of penetration of various agents are relatively slower than at other biologic barriers, they conform qualitatively to the general principles governing this transport process. In humans, no evidence of active transport processes has been obtained even though various inorganic ions can traverse the skin. This might be anticipated since the horny layer is really dead tissue. But the point that needs emphasis is that, even though the skin is an effective barrier against the transport of almost all substances, letting no molecule through readily, *it is a perfect barrier to very few substances.* Even a heavy metal like mercury can be absorbed to some degree through the skin. Indeed, absorption through the skin represents one of the most common routes by which poisoning in man and animals occurs following accidental exposure to foreign chemicals. For example, many insecticides, particularly those containing parathion, malathion or nicotine, may cause serious poisoning as a result of percutaneous absorption following inadvertent contamination of the skin or even clothing.

When drugs are purposely applied to the skin, or for that matter to any external mucous membrane (nasal drops, intravaginal jellies and the like), they are ordinarily expected to produce their desired effects only in the local area of administration. Little thought is usually given to the fact that the skin is not an *absolute* barrier and that there may be absorption of the drug leading to systemic effects, sometimes of a serious nature. For example, tannic acid, once widely used in the treatment of burns, was abandoned during World War II when it was discovered that it produces toxic effects on the kidney. Some of the preparations presently available for decreasing the pain of sunburn contain local anesthetics. Again, if these preparations are not used as directed and are placed over large areas of the body, the quantity of local anesthetic absorbed through the skin may prove harmful. Of course, any time the skin is broken by cuts or wounds, it no longer retains its barrier function in the injured area, and substances can be readily absorbed through the exposed tissues underlying the epidermis.

Absorption from the Respiratory Tract

As air is inhaled, it passes first into the *pharynx,* a region common to both the respiratory and gastrointestinal tracts. From there it moves into the *trachea,* the principal air tube of the vertebrate respiratory system, and then into the *bronchi,* the major branches connecting the trachea with the lungs. Food and water are normally prevented from entering the air tube by the *epiglottis,* a flap which covers the opening into the trachea upon swallowing. Within the lungs the bronchial tubes subdivide into the finer *bronchioles,* whose branches communicate with the *alveoli* (Fig. 5-8).

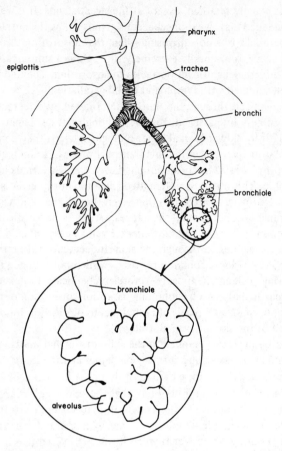

FIGURE 5-8. Respiratory apparatus.

It is the anatomic structure and organization within the lung of these minute, sac-like chambers, the alveoli, which enable the lung to carry out its primary function of rapidly supplying oxygen to the body and removing carbon dioxide.

The pulmonary alveolus is lined with a single layer of flat epithelial cells forming an extremely thin barrier between alveolar air and an interstitium richly supplied with capillaries. The alveolar epithelium and capillary wall are so closely associated that the total air-blood barrier is only 0.5 to 1 μ thick (Fig. 5-9). This is quite different from the space separating the epithelial cells of the intestinal villus from their underlying capillaries, or from the space separating the surface of the skin from the dermal layer, which are about 40 and 100 μ, respectively. In man, the number of alveoli in the lungs is estimated to be from 300 to 400 million, providing a total surface area of about 200 m². Of equal importance to absorption is the fact that the pulmonary vasculature is functionally structured to ensure the rapid removal of material which has crossed this huge surface. First, the pulmonary capillaries have a surface area of

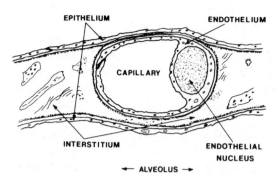

FIGURE 5-9. *Alveolar capillary membranes. (After F. N. Low,* Anat. Rec. *139:105, 1961.)*

about 90 m². Second, all the blood coming from the right side of the heart passes through the lungs, and since the same volume of blood is ejected by both sides of the heart, the lungs receive in one minute an amount of blood equal to that passing through the remainder of the entire body in the same interval. All these factors combine to make the lungs the most effective absorptive area of the body.

As air is inhaled its water content quickly increases, and it becomes virtually saturated by the time it reaches the alveoli. Thus the normal external environment at the primary absorptive surface is really not dry air but moisture-laden air. This is of physiologic importance since it prevents the loss of considerable amounts of water from the body upon expiration. In humans, only about 400 cc of water per day are lost to the environment through the lungs. In animals that have no sweat glands, like the dog, or in man when body temperature is elevated and respiratory rate is increased, there is a compensatory increase in water loss from the lungs to assist in regulating body temperature.

The cellular membrane in the alveolus or elsewhere is not a barrier to diffusion of gases into or out of a cell, since gases as a rule are small molecules of relatively high lipid solubility. Thus, materials inhaled as gases or as vapors of volatile liquids almost instantaneously cross the alveolar epithelium and enter the blood when they are in higher concentrations in the alveolar air than in the blood. This extremely rapid absorption is a desirable feature for gases like nitrous oxide and cyclopropane or volatile liquids like ether when they are used to produce general anesthesia, but it can be disastrous when the inspired air contains poisonous gases or vapors like carbon monoxide or gasoline fumes.

Chemicals can also be inhaled as aerosols, which are liquid droplets or solid particles so small that they remain suspended in air for some time instead of settling out quickly under gravitational pull. Once within the respiratory tract, these suspended particles are deposited along its various segments as the current of air in which they are moving causes them to impact on the tissue. The deposition, or *impaction,* occurs principally at the points where the pulmonary tree branches and the airstream changes course, since the tendency of a particle is to continue moving in its original direction. Particle size largely determines the site of impaction; the smaller the particle, the deeper into the pulmonary system it is drawn before being deposited. Particles larger than 10 μ in diameter are usually completely removed before leaving the nasal passages, and those larger than 2 μ rarely reach the alveolar sac. Pollens, smoke, industrial dusts and fumes, bacteria, viruses and various aerosol preparations used in the treatment of asthma are examples of substances with particle sizes below 10 μ in diameter.

The reactions produced by the deposited particles depend on their solubility and on whether they reach the alveolus. Soluble chemicals can be absorbed anywhere along the respiratory tract in accordance with the principles governing passive diffusion. The smaller the particle size, the greater the rate of solution of the chemical and the greater its rate of absorption. Also, the smaller the particle is in size, the greater the likelihood of its reaching the alveoli, where conditions are most conducive to absorption. Insoluble particles are dangerous only if they reach the alveoli.

The upper respiratory tract is lined as far down as the end of the bronchioles with mucus-secreting epithelial cells bearing many cilia. The constant movement of these hair-like processes propels the mucous secretions and any insoluble particles deposited on them toward the nose and mouth and, in this way, rapidly clears the bronchial epithelium. Insoluble particles reaching the alveolus are in part transported, by some unknown means, to the base of the ciliated epithelium in the bronchioles and are excreted by the ciliary movement. Removal by the phagocytic white blood cells (cf. p. 61, Pinocytosis) present in the alveoli or other lung tissue is also a mechanism by which the lung rids itself of insoluble material reaching the alveolus. When the airborne concentration of particles is low — less than about ten particles per cubic centimeter of air — the lungs can completely eliminate the insoluble material by these two mechanisms. As a consequence, only a minute quantity of the total particulate material inhaled during a lifetime is retained in the normal, healthy lung. But as the particle concentration in the air increases, the capacity for elimination is overtaxed and some of the particles are retained in the tissue. A small decrease in the lung's capacity to rid itself of solid particles can lead to a great increase in the quantity retained. This may explain the several lung diseases which frequently afflict miners exposed to relatively high concentrations of mineral dust in their work. In this connection it is also interesting to note that cigarette smoke consists primarily of particles measuring less than 1 μ in diameter. Comparison of the number of particles in inhaled and exhaled cigarette smoke has shown that 82 per cent of the particles are retained when the smoke is held for 5 seconds in the lungs. The ability of the lung to rid itself of these particles is then related to whether its capacity is sufficient to keep up with the rate of smoke entry. Some of the vapors contained in cigarette smoke slow down the ciliary action of the bronchial epithelium, and this may work against the lung, decreasing its capacity to rid itself of particulate matter by ciliary excretion.

Absorption From Subcutaneous Sites

Subcutaneous injections of drugs bypass the barrier of the epidermis since they are placed below the dermis directly in contact with channels into the general circulation. Thus, in a sense, we have already discussed some aspects of subcutaneous absorption when we indicated that once substances pass through the epithelial cells separating the external environment from the internal environment, they enter into the immediate vicinity of blood and lymph capillaries. At subcutaneous sites, just as on the *inside* of the epithelial barrier, the hindrance to entry into the systemic circulation is the wall of the capillary (Fig. 5-10). It is composed of *endothelial* cells, and it is the endothelial tissue which forms the barrier to solute movement into as well as out of the circulation.

The rates at which all substances penetrate endothelial tissue at all sites except the brain are far in excess of those at which these same materials cross epithelial tissue. Even large macromolecules like protein can make their way into and out of capillaries, albeit relatively slowly. The reason for this increased permeability will be discussed more fully in the section on distribution. But as a rule, the rates of absorption into capillaries are determined for lipid-soluble substances by their oil/water partition coefficients and for lipid-insoluble substances by their molecular size.

The rate of capillary blood flow is the major factor in determining rate of entry into the circulation. The more vascular the subcutaneous area, the greater the rate of absorption. Removal from the site of injection by way of the lymph plays only a minor part in the total absorption of smaller molecules, since the flow of lymph is

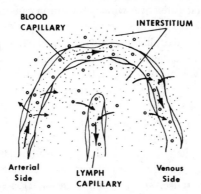

BLOOD CAPILLARY
INTERSTITIUM
Arterial Side
LYMPH CAPILLARY
Venous Side

FIGURE 5-10. Movement of substances into and out of capillaries (highly idealized). Fluid, solutes and macromolecules like proteins leave the blood capillary on the arterial side and enter intercellular fluid and tissue cells. At the venous side, fluid, solutes and some protein enter the blood capillary. Solutes, fluid and particularly proteins are also returned to the circulation by way of the lymph capillary. The proteins and macromolecules are represented as small circles (○) and the fluid and solutes of blood and tissue as dots (·). Arrows show direction of flow. (After A. W. Ham, Histology. Philadelphia: Lippincott, 1965.)

so slow compared to that of blood. However, lymphatic absorption is significant in the case of larger molecules such as proteins.

This dependence of rate of absorption on rate of blood flow makes it possible to change the rate at which a drug enters the circulation following subcutaneous injection. This can be done by changing either the rate of blood flow through the area of administration or the rate at which the drug is exposed to capillary surfaces. For example, when a local anesthetic is injected subcutaneously around a tooth on which work is to be performed, the dentist wishes to retard absorption and keep the anesthetic in the local area as long as possible. Therefore, he uses a preparation which, together with the local anesthetic, contains an agent capable of decreasing the diameter of the blood vessels at the site of injection. Under these conditions, the local anesthetic is carried away more slowly since less blood is flowing through the area in a given period compared with the flow when the vessels are not constricted.

It is also sometimes desirable to decrease the rate of absorption from subcutaneous injections, even when the drug is being given to produce its effects systemically. In these instances, special preparations are used which release small amounts of drug continuously over a period of time. Some insulin is prepared in this way so that the diabetic patient need use only a single injection during a day to obtain a long-lasting effect. Certain hormones can also be incorporated into a compressed pellet form and implanted subcutaneously. These pellets resist rapid disintegration in the fluid at the subcutaneous site, but minute amounts of the hormone go into solution very slowly, and a single administration sometimes lasts as long as five to six months.

Increasing the rate of absorption from a subcutaneous site is usually achieved by increasing the total surface area over which absorption can occur. Gentle massage following administration may spread the solution over a wider area so that the drug comes in contact with more capillaries. However, the lateral spread of an injected solution is limited by the connective tissue present in the subcutaneous area, and ordinarily only a small volume of solution, 0.5 to 2.0 ml, can be comfortably injected. So when the subcutaneous route is used for administration of large fluid volumes, special means must be used to overcome the resistance of the connective tissue. This is done with an enzyme, hyaluronidase, which breaks down the connective tissue matrix and allows the fluid to spread over larger areas.

Rapid absorption and the relative ease with which subcutaneous injections can be given, compared with intramuscular or intravenous injections, account for the frequent use of the subcutaneous route for drug administration. However, many drugs are too irritating to tissue or produce too much pain to be given in this way, and their injection may even lead to the formation of sterile abscesses (abscesses free of living microorganisms). Infections also occur more readily after subcutaneous than after intravenous injection. Nevertheless, the subcutaneous route offers an advantage over the intravenous one in that the rate of absorption from the subcutaneous site can be retarded when immediate adverse reactions occur in response to the administration of a drug. Once a drug has been given intravenously, it cannot be recalled. But after subcutaneous administration, as well as in some intramuscular administrations, it is possible to place a tourniquet between the site of injection and the heart and thereby block the superficial venous and lymphatic flow from the area. This is also the technique used to slow the rate at which venoms reach the general circulation following bites from poisonous snakes or insects.

Absorption From Intramuscular Sites

Intramuscular injections are usually made into the muscles of the buttock, the lateral side of the thigh or the upper arm. Thus drugs are introduced into areas that lie below the skin and subcutaneous tissue. The intramuscular route permits the administration of more irritating drugs and of large volumes of solutions than can be tolerated subcutaneously.

The barrier to absorption from muscles is also the capillary wall. Qualitatively, the permeability of the muscle capillaries is hardly different from that of subcutaneous capillaries. Therefore, all that was said about absorption from subcutaneous sites applies equally to absorption from intramuscular sites. The rates of absorption from both areas also appear to be about the same when the muscles are at rest. But during activity, the blood flow through the muscles may increase markedly as additional vascular channels are opened. During exercise, since rate of absorption is dependent on rate of blood flow, drugs would gain access to the general circulation more rapidly from intramuscular than from subcutaneous sites.

The intramuscular route, like the subcutaneous route, can be used to introduce drugs into the body slowly as well as rapidly. This is accomplished by altering the physical state of the drug so that, after it is deposited in the muscle, it goes into solution gradually, making small fractions of the dose available for absorption over an extended period. For example, special microcrystalline suspensions of penicillin, when injected intramuscularly, dissolve so slowly that a single injection may provide adequate penicillin therapy for a few days. Such preparations, called *depot preparations,* are convenient for patient as well as physician, since they eliminate the necessity and discomfort of frequently repeated injections.

Intravenous Administration

The placement of a drug into the bloodstream, usually into a vein of the arm, ensures that the entire quantity of drug administered is available for distribution to its site(s) of action. This procedure obviously has certain advantages over other routes of administration which necessitate absorption before distribution. But at the same time, the immediate availability of a drug given intravascularly entails certain hazards. And the procedure of injection itself, regardless of the nature of the drug, presents certain dangers worthy of consideration.

The intravenous route of drug administration is of greatest value in emergencies when speed is vital. Another advantage is that the amount of drug administered can be controlled with an accuracy not possible by any other procedure. Administration by a route which requires absorption never guarantees that all the drug given will be absorbed, even though there is the potential for complete absorption from the site. The intravenous route may also be used for drugs which are too irritating to be injected into other tissues without causing undue pain and tissue damage. An example is nitrogen mustard in the treatment of cancer. The irritating drug is quickly diluted by the blood, and the vessel wall is relatively insensitive to damage. Drugs that would be destroyed by chemical reactions before reaching the bloodstream are also given intravenously. Obviously, whole blood or blood plasma would be effective only when given directly into the vascular system. Intravenous administration is also the route of choice when blood circulation is so poor that the rate of absorption from tissue sites would be extremely uncertain.

Once a drug has been injected into the bloodstream there is no retreat, in contrast to the various techniques that can be used to slow absorption from intramuscular or subcutaneous sites or to remove a drug physically from the gastrointestinal tract. From this standpoint, the intravenous route is the least safe method of drug administration. However, if injections are made slowly, the danger can be largely averted. It takes about 1 minute for a complete circulation of blood in the normal individual and about 10 to 15 seconds for material injected in the arm to proceed through the heart to the brain. Thus, if injections are made over a period of at least 1 minute, it may be possible to discontinue further administration in patients in whom adverse reactions, such as loss of consciousness, occur within 15 to 30 seconds.

Rapid intravenous injections may produce deleterious effects which are unrelated to the effects of the injected drug, since they occur with pharmacologically inert substances as well. These effects usually involve the respiratory and circulatory systems and are seen as shallow and irregular breathing, precipitous fall in blood pressure and stoppage of the heart. They are probably associated with the fact that the material in the rapidly injected solution arrives at the heart as a relatively concentrated solution, since too much is placed in the bloodstream at one time to permit dilution in the circulating blood volume. Still other dangers attend intravenous injections, such as the inadvertent administration of particulate matter or air, which can produce serious complications. This route should be reserved for those instances when it is specifically indicated.

General Considerations

The oral route is the safest, most convenient and most economic method of administering drugs. However, the daily fluctuations of the gastrointestinal environment produced by food, combined with the dependence of absorption on the rate of gastric emptying, make it the most unpredictable and slowest of the commonly used routes in terms of both amount and rate of drug absorption. Moreover, this route cannot be used for drugs which are susceptible to alteration by the chemical processes involved in digestion. Thus a protein drug like insulin, which is destroyed by the enzymes normally secreted to digest food protein, must be given by a parenteral route despite daily need of long duration. The economy of oral administration also becomes questionable at times for those drugs which are rapidly destroyed by chemical reactions in the liver. Since all the drug absorbed from the stomach and small intestine passes through the liver on its way to the general circulation, larger amounts may be required to ensure an adequate biologic effect.

Drugs administered by the other enteral routes, sublingually and rectally, are not changed by the digestive processes and also avoid passage through the liver before reaching the systemic circulation. However, the sublingual route is restricted in usefulness to readily soluble drugs and, like the oral route, is dependent on the patient's cooperation. Rectal administration can be used in noncooperative or unconscious patients, but it has the disadvantage that retention is frequently unpredictable.

The administration of drugs at other epithelial barriers is usually limited to specific agents or effects. Application to the skin is used today only when a local drug effect is desired. Administration by way of the respiratory tract is used in the general population for gaseous and volatile agents, either for stimulation of respiration (oxygen) or production of general anesthesia. The rapidity of absorption by the lung makes specific therapy by inhalation a useful means of self-treatment in acute attacks of asthma, however.

Subcutaneous and intramuscular administration provide for relatively rapid absorption of drugs since they bypass the epithelial barrier. Absorption from these sites is also more predictable and less variable than from the alimentary canal. The environment at the sites of injection is kept relatively constant, and rates of absorption usually vary only with rates of blood flow through the subcutaneous tissue or muscle. At rest, the rate of absorption following subcutaneous administration is not much slower than that from sites of intramuscular injection, and the latter usually provides more rapid absorption only during muscular activity. Irritating drugs cannot be given by either of these routes, although muscle is less sensitive to damage than is subcutaneous tissue. Both the subcutaneous and intramuscular sites may be used as depots for sustained therapy with appropriate preparations of drugs which are slowly released for solution and absorption. The main disadvantage of both the subcutaneous and intramuscular routes of administration, in common with all routes requiring injection, is the need for special equipment, skill and a suitably prepared form of absolutely sterile medication.

The intravascular route completely eliminates the process of absorption and thus represents the most rapid means of introducing drugs into the body. This route has its greatest value in the treatment of emergencies and when absolute control of the amount of drug administered is essential. It is the most hazardous route, since there can be no recall once the drug is given. Intravascular injections require the greatest amount of skill and the most careful attention to the preparation of the injected material. Introduction of particulate matter or air may produce embolism — the obstruction of blood vessels to essential organs — which may prove fatal. Infections introduced by intravenous injections may also be more widespread than those resulting from injections at other sites. Drugs should never be introduced directly into the bloodstream unless specifically indicated.

DISTRIBUTION

Once a solute has reached the bloodstream, the principal pathway for its distribution, it usually must traverse one or more biologic barriers in order to reach its ultimate site of action. Its accessibility to this site is determined initially by its ability to cross the capillary wall, then by the blood flow through the site and, finally, if the drug acts intracellularly, by its rate of passage across cells. Thus the sequence of movement of a solute in the process of its distribution is the *reverse* of that involved in its absorption.

Since the capillary is the initial barrier to distribution, its permeability characteristics will be our first concern. We shall then examine the general factors which influence the amount of drug eventually reaching its site of action. Finally, special attention will be directed to the singular aspects of passage of drugs into the brain and across the placenta into the fetus.

Capillary Permeability

The tissue covering the surface of internal cavities of the body is *endothelium*. The individual cells comprising the endothelium overlap each other at their margins but are not as closely approximated as are epithelial cells. In the capillaries, this lining is one cell thick and is continuous throughout the closed passages. However, in the liver, the smallest channels of the circulation, called *sinusoids,* are even simpler than capillaries. These sinusoids lack a complete endothelial lining, and their walls are, at least in part, nonexistent.

We have previously noted that small lipid-soluble molecules like gases pass into, and consequently out of, the capillary so expeditiously that equilibrium on both sides of the vessel wall is reached almost instantaneously. The same can be said of nongaseous lipid-soluble materials, the lipid/water partition coefficient being the most important factor in determining differences in rates among compounds. In fact, the rate at which any molecule diffuses across the capillary endothelium at all sites except the brain is greater than its rate of passage across epithelial tissue. At both types of tissues this diffusion occurs across the *cellular membrane* and not between cells. Thus, whether there is greater separation between endothelial cells than between epithelial cells becomes a moot point with respect to the observed differences in rates of penetration of lipid-soluble substances across these two barriers. Rather, these differences may be attributed to disparities in the rates at which an absorptive surface is made available to a molecule within the capillary compared with that at epithelial tissues. The solutes in the blood are flowing within minute tubes, only 1/90 to 1/200 mm in diameter, completely surrounded by endothelium whose entire surface is conducive to diffusion. The flow of blood within these tiny channels affords many more opportunities for molecules of solute to collide with permeable surfaces than are provided for molecules within the intraluminal contents of the intestine, for example. This situation is somewhat analogous to the differences in rates of absorption between the stomach and small intestine: it is the huge difference in the area of available absorptive surface that gives the intestine the much greater capacity for absorption of all materials.

Water-soluble molecules, and water itself, also readily traverse the capillary wall, but at rates slower than compounds with lipid solubility. Molecular size is the major determinant of the rate of transcapillary movement: the smaller the water-soluble molecule, the faster its rate of diffusion. But even relatively large molecules like proteins are able to penetrate the capillary endothelium very slowly. The hypothetical existence of pores penetrating the cell membrane might explain these phenomena. Yet none have been seen, even though the electron microscope can detect pores of the diameter needed to accommodate proteins. However, in the case of water-soluble molecules, the gaps that exist *between* endothelial cells have indeed been shown to serve as passageways from the circulation to the extravascular spaces. Furthermore, capillary permeability can be increased by an agent such as histamine, which acts directly on the endothelial cells to enlarge the gaps between them. Thus the difference between the organization of individual cells of the endothelial and epithelial barriers does have some functional significance.

Relatively small water-soluble molecules cross the capillary at rates directly proportional to their concentration gradients and as if they were simply diffusing in water. In contrast, the driving force for movement of the large water-soluble substances appears to be the hydrostatic pressure exerted by the blood. The pressure of the blood on the arterial end of the capillaries is normally higher than that at the venous end. It is this pressure gradient between the two ends of the capillary bed that largely accounts for the transcapillary movement of high-molecular-weight compounds like protein. Since the pressure gradient normally fluctuates and may also be influenced by various drugs, the permeability of the capillary is characteristically dynamic and continually subject to change. Whereas the rate of movement of macromolecules is strongly dependent on the hydrostatic pressure in the capillary lumen, the actual mechanism of their transfer across the capillary remains in doubt. Pinocytosis has been suggested as a possibility on the basis of microscopical studies that revealed the presence of vesicles at either margin of the endothelial membrane.

In the liver and kidney the capillaries present less of a barrier to the movement of molecules of all sizes than do capillaries elsewhere. These differences are important since they serve the functions of these organs: the kidney is the organ chiefly responsible for the excretion of water-soluble compounds; the liver not only manufactures many proteins for use by the body, but also receives most substances absorbed from the small intestine before they are distributed. In the kidney the increase in permeability is primarily one of rate rather than kind of material transferred. Two factors contribute to this increase. First, the capillaries associated with the initiation of urine formation contain large pores in the *membrane of the endothelial cell* itself; these pores are readily visualized by means of the electron microscope. Second, the hydrostatic pressure within these capillaries is very high compared with many other capillary beds. It is this force which is responsible for the increased rates of solute movement, since diffusion is supplemented by transcapillary *filtration* through the pores. In the liver the increased permeability relates mainly to the greater rate of translocation of large molecules. Blood from both the heart and the portal vein draining the intestine courses through the hepatic *sinusoids* before being returned to the heart by the hepatic vein. Since these sinusoids lack a complete endothelial lining, large molecules, even large proteins, can enter and leave the blood flowing through the liver more readily than the blood flowing through other tissues of the body.

Magnitude of Distribution

It is clear from the foregoing that the blood capillary is a relatively effective barrier only to large molecules. Therefore, when a macromolecular compound is injected intravascularly, it is almost completely retained in the extracellular fluid of the circulation — the plasma — since its size also precludes entry into the blood cells. The action of the heart and the turbulence of the uneven blood flow through various vessels quickly mixes the agent with the circulating plasma. In the average 70-kg man the volume of plasma is approximately 3 liters, a little more than half of the whole blood volume. So within a very few minutes the quantity of drug originally entering the circulation is diluted into this volume of fluid. We can say, then, that a drug which is unable to cross the capillary wall has an *apparent volume of distribution* equal to plasma-water (Fig. 5-11).

The volume of distribution of a drug capable of readily traversing the capillary endothelium will, explicitly, be greater than that of plasma-water. Let us, for the moment, specify an ideal situation in which the drug is (1) a free solute, unbound to any tissue components; (2) unchanged by any chemical reactions of the body; and (3) not eliminated during the period of distribution. When such an agent enters the circulation, either by direct placement or following absorption, it also will be mixed into plasma-water. But as this dilution is taking place, the concentration gradient in the plasma will drive the drug across the capillary wall. It will diffuse at a rate consistent with its molecular size, lipid solubility and degree of ionization. Let us also assume, for the present, that the permeability characteristics of capillaries are identical all over the body. Then, since all tissues are supplied with capillaries, the drug will be distributed from the plasma to the extracellular fluid of *all* parts of the body. This movement of drug into the interstitial water of the tissues will continue until there is no longer a gradient between the inside and outside of the capillaries supplying the tissues. Obviously, however, the *rate* at which the drug concentration in the extracellular fluid of a particular site reaches this point of equilibrium will depend on the number of capillaries coursing through it. The richer the vascularity, the greater the blood flow and the more rapid the distribution of drug from plasma to the extravascular interstitial fluid. Table 5-5 shows average rates of blood flow through some organs of the body in relation to their mass. These data indicate that a drug will appear in the extracellular fluid of organs like the liver, kidney and brain more rapidly than in that of tissues like muscle.

Yet eventually, assuming our ideal conditions, the concentration of drug in *all* extracellular water, including plasma-water, will reach the *same* level. When this equilibrium is attained, the quantity of drug that originally entered the bloodstream will be diluted into about 12 liters, the sum of the extravascular interstitial fluid (about 9 liters in the adult male) plus the volume of plasma-water. Hence, a drug which can readily leave the capillaries but which cannot enter cells will have an

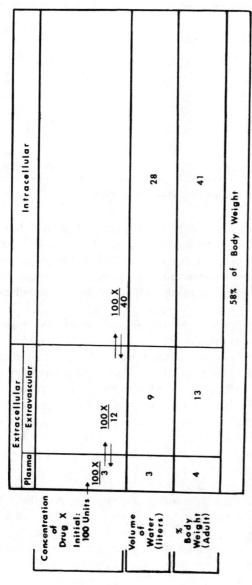

FIGURE 5-11. Distribution and concentration of a drug in the various fluid compartments of the body in relation to its permeability characteristics. The values for water content of the plasma and extracellular and intracellular compartments are only approximate. These figures do not include the inaccessible water in bone, or the water in the cavities of the stomach, intestine, and tracheobronchial tree, in the cerebrospinal fluid or in the anterior chamber of the eye (total 7 to 10 per cent).

Table 5-5. Blood Flow to Various Organs and Tissues[a]

Tissue	Blood Flow (liters/min)	Tissue Mass (% of total body weight)
Blood	5.4	8.0
Rapidly perfused		
Brain	0.75	2.0
Liver	1.55	3.5
Kidney	1.2	0.5
Heart (musculature)	0.25	0.5
Less rapidly perfused		
Muscle	0.8	48.0
Skin	0.4	6.5
Poorly perfused		
Fat	0.25	14.0
Skeleton	0.2	17.0

[a]The values in this table are to be considered as approximations only.

apparent volume of distribution equal to the total extracellular fluid. Ions such as iodide and bromide or water-soluble molecules the size of sucrose or larger remain, for the most part, distributed within extracellular fluid. And drugs that are so poorly absorbed from the gastrointestinal tract that they must be administered by a route which bypasses epithelial tissues are usually largely confined to this volume of distribution.

If the drug is capable of traversing the cell membrane, it will move from the extracellular space into the fluid within the cell. Assuming no active transport process is involved, the transfer across the cell wall will proceed until the intracellular drug concentration is the same as that outside the cell. Since the permeability characteristics of the cellular membrane are about the same for all cells, it follows that the concentration of the drug will be further diluted by a volume equal to that of the total intracellular water of all cells, approximately 28 liters. Consequently, a drug which can readily pass all biologic barriers will have an apparent volume of distribution equal to the total water content of the body, about 40 liters. Recognizably, all highly lipid-soluble drugs have this type of distribution.

It is both customary and convenient to express the extent of drug distribution, as we have above, in terms of the water content of compartments of the body which are anatomically and functionally distinct, i.e., vascular fluid, extracellular fluid and intracellular fluid (see Fig. 5-11). This convention, however, is based on an idealized situation, and as such is an oversimplification, ignoring many known variables while incorporating a number of assumptions that may or may not be correct. Nonetheless, this general treatment permits drawing some valid and important conclusions about the distribution of drug from the circulation. First, the quantity of drug reaching an extravascular site of action represents only a *small* fraction of the total amount of drug administered. And the more readily diffusible the drug, the smaller the fraction likely to reach its receptor, whereas the greater will be its distribution to parts of the body not involved with the production of the desired biologic effects. Thus the very nature of the process for getting the vast majority of drugs to their respective sites of action is responsible for dispersing them throughout the tissues of the body.

Binding of Drugs to Plasma Proteins and Other Tissue Components

One of the assumptions made in developing the general picture of the distribution of drugs is that the drug remains as a solute in the fluid of various compartments of the body. Obviously, the rate of movement of a drug across biologic barriers is determined by its *own* physicochemical properties only when it exists as an independent entity. This ideal behavior is characteristic of very few drugs. The same kinds of bonds that are formed when a drug interacts with its receptor can be formed between drug molecules and other macromolecular tissue components. The major difference, of course, is that the drug-receptor combination leads directly to a sequence of events measurable as a biologic effect, whereas binding with a nonreceptor substance does not. The binding sites that do not function as true receptors are frequently referred to as *secondary receptors, silent receptors* or *sites of loss.* The last is the most appropriate designation, since the molecules of a drug that are bound to the nonreceptor macromolecule are neither free to move to a site of action nor free to produce a biologic effect. The importance of these interactions with sites of loss will depend on how much drug is bound and on the strength, or reversibility, of the bond formation.

Binding of drugs to tissue constituents can occur at sites of absorption, within the plasma or at extravascular sites following egress from the bloodstream. For example, in the intestine the positively charged quaternary ammonium compounds are strongly bound to highly negatively charged groups of the mucus secreted into the lumen. The large quantities of mucus normally present can act as sites of loss for a considerable quantity of the positively charged molecules and thereby decrease the effective concentration gradient of the drug. This binding has been shown to account in part for the incomplete absorption of quaternary ammonium drugs and for the fact that, to produce equal effects, larger quantities must be administered orally than parenterally. However, the proteins of plasma appear to be the most common site for drug binding, probably because this binding can be so readily detected.

Albumin, the principal protein of plasma, is also the protein with which the greatest variety of drugs combine. Antibiotics such as penicillin, tetracycline and streptomycin, as well as drugs like aspirin, the barbiturates and the sulfa preparations, among many others, exist in plasma to a greater or lesser extent as a reversibly bound albumin complex. But how much and how strongly any drug will be bound to albumin is a property of the drug inherent in its molecular structure; the tendency to bind with protein — its affinity for protein — is a constant for a given drug. And since we are dealing with a reversible reaction:

$$\text{Free drug} + \text{Protein} \rightleftharpoons \text{Drug-protein complex}$$

the law of mass action is applicable. The fraction of drug that is bound will be in equilibrium with the fraction of drug that is free. Ordinarily, the protein concentration of plasma is fixed, and therefore the fraction of drug that is free to leave the plasma is determined only by the concentration of drug and strength of the binding. At low drug concentrations, the stronger the bond between the drug and protein, the smaller the fraction that is free. As drug concentration increases, the concentration of free drug also gradually rises until all the binding capacity of the protein has been saturated. At this point, any additional drug will remain unbound.

How does this binding to plasma protein influence the distribution of a drug to its site of action? Binding to protein, by decreasing the concentration of free drug in the circulation, lowers the concentration gradient driving the drug out of the circulation and slows its rate of transfer across the capillary. As the drug leaves the circulation, the protein-drug complex begins to dissociate and more free drug is available for diffusion. Thus as long as the binding is reversible, it does not prevent the drug from reaching its site of action but only *retards* the rate at which this occurs. Furthermore, as the drug is eliminated from the body, more can be dissociated from the protein complex to replace what is lost. In this way, plasma-protein-binding can act as a reservoir to make a drug available over a longer period. For example, some sulfa drugs are strongly bound to protein and are eliminated slowly in the urine, since only the fraction that is free can diffuse out of the capillaries. Consequently, these compounds remain in the body and are effective for longer periods than those sulfa drugs which have lower affinities for protein. Suramin, a drug used in the treatment of the protozoal infection trypanosomiasis, is an example of an agent still more firmly bound to plasma proteins. It is likewise very slowly eliminated in the urine, but unlike the sulfa drugs, suramin is not distributed to intracellular water and is not appreciably altered by the chemical reactions carried out by the body. These factors combine to yield therapeutically effective levels of suramin for extended periods, sometimes as long as three months, following a single intravenous injection.

Other tissues of the body can also act as reservoirs for drugs, but usually the *sites where drugs accumulate are not those where they exert their pharmacologic effect.* For example, tetracycline may be stored in bone and the insecticide DDT in fat. These stored drugs are in equilibrium with the drug in plasma and are returned to plasma as the plasma concentration decreases upon elimination of the drug from the body. However, the rate of release from the storage depots in the case of these two agents is ordinarily too slow to provide enough circulating drug to produce biologic effects. Consequently, this type of storage represents a site of loss rather than a depot for continued drug action. A classic example of binding to tissue components is provided by the interaction of chloroquine with nucleic acids of the cell nucleus. The drug may achieve a concentration in the liver 200 to 700 times the plasma concentration. When chloroquine is used to treat malaria, the liver represents a site of loss which must be saturated before plasma levels adequate for antimalarial therapy can be reached. In contrast, this accumulation of chloroquine in the liver becomes therapeutically useful in amebiasis when the intestinal infestation has spread to the liver.

It follows that the binding of a drug to nonreceptor tissue components generally means that more drug has to be administered initially in order to ensure its availability to its site of action. When the phenomenon of binding is added to the generalized

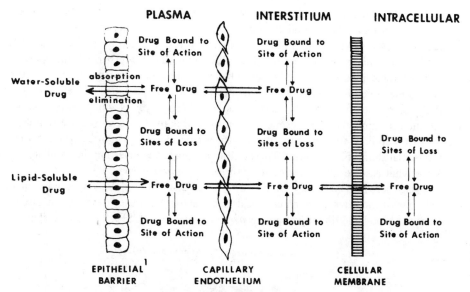

FIGURE 5-12. Factors influencing the amount of drug that will reach a site of action following absorption and distribution. In the plasma and interstitium, functionally important small ions or proteins may be sites of action; in the interstitium, the cell membrane may also be a site of action for drugs acting by receptor or nonreceptor mechanisms. Intracellular sites of action may be receptors or identifiable cellular components.

---

[1]The capillary endothelial barrier is not included on the other side of the epithelial barrier for the sake of clarity. Obviously, drugs which are absorbed through an epithelial barrier must also pass through the capillary endothelium before entering the plasma.

dispersal of drug inherent in the process of distribution, it becomes obvious that the amount of drug in the tissue or site where it acts is, indeed, a very small portion of what was originally introduced into the body (Fig. 5-12).

Distribution From Blood to Brain

It has been stated several times that capillaries in the brain do not permit substances to leave the blood as readily as do capillaries elsewhere in the body. Actually, this decreased permeability pertains only to the *diffusion of water-soluble or ionized* molecules. Lipid-soluble substances diffuse across brain capillaries at rates determined by their lipid/water partition coefficients, just as at other capillary barriers. In fact, since the brain receives one-sixth of the total amount of blood leaving the heart, lipid-soluble drugs are distributed to brain tissue very rapidly compared with a tissue such as muscle. Water-soluble materials for which active transport processes exist, such as glucose and amino acids, also gain rapid access to brain cells.

A factor that may contribute to the sluggish diffusion of water-soluble materials from capillary to brain tissue is the organization of the endothelium itself. The endothelial cells of brain capillaries appear to be more firmly joined to one another than is characteristic of other capillary endothelium. Even so, the increased resistance to the passage of water-soluble and ionized materials arises primarily from the fact that the brain capillaries do not communicate directly with the interstitium. Interposed between the capillary endothelium and the extracellular space of the brain is another membrane which is very closely attached to the capillary wall. Certain cells within the brain connective tissue, the astrocytes, have long processes which form sheaths around the capillaries. As a result, substances leaving the blood must traverse not only the capillary endothelium, but also the astrocytic sheath in order to reach the interstitial fluid of brain tissue. This additional membrane investing the capillary is really what is sometimes referred to as the *blood-brain barrier*.

Passage across the capillary directly into the interstitial fluid, however, represents only one of the ways in which chemicals can reach brain tissue. Materials can also leave the blood and directly enter the *cerebrospinal fluid* (CSF). The CSF system

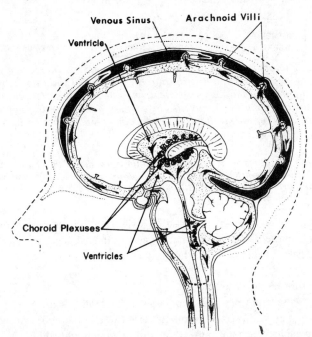

FIGURE 5-13. Circulation of cerebrospinal fluid (CSF). Channels through which CSF flows are exaggerated, and structures of the brain are not drawn to scale. The choroid plexuses are tufts of small capillary vessels much like renal glomeruli. The CSF elaborated into the centrally located ventricles (lateral and third) flows downward to the lower ventricle. Fluid is added by the choroid plexus of the lower ventricle (fourth) and then flows either downward to bathe the spinal cord or upward to bathe the convexities of the brain. The fluid finally reaches the arachnoid villi, where it drains into the great venous sinuses. The quantity of CSF in the ventricles and subarachnoid spaces is usually between 125 and 150 ml.

bathes the surfaces of the brain and spinal cord, functioning as a protective layer to cushion the delicate tissue against trauma. The CSF thus represents a third fluid compartment within the brain, the other two being the extravascular extracellular and intracellular fluid compartments. Cerebrospinal fluid is formed in the brain itself, primarily within its cavities, or *ventricles* (Fig. 5-13). From these ventricular sites of formation the CSF circulates to the spaces surrounding the surfaces of the brain and spinal cord, and from these spaces the bulk of the fluid flows directly into the venous drainage system of the brain. Since most of the CSF does not recycle, there is constant need for its regeneration. A specialized vascular organ within each ventricle, the *choroid plexus*, functions in this capacity. It is located between the blood capillary wall and the ventricle and is lined on its ventricular side with epithelial cells. These cells have the same provisions for solute transport as do other epithelial barriers, including active transport processes. Consequently, the transfer of chemical substances from the blood across the choroid plexus into the CSF has the character-istics of passage across epithelium rather than those across simply endothelium. Once in the CSF, material can enter brain tissue at rates typical of passage from interstitial fluid across cell membranes. In this manner the CSF provides a gateway for sub-stances to reach the intracellular spaces of the brain as well as a pathway for solutes to be returned to the venous system (Fig. 5-14). The juxtaposition of epithelial tissue

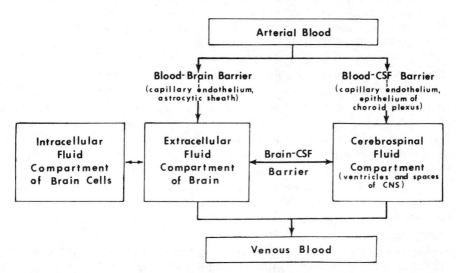

FIGURE 5-14. *Structural and functional relationships of the blood supply, cerebrospinal fluid and extracellular and intracellular fluid compartments of the brain. A drug may enter the brain by crossing either the blood-brain barrier or the blood-CSF barrier. Material entering by the blood-CSF barrier must cross an additional barrier, the brain-CSF barrier, in order to reach the extracellular fluid compartment of the brain. Material can only enter and leave the intracel-lular fluid compartment by the extracellular fluid compartment. Materials are returned to the venous blood from either the extracellular fluid compartment or the CSF fluid compartment.*

between the blood-CSF barrier and the investment of the blood capillary by a cellular sheath at the blood-brain barrier together account for the slow diffusion of water-soluble materials into brain tissue.

Drainage of the major portion of the CSF directly into venous blood effectively makes the CSF an undirectional route for solute movement — only into the brain. However, a small portion of the CSF is formed from material returning to the ventricle from the extracellular fluid. This is important from a pharmacologic viewpoint, since some drugs are actively transported by the choroid plexus *out of* the CSF back into the blood. One such drug is penicillin. Because this water-soluble drug also enters the brain and CSF very slowly, as would be expected, it is not ordinarily as effective an antibiotic in the treatment of infections in this region of the body as it is elsewhere.

The slow rate of entry of water-soluble drugs into the brain has still other pharmacologic consequences. As the example of penicillin illustrates, a drug intended for action in the brain must have solubility characteristics which permit its distribution to this site. Conversely, water-soluble drugs may be used purposely when it is desirable to exclude effects on the brain. For example, atropine has lipid solubility and readily enters brain tissue, where it has some pharmacologic activity. However, when atropine is used in the treatment of peptic ulcer, its action within the brain may be undesirable. This side-effect can be avoided by substituting a highly water-soluble agent which has pharmacologic effects outside the brain similar to those of atropine. Some quaternary ammonium agents, which are completely ionized substances, adequately fulfill these conditions.

Distribution From Mother to Fetus

The same pathways that serve to supply the fetus with the substances necessary for development and growth and that act to remove waste material also provide the means by which drugs interchange between the maternal and fetal circulations. This mutual exchange takes place primarily in the placenta, which connects the embryo or fetus with the maternal uterine wall (Fig. 5-15). Within the placenta are relatively large cavities, sinuses, into which the maternal arterial blood empties and from which veins arise to carry blood back to the mother. Fetal capillaries are contained in finger-like processes, villi, protruding into the blood sinuses. Thus, maternal and fetal blood do not mingle, and solute transfer takes place across the epithelial cells of the villi and the endothelium of the fetal capillaries. Material reaching the fetal capillaries is carried to the fetus by the umbilical venous blood, and material to be transferred from fetus to mother returns to the villi by the umbilical arterial blood.

The characteristics of drug diffusion from maternal blood to fetal blood in the capillaries of the villi are very similar to those of passage across any epithelial barrier. Lipid-soluble materials readily move from mother to fetus in accordance with lipid/water partition coefficients and degree of ionization. Water-soluble drugs move much more slowly and in inverse proportion to their molecular size. The rate and direction of this exchange is dependent on the concentration gradients and the rate of delivery to the intervillous spaces and villi.

As indicated above, drug distribution from mother to fetus begins with diffusion of

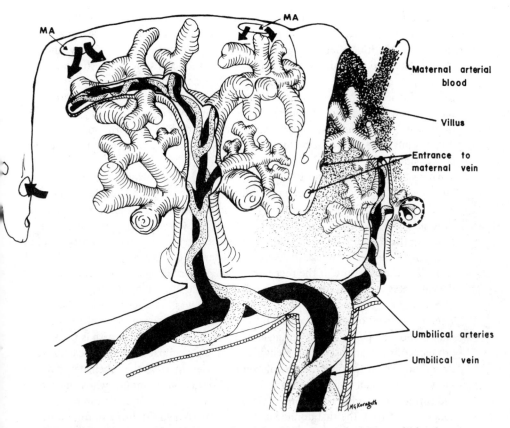

MA

MA

MA

Maternal arterial
blood

Villus

Entrance to
maternal vein

Umbilical arteries

Umbilical vein

MG Karaguth

FIGURE 5-15. Relationship of maternal and fetal blood vessels. Maternal blood from the uterine arteries (MA) enters a pool (intervillous space) where it is exposed directly to the epithelial membranes of the fetal villus. Materials from the maternal blood cross the villous membrane and enter fetal capillaries, from which they are carried to the fetus by the fetal placental veins which converge into the umbilical vein. Materials to be transferred from the fetal circulation to maternal blood are brought to the fetal side of the placenta by the umbilical arteries. Maternal blood from the intervillous space drains into the maternal uterine veins to be returned to the maternal systemic circulation.

the drug across the villous membrane into the fetal blood capillary. The drug is then carried to the fetus by way of the umbilical vein and finally becomes available for distribution to the various fetal organs and tissues. It is obvious from this pattern of distribution that the cord venous blood will reach equilibrium with maternal blood much more rapidly than will be true for the various tissues of the fetus. It has been estimated that the fastest equilibrium possible between maternal blood and fetal tissues is about 40 minutes, even when the maternal blood has a constant level of a drug over a period of time. The rate of maternal blood flow to the placenta limits the availability of the drug to the fetus. This explains why a wakeful infant can be delivered to an anesthetized mother provided the delivery takes place within about 15 to 30 minutes after drug administration. If the quantity of drug used to anesthetize the mother is within therapeutic range and the delivery takes place quickly, the fetus is never likely to have blood levels sufficient to produce a state of anesthesia. However, if a drug is administered many hours before delivery, the fetus may, indeed, acquire sufficient drug to produce effects. For example, the newborn infant may remain drowsy for 12 to 24 hours following delivery, if delivery is delayed for 2 to 3 hours after the mother has been deeply anesthetized with a barbiturate. Also, pinpoint pupils have been observed in infants born to mothers who received morphine during labor.

Whereas a single administration of a drug may not necessarily lead to pharmacologic effects in the fetus, frequent administration during gestation may produce adverse effects. Infants born to mothers addicted to drugs like morphine or heroin show all the withdrawal symptoms that addicts show when they, too, are no longer receiving these agents. Typical pharmacologic effects are observed in newborn infants which indicate that other agents like tranquilizers also gain ready access to the fetus. Moreover, the exposure of the pregnant female to certain agents, particularly during the early stages of fetal development, has been linked to the production of defects of one or more of the infant's organ systems. This was first recognized in the 1930's when malformed offspring were born to women who had been exposed to x-ray irradiation of the pelvic region during early pregnancy. Today's concern is the effect of products of nuclear fission in the environment, e.g., radioactive cesium, calcium and strontium, which readily cross the placental barrier. In 1940 the rubella virus was shown to be capable of producing serious malformations in infants whose mothers had suffered even mild infections of German measles in the first trimester of pregnancy. But it took the thalidomide disaster of 1960–1962 to bring to full awareness the fact that ordinary drugs can be most harmful to the fetus even though they have little potential for adverse effects in the adult individual. In some cases adverse effects of a drug on the fetus may not become apparent until the offspring have themselves reached adulthood. This has recently been shown to be the case for diethylstilbesterol (DES), a once widely used estrogen. Large doses of estrogens were used in the past in the unsubstantiated belief that this might prevent threatened abortion. Since DES, in contrast to the natural estrogens, was orally effective as well as cheap and plentiful, it was the drug usually administered. In the early 1970's, an increased incidence of vaginal carcinoma was discovered in the female offspring of women who had received DES during the first trimester of pregnancy – a time when the fetal reproductive system is developing. The uncertainty of the risk to the human embryo that may be associated with the use of any drug certainly dictates that all unnecessary medication be avoided during pregnancy and particularly during the first trimester.

REMARKS

In this chapter we have gained some insight into the ways in which absorption and distribution influence the accessibility of a drug to its site of action. The rates at which both processes take place will, of course, determine not only how much drug is made available but also how quickly the action will be seen after drug administration — the *onset* of drug action. However, while absorption and distribution are going forward, other processes are also in operation, namely those involved in removing the drug from its site of action. In the next chapter we shall consider how drugs are eliminated, so that we can put all the processes together in proper perspective and determine their combined effects on the entire course of drug action.

GUIDES FOR STUDY AND REVIEW

What distinguishes *enteral* from *parenteral* routes of absorption?

What distinguishes drug administration for local effects from administration for systemic effects? How may drugs be administered for local effects?

From the standpoint of absorption, what distinguishes the subcutaneous, intramuscular and intravenous routes from the oral route of administration? What are the advantages and disadvantages of each of these routes?

How does the blood flow influence the rate of absorption from different sites of drug administration? What is the role of the lymphatic system in drug absorption?

Which routes of administration avoid exposure of the drug to the liver before its exposure to the general circulation? Why is the initial exposure of a drug to the liver an important factor in the overall pharmacologic effect of some drugs?

What are the factors that modify the gastric absorption of a drug? Why is the rate of gastric emptying a primary determinant of the overall rate of drug absorption following oral administration?

Why is absorption usually greater from the intestine than from the stomach in the case of basic drugs? in the case of acidic and neutral drugs?

When are rates of disintegration and dissolution of solid dosage forms determinants of the rate of drug absorption? of pharmacodynamic effects?

How can the rate of absorption of the drug in solution be altered intentionally for a drug given orally? subcutaneously? intramuscularly?

How are rates of disintegration and dissolution of solid dosage forms modified? Does a change in particle size always affect dissolution rate? absorption rate? How can drugs that are susceptible to chemical alteration in the stomach be protected?

For what types of drugs or clinical situations is the "sustained-release" preparation a useful dosage form for oral administration? for subcutaneous administration? for intramuscular administration? Why are "sustained-release" preparations unsatisfactory in some people at certain times?

What environmental and physiologic factors in addition to pH can modify oral absorption?

When would it be advantageous and feasible to use the sublingual route for drug administration? The rectal route?

How does drug absorption from the skin compare qualitatively and quantitatively with absorption at other epithelial barriers?

Why does drug administration by inhalation closely resemble intravenous drug administration in terms of the rapidity with which the drug enters the general circulation?

How do drug solubility and particle size influence the site and extent of absorption of drugs inhaled as solids?

What distinguishes the process of distribution from that of absorption?

What do we mean by "apparent volume of distribution?" What is the approximate fluid volume of the major compartments into which the body is conveniently divided?

What factors determine the rate and volume of distribution of different types of drugs? What factors determine the rate of distribution of a particular drug to various organs and tissues?

How do differences in capillary permeability affect drug distribution to various organs and tissues?

How does binding to plasma proteins influence the rate of drug distribution to various tissues and organs? Does binding to plasma proteins alter the actual volume of distribution of the unbound drug? Does binding to plasma proteins alter the rate of drug elimination? If so, how? Does binding to sites of loss (or secondary receptors) other than plasma proteins alter the calculated apparent volume of drug distribution? How?

How are drugs transferred from the blood to the brain?

What are the factors that tend to keep many drugs from the tissues of the central nervous system (CNS)? What factors tend to make the rate of distribution of some drugs more rapid to tissues of the CNS than to tissues like muscles? Which types of drugs gain ready access to the CNS and which do not?

How are drugs transferred between the mother-to-be and the fetus? Why can a wakeful infant be delivered to an anesthetized mother when the delivery takes place within about 15 to 30 minutes of drug administration?

SUGGESTED READING

Alsing, J., and Way, E.L.   Placental Transfer of Drugs. In B.N. La Du, H.G. Mandel, and E.L. Way (eds.), *Fundamentals of Drug Metabolism and Drug Disposition.* Baltimore: Williams & Wilkins, 1971.

Binns, T.B. (ed.).   *Absorption and Distribution of Drugs.* Baltimore: Williams & Wilkins, 1964.

Butler, T.   The Distribution of Drugs. In B.N. La Du, H.G. Mandel, and E.L. Way (eds.), *Fundamentals of Drug Metabolism and Drug Disposition.* Baltimore: Williams & Wilkins, 1971.

Davidson, C.   Protein Binding. In B.N. La Du, H.G. Mandel, and E.L. Way (eds.), *Fundamentals of Drug Metabolism and Drug Disposition.* Baltimore: Williams & Wilkins, 1971.

Levine, R.R.   Intestinal Absorption. In J.L. Rabinowitz and R.M. Myerson (eds.), *Absorption Phenomena.* New York: Wiley, 1972.

Levine, R.R., and Pelikan, E.W.   Mechanisms of drug absorption and excretion. *Annu. Rev. Pharmacol.* 4:69, 1964.

Levy, G.   Kinetics and Implications of Dissolution Rate Limited Gastrointestinal Absorption of Drugs. In E.J. Ariens (ed.), *Physico-Chemical Aspects of Drug Action, Proceedings of the Third International Pharmacological Meeting,* Vol. 7. Oxford, Eng.: Pergamon, 1968. P. 33.

Rall, D.   Drug Entry into Brain and Cerebrospinal Fluid. In B.N. La Du, H.G. Mandel, and E.L. Way (eds.), *Fundamentals of Drug Metabolism and Drug Disposition.* Baltimore: Williams & Wilkins, 1971.

Schanker, L.   Drug Absorption. In B.N. La Du, H.G. Mandel, and E.L. Way (eds.), *Fundamentals of Drug Metabolism and Drug Disposition.* Baltimore: Williams & Wilkins, 1971.

6. HOW THE ACTIONS OF DRUGS ARE TERMINATED

The processes of absorption and distribution determine not only how but also how quickly a drug will reach its site of action; they determine the *speed of onset* of drug effect. If nothing else happened to a drug after it entered the body, its action would continue indefinitely. Although this would be advantageous in chronic diseases such as epilepsy or diabetes, it would not be so in most other illnesses. But the interactions between a drug and the body are not confined to the changes which the drug brings about in the living organism; the body also acts on the drug. The same processes which the body normally utilizes to eliminate waste products associated with its growth and maintenance, or to stop the actions of chemicals that it has synthesized, e.g., hormones, also put an end to the actions of drugs introduced into the body. The processes of *excretion* and *biotransformation* and, to a lesser extent, *tissue redistribution* terminate the actions of drugs by removing them from their sites of action.

Excretion is the process whereby materials are removed from the body to the external environment. Biotransformation, or metabolism as it is frequently called, is the process by which chemical reactions carried out by the body convert a drug into a compound different from that originally administered. Tissue redistribution, as the term implies, is the removal of a drug from the tissues where it exerts its effect to tissues unconnected with the characteristic pharmacologic response. The combined rates at which these processes occur determine the *duration of action* of a drug.

We shall start our discussion of how the body acts to terminate the action of a drug by considering the process of excretion; this process, by removing the drug from the body, almost always puts an end to the action of a drug. Next, in the section on biotransformation, we shall be primarily concerned with general principles and deal only cursorily with the many chemical reactions which drugs undergo in the body. We shall see that the process of biotransformation does not necessarily lead to the immediate cessation of drug effect, yet it generally yields products that are more readily excreted than are the parent compounds. The topic of the influence of tissue redistribution on the termination of drug effects is deferred to Chapter 8, in which its discussion will be more pertinent.

117

EXCRETION

In the process of excretion the direction of movement of a drug is just the opposite of that involved in getting a drug to its site of action — it is the reverse of distribution and absorption. For excretion involves movement of a drug from the tissues back into the circulation and from the bloodstream back into those tissues or organs separating the internal from the external environment. Thus, we need formulate no new principles to understand the process of excretion; we need only reconsider the principles that generally govern movement of materials across biologic barriers in terms of some additional anatomic structures.

The lung is the major organ of excretion for gaseous substances, and agents remaining as gases in the body are almost completely eliminated by this route. Agents that can be volatilized at body temperature are also excreted in the expired air to a greater or lesser extent, depending on their volatility. Indeed, so much of the foul-smelling liquid drug paraldehyde is eliminated through the lungs that it finds limited use, even though pharmacologically it is a desirable agent for inducing sleep. Some alcohol is also excreted in expired air; this is the basis for the medicolegal test commonly used to determine whether an individual has ingested alcohol and to aid in the diagnosis of drunkenness.

Nonvolatile, water-soluble drugs can leave the body by way of any of the media discharged to its external surface. Sweat, tears, saliva, nasal excretion and the milk of the lactating mother are all examples of fluids in which drugs may be excreted. The amount excreted by any of these routes ordinarily represents only a minor fraction of the total amount of drug eliminated from the body. Yet in the case of milk, even a small content of drug may be of considerable consequence to the suckling infant. However, the most important vehicle by far for the excretion of nonvolatile, water-soluble drugs is the urine; there are many instances in which a drug or the product of its biotransformation or both are excreted almost entirely by this route.

The alimentary canal is the next most important route of excretion of nonvolatile agents, and not just for drugs incompletely absorbed following oral administration. Drugs may enter the alimentary canal along its entire length from the mouth to the rectum in any of the fluids secreted into it. If the drug entering the gastrointestinal tract is not readily reabsorbed, it leaves the body in the feces. However, the liver, through its secretion of bile into the small intestine, contributes the major portion of material excreted in this manner. We shall confine our detailed discussion to the two major organs of excretion of water-soluble drugs — the kidney and the liver.

Excretion of Drugs by the Kidney

The volume and composition of the body fluids are kept remarkably stable despite the daily fluctuations imposed by the intake of water, food and other materials, and by the many substances produced by the body itself. To maintain these relatively constant conditions — homeostasis — the body has to rid itself of materials it cannot use or that are present in excess, while conserving substances essential for its very existence and well-being. In this regulation of homeostasis, the kidney plays a very significant and strategic role. As a major organ of the excretory system, it is responsible for eliminating the majority of the nonvolatile, water-soluble substances pro-

Table 6-1. Electrolyte Composition of Normal Blood Plasma

Constituent	Concentration in Plasma (mEq/liter)
Cations	
Sodium (Na^+)	142
Potassium (K^+)	4
Calcium (Ca^{++})	5
Magnesium (Mg^{++})	2
Anions	
Chloride (Cl^-)	101
Bicarbonate (HCO_3^-)	27
Phosphate ($HPO_4^=$)	2
Sulfate ($SO_4^=$)	1
Organic acids	6
Protein	16

duced or acquired and not needed by the body. But at the same time that the kidney is performing its excretory function, it must also carry out its additional functions: (1) to maintain a constant volume of circulating blood and regulate the fluid content of the body as a whole; (2) to regulate the **osmotic pressure** relationships of the blood and tissues; and (3) to adjust the relative and absolute concentrations of normal constituents of the plasma (Table 6-1). To carry out these functions simultaneously, the kidney cannot be just a waste-disposal unit. It must be, and is, an organ of functional selectivity, capable of handling individually and according to need the many substances brought to it by the blood. Thus the kidneys, as the "master chemists of the internal environment,"[1] are able to regulate and maintain the constancy of the volume and composition of the body's fluids because they are capable of elaborating a urine of variable volume and composition. And nowhere is it more clearly evident than in the kidney that function is related to structure.

Anatomic Considerations

The human kidney is a bean-shaped organ about six inches long, composed of a cortex, or outer layer; a medulla, or middle layer; and a central cavity called the pelvis (Fig. 6-1). The funnel-shaped pelvis is continuous with the ureter, the long tube connecting the kidney to the bladder.

The functional unit of the kidney is the nephron. Each nephron consists of a long, unbranched, tortuous tubule originating in the kidney cortex as a closed-ended structure known as *Bowman's capsule*. This capsule envelops a tuft of capillaries called a *glomerulus*. The tubule leading from Bowman's capsule, but continuous with it, is divided into four segments: (1) the proximal segment or proximal convoluted tubule; (2) the loop of Henle; (3) the distal segment or distal convoluted tubule; and (4) the collecting tubule. A single layer of epithelial cells lines the lumen of the nephron throughout its entire length.

[1] Attributed to Homer W. Smith (1895–1962), a famous American renal physiologist.

A

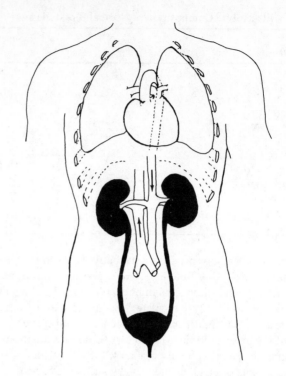

B

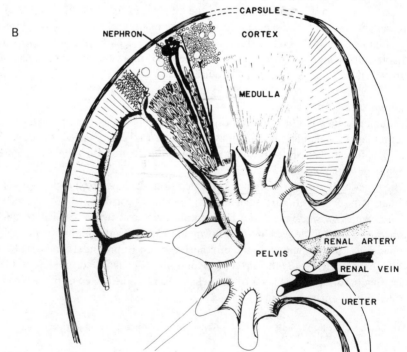

C

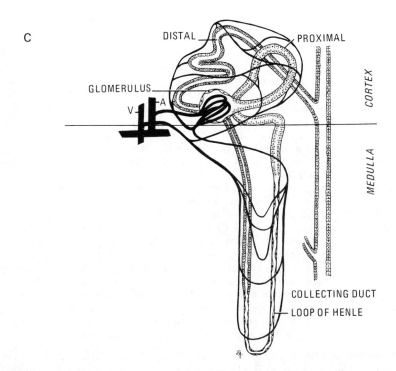

DISTAL

PROXIMAL

CORTEX

GLOMERULUS

V — A

MEDULLA

COLLECTING DUCT

LOOP OF HENLE

FIGURE 6-1. Anatomy of the kidney. (A) Position of the kidneys in relationship to blood vessels and ureters. (B) Gross structure of the kidney, showing relationship of cortex, medulla, pelvis and ureter. The position of a nephron with a long loop of Henle (greatly enlarged) is also indicated. In humans, about 20 per cent of the nephrons extend from the cortex to the papilla. Other nephrons have shorter loops of Henle penetrating to varying depths within the medulla; still other nephrons lie wholly within the cortex. (C) A nephron with a long loop of Henle. The glomerulus and the proximal convoluted, distal convoluted and collecting tubules lie within the cortex. The loop of Henle lies within the medulla, and the collecting duct courses from the cortex through the medulla to the pelvis. The long capillary loop paralleling the loop of Henle is known as the vasa recta.

Bowman's capsule, created by the invagination of the dilated blind end of the tubule, forms a double-walled enclosure around the glomerular capillaries, the space between the walls of the capsule being continuous with the lumen of the tubule. We may picture the glomerulus then as being surrounded by the capsule in the same way as a fist would be if it were pushed into a large, partially inflated balloon. But the capsule does not represent merely a pouch to receive the capillaries. The inner wall of capsular epithelium has numerous projections which completely cover the fifty or more loops of the glomerular capillaries, much as a finger is covered by a glove. This close contact of capillary and capsule, and the fact that the capsular and capillary lumen are each lined by a single layer of cells, make the biologic barrier between a capillary and the lumen of Bowman's capsule exceedingly thin; normally the total thickness is only about 0.001 mm.

The proximal segment of the tubule lies within the cortex in the vicinity of the capsule and coils back on itself in a much more complicated fashion than is shown in Figure 6-1. The tubule then proceeds in a straight line for a variable distance into the medulla of the kidney before making a sharp bend and returning to the cortex; this narrow, hairpin-shaped structure is the loop of Henle. The segment distal to the loop of Henle, the distal convoluted tubule, also coils back on itself repeatedly, as its name implies, before emptying into the collecting duct by way of the collecting tubule. The collecting duct then courses straight through the medulla and empties into the renal pelvis. The collecting ducts, the ureter and the urinary bladder are the channels between the nephron and the external environment. They provide a clear path for urine, the fluid formed in the kidney, to pass to the outside of the body. The inside of the tubule itself may be considered a part of the external environment.

It is estimated that there are about one million nephrons per kidney and that the total length of the tubules of both kidneys is in the order of 75 miles! This huge surface area and the thinness of the barrier separating the tubular lumen from the internal environment make it obvious that the kidneys are ideally structured to provide maximum contact between the external and internal environments of the body. But in order to serve the body effectively, the kidney must also be able to obtain readily from blood the substances to be eliminated and to return to the blood the essential materials that must be conserved. And the manner in which blood is supplied to the kidney is admirably geared to these functions.

The arteries leading from the heart to the kidney are short and wide, permitting a large supply of blood to reach the kidney at a high hydrostatic pressure. Between one-fourth and one-fifth of the blood pumped out of the heart at every beat is routed through the kidney. This means that a volume of blood equal to the total blood volume of the body is made available to the kidneys about every four to five minutes (cf. p. 104, Table 5-5).

Upon entering the kidney, the renal artery branches into smaller and smaller arteries, and these in turn subdivide into arterioles. Each Bowman's capsule is supplied with one of these arterioles, referred to as the *afferent arteriole*.

The network of capillaries — the glomerulus, formed by the subdivision of the afferent arteriole — has several distinguishing characteristics with respect to structure and location which are of functional importance. First, as we have seen, the endothelium of the glomerular capillary contains large pores which readily permit passage of all plasma constituents except macromolecules like protein (cf. p. 101). By discriminating against the passage of blood constituents only on the basis of molecular size, the glomerular endothelium resembles an artificial porous structure. And, in common with other porous filters, the force which determines the rate of filtration is pressure; in the case of the glomerulus this pressure is supplied by the work of the heart. The hydrostatic pressure within the glomerulus, the porous nature of the endothelium and the thinness of the total barrier between capillary and capsular lumen provide for rapid movement out of the capillary and into the capsule of all plasma constituents but proteins. This filtrate of plasma, lacking only the plasma proteins, is termed an *ultrafiltrate*. That the formation of this ultrafiltrate is rapid is evidenced by the fact that as blood passes through the glomerulus, one-fifth of its volume is filtered. The high head of pressure which forces this fluid out of the glomerular capillaries also prevents its reentry into the capillary bed. But nearly all this fluid is recaptured by the bloodstream through a *second set of capillaries*. For another feature of the glomerulus is that it is the first of two capillary beds between the arterial supply and venous drainage of the kidney. The vessel leaving the glomerulus is not a venule but an *efferent arteriole*. It subdivides into another network of capillaries nestling around the tubules of the nephron and forming their blood supply. It is only after passing through this second capillary bed that blood enters the venous side of the circulation to be returned to the heart (see Fig. 6-1).

Thus the unique characteristics of the glomerulus readily provide the means whereby the kidney can easily obtain everything from the blood — the delivery system of the body — that needs to be eliminated. The enormous surface area of the tubules and their intimate contact with blood capillaries throughout their length afford the opportunities necessary to return to the body those substances which cannot be considered superfluous. All these factors combine to make the kidney ideally suited for its role as the guardian of the body's economy. Now let us turn our attention to how the dichotomous functions of reabsorption and excretion can be carried out simultaneously by the kidney and, moreover, on a very selective basis. An understanding of these functions is essential for understanding not only how the kidney eliminates drugs from the body, but also how drugs act on the kidney. The renal mechanisms which normally account for the formation and final composition of voided urine are identical with those which account for the rate and extent of the urinary excretion of drugs.

Formation of Urine

In the average, healthy adult, about 1,200 ml of blood (650 ml plasma) are delivered each minute to the glomeruli of the two kidneys. Of this volume, about one-fifth, or 130 ml per minute, appears in Bowman's capsule as an ultrafiltrate of the plasma. This amounts to about 180 liters of fluid per day being presented to the kidneys for processing. Since all the plasma constituents except proteins and protein-bound compounds pass through the glomerulus, the filtrate contains indispensable substances like water, ions, glucose and other nutrients, in addition to disposable waste materials such as phosphate, sulfate and urea, the end products of protein metabolism. Urine formation begins indiscriminately and lavishly. This is essential, however, if the fluids of the body are to be subjected to a purification process by the kidney. But it would spell rapid and total disaster through exhaustion of body resources were it not for

Table 6-2.   Quantitative Aspects of Urine Formation[a]

Substance	Per 24 Hours				Per cent Reabsorbed
	Filtered	Reabsorbed	Secreted	Excreted	
Sodium ion (mEq)[b]	26,000	25,850		150	99.4
Chloride ion (mEq)	18,000	17,850		150	99.2
Bicarbonate ion (mEq)	4,900	4,900		0	100
Urea (mM)[b]	870	460[c]		410	53
Glucose (mM)	800	800		0	100
Water (ml)	180,000	179,000		1,000	99.4
Hydrogen ion			Variable	Variable[d]	
Potassium ion (mEq)	900	900[e]	100	100	100[e]

[a]Quantity of various plasma constituents filtered, reabsorbed and excreted by a normal adult on an average diet.
[b]See Glossary for explanation of **mEq** and **mM.**
[c]Urea diffuses into, as well as out of, some portions of the nephron.
[d]pH of urine is on the acid side (4.5–6.9) when all bicarbonate is reabsorbed.
[e]Potassium ion is almost completely reabsorbed before it reaches the distal nephron. The potassium ion in the voided urine is actively secreted into the urine in the distal tubule in exchange for sodium ion.

the fact that more than 99 per cent of the original filtrate is reabsorbed and returned to the body (Table 6-2). Under normal conditions, the total quantity of water and solutes lost daily in the urine is equal to that acquired by the body, minus only the amounts excreted through other routes.

It is obvious, however, that the processes responsible for reabsorption from the renal tubules can have little in common with the mechanism involved in the first step of urine formation. Glomerular filtration, the process primarily responsible for excretion, is a physical process dependent for its operation on energy derived from the work of the heart. As such, it is selective only with respect to the molecular size of the substances filtered. On the other hand, the movement of solutes out of the tubular urine, across the tubular epithelial cells and through the interstitium back into the circulation involves physicochemical processes. The driving force for this movement is either a concentration gradient or the energy derived from the work of the renal tubular cells. Thus, passive diffusion and active transport across the tubular epithelium account for the changes in the composition of the ultrafiltrate after it leaves Bowman's capsule. The selectivity of this solute movement is determined by the same principles that govern solute movement at other biologic barriers. And the availability of a huge absorptive surface area in close contact with the circulation provides the conditions essential for these transport processes to operate at maximum efficiency.

The transport processes that permit cells, in general, to accumulate vital substances against concentration gradients also allow the tubular epithelial cells to reclaim these same essential solutes from the tubular urine (cf. pp. 66–67). Thus, nutrients such as

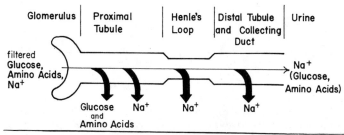

FIGURE 6-2. Sites of active transport of glucose, amino acids and Na⁺. Glucose and amino acids are excreted only when the amount filtered exceeds saturation levels of active transport mechanisms. Na⁺ is excreted in direct proportion to intake. In this figure, as in Figures 6-3 to 6-6 and 6-9, the heavy arrows indicate active transport processes and the light arrows, passive diffusion.

glucose, amino acids and some vitamins are salvaged from the tubular urine by active transport, a mechanism indispensable to their return to the body since their physicochemical properties preclude effective passive diffusion. Glucose, for example, under normal conditions is completely reclaimed from the urine in the proximal convoluted tubule. Glucose appears in the voided urine only when the quantity delivered to the kidneys is greater than that which saturates the active transport process, a situation that may occur following a meal rich in carbohydrates or in patients with diabetes mellitus (Fig. 6-2).

The process of greatest consequence to the final composition of voided urine is the active transport of sodium ion (Na⁺), which may take place along the entire length of the tubule and collecting duct (see Fig. 6-2). Not only is this ion the principal solute of the ultrafiltrate (see Table 6-2), but its active removal from the filtrate is also largely responsible for the reclamation of water and a number of other important urinary constituents. Thus, by following the transport of Na⁺ as the filtrate flows through the various segments of the nephron, we can also survey the changes in urinary volume and content of chloride, bicarbonate, hydrogen and potassium ions as well as urea (Figs. 6-2 to 6-6).

THE PROXIMAL TUBULE. The active reabsorption of Na⁺ begins in the proximal convoluted tubule. By the time the tubular urine reaches the loop of Henle, about 80 per cent of the Na⁺ originally filtered at the glomerulus has been returned to the circulation. The removal of so much solute would make the ultrafiltrate extremely hypotonic with respect to its surroundings. But the isotonicity of the filtrate is maintained throughout the proximal segment by the concomitant removal of water. The proximal epithelium is freely permeable to water, and water passively diffuses out of the tubular lumen back into the circulation in proportion to the amount of solute reabsorbed. Thus it is the active transport of solute, principally Na⁺ and to a lesser extent glucose and other actively transported constituents of the ultrafiltrate, that sets the stage for the removal of water. The osmotic pressure gradient developed by the removal of solute forces water to diffuse along this gradient so rapidly that the tubular fluid and the fluid of its surrounding tissues maintain approximately the same osmotic conditions (Fig. 6-3).

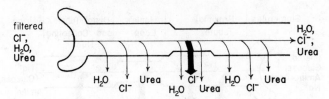

FIGURE 6-3. Sites of passive diffusion of water, Cl⁻ and urea along osmotic gradients established by active transport, particularly of Na⁺. In the presence of antidiuretic hormone (ADH), water is excreted in direct proportion to intake (pp. 131-132). In the absence of ADH, water is not reabsorbed in distal tubule and collecting duct. In the loop of Henle, water is reabsorbed only in the descending limb, since the ascending limb is water impermeable. Chloride ion is passively reabsorbed in the proximal and distal convoluted tubules and in the collecting duct but is actively transported out of the ascending limb of the loop of Henle. Between 50 and 60 per cent of the urea is reabsorbed; the remainder is excreted. Cl⁻ is excreted in amounts nearly equivalent to Na⁺ in order to maintain electroneutrality.

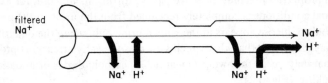

FIGURE 6-4. Acidification of urine by active reabsorption of Na⁺ in exchange for H⁺ secreted into tubular urine.

The electroneutrality of the filtrate must also be maintained. Therefore a major portion of the Na^+ reabsorbed is accompanied by an equivalent quantity of anion, principally Cl^- (see Fig. 6-3). The remainder of the actively reabsorbed Na^+ is indirectly responsible for the reabsorption of another anion, HCO_3^-. Bicarbonate ion is an essential factor in the transfer of carbon dioxide from cells to expired air and in the regulation of the pH of body fluids. Since the HCO_3^- is limited in quantity in the body, the kidney must conserve whatever HCO_3^- enters the tubule by filtration. The renal epithelium is relatively impermeable to HCO_3^-. However, in the presence of hydrogen ion, HCO_3^- is readily converted to water and carbon dioxide:

$$H^+ + HCO_3^- \rightleftharpoons H_2CO_3 \rightleftharpoons H_2O + CO_2$$

The H^+ is obtained from the tubular epithelial cell and is secreted into the tubular urine in exchange for Na^+ (Fig. 6-4). The carbon dioxide that is liberated by the reaction of H^+ and HCO_3^- readily diffuses back across the renal epithelium. Within the tubular cell the reverse process occurs, and carbon dioxide is rapidly hydrated with the help of the enzyme *carbonic anhydrase*, which catalyzes this hydration:

$$CO_2 + H_2O \rightleftharpoons H_2CO_3 \rightleftharpoons H^+ + HCO_3^-$$

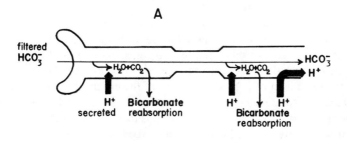

A

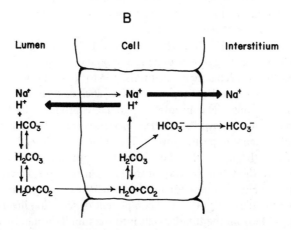

B

FIGURE 6-5. Sites and mechanisms of bicarbonate reabsorption and acidification of urine. (A) Hydrogen ion secretion in exchange for Na⁺ takes place in proximal and distal tubules. Under normal conditions urine is acidic, so all bicarbonate is reabsorbed and excess H⁺ is excreted in urine. Bicarbonate ion is excreted only when the body has to readjust pH to account for excess of base. (B) Bicarbonate is reabsorbed as CO_2, which is formed from carbonic acid. In the tubular cell CO_2 is hydrated, catalyzed by carbonic anhydrase. This process yields additional H⁺ for secretion into the tubular urine, while the HCO_3^- formed is returned to the circulation along with actively transported Na^+.

The carbonic acid formed then ionizes to yield HCO_3^-, which combines with Na^+ and is returned to the extracellular fluid and circulation as $Na^+HCO_3^-$. This ionization also provides an additional source of H^+ for continued secretion into the tubular urine. The overall result of these reactions is the reabsorption of Na^+ with an equivalent amount of HCO_3^- (Fig. 6-5). The removal of HCO_3^- is also responsible, in part, for the ultrafiltrate becoming more acid than the plasma from which it was derived.[2]

Immediately after filtration, the concentration of each of the constituents of the ultrafiltrate is identical with its concentration in plasma. As water leaves the tubular

[2]HCO_3^- is considered a base by definition, since it can accept the proton H^+.

urine, however, the constituents of the glomerular filtrate tend to become more concentrated. As higher concentration gradients are established between the tubular urine and the fluids of its surroundings, the gradients furnish the force necessary for passive diffusion of solutes across the tubular cell and back into the blood. This is the mechanism by which urea returns to the body (see Fig. 6-3) and probably also explains the movement of potassium ion out of the proximal tubule (Fig. 6-6). (The exact mechanism for potassium ion reabsorption is unknown.) Thus, as a result of the active transport of Na^+ and the mechanisms that this process sets in motion, the tubular urine delivered to the loop of Henle is essentially isosmotic with plasma. However, although most of the constituents are present in the same concentration as they are in plasma, the total content and volume of the tubular fluid are only 20 per cent of that which left the glomerulus.

In addition to secreting H^+ (in exchange for Na^+), the cells of the proximal tubule are also capable of secreting several organic compounds from the blood into the tubular urine. There are two separate mechanisms, one for the transport of organic acids, such as uric acid, and the other for organic bases, such as thiamine. Since this movement into urine is against the concentration gradients produced by the normal removal of water from the glomerular filtrate, these processes are active transport mechanisms, requiring cellular energy to perform work. The solutes remaining in the plasma after its passage through the glomerulus (only one-fifth of the blood entering the glomerulus is filtered) come to the tubule by way of the efferent arteriole. Passive diffusion along concentration gradients accounts for solute movement out of plasma into the interstitium and the tubular cells; the active component of secretion involves only the movement of solute from the tubular cells into the tubular urine. However, these two secretory systems, unlike the system for H^+ secretion, play only a minor role in the formation of urine in healthy individuals.

Active tubular reabsorption of Na^+ continues throughout the remainder of the nephron. If the reabsorption of water always followed passively in response to this active transport of Na^+, the urine would continue to decrease in volume but would remain isosmotic during its entire passage along the tubule. This would permit the kidney little scope in accommodating the needs of the body and the dietary intake. So at some point before urine reaches the ureters, the reabsorption of water and Na^+ must become independent of each other to allow for excretion of **hypertonic** or **hypotonic** fluid, as physiologic conditions warrant. The mechanisms responsible

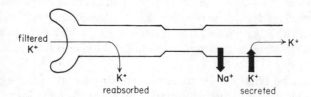

FIGURE 6-6. Origin of excreted potassium ion (K^+). K^+ is almost completely reabsorbed in proximal tubule. All K^+ excreted in the urine is apparently secreted in the distal tubule in exchange for Na^+.

for the production of a hypertonic urine reside in nephrons whose long loops of Henle course through the medulla and approach the tip of the papilla, whereas those responsible for a hypotonic urine are associated with the distal convoluted tubule and collecting duct.

THE LOOP OF HENLE. Only animals that possess a loop of Henle are capable of producing a concentrated urine, and only mammals and some birds have this unique hairpin-like structure. The essential factors in the ability to elaborate a urine hypertonic to the body fluids are (1) the special anatomic arrangement of those loops of Henle that descend deep into the medulla; (2) the *permeability* of the descending limb to both water and sodium chloride; (3) the *impermeability* of the ascending limb to water despite its active transport of Na^+ and Cl^-; and (4) the concentration of total solutes in the interstitial fluids of the medulla, which makes this region hypertonic to normal plasma and other body fluids.

The parallel descending and ascending limbs of long loops of Henle lie very close to each other over their entire course deep into the medulla. They are also in very close proximity to the corresponding limbs of parallel loops of a blood capillary (see Fig. 6-1). The narrow interstitial space which intervenes between these structures is conducive to the rapid exchange of water and solute from one to another of these four tiny tubes. The anatomic arrangement of the loop of Henle and its parallel capillary has still another important feature: it places tubules in which the flow of fluid is in opposite directions in close juxtaposition. In the descending limbs of both Henle's loop and the capillary, fluid flows from the cortex toward the pelvis; in the corresponding ascending limbs, the flow of fluid is back to the cortex. As a consequence, the events transpiring in one limb of the loop affect the composition of fluid in the other limb. The term *countercurrent exchange* is given to a system in which the exchange of solute or water (or heat) occurs between fluids flowing in opposite directions within the closely approximated limbs of a loop.

Although the epithelial lining of the entire loop of Henle contains only a single layer of cells, the architecture of the cells in the descending limb is different from that in the ascending limb. The epithelial cells in the descending segment are flat and permit the passive diffusion of water together with solutes. In the ascending limb the cells are thicker and resist the passage of water. Thus the descending limb of the loop of Henle is permeable to both water and Na^+, whereas the ascending limb is relatively impermeable to water but actively transports Na^+. The cells of the ascending limb of the loop of Henle are also functionally different in another respect from those of the descending limb and from those throughout the nephron: *they are capable of actively transporting Cl^-*. Indeed, it appears that the active transport of Cl^- is the process in the ascending limb that is primarily responsible for the reabsorption of sodium chloride in this segment.

In the kidney cortex, both the proximal and distal tubules are in contact with interstitial fluid which is isotonic with the plasma entering the kidney and with body fluids in general. However, this condition does not persist throughout the medulla. Instead, the concentration of total solutes, mainly sodium chloride, in the interstitial fluid of the medulla progressively increases from the cortex to the pelvis (Fig. 6-7).

Thus the interstitial fluid at the junction of the cortex and medulla is isotonic, but it becomes increasingly more hypertonic and reaches its greatest hypertonicity in the deepest portion of the medullary tissue. At this deepest point the sodium chloride concentration may be two to three times that in other body fluids. As a result, the loop of Henle and its parallel capillary are exposed to a gradually changing fluid environment as they course through the medullary tissue from the cortex to the end of the medulla and back again. The collecting duct, which passes through the medulla

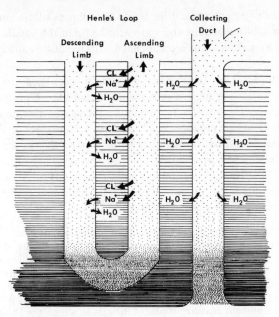

FIGURE 6-7. Representation of progressively increasing hypertonicity of medullary interstitium and its effect on concentration and dilution of tubular urine. Tonicity of all fluids in medullary interstitium and in urine of loop of Henle and collecting duct increases from cortex to pelvis. Water leaves collecting duct only in the presence of antidiuretic hormone. (Modified and redrawn from R. F. Pitts, The Physiological Basis of Diuretic Therapy, *1959. Charles C. Thomas, Publisher, Springfield, Illinois.)*

on its way to the ureter, is also subjected to progressively increasing hypertonic surroundings.

Now let us see how these factors influence the events that occur within the loop of Henle. As the isotonic tubular urine enters the descending limb, it comes into contact with the more hypertonic fluids of the interstitium. This difference in tonicity creates an osmotic gradient, and water passively diffuses out of the permeable epithelium into the tissue space to achieve equilibrium. Thus the fluid entering the system at the upper end of the descending limb becomes more concentrated as it approaches the bend in the hairpin. This movement of water from the descending limb into the interstitium would tend to dilute the interstitial fluids were it not for the countercurrent aspects of the hairpin-like structure. For as the water is leaving the descending limb, Cl^- (with Na^+) is being actively transported out of the ascending limb. And since the ascending limb is water-impermeable, the Cl^- moves out accompanied only by Na^+. Thus this addition of sodium chloride to the interstitium maintains hypertonicity (Fig. 6-8).

This active transport of ions by the ascending limb has an additional influence on the fluid flowing within the descending limb. Active transport of Na^+ can take place throughout the length of Henle's loop, but within the descending limb the active transport outward is offset by sodium chloride diffusing through the permeable membrane into the lumen, the driving force being the hypertonicity of the interstitium.

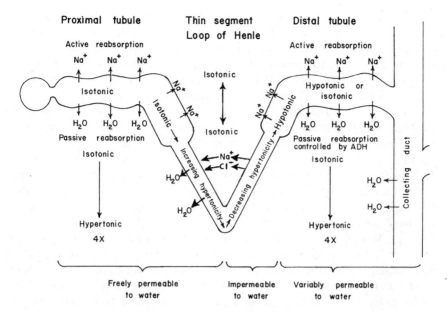

FIGURE 6-8. Functional organization of nephron in relation to reabsorption of Na⁺ and water and to formation of hypotonic and hypertonic urine. (Modified and redrawn from R. F. Pitts, The Physiological Basis of Diuretic Therapy, 1959. Charles C Thomas, Publisher, Springfield, Illinois.)

Two factors, then, account for the increasing hypertonicity of the fluid in the descending limb: (1) the passive movement of water into the interstitium, and (2) the passive diffusion of sodium chloride into the tubular lumen. And because of these two factors, the fluid in the lumen of the limb at any point along its descent approaches equilibrium with its immediate environment (see Fig. 6-8).

The fluid entering the ascending limb is exceedingly hypertonic and has a high content of sodium chloride. But as the tubular fluid flows toward the cortex it becomes progressively less hypertonic and more dilute; the fluid is constantly losing Na⁺ and Cl⁻, but the thicker epithelium prevents the passage of water. This continued loss of solute without a proportional reabsorption of water yields a somewhat hypotonic fluid by the time the ascending limb reaches the cortex and the distal convoluted tubule.

The blood that perfuses the elongated capillary loop paralleling the loop of Henle reinforces the function of the latter in maintaining the hypertonicity of the interstitium. As the isotonic blood enters the medulla and flows through the descending capillary limb, it is brought to osmotic equilibrium with its hypertonic surroundings by the passive diffusion of Na⁺ and Cl⁻ into the capillary lumen. But as the blood returns to the cortex, it redelivers this Na⁺ and Cl⁻ to the interstitium, again in order to maintain its osmotic equilibrium. The blood entering the cortex is isotonic or only slightly hypertonic. Thus, in consequence of a countercurrent exchange system, the blood does not remove the solute that is essential for the maintenance of the hypertonicity of the medullary tissues. Actually, the *net* reabsorption of Na⁺ and Cl⁻ from the tubular urine as it flows through the loop of Henle is very small and probably takes place only in the terminal part of the ascending limb.

The tubular urine leaving the loop of Henle and entering the distal convoluted tubule is hypotonic to the plasma and fluids in the cortex. Moreover, the net loss of sodium chloride and water from the urine during its passage through the loop accounts for only a small portion of their total reabsorption. One may well ask at this point, "How can a loop of Henle be essential for the production of a hypertonic urine when the fluid that leaves it is hypotonic and little decreased in volume and content of solute?" The answer is that Henle's loop serves the special purpose of establishing and maintaining the hypertonic gradient in the medullary interstitium that is essential for the final concentration of urine in the collecting duct.

DISTAL CONVOLUTED TUBULE AND COLLECTING DUCT. Active reabsorption of Na^+ continues throughout the remainder of the nephron and collecting duct. Again, as in the more proximal segments, Cl^- accompanies most of the Na^+ that is reabsorbed. In the distal tubule some of the Na^+ also exchanges for H^+, and this accounts for the removal of any HCO_3^- that may have escaped previous reabsorption (see Fig. 6-5). Thus, this $Na^+ - H^+$ exchange determines the final pH of the voided urine. However, in the distal segment, unlike the situation in the proximal tubule, Na^+ can also exchange for another cation, K^+. Since most of the latter is completely removed from the tubular urine before it reaches the loop of Henle, this secretion of K^+ in exchange for Na^+ in the distal tubule accounts for almost all the K^+ that is excreted (see Fig. 6-6).

Much of what else happens to the tubular urine in the distal segment, collecting tubule and duct depends on whether water is able to diffuse passively along the gradients established by Na^+ transport. For in these segments, unlike the proximal segment and loop of Henle, the permeability characteristics of the tubular epithelium are not constant with respect to water. Here the removal of water from the tubular fluid is dependent on the presence of a hormone, *antidiuretic hormone (anti,* against"; L. *diureticus,* "to make water through"). This hormone, referred to as ADH and also vasopressin, is produced by the posterior lobe of the pituitary. In the absence of ADH, the epithelium of the distal segment and collecting ducts is relatively *impermeable* to water; as Na^+ and other solutes are removed, water is unable to follow passively along the established osmotic gradients. As a result, in the absence of ADH, the slightly hypotonic fluid delivered to the distal segment by the loop of Henle becomes more and more dilute as solutes unaccompanied by water are reabsorbed. Thus, when ADH secretion is completely suppressed, as it would be in overhydration, as much as 15 per cent or more of the water of the original glomerular ultrafiltrate may escape reabsorption and be voided as a hypotonic urine.

The distal tubule and collecting duct become increasingly permeable to water as the levels of circulating ADH are increased, and then water is reabsorbed together with solute. In the distal convolution, which lies completely within the isotonic cortex, water will be reabsorbed in proportion to the solute absorbed, just as it is in the proximal segment. The urine entering the collecting duct will be isotonic with plasma and much reduced in volume. As the collecting duct courses through the medulla, water will diffuse out of the tubular lumen in response both to the continued reabsorption of Na^+ and to the steeper osmotic gradients established and maintained by the loop of Henle. And now the necessity of this unique structure for the formation of a hypertonic urine becomes fully apparent. For, although only one-fifth of the nephrons have long medullary loops, the urine formed in *every* nephron is affected by the medullary hypertonicity during its passage through the collecting ducts.

Thus, three basic factors are necessary to convert the isotonic urine of the glomerular filtrate to a concentrated urine: (1) the active reabsorption of the major urinary solutes, particularly sodium and its attendant anions; (2) the presence of ADH; and (3) a hypertonic medullary interstitium maintained by the activities of the loop of Henle. And in normal individuals on a balanced diet, the voided urine is hypertonic; it is decreased in volume and content of essential solutes to less than 1 per cent of what was originally filtered at the glomerulus.

Renal Excretion of Drugs

GLOMERULAR FILTRATION AND TUBULAR REABSORPTION. As blood flows through the glomerulus, any drug that is free in the plasma will be filtered together with other plasma constituents. Only drugs bound to protein or drugs of excessively large molecular size will be retained in the bloodstream. Since the epithelial lining of the renal tubules is like any other epithelial barrier, reabsorption of drugs from the glomerular filtrate is governed by the familiar principles of biotransport. As we have seen, the conservation and removal of water in the normal formation of urine creates concentration gradients in favor of solute movement out of the tubular urine. Thus, drugs will passively diffuse back into the circulation in accordance with their lipid/water partition coefficients, degree of ionization and molecular size (Fig. 6-9).

When the glomerular filtrate enters the proximal tubule its pH is the same as that of plasma, 7.4. However, the pH of the voided urine may vary from 4.5 to 8.0, depending on the amount of H^+ secreted and the quantity of HCO_3^- reabsorbed. Normally the urine is somewhat more acidic than plasma as a result of the secretion

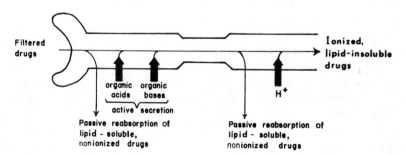

FIGURE 6-9. Excretion of drugs. Lipid-soluble and nonionized drugs are passively reabsorbed throughout tubule. In distal segments, the secretion of H^+ favors reabsorption of weak acids (less ionized) and, conversely, excretion of weak bases (more ionized). Active secretion of organic acids and bases occurs only in proximal segment.

of H^+ into the distal tubule. This increased acidity of the tubular urine profoundly affects the rate of reabsorption of weak electrolytes (cf. pp. 59–63). The nonionized forms of weak electrolytes, being more lipid soluble, may readily diffuse back into the circulation, whereas the ionized or charged forms are "trapped" in the tubular urine and excreted. Let us consider, for example, the weak electrolyte salicylic acid. In plasma, at pH 7.4, more than 99.9 per cent of salicylic acid exists in the ionized, water-soluble form, with only a very small fraction as the nonionized, freely diffusible species:

Undissociated salicylic acid $\rightleftharpoons$ Salicylate ion + H^+

At pH 7.4   0.01%   99.99%   99.99%

Both the salicylate ion and salicylic acid are filtered across the glomerulus. As water is removed from the glomerular filtrate, a concentration gradient is established between the urine and plasma, and some salicylic acid diffuses back into the blood. Acidification of the urine depresses the ionization of salicylic acid, since:

$$\frac{[\text{Salicylate ion}] \times [H^+]}{[\text{Undissociated salicylic acid}]} = \text{A constant}$$

Thus the increase in $[H^+]$ concentration drives the equilibrium to the side of undissociated salicylic acid, thereby increasing the fraction of the more lipid-soluble, nonionized form. The higher concentration gradient of the undissociated species so established favors more rapid reabsorption, and consequently the rate of salicylic acid excretion is reduced. Conversely, an alkaline urine promotes the urinary excretion of salicylic acid. In fact, practical use is made of these effects of pH on drug excretion in the treatment of poisoning with certain weak acids, such as phenobarbital. Sodium bicarbonate may be administered in order to produce an alkaline urine and hasten elimination of the drug. Obviously, for weak bases an alkaline urine retards excretion and an acidic urine enhances urinary elimination.

TUBULAR SECRETION. Whereas active reabsorption is known to play a significant part in the conservation of many compounds that are essential to the body's economy, carrier-mediated processes account for the reabsorption of only small quantities of a few drugs or nonessential substances. In contrast, the mechanisms responsible for active tubular secretion of organic compounds are of minor consequence in the normal formation of urine, but are important processes for the excretion of a number of drugs. Examples of drugs handled in this fashion are acids such as penicillin, phenylbutazone and salicylic acid, and bases such as quinine and quaternary ammonium compounds.

Since only two transport processes appear to be responsible for almost all the secretion that does occur, this may at times place restrictions on the transport of substances sharing the same system. Thus when blood coming to the tubule contains more than one of the organic acids which can be secreted, these compounds will compete with each other for binding sites on the same carrier. If the total quantity of acids to be secreted is in excess of available carrier, the rates of secretion of the individual anions will be decreased compared with their rates in the absence of each other. For example, when the amount of circulating uric acid is above normal, as it is in gout, small quantities of salicylic acid will inhibit the excretion of the former by competing for the same active secretory system.

The extent to which the organic acids or bases are eliminated in the urine following secretion is dependent on their degree of ionization within the tubular urine. Secretion of the quaternary ammonium compounds is tantamount to urinary elimination, since these agents are fully ionized regardless of the pH of the urine. Organic acids, such as penicillin, also are highly ionized in the urine and therefore undergo little reabsorption.

RATE OF DRUG EXCRETION. The rate at which a drug will be eliminated in the urine is the net result of the three renal processes: glomerular filtration, tubular secretion and tubular reabsorption. The rates of glomerular filtration and tubular secretion are dependent on the rate at which a drug is presented to the kidney — on its concentration in plasma. The rate of reabsorption by the tubules is dependent on the concentration of drug in the urine. For glomerular filtration, it is the concentration of free drug in the plasma that is important, since protein-bound drug cannot be filtered. On the other hand, the extent of protein binding, as long as it is reversible, makes little difference in the rate of elimination of those agents which can be secreted. The fraction of drug that is bound in plasma is in equilibrium with the fraction of drug that is free. As the latter is removed by secretion, the protein-drug complex dissociates very rapidly, and more free drug diffuses out of the plasma and is made available to the secretory process. Thus it is the concentration of both free and bound drug in plasma that is important in determining the rate of tubular secretion.

Determinations of the rates at which certain drugs are excreted by the kidney have proved to be extremely useful procedures for diagnosing the functional status of this organ. For example, if we wish to assess the competence of the glomeruli, we need a means of measuring the volume of plasma that the glomeruli are capable of filtering in a given period. A simple way of obtaining this information is to determine the rate at which a foreign compound present in the plasma appears in the urine. The compound used as a yardstick of glomerular competence would have to satisfy the following requirements: (1) it must be freely filterable in the glomeruli, i.e., it must not be bound to plasma protein; (2) it must be neither reabsorbed nor actively secreted into the tubular urine; (3) it must be nontoxic and have no direct or indirect pharmacologic effect on renal function; (4) it must remain chemically unaltered during its passage through the kidney; and (5) it must be a chemical that can be accurately determined in both urine and plasma. The polymeric carbohydrate inulin meets all these requirements. It is freely filterable by the glomeruli; it can reach the urine only by glomerular filtration; and all the inulin filtered is excreted, since it is not reabsorbed in its passage through the tubules. Therefore, following inulin administration, the amount recovered in the urine in a given interval is equal to the amount filtered by the glomeruli in that same period. For example, if 10 mg is the amount of inulin recovered in the voided urine in 10 minutes, then inulin is being filtered in the glomeruli at the rate of 1 mg per minute.

The next question we need to answer in order to determine the efficiency of the glomeruli is, "How many milliliters — what volume — of plasma have to be filtered each minute to yield the amount recovered per minute in the urine?" The answer can be obtained very easily by taking a sample of blood during the time the urine is being collected and determining how much inulin is present per milliliter of plasma. If we find the plasma concentration to be 0.008 mg per milliliter, then clearly, 125 ml of plasma must be filtered each minute to provide the 1 mg excreted by the kidney per minute:

$$\frac{\text{Amount excreted in urine per minute}}{\text{Amount in plasma per milliliter}} = \text{Number of milliliters of plasma filtered}$$
$$\text{per minute}$$
$$\text{(Equation 1)}$$

$$\frac{1 \text{ mg/min inulin in urine}}{0.008 \text{ mg/ml inulin in plasma}} = 125 \text{ ml/min, volume of plasma filtered}$$

Quantitative data on kidney function obtained in this manner are termed a *renal plasma clearance study*. And renal plasma clearance is defined as the volume of plasma needed to supply the amount of a specific substance excreted in the urine in 1 minute. A substance like inulin, which not only is completely filterable but is neither reabsorbed nor secreted by the tubular cells, has a renal plasma clearance identical to the rate at which it is filtered by the glomeruli. Thus the clearance of a substance such as inulin measures the *glomerular filtration rate* (GFR), but it must be remembered that GFR is expressed in milliliters per minute. In the average healthy adult male the GFR is about 130 ml per minute, indicating that 130 ml of plasma are filtered by the glomeruli each minute. This value was established using the procedures just described; similar procedures are used clinically to assess glomerular function in patients.

Renal plasma clearance is usually calculated as follows:

$$\text{Clearance (ml/min)} = \frac{U \times V}{P} \qquad \text{(Equation 2)}$$

where U is the concentration of the test substance per milliliter of urine, V is the volume of urine excreted per minute and P is the concentration of test substance per milliliter of plasma. In our example above, the volume of urine collected in 10 minutes was 10 ml. Thus $V = 1$ ml/min and $U = 10$ mg/10 ml, or 1 mg/ml. Then:

$$C = \frac{1 \text{ mg/ml} \times 1 \text{ ml/min}}{0.008 \text{ mg/ml}} = 125 \text{ ml/min}$$

Whereas Equations 1 and 2 are mathematically identical, the latter indicates not only the functional capacity of the glomeruli but also the kidney's ability to concentrate urine by removal of water. Comparison of the milliliters of plasma cleared with the milliliters of urine voided in 1 minute yields direct information of the amount of water reabsorbed during passage through the tubule. In our example, 124 ml of each 125 ml filtered were absorbed. And simple arithmetic shows that continued excretion at the rate of 1 ml per minute will lead to a daily output of urine of 1,440 ml.

Certain organic acids, such as para-aminohippuric acid (PAH), are secreted so rapidly and efficiently by the renal epithelium that they are almost entirely removed from the plasma in a single passage through the kidney. (Obviously, this can occur only when the plasma levels are low enough to insure that the carrier transport system is not over-loaded.) These acids are also not reabsorbed to any significant degree. A substance like PAH can then be used in clearance studies to obtain information about the total amount of plasma flowing through the kidneys. The term *clearance* is used here to mean exactly what it did in the case of the clearance of inulin: the amount of plasma needed to supply the amount of a specific substance excreted in the urine in 1 minute. Then, if the kidneys extract all of a compound that is delivered to them by the blood, the clearance of that substance is equal to the volume of plasma flowing through the kidneys per minute. By measuring the concentration of PAH per milliliter of urine (U), the volume of urine excreted per minute (V) and the concentration of PAH per milliliter of plasma (P), and then applying Equation 2, we obtain the renal clearance of PAH in milliliters per minute. This clearance of PAH represents the rate of plasma flow through the kidneys. The average renal plasma flow in the normal, healthy adult male is about 650 ml per minute.

The determination of the renal plasma clearance of any drug can give some insight into the mechanisms by which the drug is excreted when this clearance is compared with the normal glomerular filtration rate, i.e., 130 ml per minute as obtained for inulin. If the concentration of drug not bound to plasma proteins is used to calculate its renal plasma clearance, an expression of the *excretion ratio* is obtained:

$$\text{Excretion ratio} = \frac{\text{Renal plasma clearance of drug (ml/min)}}{\text{Normal GFR (ml/min)}}$$

A ratio of less than 1.0 indicates that the drug is filtered, perhaps also secreted, and then partially reabsorbed. A substance such as glucose has an excretion ratio of zero since it is completely reabsorbed in the healthy individual. A value greater than 1.0 indicates that secretion, in addition to filtration, is involved in the excretion. Obviously, the greatest excretion ratio, about 5, would be obtained with a substance like PAH.

Excretion of Drugs by the Liver

Each day the liver secretes 0.5 to 1 liter of bile into the duodenum through the common bile duct (Fig. 6-10). This secretion, in particular the bile acids which it contains, is functionally important for the digestion and absorption of fats. Normally, about 80 to 90 per cent of the bile acids secreted are reabsorbed from the intestine and transported through the portal blood back to the liver to be available again for secre-

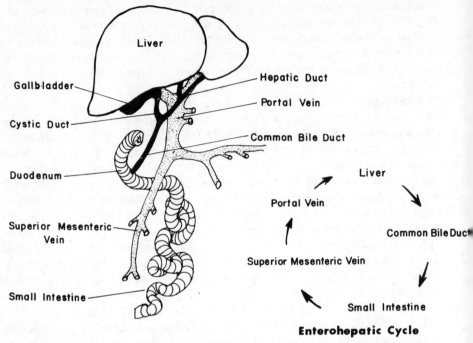

FIGURE 6-10. Relationships of the biliary ducts and blood supply to liver and intestine. Bile, containing bile acids, is discharged into the duodenum. The bile acids are reabsorbed from the small intestine and returned to the liver by way of the superior mesenteric and portal veins.

tion. Thus the major portion of the daily output of bile acids is conserved through this portobiliary circulation, or *enterohepatic cycle*; only a small daily deficit has to be replaced by the body.

Large quantities of bile are discharged into the duodenum in response to food intake, and the total quantity of bile acids available is recirculated twice during digestion of a single meal. During this digestion period, the concentration of bile acids in the bile duct or blood vessels draining the intestine is frequently higher than that in the hepatic fluids or intestinal contents, respectively. Also, the bile acids exist largely as ionized solutes. Therefore, passive diffusion alone could hardly account for their secretion into bile or their almost complete reabsorption from the intestine against high concentration gradients. But in both liver and intestinal epithelial cells there is an active transport system which ensures that adequate supplies of bile acids can be cycled between liver and intestine.

Many drugs are also excreted by the liver into bile. However, the majority of agents reaching the small intestine in this way are not subsequently excreted in the feces. They are almost completely reabsorbed because their physicochemical properties are favorable for passive diffusion across the intestinal barrier. These agents then remain in the enterohepatic cycle until they are excreted in the urine. For example, the presence of an enterohepatic cycle has been shown to have a marked influence on the persistence of glutethimide (Doriden) in the body. Glutethimide, an agent with pharmacologic actions similar to those of the barbiturates, is only slowly eliminated in the urine of normal animals. However, the rate of urinary elimination of glutethimide was increased four-fold in animals in which the bile duct was diverted and prevented from emptying its contents into the small intestine.

Certain organic acidic and basic drugs are actively transported from liver into bile by mechanisms very similar to those that secrete these same substances into the tubular urine. Protein-bound drug is fully accessible to this biliary active transport system, as it is in renal tubular secretion. Unlike the bile acids, however, the acidic and basic drugs do not recycle. No active transport process appears to be available within the intestine for the absorption of foreign organic acids, and the physicochemical properties of both the acids and bases are not conducive to absorption by passive diffusion. Bases such as the quaternary ammonium compounds are fully ionized, and the organic acids are ionized to an even greater extent at intestinal pH than at urinary pH's. Thus the active transport of the acidic and basic drugs from the liver into bile becomes an effective means of eliminating them from the body by way of the feces.

The active biliary transport of these foreign organic acids has also found practical application, particularly in diagnostic tests of liver function. The compound most frequently used for this purpose is the dye sulfobromophthalein, a synthetic organic acid. In the average individual with a normally functioning liver, most of the dye is excreted into the intestine within 30 minutes after intravenous administration. Whether liver function is normal or depressed is indicated by the amount of dye remaining in a sample of blood withdrawn 30 minutes after the beginning of the test.

BIOTRANSFORMATION

The interaction between a drug and the living organism in which the body brings about a chemical change in the drug molecule is variously referred to as *detoxification, drug metabolism* or *biotransformation.* The term *detoxification* has historical significance; the first foreign agents shown to be chemically altered by the body were indeed converted into substances of less potential toxicity. This term has been largely discarded since it is now apparent that the chemical reactions of the body can at times yield compounds of greater toxicity than the parent drugs. The term *metabolism*, as it was originally used, designated the process by which food, on the one hand, is built into living matter (anabolism) and living matter, on the other, is broken down into simple products within a cell or organism (catabolism). Metabolism is the sum of the chemical changes in living cells by which energy is provided for vital processes and activities and new materials are produced and assimilated for growth and maintenance. The chemical reactions that drugs undergo in the body do not ordinarily provide such energy or new materials. Thus the term *biotransformation* is preferable to *drug metabolism* for describing the chemical aspects of the fate of foreign compounds which are not normally considered under carbohydrate, protein, fat, vitamin, hormone or mineral metabolism.

Before considering the general aspects of the many reactions responsible for the chemical alterations of drugs and the pharmacologic significance of these biotransformations, let us briefly discuss the means by which they are brought about.

The Mediators of Biotransformation

The chemical alterations of drugs, like the chemical changes taking place in normal metabolism, are not spontaneous reactions: they are not like the neutralization of hydrochloric acid by sodium bicarbonate, but rather like that of the interaction between hydrogen and oxygen. At room temperature the reaction between the gases cannot be appreciably detected; introduction of a catalyst (platinum powder) produces an instantaneous union of the gases to give water. In a completely analogous fashion, drug biotransformations, like the normal metabolic processes, are all *catalyzed reactions*. They take place only in the presence of *enzymes,* the protein catalysts which accelerate the action but remain apparently unchanged in the process.

The word *enzyme* occasionally denotes more than just a catalytic protein. Many enzymes require nonprotein organic compounds called *prosthetic groups,* or *coenzymes,* which play an intimate and frequently essential role in catalysis. Ordinarily, the term *prosthetic groups* is reserved for groups which are bound firmly to the protein and cannot be readily removed without destroying the enzyme, whereas *coenzymes* refer to dissociable entities necessary for the reaction. Some enzymes also require small ions, such as Mg^{++}, for full catalytic activity. We shall use the term *enzyme* to refer to the whole enzyme system, thereby including all the *cofactors* necessary for optimum activity.

Mode of Action of Enzymes

Enzymes, like receptors, produce their activity by combining reversibly with the substances on which they act — by combining with their *substrates.* Moreover, the forces responsible for this enzyme-substrate binding are the same as those which account for drug-receptor interactions: ionic bonds, hydrogen bonds and Van der Waals attractive forces. The consequence of this binding is also comparable to that of the drug-receptor interaction, since the combination of enzyme and substrate initiates a sequence of events that leads to the appearance of end products of the reaction.

$$\text{Enzyme } + \text{Substrate} \rightleftharpoons \text{Enzyme-substrate complex} \quad \text{(Equation 3)}$$

$$\text{Enzyme-substrate complex} \rightleftharpoons \text{Enzyme } + \text{ Products of enzyme action}$$
$$\text{(Equation 4)}$$

Enzymes show specificity for the substances upon which they act, and this specificity is also akin to that of receptors and the drugs with which they combine. The specificity of both types of interaction arises from the number and kinds of bonds formed and the spatial configuration of the "active sites" for bond formation on the surface of the macromolecule (Figs. 6-11, 6-12). In fact, the principle of the "lock

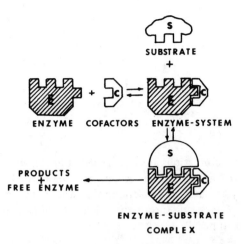

FIGURE 6-11. Schematic diagram of the interaction of substrate with an enzyme requiring a cofactor. For some enzymes, the step involving the combination with cofactor or activating metal is not needed. (Modified from W. D. McElroy, Q. Rev. Biol. 22:25, 1947.)

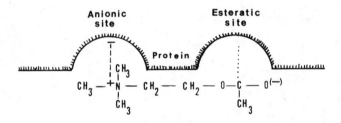

FIGURE 6-12. Interaction of acetylcholine with the enzyme acetylcholinesterase. There are two active sites for binding on the enzyme: the anionic site and the esteratic site. At the anionic site an ionic bond is formed between the positively charged nitrogen and a negatively charged group of the enzyme. At the esteratic site the ester bond is actually split. (Modified from I. B. Wilson, Fed. Proc. 18:752, 1959.)

and key" fit between a chemical compound and the active sites of an enzyme was outlined by Emil Fischer several years before its adaptation by Ehrlich into his concept of receptors.

Although nearly all the individual reactions of normal metabolism are catalyzed by separate enzymes, few of the enzymes are absolutely specific for their particular substrates. Most can also act on structural analogues of their physiologic substrates — on drugs. For example, the enzyme in muscle or nervous tissue which acts on acetylcholine also acts on the drug methacholine, but at a slower rate. Methacholine differs from acetylcholine only by the addition of a methyl group:

$$CH_3-\underset{\underset{CH_3}{|}}{\overset{\overset{CH_3}{|}}{N^+}}-CH_2-\underset{\underset{CH_3}{|}}{CH}-O-\underset{\underset{CH_3}{|}}{C}=O$$

Many other biotransformations are also carried out by enzymes of moderate specificity which catalyze similar reactions of normal metabolism. However, a few enzymes show less specificity by catalyzing reactions of a variety of physiologic substrates and drugs, whereas others lack true specificity and act on a diverse group of drugs but on few physiologic substrates.

Enzyme Kinetics

The rate of a chemical reaction is understood to mean the rate at which the concentrations of reacting substances vary with time. And according to the law of mass action, the rate of any reaction is proportional to the concentrations of the reactants present at any given time. It follows that the velocity of an enzymic process should

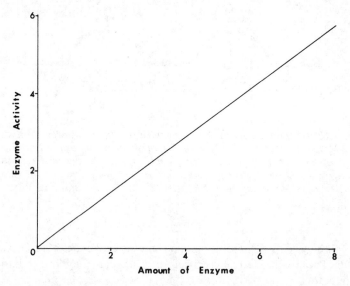

FIGURE 6-13. *Effect of enzyme concentration on enzyme activity when the substrate concentration remains constant. Units are arbitrary. Such data may be obtained in vitro by determining the quantity of end product formed per unit time in mixtures containing different amounts of enzyme, e.g., the amount of para-aminobenzoic acid (or diethylaminoethanol) formed by hydrolysis of the local anesthetic procaine, using varying amounts of plasma as the source of enzyme.*

be proportional to the concentrations of enzyme and substrate. In fact, when the concentration of substrate is held constant, it can be shown that within fairly wide limits the speed of an enzyme reaction is proportional to the enzyme concentration (Fig. 6-13). However, only in certain instances does the speed of an enzyme reaction parallel the substrate concentration when the enzyme concentration is held constant. This relationship exists at low and intermediate substrate concentration. But at higher levels of substrate, the rate of enzyme action stops increasing and becomes virtually independent of the concentration of substrate (Fig. 6-14).

The curve in Figure 6-14 is similar to the curve in Figure 4-8 (p. 64), which depicts the rate of facilitated diffusion as a function of the concentration of solute. The reason why the rate of enzyme action does not increase beyond a certain level of substrate is also very much like the reason for the limited capacity of the facilitated diffusion process. When a substrate molecule combines with a molecule of enzyme, there is an interval (even though this may be measured in milliseconds) before the enzyme-substrate complex dissociates and the reaction products are freed. Following this interval the enzyme molecule is ready to combine with another molecule of substrate. By the mass action interpretation, the more abundant the substrate molecules, the less time required to form the substrate-enzyme complex. But at constant temperature and other fixed conditions, the *rate of dissociation* of the complex is independent of substrate concentration and is the same for all substrate concentrations. So at or above a certain substrate level, the enzyme is operating at full speed because the intervals when it is unused become negligible. On this basis, an additional rise in sub-

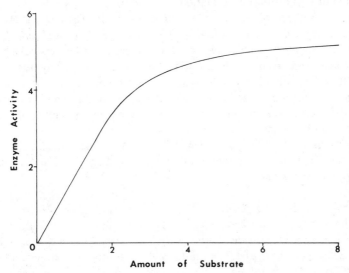

FIGURE 6-14. Effect of substrate concentration on enzyme activity when the enzyme concentration remains constant. Such data may be obtained in vitro by determining the quantity of end product formed per unit time in mixtures containing different amounts of substrate.

strate levels does not lead to an increase in rate of reaction. The rate-limiting step is the rate of dissociation of the enzyme-substrate complex.

A reaction is said to be a *monomolecular* or *first-order reaction* when only one substance is reacting and when the reaction velocity is proportional to the concentration of this substance. In the intact organism the concentration of enzyme usually remains constant, so that only the changing substrate concentration influences the rate of metabolism or biotransformation. Therefore, when the substrate concentration is low and active sites on the enzyme are available for occupancy, the enzyme reaction is like a first-order reaction even though two reactants have to combine. At high substrate concentrations, when the enzyme is saturated, the velocity of the reaction becomes almost constant. Since it is no longer dependent on the concentration of reactants, it is said to be a *zero-order reaction.*

It will be recalled that the term *enzyme* refers to the complete enzyme system, i.e., the protein as well as any cofactors necessary for activity. Therefore the failure of a reaction to increase in rate with an increase in substrate concentration — zero-order kinetics — may occur not only when the enzyme is saturated, but also when the supply of a cofactor is insufficient.

Most drugs are administered therapeutically in amounts which lead to concentrations well below the saturation levels of their enzyme system; their rate of biotransformation is proportional to drug concentration. However, in later discussions we shall note a number of instances in which the rate of biotransformation may be constant and independent of the concentration of drug in the body.

Chemical Pathways of Biotransformation

Most drugs are subject to chemical alteration by the body. The few that are not, such as the diuretic agent chlorothiazide, Diuril, are said to be *biochemically inert* although they are pharmacologically active. Chemical alterations can take place in many tissues and organs. In the intestine, for example, drugs may be biotransformed either within the epithelial cell or by normal digestive enzymes or enzymes of the symbiotic microorganisms present in the intestinal lumen. Biotransformation may also occur in the plasma, kidney and brain; but by far the greatest number of chemical reactions occur in the liver.

The reactions in which drugs are chemically altered by the body are many and varied. They can, however, be divided into two main categories: *synthetic reactions* and *nonsynthetic reactions.*

Synthetic Reactions or Conjugations

The synthetic reaction, or *conjugation,* involves the chemical combination of a compound with a *molecule provided by the body.* The latter, known as the conjugating agent, is usually a carbohydrate, an amino acid or a substance derived from these nutrients. The tendency for a particular compound to combine with a given conjugating agent depends only on its possessing an appropriate group or "center for

---

[3] Another conjugation reaction involves the addition of the amino acid cysteine to aromatic or halogenated hydrocarbons. The types of compounds undergoing this process are few in number, and therefore the process will not be considered further. The conversion of cyanides to thiocyanide is also considered a conjugation process.

conjugation," such as carboxyl ($-COOH$); hydroxyl ($-OH$), amino ($-NH_2$) or sulf-hydryl ($-SH$).[3] Thus any compound, whether a drug or a normal body constituent, may participate in a conjugating reaction as long as it possesses one of the necessary centers for conjugation. When the parent molecule does not possess such a functional group, it may acquire one as a result of a nonsynthetic reaction; the metabolite, or end product of the nonsynthetic reaction, then undergoes further biotransformation by conjugation. For example, benzene contains no center for conjugation but acquires one when it is converted by the body to phenol; phenol, by virtue of the hydroxyl group it has acquired, is then conjugated.

Since mere possession of a center for conjugation determines the occurrence of a particular synthetic reaction, it is obvious that a wide variety of compounds may act as substrates for the enzyme of a specific conjugation process. Thus all the enzymes of the synthetic reactions are specific only with regard to certain reactive groups in compounds; compounds with similar centers of conjugation may or may not be structurally related in other respects.

The small number of chemical centers that can enter into conjugation places a limit on the number of synthetic reactions that are possible. Of the dozen or so that are known to occur in animals and insects, the following are the primary synthetic pathways of biotransformation in humans: glucuronide synthesis; glycine and glutamine conjugations; acetylation; sulfate conjugation; and methylation (Table 6-3).

The features common to all the synthetic reactions are worthy of emphasis. First, these reactions require that energy and a conjugating agent be supplied by the body. Second, none of the reactions is confined to drugs; a number of substances formed in the normal metabolic processes also undergo conjugation. Almost without exception, these synthetic reactions change drugs and normal metabolites into compounds that are, respectively, pharmacologically and biologically *inactive*. Moreover, the conjugated metabolites are almost invariably less lipid soluble than the parent compounds; practically all conjugated compounds are relatively strong acids — strong in the sense that they are highly ionized. Thus, ordinarily the conjugation processes lead not only to inactivation of drugs but also to their more rapid elimination in the urine and feces, since the end products are less likely to be reabsorbed. The limited number of conjugation reactions and the small number of chemical centers which can participate in them make it relatively easy to predict the reactions that will occur with given agents. If a drug carries one of the centers for conjugation, some conjugation always takes place; only the extent of the reaction is unpredictable. Moreover, a compound may be excreted as several different conjugates if one or more of its groups can serve as the center for conjugation for more than one reaction, e.g., salicylic acid or chloramphenicol (Table 6-3).

GLUCURONIDE CONJUGATION. These are the most frequently occurring reactions because several of the chemical groups commonly encountered in the structure of drug molecules can act as centers for conjugation. Also, the general availability of glucose, the carbohydrate from which glucuronic acid is derived, provides an ample supply of the conjugating agent. The functional groups may be an *amino* ($-NH_2$), a *carboxyl* ($-COOH$), a *sulfhydryl* ($-SH$) or a *hydroxyl* ($-OH$), either phenolic (attached to a ring structure) or alcoholic (attached to a straight-chain organic compound). The conjugating agent is glucuronic acid, $C_6H_{10}O_6$, derived from glucose.

Table 6-3.   Examples of Conjugation, Oxidation, Reduction and Hydrolysis of Drugs in Humans

Reaction	Drugs Biotransformed	Naturally Occurring Compound Metabolized
Conjugation		
Glucuronide synthesis	Salicylic acid Morphine Meprobamate (Equanil, Miltown) Chloramphenicol (Chloromycetin)	Bilirubin Thyroxine
Glycine synthesis	Salicylic acid Benzoic acid Nicotinic acid	Bile acids
Acetylation	Sulfonamide drugs Para-aminosalicylic acid Aminopyrine (Pyramidon)	Choline
Sulfate conjugation	Phenol Chloramphenicol	Steroids
Methylation	Nicotinamide Pyridine Quinidine	Histamine Epinephrine
Oxidation		
Microsomal enzymes	Phenobarbital Phenytoin (Dilantin) Meprobamate Meperidine (Demerol) Quinine Phenacetin (Acetophenetidin) Aminopyrine Codeine Morphine Chlorpromazine Parathion	Steroids
Nonmicrosomal enzymes	Ethanol Methanol Acetaldehyde Caffeine Isoproterenol (Isuprel)	Vitamin A Xanthine Epinephrine Serotonin
Reduction		
Microsomal enzymes	Prednisolone Chloramphenicol Nitrobenzene	Cortisone
Nonmicrosomal enzymes	Chloral hydrate	
Hydrolysis		
	Procaine (Novocain) Lidocaine (Xylocaine) Aspirin Methantheline (Banthine)	Acetylcholine

Salicylic acid, with both a hydroxyl and a carboxyl group, can combine with glucuronic acid in two ways[4]:

salicylic acid (SA) → ether glucuronide of SA

or

SA → ester glucuronide of SA

Other examples of compounds that undergo this synthesis with glucuronic acid are given in Table 6-3. Some drugs, such as phenobarbital, are also eliminated as glucuronides, but only after they have acquired a center for conjugation through nonsynthetic reactions. Aspirin is first rapidly biotransformed to salicylic acid and then is eliminated as conjugates of the latter.

The glucuronides are rapidly eliminated in the urine, being highly ionized and water soluble. They are also secreted in the bile; however, this action does not always lead to their elimination in the feces. The enzymes of the bacteria normally present in the intestine can remove the glucuronic acid from the parent compound, and, if the latter is lipid soluble, it will be reabsorbed. The establishment of an enterohepatic cycle will of course prolong the presence of the drug in the body. The sedative drug glutethimide (Doriden) and phenolphthalein, a cathartic drug, show this type of behavior.

AMINO ACID CONJUGATION. Several amino acids may serve as conjugating agents, but only in reactions with compounds which possess a *carboxyl group, —COOH*. In humans the amino acids utilized in these reactions are glycine and glutamine. We may again use salicylic acid to exemplify this type of conjugation:

SA   glycine   salicyluric acid

The amino acid conjugates, like the glucuronides, are for the most part more water soluble than their parent compounds and, therefore, are more readily excreted in the urine. They are not secreted into the bile to any significant extent.

[4]Throughout this text, the diagrams of chemical reactions show only the overall process. All the chemical reactions involved in conjugation and in many of the nonsynthetic reactions are much more complicated than the simple diagrams indicate.

ACETYLATION. This is really the converse of amino acid conjugation, since in acetylation a foreign amino group is conjugated with an acid provided by the body. Acetylation is the primary route of biotransformation for the sulfonamide drugs, thus:

$$NH_2\text{-benzene ring-}SO_2NH_2 \quad + \quad HOOC-CH_3 \quad \longrightarrow \quad NH-CO-CH_3\text{-benzene ring-}SO_2NH_2$$

sulfanilamide   acetic acid   acetylsulfanilamide

The acetylation of sulfonamides exemplifies two important points: (1) a decrease in lipid solubility does not necessarily mean an increase in water solubility, and (2) biotransformation does not always lead to the production of a less toxic agent. The acetyl derivatives of a number of the first clinically useful sulfonamides are not only less lipid soluble, but also less water soluble than their parent compounds. For example, the solubility of sulfathiazole is 98 mg per 100 ml water at 37°C, whereas its acetylated compound is soluble to the extent of only 7 mg per 100 ml. The sulfonamides and their acetylated derivatives are also less soluble at acid pH. Therefore, injury to the urinary tract may result from the precipitation of the conjugated sulfonamide within renal passageways as the kidney concentrates the urine and it becomes more acid.

SULFATE CONJUGATION. The reaction of sulfate (derived from sulfur-containing amino acids such as cystine) with hydroxyl groups and certain compounds containing an amino group is frequently called ethereal sulfate synthesis. A typical example is:

$$\text{benzene ring-}OH \quad \xrightarrow{\text{sulfate}} \quad \text{benzene ring-}O-\overset{\overset{O}{\|}}{\underset{\underset{O}{\|}}{S}}-OH$$

phenol   phenyl sulfate

The ethereal sulfates appear to be more water soluble than their parent compounds and are readily excreted in the urine.

METHYLATION. A methyl group, $-CH_3$, derived from the amino acid methionine can be transferred from the conjugating agent to a phenolic hydroxyl group (an $-OH$ attached to a ring) or to various amines, and even to nitrogen contained within a ring structure. This reaction is an important physiologic process, accounting for the conversion of norepinephrine[5] to epinephrine:

HO—⟨⟩—OH CH—CH$_2$—NH$_2$ ⟶ HO—⟨⟩—OH CH$_3$ CH—CH$_2$—NH

norepinephrine   epinephrine

as well as being one of the major pathways of inactivation of either norepinephrine or epinephrine:

HO—⟨⟩—OH CH$_3$ CH—CH$_2$—NH ⟶ CH$_3$O—⟨⟩—OH CH$_3$ CH—CH$_2$—NH

epinephrine   metanephrine

Other important endogenous compounds are also methylated, including histamine and the hormones estradiol and thyroxine.

The biotransformations of exogenous compounds, such as nicotinamide, are examples of the addition of the methyl group to a nitrogen contained within a ring, viz.:

nicotinamide   N-methylnicotinamide[6]

The attachment of a methyl group to the ring nitrogen creates a quaternary ammonium compound which is completely ionized and therefore poorly reabsorbed from the tubular urine.

Nonsynthetic Reactions

In nonsynthetic reactions the parent drug itself is chemically altered by oxidation, reduction, hydrolysis[7] or a combination of these processes. Usually these nonsynthetic reactions represent only the first stage of biotransformation. The second stage encompasses all the conjugation reactions of the metabolites formed in the nonsynthetic processes. Since most drugs undergo two-stage biotransformation, the end

[5] The designation *nor* is from the German meaning "nitrogen without a radical"; in this case, norepinephrine is epinephrine without the radical —CH$_3$ attached to the nitrogen atom.
[6] The *N* indicates that the methyl group is attached to the nitrogen.
[7] *Oxidation* is a chemical reaction in which oxygen is added to a compound or, by extension, the proportion of oxygen in a compound is increased by removal of other groups.
   Reduction is the opposite of oxidation, i.e., the removal of oxygen or an alteration which leads to a decrease in the proportion of oxygen in a compound.
   Hydrolysis refers to the cleavage of a compound by the addition of water.

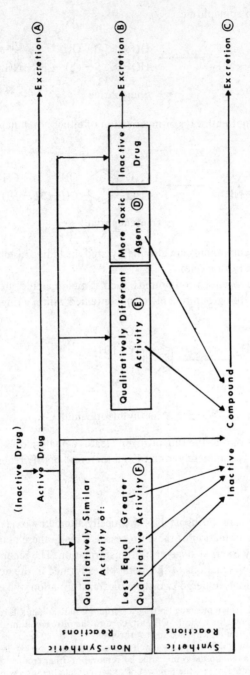

FIGURE 6-15. Effect of biotransformation on the pharmacologic activity of a drug in the body. The original drug administered may be either an active or an inactive drug. The inactive drug is first converted to an active one. An active drug may be excreted unchanged (A) or biotransformed by a nonsynthetic reaction and excreted without additional chemical alteration (B). The active drug may also be conjugated directly and excreted as the conjugate (C).

Alternatively, the active drug may undergo a nonsynthetic reaction, and the products of this reaction may be conjugated and excreted as the conjugate (C). The nonsynthetic reaction may yield a more toxic agent (D), an agent with qualitatively different activity (E) or an agent with quantitatively different activity either less, equal to or greater than that of the parent compound (F).

150

Table 6-4. Changes in Pharmacologic Activity Produced by Biotransformation

Drug	Activity of Drug	Metabolic Reaction	Activity of Metabolite
Chloroguanide	Inactive	Oxidation	Antimalarial
Parathion	Inactive	Oxidation	Toxic agent (insecticide)
Codeine	Analgesic	Oxidation	More potent analgesic
Phenacetin	Analgesic	Oxidation	More potent analgesic
Aspirin	Analgesic	Hydrolysis	Equally potent analgesic
Mesantoin	Antiepileptic	Oxidation	Antiepileptic but more toxic
Phenylbutazone (Butazolidin)	Antirheumatic and uricosuric[a]	Oxidation	Metabolite I — antirheumatic;
		Oxidation	metabolite II — uricosuric
Methanol	Depressant	Oxidation	Different activity but more toxic

[a]Antirheumatic: effective in the treatment of acute rheumatic fever; uricosuric: increasing the excretion of uric acid in the urine.

products of the nonsynthetic reactions are generally not eliminated from the body as such, even though they are usually less lipid soluble than their parent drugs; they are excreted only after conjugation (Fig. 6-15). Again, unlike the products of the conjugation reactions, the products of the first stage of biotransformation are not always pharmacologically inactive. Indeed, instead of inactivating an agent, the non-synthetic processes may *convert an inactive drug into an active agent or change an active drug into another pharmacologically active compound* (Fig. 6-15). If the latter change takes place, the metabolite may have (1) a qualitatively similar activity but be less, equally or more active[8]; (2) a qualitatively different type of activity; or (3) a greater toxicity. For instance, codeine is partially biotransformed to morphine, a drug with similar but greater activity than codeine.[9] On the other hand, salicylic acid, the metabolite of aspirin, has activity both similar and equal to its parent drug. Table 6-4 lists some of the many known examples of biotransformation which lead to changes in activity of the administered drug.

The rate of change of an active drug into another active drug has an important bearing on the pharmacologic activity manifested. If the biotransformation is rapid, the pharmacologic effect will be largely that of the metabolite. If the transformation is slow, the observed effect may be that of both the parent drug and the metabolite.

[8]Here, quantitative difference refers to the effects produced by equal amounts of drug, i.e., a more active drug produces a greater intensity of effect when given in the same amount as a less active agent.

[9]The pharmacologic activity of codeine is not that of morphine, however, since codeine is excreted in the urine more rapidly than it is converted to morphine.

Table 6-5.   Comparison of Synthetic and Nonsynthetic Drug Biotransformations

Synthetic Reactions	Nonsynthetic Reactions
A. TYPE OF REACTION	
Determined by functional group	Determined by functional group
Limited number	Wide variety
Relatively predictable	Relatively unpredictable
B. METABOLITE	
Almost always less lipid soluble	Usually less lipid soluble
Almost always pharmacologically inactive	May have less, equal, greater or different activity
C. REACTIONS CATALYZED BY NONMICROSOMAL ENZYMES	
All except glucuronide conjugation	Most hydrolyses; some oxidations and reductions
No stimulation of rate of biotransformation by other drugs	No stimulation of rate of biotransformation by other drugs
D. REACTIONS CATALYZED BY MICROSOMAL ENZYMES	
Only glucuronide conjugation	Most oxidations and reductions; some hydrolyses
Rate of reaction stimulated by drugs	Rate of reactions stimulated by many agents

Whether a particular compound is amenable to oxidation, reduction or hydrolysis depends, as it does in the synthetic reactions, on the presence of an appropriate functional group or chemical structure. However, the mere presence of such a group in a drug does not mean that it will undergo one of the nonsynthetic reactions. Consequently, the reactions of the first stage of biotransformation are much less predictable than those occurring in the second stage. These similarities and differences between the synthetic and nonsynthetic reactions are summarized in Table 6-5.

The reactions classified as nonsynthetic are many and varied, but they may be categorized on the basis of the type of enzyme involved. One group consists of reactions mediated by enzymes of moderate specificity whose substrates may be either foreign compounds or substances normally present in the body. Most hydrolyses and a few, but important, oxidations and reductions fall into this group. The vast majority of oxidations and reductions comprise the second category of reactions; these reactions are catalyzed by enzymes which *lack specificity* and which, with few exceptions, are concerned *entirely with drug biotransformation* and not with normal metabolism. These remarkable enzymes of drug biotransformation are known as the *microsomal enzymes.*

MICROSOMAL ENZYMES. The microsomal enzymes are located predominantly in liver cells, where they are associated with a subcellular component, the endoplasmic reticulum. This reticulum is a network of lipoprotein tubules extending throughout the cytoplasm and continuous with the cellular and nuclear membranes. Electron microscopy has revealed that part of the surface of this endoplasmic network is

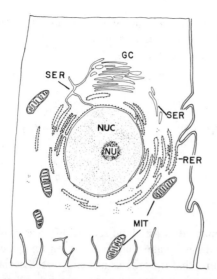

FIGURE 6-16. A cell, showing the smooth and rough endoplasmic reticulum.
(Ser: *smooth endoplasmic reticulum;* GC: *Golgi apparatus;* RER: *rough endo-plasmic reticulum;* MIT: *mitochondria;* NU: *nucleolus;* NUC: *nucleus.)*

smooth and the remainder is "rough," being studded with ribonucleoprotein granules called ribosomes (Fig. 6-16). The rough-surfaced cellular fraction contains the enzymes involved in protein synthesis. The enzymes that can metabolize drugs are associated primarily with the smooth-surfaced endoplasmic reticulum. Experimentally, when liver (or other) cells are ruptured by homogenization, the endoplasmic reticulum is fragmented. The fragments can then be separated from other parts of the cell by differential centrifugation. The sediment obtained after very high-speed centrifugation is known as the microsomal fraction; it contains the smooth-surfaced fragments and their associated drug-metabolizing enzymes, or microsomal enzymes.

Although the microsomal enzymes lack specificity and are capable of metabolizing substances of widely different structure, they can *only catalyze reactions of compounds which are lipid soluble.* In fact, this requirement for lipid solubility may explain the apparent paradox of a component of living cells being able to biotransform foreign compounds but being largely unable to promote similar reactions of natural metabolites. For example, the lipid-soluble drug amphetamine is biotransformed by the microsomal enzyme system:

$$\text{amphetamine} \longrightarrow \text{phenylacetone} + NH_3$$

amphetamine   phenylacetone   ammonia

On the other hand, the less lipid-soluble natural amine tyramine is not altered by microsomal enzymes but undergoes a similar reaction in the presence of a nonmicrosomal enzyme, monoamine oxidase:

$$HO-\langle ring \rangle-CH_2-CH_2-NH_2 \longrightarrow HO-\langle ring \rangle-CH_2-\underset{H}{\overset{}{C}}=O + NH_3$$

tyramine   benzylaldehyde   ammonia

Like amphetamine, many drugs are lipid soluble, whereas most natural substances are less lipid soluble and more water soluble than their foreign counterparts. It has been suggested, therefore, that the microsomal enzymes, associated as they are with a lipoprotein cellular component, are themselves protected by a lipid barrier which restricts diffusion of hydrophilic compounds. This view has been corroborated by the fact that *all* oxidative and reductive activity is lost following attempts to obtain the microsomal enzymes in soluble form, freed from the structures to which they are bound. Enzymes of nonmicrosomal origin *can* be prepared as soluble cell fractions which retain their catalytic activity.

There is one microsomal enzyme system which has been prepared as a soluble cell fraction, and this system has some additional properties which are equally unique. First, this enzyme system mediates the glucuronic acid conjugation — the only synthetic reaction carried out by a microsomal enzyme system. Second, the microsomal enzymes involved in glucuronide syntheses are different from almost all the other microsomal enzymes, in that they can form glucuronides with a wide range of *natural metabolites,* e.g., bilirubin, as well as foreign substances. All the other microsomal enzymes are concerned with oxidation and reduction, and their substrates are almost exclusively drugs (cf. Table 6-3).

OXIDATION. Oxidation is one of the most general biochemical reactions of foreign compounds because there are so many ways in which a compound can be oxidized (see Table 6-3). The oxidative transformations catalyzed by the microsomal enzyme systems include (1) the addition of a hydroxyl group to a ring structure or to a side-chain attached to a ring; (2) the removal of a methyl ($-CH_3$) or an ethyl ($-C_2H_5$) group from an oxygen, nitrogen or sulfur atom of a compound; (3) the replacement of an amine group ($-NH_2$) by oxygen; and (4) the addition of oxygen to a sulfur or nitrogen and a variety of other processes. Specific examples of these reactions are illustrated in Figure 6-17.

The oxidations catalyzed by nonmicrosomal enzymes are less varied than those of the microsomal fraction but are important reactions of many naturally occurring substances as well as of drugs. The enzymes that oxidize the nutritionally essential

1. Side-chain hydroxylation

pentobarbital

2. Ring hydroxylation

phenobarbital

3. Removal of methyl group from ring nitrogen

mephobarbital   phenobarbital

4. Removal of ethyl group from oxygen

phenacetin   acetaminophen (Tylenol)

5. Oxidation of an amine

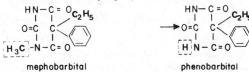

aniline

6. Removal of -NH$_2$ group

amphetamine

7. Replacement of sulfur by oxygen

FIGURE 6-17. Oxidative reactions catalyzed by microsomal enzyme systems.

155

vitamin A also catalyze the reactions of various foreign alcohols and aldehydes:

$$CH_3OH \longrightarrow HCHO \longrightarrow HCOOH$$

methyl   formaldehyde   formic
alcohol   acid

$$CH_3CH_2OH \longrightarrow CH_3CHO \longrightarrow CH_3COOH$$

ethyl   acetaldehyde   acetic
alcohol   acid

The oxidation of amines to aldehydes can also be catalyzed by nonmicrosomal soluble enzymes, such as monoamine oxidase or diamine oxidase. Their substrates include compounds normally found in the body, e.g., epinephrine, tyramine and histamine, as well as drugs like isoproterenol. Xanthine oxidase, the nonmicrosomal enzyme responsible for converting the purine bases of nucleic acids into uric acid, also catalyzes the oxidation of caffeine and other foreign xanthines.

REDUCTION. A typical example of reduction as the reversal of oxidation is the conversion of the sedative-hypnotic drug chloral hydrate to trichloroethanol, a reduction catalyzed by the same enzyme which oxidizes ethanol:

chloral hydrate   trichloroethanol

The addition of hydrogen to double bonds, particularly in the metabolism of some steroid hormones, is another example of reduction carried out by nonmicrosomal enzymes. On the other hand, the enzymes of the microsomal fraction are concerned primarily with the addition of hydrogen to nitrogen atoms of foreign compounds, e.g.:

nitrobenzene   aniline

HYDROLYSIS. Hydrolysis as a mechanism of biotransformation of drugs occurs only in compounds with as ester linkage:

$$\overset{O}{\overset{\|}{-C-O-}}$$

or an amide linkage:

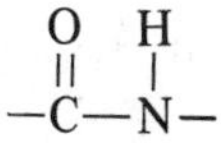

$$\underset{\overset{\displaystyle O}{\shortparallel}}{-C}-\underset{\overset{\displaystyle H}{|}}{N}-$$

When an ester is hydrolyzed by an esterase, an alcohol (phenolic or straight chain) and an acid are formed; when an amide is acted upon by an amidase, the products are an amine and an acid. For example:

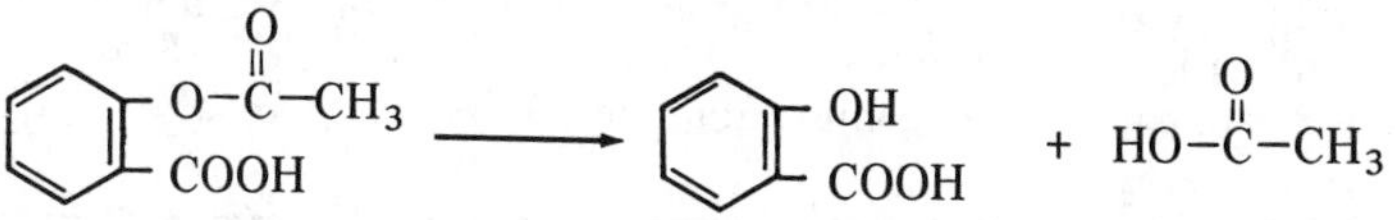

aspirin   salicylic acid   acetic acid

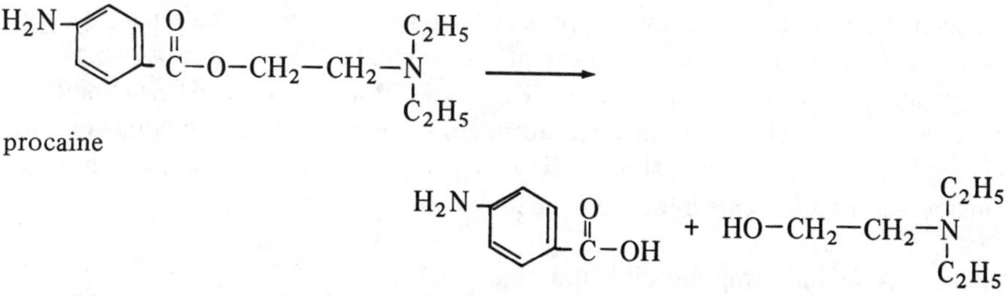

procaine

para-aminobenzoic acid (PABA)   diethylaminoethanol

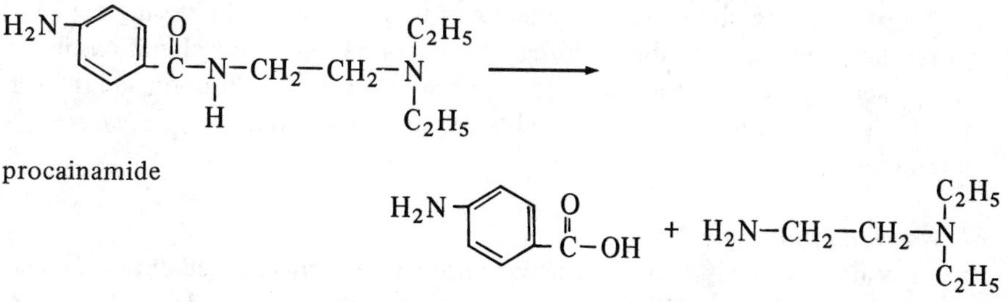

procainamide

PABA   diethylaminoethylamine

The esterases are found in blood plasma, liver and many other tissues, primarily in the nonmicrosomal soluble fraction. The amidases are also nonmicrosomal enzymes and are found principally in the liver but not in blood plasma.

Major Pathways of Biotransformation

We have seen that a single compound such as salicylic acid can be conjugated in at least three different ways. Salicylic acid may also undergo several oxidative reactions,

Table 6-6.   Major Route of Biotransformation of Some Common Functional Groups

---

Hydroxyl (−OH)
   Alcohols (straight chain, i.e., aliphatic): oxidation; glucuronide conjugation
   Phenols (ring structure, i.e., aromatic): glucuronide conjugation; sulfate conjugation; methylation
Carboxyl (−COOH)
   Aliphatic: oxidation; glucuronide conjugation
   Aromatic: glycine conjugation; glucuronide conjugation
Amino (−NH$_2$)
   Aliphatic: deamination (removal of amino group and formation of aldehyde); glucuronide conjugation
   Aromatic: acetylation; glucuronide conjugation; methylation
Aromatic rings: hydroxylation

---

and these metabolites may be conjugated as well. Since so many drugs are similar to salicylic acid in possessing several groups which can be chemically altered by enzymic activity, they too give rise to a variety of end products. Usually, one or two pathways account for the major metabolic alterations. For salicylic acid, the conjugates with glycine and glucuronic acid are the major metabolites. Although it is not always possible to predict which reactions will take place, Table 6-6 lists the most probable major reactions of some important functional groups.

Factors Affecting Drug Biotransformation

We saw earlier that the rate of biotransformation of drugs is influenced only by changing the substrate concentration since, under normal conditions, the concentration of enzyme is usually constant. There are, however, several factors which alter the activity of enzymes, and these are tantamount to decreasing or increasing the concentration of enzyme available for drug biotransformation. These alterations in enzyme activity are pharmacologically important because the duration and intensity of action of many drugs are determined largely by the speed at which they are biotransformed.

Enzyme Inhibition

Enzymes are true catalysts in that they are not appreciably changed during a reaction, but as proteins they are subject to decomposition in the body. Under normal conditions the rate of enzyme production equals its rate of destruction. Obviously, however, any abnormal condition, such as malnutrition or disease, that decreases the overall rate of protein synthesis may also result in decreased availability of enzymes. Since the liver plays such an important role in protein synthesis as well as in metabolism, malfunction of this organ frequently depresses drug biotransformation.

To catalyze a reaction, an enzyme must be able to combine with its substrate. Therefore, any agent that interferes with a substrate's access to active binding sites will also decrease the rate of metabolism, even when the concentration of enzyme is normal. A decrease in metabolic rate of a given substrate is said to be *competitive inhibition* when the interfering agent is (1) a compound which is itself a substrate for the enzyme, or (2) a compound which undergoes no catalytic change but which combines reversibly with the active sites of the enzyme by virtue of its structural similarity to the substrate. Methacholine is an example of a substrate that competes with acetylcholine for the active sites on the enzyme cholinesterase (cf. p. 141). The second type of competitive inhibition is exemplified by the action of amphetamine. As we have seen, amphetamine is not biotransformed by monoamine oxidase, but it can inhibit the metabolism of tyramine, a natural substrate of this enzyme. These competitive interactions may be represented as follows:

$$E + S_1 + S_2 \rightleftharpoons ES_1 + ES_2 \rightleftharpoons E + P_1 + P_2 \quad \text{(Equation 5)}$$

$$E + S_1 + I \rightleftharpoons ES_1 + EI \rightleftharpoons E + P_1 + I \quad \text{(Equation 6)}$$

Where E is enzyme, S_1 and S_2 are substrates, I is a nonsubstrate and P_1 and P_2 are the end products of the metabolism of S_1 and S_2, respectively.

In Equation 5, S_1 may represent acetylcholine, the natural substrate of cholinesterase (E), and S_2 may be the drug substrate, methacholine, which can bind to the same active sites on the enzyme as acetylcholine. In Equation 6, S_1 may be tyramine, the endogenous substrate of monoamine oxidase, and I may be amphetamine, which combines with the active sites of this enzyme even though this combination does not lead to biotransformation of the drug.

In both cases, the effect of two agents competing for the same quantity of enzyme is to reduce the rate of metabolism of the primary substrate, S_1, as predicted by the law of mass action. First, the degree of inhibition produced is dependent on the concentration of the primary substrate, S_1, relative to the concentrations of either S_2 or I. The greater the number of molecules of S_1 present in the total number of molecules capable of combining with active sites, the greater the possibility that a molecule of S_1 will complete the binding reaction. Then, since the rate of metabolism is proportional to substrate concentration, increasing the ratio of S_1 to either S_2 or I will decrease inhibition. A sufficiently high ratio of S_1 to either S_2 or I will force almost complete occupancy of active sites by S_1 despite the presence of either S_2 or I (Fig. 6-18). Thus *competitive inhibition can be overcome by a large enough concentration of substrate.* Of course the extent of inhibition is also determined by the relative rates of dissociation of the complexes formed, i.e., on the rates of dissociation of ES_1, ES_2 or EI. The rates of dissociation of all three complexes must be sufficiently rapid to make free, unoccupied sites available for continuous combination with molecules of S_1.

Inhibition of metabolism may also be brought about by an agent unrelated in structure to the substrate but capable of combining with the enzyme in such a way as to prevent the formation of an enzyme-substrate complex. This is termed *noncompetitive inhibition.* Many heavy metals, such as mercury, lead or arsenic, and the organic phosphate insecticides are typical noncompetitive inhibitors. Since noncompetitive inhibitors do not combine with the enzyme in the same manner as the substrate, an excess

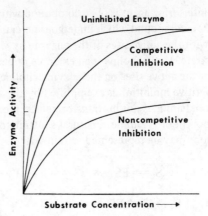

FIGURE 6-18. Effect of inhibitors on enzyme activity. The rate of the catalyzed reaction is plotted as a function of substrate concentration when the amount of enzyme is constant and the concentration of each of the inhibitors is also constant.

of substrate cannot displace the inhibitor from the enzyme surface. Noncompetitive inhibition may be reversible or irreversible; the important point is that the concentration of substrate does not influence the reversibility or the degree of inhibition (see Fig. 6-18). When the action of a noncompetitive inhibitor is irreversible, the enzymic activity is destroyed and new molecules of enzyme must be synthesized before full enzymic activity is restored.

The inhibition of enzyme activity has pharmacologic significance aside from decreasing the rate of drug biotransformation and prolonging the duration of drug action. In certain pathologic conditions the inhibition of specific normal metabolic processes appears to be beneficial. Under these circumstances, a chemical that can inhibit the appropriate enzyme system is a useful therapeutic agent; its receptor is the enzyme and not a hypothetical macromolecular tissue component. Enzyme inhibitors that are therapeutically useful drugs include inhibitors of cholinesterase, monoamine oxidase, carbonic anhydrase and xanthine oxidase.

Enzyme Stimulation

The remarkable enzymes of the microsomal fraction of cells possess yet another unique characteristic: their ability to metabolize certain compounds can be *stimulated* or *increased* by the prior administration of a large variety of chemical substances. Various therapeutic agents, pesticides, herbicides, food additives and carcinogenic compounds, already numbering in the hundreds, have been shown to increase the rate of their own biotransformation or that of other foreign agents and even normal body constituents. More compounds are constantly being added to the list. However, there appears to be no relationship as yet between either pharmacologic activity or structure and the ability of this diverse group of agents to stimulate microsomal enzyme activity. The only property that most of the stimulating compounds appear to share is that of lipid solubility. Table 6-7 lists some of the agents known to stimulate drug

Table 6-7. Agents Stimulating Microsomal Enzyme Activity in Humans and the Compounds Whose Biotransformation Is Affected

Stimulating Agents (pretreatment)	Compounds Whose Rate of Biotransformation Is Increased
Phenobarbital	Phenobarbital (sedative)
	Dicumarol (bishydroxycoumarin) (anticoagulant)
	Warfarin (Coumadin) (anticoagulant)
	Phenytoin (antiepileptic)
	Griseofulvin (antifungal agent)
	Digitoxin (increases performance of the failing heart)
	Bilirubin (naturally occurring breakdown product)
	Cortisol (naturally occurring hormone)
	Testosterone (male sex hormone)
Phenylbutazone (Butazolidin)	Phenylbutazone (antirheumatic agent)
	Aminopyrine (Pyramidon) (nonnarcotic analgesic)
	Cortisol
Tetrachlorodiphenylethane (DDD) (insecticide)	Cortisol
Meprobamate	Meprobamate (sedative)
Glutethimide (Doriden)	Glutethimide (sedative-hypnotic)
	Warfarin
Phenytoin	Cortisol
Griseofulvin	Warfarin
Cigarette smoke	3,4-Benzpyrene (carcinogenic compound)
	Nicotine

biotransformation in humans and some of the substances whose metabolism is affected.

How is this enhancement of enzymic activity brought about? The evidence suggests that it is the consequence of an augmented rate of *protein synthesis*; the agents act to *induce* enzyme production. An increase in the quantity of smooth endoplasmic reticulum, the cellular fraction associated with microsomal enzymes, is seen in electron micrographs of liver cells from animals pretreated with agents, such as phenobarbital, which stimulate enzyme activity. Also, pretreatment with phenobarbital in the presence of compounds like puromycin, which prevent protein synthesis, does not lead to increased enzyme activity or increased quantities of endoplasmic reticulum. Moreover, the compounds that produce an increase in drug biotransformation do not enhance the activity of enzymes when added to an incubation mixture in vitro; this phenomenon can be evoked only in the intact animal. And the elapsed time between the start of drug pretreatment and the appearance of stimulated drug metabolism corresponds to known rates of protein synthesis. When the administration of the compound that stimulates the production of enzyme is discontinued, the rate of enzyme synthesis slowly returns to its pretreatment level. Thus, prior administration of a variety of foreign agents may accelerate drug biotransformation, as well as metabolism of normally occurring substances, by increasing the total quantity of microsomal enzymes. The term *enzyme induction* has been given to this unusual process.

An example of how a drug may stimulate its own biotransformation is illustrated in Figure 6-19 for benzpyrene. Weanling rats were given a single injection of benzpyrene at two different doses. The animals were sacrificed at intervals over the course of six days, and the benzpyrene-metabolizing activity of their livers was determined in vitro. Stimulation of enzyme activity was evident for both doses at the earliest time of testing, the large dose producing a stimulation of greater intensity and longer duration. Benzpyrene is a major coal tar carcinogen and is found in tobacco smoke, and cigarette smoke has also been shown to increase the rate of biotransformation of benzpyrene in humans. Although fortuitous, this may be advantageous, since the source of the carcinogen may help to decrease its own potential toxicity.

Phenobarbital has been shown to increase the rate of biotransformation of a wide variety of drugs in humans as well as in animals. One of the agents affected by phenobarbital is dicumarol (bishydroxycoumarin), a drug used to decrease the clotting ability of blood in patients prone to form clots too readily. Dicumarol is itself a good example of a drug which produces its pharmacologic action by inhibition of an enzymic process. It interferes with the liver's normal synthesis of clotting factors, particularly the synthesis of prothrombin. The dose of dicumarol needed to lower the clotting ability of blood to an appropriate level is adjusted for each patient

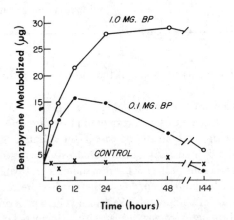

FIGURE 6-19. Stimulation of the biotransformation of a drug produced by prior administration of the same drug. A single injection of benzpyrene (BP), either 0.1 mg or 1.0 mg, was administered to two groups of rats. Animals were sacrificed at intervals over the course of six days, and the benzpyrene-metabolizing activity of their livers was determined in vitro. Each point is the average from two rats. (From A. H. Conney, E. C. Miller and J. A. Miller, J. Biol. Chem. 228:753, 1957.)

according to his particular requirements. This is done by monitoring the patient's blood prothrombin concentration, or *prothrombin time,* until a dose is found which yields the desired effects. Once established, the dose is maintained. Figure 6-20 illustrates what happens when phenobarbital is given to a patient who is receiving such a maintenance dose of the anticoagulant. In the presence of phenobarbital, the plasma concentration of dicumarol falls, indicating an increased rate of destruction of the latter, and the prothrombin time decreases (blood is clotting more rapidly), indicating a diminution of anticoagulant activity. If additional dicumarol were given during phenobarbital administration, the concentration of the anticoagulant might become much too high were the barbiturate to be discontinued. Excessive dosage of an anticoagulant can lead to internal hemorrhage. On the other hand, if phenobarbital administration were continued and the dose of dicumarol were not increased to counteract the effect of enzyme induction, the value of the anticoagulant therapy might be nullified.

Whenever microsomal enzymes convert a drug to an inactive metabolite, the consequences of enzyme induction will be decreased therapeutic activity, as in the case of dicumarol. However, we have seen that an inactive drug may be changed to an active agent or an active drug may be converted to a compound of greater or different pharmacologic activity. In such cases the increase in microsomal enzyme activity by the concomitant use of another drug may lead to enhanced pharmacologic effect or even to toxicity. For example, the insecticide malathion is an inactive compound; its toxicity in insects as well as in humans is contingent on its conversion to the active metabolite malaoxon. Malathion's usefulness as an insecticide depends on the fact that malaoxon is more stable in insects than in mammals. In humans, the inactive drug is not only activated by microsomal enzymes but is also rapidly inac-

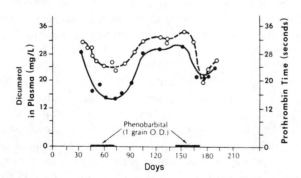

FIGURE 6-20. Effect of phenobarbital on plasma levels of dicumarol (bishydroxy-coumarin) (●) and on prothrombin time (○) in a human subject (dose of dicumarol: 75 mg per day). Phenobarbital was administered (60 mg once daily) during the period indicated by heavy marks on the abscissa. (Redrawn from S. A. Cucinell, A. H. Conney, M. Sansur and J. J. Burns, Drug interactions in man: I. Lowering effect of phenobarbital on plasma levels of bishydroxycoumarin [Dicumarol] and diphenylhydantoin [Dilantin]. Clin. Pharmacol. Ther. 6:420–429, 1965.)

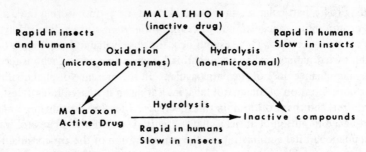

FIGURE 6-21. Biotransformation of the insecticide malathion in human and insect hosts. (Modified from T. A. Loomis, Essentials of Toxicology. Philadelphia: Lea & Febiger, 1970.)

tivated by nonmicrosomal hydrolysis (Fig. 6-21). The latter process reduces the quantity of insecticide available for oxidation to the toxic metabolite. The insecticide may become more harmful to humans, however, if microsomal enzyme activity has been stimulated.

Although the microsomal enzyme systems are largely confined to reactions involving foreign substances, they do participate in the metabolism of some important normal body constituents. The steroid hormones are normal substrates for nonsynthetic reactions, and substances like bilirubin and thyroxine are natural substrates for glucuronide conjugation, the one synthetic enzyme system catalyzed by the microsomal fraction of cells. Many experiments in animals and some few in human subjects indicate that the metabolism of normal body constituents can also be accelerated by various inducers of the microsomal enzymes. In addition, androgens, estrogens, progestational steroids and other hormones influence drug action in animals by altering the activity of the microsomal enzyme systems. Clearly, the phenomenon of enzyme induction and the possibilities it creates for interactions among foreign agents and between drugs and naturally occurring substances have far-reaching significance.

Enzyme induction may not only have widespread implications for chronic drug therapy with single or multiple drugs but may also have some useful applications. One such is the stimulation by phenobarbital of the glucuronide-synthesizing system in newborn infants. The newborn offspring of most species, including the human, have low levels of microsomal enzymes; these enzymes develop slowly during the first weeks after birth. Some newborn infants suffer from a condition known as congenital nonhemolytic jaundice, in which there is an excessive amount of circulating bilirubin. As a consequence of the defective glucuronide-synthesizing system, the bilirubin remains unconjugated and is very slowly excreted; the water-soluble glucuronide accounts for most of the elimination of bilirubin. When small quantities of phenobarbital are given to these jaundiced infants, the bilirubin concentration of the blood declines and the jaundice disappears. The bilirubin concentration rises to its pretreatment levels when phenobarbital administration is stopped but declines again upon reinstitution of therapy. Many human illnesses are expressions of inborn errors of normal metabolic processes. Only intensive investigation will determine whether it will be possible to correct such diseases by the administration of appropriate enzyme inducers.

SYNOPSIS

The actions of drugs in the body are terminated mainly by biotransformation and by excretion through the kidneys and liver. The elimination of most drugs depends on these processes acting in concert. The great majority of drugs are lipid-soluble chemicals which readily cross biologic barriers. This solubility characteristic permits their easy access to sites where they may produce a pharmacologic effect. It would lead equally to their indefinite retention in the body if means were not available to convert them into less lipid-soluble materials since lipid-soluble drugs are not excreted to any significant degree by the kidney or the liver. However, the reactions that drugs undergo during biotransformation yield products which are almost invariably less lipid soluble than their parent compounds. It is significant, too, that the enzymes which catalyze the greatest number and variety of drug biotransformations — the microsomal enzymes — act only on lipid-soluble substrates.

The principal route for drug excretion is by way of the kidney, although drugs may be excreted in any media eliminated from the body. Urinary excretion of drugs begins with glomerular filtration of any drug that is not bound to plasma proteins. The final concentration of the product in the voided urine is determined by how much is passively reabsorbed in its passage through the renal tubules. Active tubular secretory mechanisms account for the rapid elimination in the urine of certain organic acidic or basic drugs.

Most drugs undergo chemical alteration by the body, being biotransformed by either a nonsynthetic reaction or a conjugation process or a combination of the two. All these reactions are catalyzed by enzymes, many of which also catalyze normal metabolic processes. By far the most important enzymes of drug biotransformation are those of the microsomal fraction of cells. The activity of all enzymes involved in drug biotransformation may be decreased or inhibited by pathologic conditions or chemical agents. The stimulation of enzyme activity through chemical induction of protein synthesis is known at present only for microsomal enzyme systems.

Drugs may be biotransformed into inactive metabolites by either synthetic or nonsynthetic reactions. The nonsynthetic reactions can also convert an inactive drug into an active agent or an active agent into another compound with less, equal, greater or different pharmacologic activity. The consequences evoked by these potential changes in activity and by the phenomenon of enzyme induction warrant careful consideration in long-term therapy with single or multiple drugs.

GUIDES FOR STUDY AND REVIEW

By what routes can drugs be excreted from the body? What is the principal route for drug excretion?

What are the renal mechanisms that normally account for the formation and final composition of voided urine? What single process is of greatest significance in determining the final composition of urine?

What kinds of material are filtered at the glomerulus? What special structural characteristics of Bowman's capsule are of great functional significance? How is the composition of the glomerular filtrate related to that of plasma?

How do the events taking place in the proximal tubule influence the composition, volume and tonicity of the urine delivered to the loop of Henle? What ions are actively absorbed in the proximal tubules? How do these active transport processes influence the reabsorption of water? of passively transferred solutes?

How is bicarbonate ion reabsorbed? What influences the rate at which H^+ is made available in the renal tubule cell? How would alteration in the rate of H^+ formation in the renal tubular cell influence the rate of reabsorption of bicarbonate ion from the tubular urine?

What special purpose does the loop of Henle serve? What are the structural and functional characteristics of the loop of Henle that account for its ability to markedly influence the tonicity of voided urine? What are the functional differences between the descending and ascending limbs? What are the differences in the volume and tonicity of the urine entering and leaving the loop of Henle?

What influences the reabsorption of water in the distal convoluted tubule and the collecting duct? What hormone plays a role in the reabsorption of water? How does the presence of this hormone influence the final tonicity of voided urine?

What are the three basic factors that are necessary to convert the isotonic urine of the glomerular filtrate to a concentrated urine? What percentage of the Na^+ filtered is normally reabsorbed? of the water? of bicarbonate ion? of urea? of glucose?

What are the mechanisms responsible for urinary drug excretion?

What are the factors that determine the rate at which drugs are filtered at the glomerulus? How does binding to plasma proteins affect this rate? Can the rate of glomerular filtration of protein-bound drug be altered by another drug that binds to plasma proteins? How can rates of glomerular filtration explain differences in the duration of action among sulfa drugs? Are there any unbound (free) drugs that cannot be filtered at the glomerulus?

How does the apparent volume of distribution of a drug affect its glomerular filtration rate?

How does rate of blood flow affect glomerular filtration? What are the factors that operate to keep filtration constant over a wide range of systemic arterial pressures?

How is glomerular filtration rate measured? What properties does a drug have to possess in order to be used to measure GFR? to measure total renal blood flow?

What factors determine whether a drug will be reabsorbed from the tubular urine? How can the rate of reabsorption of a weak acid be decreased? of a weak base be decreased? How does the process of reabsorption affect the amount of drug in voided urine?

What general types of drugs are secreted into the tubular urine? How does this process affect the amount in the voided urine?

A total of 400 mg of drug X was found in a 10-minute urine sample collection. Midway during this 10-minute interval, the plasma concentration of drug X was 25 mg% (25 mg/100 ml plasma). What is the renal plasma clearance of this drug? What is the excretion ratio of this drug? How is drug X handled by the kidney and how do you know this?

What general types of drugs are secreted by the liver into the bile? For what general types of compounds does biliary secretion become a relatively effective means of elimination from the body? In what ways are biliary secretion into the intestine and renal secretion into the tubular urine similar?

How is the chemical alteration of a drug brought about in the body? What mediates these chemical reactions? In what ways are the reactions of drug biotransformations analogous to the reactions of drugs and receptors?

What is a first-order reaction? a zero-order reaction? How does the order of a reaction relate to the rate at which a drug is biotransformed? Does the rate of biotransformation of most drugs follow first-order kinetics or zero-order kinetics?

What are some of the features common to all synthetic or conjugation reactions? What functional groups of drugs act as centers for conjugation reactions? What are the most important synthetic pathways of biotransformation in humans? Which of the conjugation reactions of drug biotransformation is the most frequently occurring and why?

How do the two basic types of drug biotransformation reactions (synthetic and nonsynthetic) compare with respect to number of different reactions possible; the rapidity with which the metabolites formed are excreted in the urine or feces; the pharmacologic activity of the metabolites formed; the number of reactions catalyzed by microsomal enzyme systems?

How may the administration of one drug affect the biotransformation of another drug? What are the characteristics of competitive inhibition and how can the effects of this type of inhibition be overcome? How does competitive inhibition differ from noncompetitive inhibition? What are the potential pharmacologic consequences of the inhibition of biotransformation of a drug?

What types of drug biotransformation can be enhanced (stimulated) by the prior administration of drugs? How is this stimulation brought about? How does this phenomenon affect the onset and duration of drug action when the metabolite formed is an inactive drug? an active drug?

SUGGESTED READING

Cafruny, E.J. Renal Excretion of Drugs. In B.N. La Du, H.G. Mandel, and E.L. Way (eds.), *Fundamentals of Drug Metabolism and Drug Disposition*. Baltimore: Williams & Wilkins, 1971. P. 119.

Conney, A.H.   Pharmacologic implications of microsomal enzyme induction. *Pharmacol. Rev.* 19:317, 1967.

Conney, A.H.   Environmental Factors Influencing Drug Metabolism. In B.N. La Du, H.G. Mandel, and E.L. Way (eds.), *Fundamentals of Drug Metabolism and Drug Disposition.* Baltimore: Williams & Wilkins, 1971. P. 253.

Gelborn, H.V.   Mechanisms of Induction of Drug Metabolism Enzymes. In B.N. La Du, H.G. Mandel, and E.L. Way (eds.), *Fundamentals of Drug Metabolism and Drug Disposition.* Baltimore: Williams & Wilkins, 1971. P. 279.

Gillette, J.R.   Metabolism of drugs and other foreign compounds by enzymatic mechanisms. *Prog. Drug Res.* 6:11, 1963.

Gottschalk, C.W.   Osmotic concentration and dilution in the urine. *Am. J. Med.* 36:670, 1964.

Kokko, J.P.   Membrane characteristics governing salt and water transport in the loop of Henle. *Fed. Proc.* 33:25, 1974.

Mandel, H.G.   Pathways of Drug Biotransformation: Biochemical Conjugations. In B.N. La Du, H.G. Mandel, and E.L. Way (eds.), *Fundamentals of Drug Metabolism and Drug Disposition.* Baltimore: Williams & Wilkins, 1971. P. 149.

Pitts, R.F. *The Physiology of the Kidney and Body Fluids,* 2d ed. Chicago: Year Book, 1968.

Plaa, G.I.   Extrarenal Excretion of Drugs. In B.N. La Du, H.G. Mandel, and E.L. Way (eds.), *Fundamentals of Drug Metabolism and Drug Disposition.* Baltimore: Williams & Wilkins, 1971. P. 253.

Smith, R.L.   The biliary excretion and enterohepatic circulation of drugs and other organic compounds. *Prog. Drug Res.* 9:299, 1966.

Symposium (various authors). Drug metabolism in man (Vesell, E.S., ed.). *Ann. N.Y. Acad. Sci.* 195:1, 1972.

Ullrich, K.J., and Marsh, D.J.   Kidney, water and electrolyte metabolism. *Annu. Rev. Physiol.* 25:91, 1963.

Weiner, I.M.   Mechanisms of drug absorption and excretion: The renal excretion of drugs and related compounds. *Annu. Rev. Pharmacol.* 7:39, 1967.

Williams, R.T.   Detoxification mechanisms in man. *Clin. Pharmacol. Ther.* 4:234, 1963.

7. GENERAL PRINCIPLES OF THE QUANTITATIVE ASPECTS OF DRUG ACTION
I. Dose-Response Relationships

Up to this point we have considered some of the fundamental principles of pharmacology on rather qualitative grounds. These principles must find expression in quantitative terms as well; only then can they provide the basis for evaluation and comparison of drug safety and effectiveness and for the rational application of drug effects to therapeutics.

One of the most basic principles of pharmacology states that the degree of effect produced by a drug is a function of the quantity of drug administered. Even the word *dose*, the term used to quantitate drugs, has this relationship implicit in its definition, since dose is the *amount of drug needed at a given time to produce a particular biologic response.* We have seen that in the living system a drug is usually present as a solute and that it can produce its characteristic effect only if it reaches its site of action or its receptor. We ought more properly to define dose, then, as the amount of drug necessary to yield an appropriate *concentration* of material at the site in the system where the interaction occurs. Usually a drug does not reach its site of action instantaneously; its rate of accessibility is determined primarily by either or both the processes of absorption and distribution. Nor does the drug's presence at its locus of action continue indefinitely; redistribution, biotransformation, and excretion operate separately or conjointly to remove it from the site and from the body. Thus, at any given moment, the concentration of drug at a site of action, and consequently the magnitude of drug effect, is a function not only of the *dose administered,* but also of *time* — the time involved in getting the drug to and from its site of action (Fig. 7-1).

Although the three properties — dose, time and effect — are interdependent, it is more expedient to quantitate the response to the administration of a drug by treating the dose-response relationship separately from the time-response relationship. Time may be eliminated from consideration of the dose-response relationship by determining the effects produced by given doses only after the observed effect has attained its maximum level. Dose is eliminated as a variable in the time-response relationship by studying the appearance and disappearance of effects following the administration of a *single* dose. In this chapter we shall examine the magnitude of drug effect (or

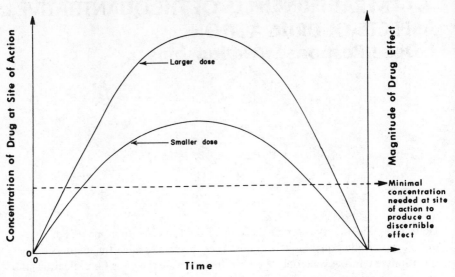

FIGURE 7-1. Theoretical curves summarizing the interrelationships of dose, time and magnitude of drug effect. Two different doses of the same drug are given at time 0. Absorption and distribution account for increase in concentration and in magnitude of effect. Elimination — i.e., redistribution, biotransformation and excretion — accounts for decrease in concentration and in magnitude of effect. These idealized curves are seen only under special conditions of drug administration. The elimination curves usually obtained are hyperbolic with concavity upward. The resultant curve of the actual amount reaching the site of action is also nonsymmetrical but is modified by many factors discussed in Chapters 9 and 10.

drug response) as a function of the dose administered. In Chapter 8, we shall turn our attention to the degree of drug effect as a function of time.

QUANTITATIVE ASPECTS OF DRUG-RECEPTOR INTERACTIONS

Application of the Law of Mass Action

As we have seen, a pharmacologic effect is considered to be the consequence of a reversible chemical, or physicochemical, reaction between a drug and a reactive entity of the living organism. The biologic reactant may be either a "receptor" or some other component of equal functional importance; in most cases it is a receptor. The product of this reaction becomes the stimulus for the events leading to the effect, which is seen as a biochemical or physiologic change or as the disappearance or appearance of clinical symptoms:

$$\text{Drug} + \text{Receptor} \rightleftharpoons \text{Drug-receptor complex} \xrightarrow{\text{Stimulus}} \text{Effect}$$

Enzymes, like receptors, produce their activity by combining reversibly with the substances upon which they act:

$$\text{Enzyme} + \text{Substrate} \rightleftharpoons \text{Enzyme-substrate complex} \longrightarrow \text{Products}$$

As was previously noted, this enzyme reaction obeys the law of mass action, the degree of the chemical reaction between enzyme and substrate being proportional to the concentrations of these reacting substances present at any given time. The rate of appearance of metabolic products is then dependent on the extent and effectiveness of the combination of substrate and enzyme — on the rate of formation of the enzyme-substrate complex. Since the substrate-enzyme and drug-receptor interactions are so similar, it should also be possible to explain the quantitative aspects of the latter on the basis of the laws governing chemical equilibrium. Thus, by analogy, the occupancy of receptors by a drug should be proportional to the dose of drug and the number of free, unoccupied receptors. Or, more properly stated, the occupancy of receptors by a drug should be proportional to the *concentration* of drug and the *concentration* of unoccupied receptors. In turn, the magnitude of a pharmacologic effect elicited by a drug should be dependent on the extent of the chemical reaction involved, i.e., it should be directly proportional to the number of receptors occupied by drug molecules.

A.J. Clark (1885–1941) is largely responsible for applying mass action principles to the concept of drug-receptor interactions and thereby providing a plausible, quantitative basis for the dose-effect phenomenon. In the simplest quantitation of the dose-effect relationship formulated by Clark, the following assumptions are made:

1. The law of mass action is applicable to a reversible reaction between one drug molecule and one receptor.
2. All receptors are identical and equally accessible to the drug.
3. The intensity of the response elicited by the drug is directly proportional to the number of receptors occupied by the drug.
4. The amount of drug which combines with receptors is negligible compared to the amount of drug to which the receptors are exposed, so that the effective drug concentration does not change during the reaction.

The relationship between dose and effect may then be derived as follows. For the reaction:

$$\underset{C \qquad (100-Y)}{\text{Drug} + \text{Free receptor}} \overset{k_1}{\underset{k_2}{\rightleftharpoons}} \underset{Y}{\text{Drug-receptor complex}}$$

where C = the concentration of drug (C is actually the concentration of unbound drug, but by assumption No. 4 it is, for all practical purposes, equal to the original concentration of drug at the site of action); and Y = the percentage of the total number of receptors occupied by drug. Thus:

$$(100 - Y) = \text{Percentage of unoccupied, free receptors}$$

Then the rate of combination of drug and unoccupied receptors is proportional to the product of the drug concentration, C, and the concentration of unoccupied receptors, $(100-Y)$:

$$k_1 C(100 - Y), \text{ where } k_1 \text{ is a constant of proportionality specific for the given reaction of combination}$$

The rate of dissociation of the drug-receptor complex is proportional to Y, the percentage of receptors occupied by drug:

$$k_2 Y, \text{ where } k_2 \text{ is the specific constant for the reverse reaction}$$

At equilibrium, when the rate of combination is equal to the rate of dissociation:

$$k_1 C(100 - Y) = k_2 Y, \text{ or}$$

$$C = \frac{k_2 Y}{k_1(100 - Y)} \qquad \text{(Equation 1)}$$

Since the ratio of two constants is itself a constant, we can substitute K_e for k_1/k_2 in Equation 1, and K_e is then the equilibrium constant of the particular reaction:

$$C = \frac{Y}{K_e(100 - Y)} \qquad \text{(Equation 2)}$$

This mathematical expression of the relationship between dose and effect takes on more meaning and clarity when it is represented in its graphic form. Such graphic representations of the quantitative aspect of drug action are called *dose-effect* or *dose-response curves*. Figure 7-2A illustrates a characteristic shape of the dose-effect curve obtained for a system in which increasing amounts or concentrations of drug produce progressively increasing intensities of response. In this example the contraction, or shortening, of the longitudinal muscle of a segment of small intestine is the response to either acetylcholine or propionylcholine, a drug structurally similar to acetylcholine. The effect is elicited by adding solutions of the drug in varying concentrations,

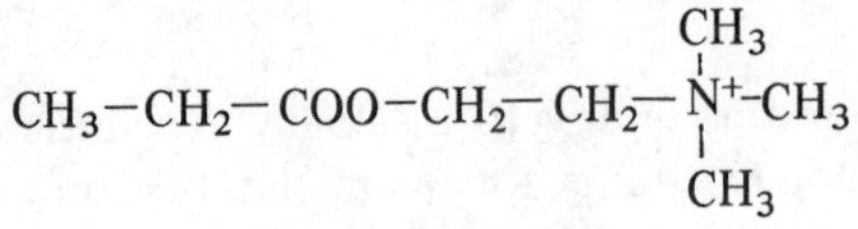

$$CH_3-CH_2-COO-CH_2-CH_2-\overset{\displaystyle CH_3}{\underset{\displaystyle CH_3}{\overset{|}{\underset{|}{N^+}}}}-CH_3$$

Propionylcholine

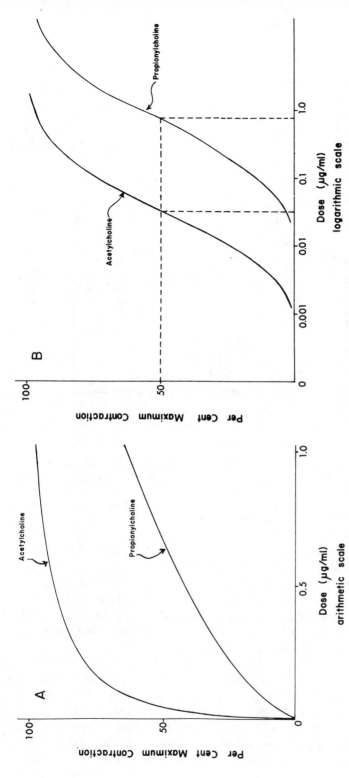

FIGURE 7-2. Dose-effect curves for the action of acetylcholine and propionylcholine on the guinea pig ileum. The ordinate shows the response of the segment of small intestine as a percentage of the maximum contraction obtainable under the conditions of the experiment. The dose of the drugs is shown on the abscissa as concentration (micrograms per milliliter). In A, a linear scale is used; in B, a logarithmic scale. The horizontal - - - in B indicates the points at which 50 per cent of the maximal effect is attained. The perpendiculars dropped from the intersections indicate the doses which produce the 50 per cent maximal response. (Modified from Gaddum's Pharmacology [revised by A. S. V. Burgen and J. F. Mitchell]. London: Oxford University Press, 1968.)

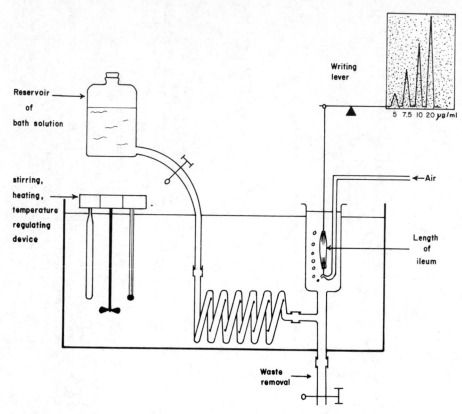

FIGURE 7-3. *Apparatus for recording contractions of the longitudinal muscle of a segment of small intestine (ileum) in response to drugs. Solutions containing drug may be added directly to the medium bathing the tissue and removed by flushing with several volumes of solution from the reservoir. Solution in tissue bath is aerated and usually kept at about 37°C.*

at different times, to the bath in which the isolated tissue is immersed (Fig. 7-3). The dose (expressed as concentration) is the independent variable and, by convention, is plotted on the horizontal scale, the abscissa; its value is not determined by any other variable and can be chosen or varied at will. The dependent variable, the effect, is plotted on the vertical scale, the ordinate. In Figure 7-2 the response to a dose of drug is expressed as the percentage of the maximum contraction which can be obtained under the conditions of the experiment.

Since the assumption has been made that the magnitude of response is a faithful indicator of the degree of receptor occupancy, the values on the ordinate are equivalent to Y of Equation 2. As the dose is increased, the pharmacologic effect (shortening of the muscle) increases in a gradual, continuous fashion. The increments in response to equal increases in dose become progressively smaller as a maximum value is approached, until further increases in dose produce no perceptibly greater effect. Obviously, the maximum response corresponds to the point at which receptor occupancy is approaching 100 per cent. Thus the relationship between dose and effect describes a hyperbolic function with concavity downward. The term *graded* is applied to this type of relationship in which the *responding system is capable of showing progressively increasing effect with increasing concentration of drug.*

The Log Dose-Effect Curve

The initial portion of the curve in Figure 7-2A, particularly for acetylcholine, is so steep that it is virtually impossible to gauge the magnitude of increase in response that corresponds to small increments in dose. This huddling together of the smaller doses is inevitable when an arithmetic scale is used to display a dose range in which the largest dose is many times that of the smallest. On the other hand, when the effect is approaching maximum, large increments in dose produce changes in response which are now too small to evaluate accurately. What we need is a way of expanding the abscissal scale used to depict smaller doses which will still permit representation of a wide dose range. Both these objectives can be achieved if the scale of doses is made logarithmic, or if the doses are converted to their logarithms.

On a logarithmic scale, if each dose is double the preceding dose, the intervals between doses are equal, since the logarithmic transformation has the property of turning multiplication into addition. The curves resulting from such a transformation are illustrated in Figure 7-2B; the values of the independent variable — dose — are plotted on a logarithmic scale, whereas the values along the ordinate remain on an arithmetic scale as in Figure 7-2A. Inspection of the two methods of graphic representation makes it clear that the logarithmic scale permits presentation of not only more detailed data in the low dose range but also a wide range of doses in a single graph. Comparison of the linear and semilogarithmic dose-response curves in Figure 7-4 shows that this is advantageous even when the range of values is narrow.

The shape of the curve obtained when the abscissal values are converted to the logarithmic scale also has certain features which are preferable to those of the hyperbola. The typical S-shaped log dose-effect curve has a center of symmetry. This midpoint represents the dose at which 50 per cent of the maximum response is elicited (Fig. 7-2B). Above the midpoint, the log dose-effect curve, like the hyperbola, slowly approaches a maximum value corresponding to the point at which the biologic system no longer has the capacity to respond. The lower end of the logarithmic curve also approaches zero asymptotically. (Reminder: there is no log value for zero.) But the middle segment of the curve is almost linear, a fact that is of practical importance since line segments lend themselves to mathematical analysis more readily than do curves. Figure 7-4 shows more clearly than Figure 7-2 how data points that represent the middle portion of the dose-effect curve can be fitted by straight lines when plotted logarithmically, but not when plotted arithmetically.

From our earlier considerations of drug-receptor interactions we know that a single receptor can react with a number of drugs, provided that each drug is structurally complementary to the receptor surface. Thus, drugs that possess similar chemical or physicochemical properties and that initiate the same selective pharmacologic response probably do so by acting on the same population of receptors. In a simple biologic system, such as the isolated small intestine, we would anticipate that

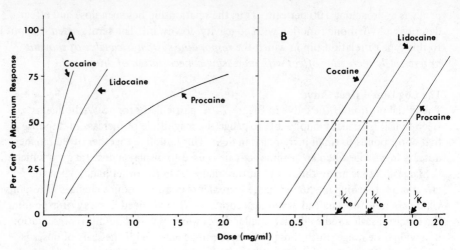

FIGURE 7-4. Arithmetic and semilogarithmic dose-effect curves of three local anesthetics. Abscissa: Concentration of drug: in A on arithmetic scale, in B on logarithmic scale. Ordinate: Response expressed as per cent of the maximal response. Local anesthetic activity was determined in guinea pigs following intracutaneous injection of different concentrations of each local anesthetic. The degree of local anesthesia was measured by determining the number of times out of 40 that a pinprick (applied to a shaved area of the back) failed to elicit a response. The horizontal dashed line in B indicates the point of 50 per cent maximal response. The perpendiculars dropped from intersections cut the abscissa at concentrations which produce the 50 per cent maximal response. The concentrations are also equivalent to the reciprocal of the affinities of the drugs for the receptor. Cocaine has the highest and procaine the lowest affinity.

drugs producing the same effect would also yield similar dose-effect curves if they acted by the same mechanism. Both graphic representations in Figure 7-2 show that about twenty times more propionylcholine than acetylcholine is required to produce a given contractile response. But only the semilogarithmic plot indicates that the dose-effect curves for the two drugs are almost identical in shape and approach the same maximal level of response. This evidence strongly supports the conclusion that both drugs act at the same receptor. Furthermore, drugs that produce the same effect by the same mechanism generally yield log dose-effect curves whose nearly linear middle segments parallel each other (see Fig. 7-4). The converse is also true, as a rule: two drugs that have nonparallel log dose-effect curves but which elicit qualitatively simiilar responses act by different mechanisms. Thus, aside from practical reasons, semilogarithmic dose-response curves are convenient devices for comparing the mechanisms by which two or more drugs produce the same end effect. And in pharmacology it is customary to use semilogarithmic dose-effect curves to evaluate the quantitative aspects of the action of a single drug or to compare the actions of several drugs.

Why do equal quantities of acetylcholine and propionylcholine produce different degrees of contraction of the isolated small intestine when both drugs act by the same mechanism and have identically shaped log dose-effect curves? And why does it require less lidocaine (Xylocaine) than procaine (Novocain), and even a smaller concentration of cocaine, to produce the same extent of local anesthesia when all three agents act at the same receptor site? These questions are readily answered by analyzing the equation for the interaction of a drug with its receptor. In deriving Equation 2, the assumption was made that the magnitude of response elicited by a drug is directly proportional to the number of receptors occupied by the drug. When effects of equal intensity are produced by several drugs acting at the same receptor, then Y — the percentage of the total number of receptor occupied — must be the same for each drug. It follows that the only way *unequal* concentrations of different drugs can produce effects of *equal* magnitude is for the constant, K_e, to have different values for each drug interacting with the receptor. This constant, which we said is the equilibrium constant for a given reaction, is then also a measure of the **affinity** of a drug for a particular receptor. It is a statement of the *effectiveness* of the inter-action of drug and receptor. The greater the affinity of a drug, the greater its propen-sity to bind with a given receptor and the greater the value of the constant, K_e. And further inspection of Equation 2 indicates that the larger the value of K_e, the smaller the concentration needed to produce the same intensity of response. Thus, when several drugs acting at the same receptor and yielding similarly shaped log dose-effect curves are compared, the position of their curves along the abscissa is indicative of their relative affinities. The curve for the drug with the greatest affinity (acting at the lowest concentration) will lie closest to the ordinate. Curves for drugs with lesser affinities for the receptor will lie farther to the right (Fig. 7-4).

A numerical expression of the affinity of a drug is also easily obtained from its log dose-response curve. When the fraction $Y/(100 - Y)$ is equal to 1, then K_e is equal to the reciprocal of the drug concentration and has the dimensions of concentration. Thus, since:

$$C = \frac{Y}{K_e(100 - Y)}$$ (Equation 2)

when $Y/(100 - Y) = 1$, then $C = 1/K_e$, or $K_e = 1/C$.

The fraction $Y/(100 - Y)$ is equal to 1 when $Y = 50$ per cent, i.e., when one-half of the receptors are combined with drug, or one-half of the maximal effect is attained. If a horizontal is drawn from the point of 50 per cent maximal response to intersect the dose-effect curve, the perpendicular from this intersection cuts the abscissa at a concentration equal to the reciprocal of affinity, or $1/K_e$. Figure 7-4 shows that the affinity of cocaine is about twice that of lidocaine and about seven times greater than procaine.

Of course, statements about the affinity of a drug or the comparative affinities of several drugs have relevance only for a particular reaction with a given receptor. A single drug may have different affinities for different receptors, and the relative affin-ities among drugs may change from receptor to receptor. Moreover, the calculated values of the affinity of a drug for its receptor must be considered only as an approximation unless the receptor is an identified or isolated entity. When a drug produces its response by interacting with a known enzyme or other macromolecule, the concentration of all the reactants can be measured, i.e., the concentration of drug and macromolecule as well as that of the drug-macromolecule complex. And then the *observed response can be determined directly by the concentration of the drug-macromolecule complex.* Obviously, however, the majority of receptors are not isolated entities but integral components of living systems which are infinitely more complex than the simple systems for which the chemical laws were formulated.

Whereas the concentration of a drug applied to a system and the consequent biologic response can both be measured very accurately, the concentration of the complex formed between drug and a postulated receptor cannot be measured by presently available methods. We already know that drugs have to traverse various biologic barriers to reach their site of action and that they may combine with non-receptor macromolecular tissue components as well as with receptors. Even in the relatively uncomplicated isolated tissue or organ preparation, there are many obstacles interposed between the drug and its site of action that may influence the quantity of drug actually entering into the combination leading to a response. Thus the quantity of drug that has produced the response can be analyzed only indirectly from the effect produced by the combination. But even though the affinity between drug and receptor cannot be accurately estimated when the receptor has not been isolated, there is little doubt that drug-macromolecule combinations obeying mass law kinetics are involved in drug action. Thus the mass action interpretation of dose-effect curves is conceptually applicable and valid.

Potency

Even though the log dose-effect curve yields only an approximation of the affinity of a drug, it nevertheless provides an accurate measure of another characteristic of a drug — its potency. Potency is determined simply by the dose needed to produce a particular effect of given intensity; like affinity, potency varies inversely with the magnitude of the dose required to produce the effect. As we have seen, the intensity of drug effect is determined by the inherent ability of a drug to combine with its receptor and by the concentration of drug at this site. Thus, potency embodies the conceptual aspects of drug-receptor interactions; it is influenced by the drug's affinity for its receptor and by factors regulating how much drug reaches the receptor, i.e., absorption, distribution, biotransformation and excretion.

Potency, unlike affinity, is a comparative rather than an absolute expression of drug activity; potency connotes the dose required to produce a particular effect *relative to a given or implied standard of reference.* For example, just knowing that 10 mg of morphine administered subcutaneously produces relief from the pain induced by a calibrated painful stimulus tells us little, by itself, about morphine's potency. It only tells us in absolute units the *dose* required to produce a given intensity of response. We find, however, that 1.5 mg of hydromorphone (Dilaudid) or 120 mg of codeine, administered by the same route, are as effective as 10 mg of morphine in relieving the pain induced by the same stimulus. We also find that the shapes of the log dose-effect curves for the three drugs are similar and reach the same maximum (Fig. 7-5). Now we can say that morphine is about seven times less potent than hydromorphone, but about twelve times more potent than codeine.

The position of the log dose-effect curves on the dose axis reflects these relative potencies. Since neither the receptors nor the exact sites involved in the action of these narcotic analgesics have been identified, no definitive explanation can be furnished for the observed differences in potencies. It is obvious, however, that differences in potencies between drugs can occur only as a result of differences in the relative affinities of the drugs for the same group of receptors or differences in the proportion of a dose ultimately reaching the receptor site(s), or both factors.

It is inappropriate to express the relative activities of two drugs in terms of potency unless they both produce their effects by the same mechanism and can exert the same maximum effect. In many instances, for example, pain of low or moderate intensity, such as toothache, is as effectively relieved by aspirin as by codeine. However, it takes about five to ten times more aspirin than codeine to achieve the same effect. On the other hand, codeine is frequently useful in obtunding severe pain,

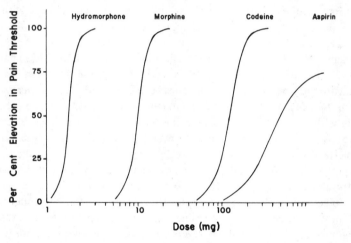

FIGURE 7-5. Log dose-effect curves, typical of those that can be obtained in healthy human males, for the analgesic action of three narcotic drugs — hydromorphine, morphine and codeine — and one nonnarcotic drug, aspirin. The ordinate shows the analgesic effect as the per cent of elevation of the pain threshold, i.e., the increase in magnitude of the painful stimulus required to elicit pain after drug administration as a percentage of the magnitude of the stimulus required to elicit the same degree of pain before drug administration. The position of the curves indicates that hydromorphone is more potent than morphine and the latter more potent than codeine, regardless of the response level at which they are compared. The different shape and maximum height of the curve for aspirin do not permit comparison with the narcotic analgesics in terms of potency. More aspirin than narcotic analgesics is required to produce the same degree of effect at lower levels of response; aspirin is incapable of producing more than a certain degree of analgesia whatever the dose.

whereas aspirin, even at the highest tolerated doses, is not (see Fig. 7-5). Aspirin and codeine act at different sites and produce their analgesic effects by different mechanisms. Although codeine is often said to be more potent than aspirin, it would be better to state that codeine and aspirin are therapeutically equivalent in some applications but that codeine has the potential for exerting a greater maximum effect.

It is important to point out that the potency of a drug is in no way related to its value, efficacy or safety. The least potent drug among agents with similar actions may be no less effective than the most potent one as long as each agent is employed in its appropriate dosage. Low potency becomes a disadvantage only when the size of the effective dose makes it difficult or awkward to administer. From the therapeutic point of view, it matters little whether the dose is 1 mg or 1 g. The only real concern is that the dose, whatever its magnitude, be both effective and safe.

Drug Antagonism

A drug whose interaction with a receptor becomes the stimulus for a biologic response is known as an *agonist*. Up to now we have taken only the overt response of a system to an agonist as evidence of a drug-receptor interaction. However, some drug-receptor combinations manifest themselves only as interactions which interfere with or prevent the formation of an agonist-receptor complex. Drugs that interact with a receptor but do not trigger the sequence of events leading to an effect are known as *antagonists*. Drug antagonism at the receptor level is analogous to enzyme inhibition and, like the latter, is readily analyzed within the framework of mass action kinetics.

Just as with enzyme inhibitors, antagonists can be classified as *competitive* or *noncompetitive* (cf. pp. 158–160). An antagonist is competitive when it combines reversibly with the same binding sites as the active drug and can be displaced from these sites by an excess of the agonist. Conversely, an antagonist is noncompetitive when its effects cannot be overcome by increasing concentrations of the agonist. The noncompetitive antagonist may produce its effect by combining either with the same sites as the active drug or with different sites in a manner that alters the agonist's capacity to combine with its own receptor sites. Even though noncompetitive antagonists cannot be influenced by increasing concentrations of the agonist, the effect of the antagonist may be reversible; in reversible, noncompetitive antagonism, the removal of the antagonist restores the system to full activity. In irreversible, noncompetitive antagonism, the receptor is destroyed and has to be resynthesized.

The quantitative aspects of drug antagonism are readily analyzed from log dose-effect curves. First let us consider the contractile response of the isolated guinea pig ileum to acetylcholine in the absence and presence of a competitive antagonist, atropine. In Figure 7-6, the curve at the left is for acetylcholine alone and that at the right, for acetylcholine when a constant amount of atropine is present in the medium bathing the isolated tissue. The two curves are identical in shape and attain the same maximum. But when atropine is present it is as if acetylcholine had become a less potent drug, since much more is required to produce responses equal in magnitude to those elicited before the addition of the antagonist. Atropine has affinity for the acetylcholine receptor and is able to combine with it. But the

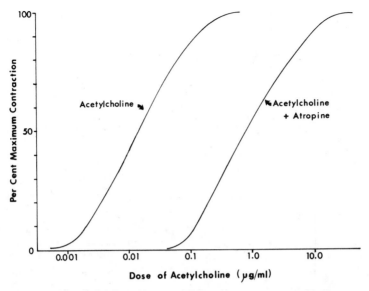

FIGURE 7-6. *Log dose-effect curves depicting competitive antagonism.*
The effect of acetylcholine on the guinea pig ileum is shown in the absence and
presence of the competitive antagonist atropine (see Figs. 7-2 and 7-3). The
ordinate shows the response as percentage of the maximum contraction obtain-
able under the conditions of the experiment. The abscissa shows the dose of
acetylcholine as concentration. The curve on the left is for acetylcholine alone;
that on the right, for acetylcholine in the presence of a constant concentration
of atropine (0.0002 µg per milliliter).

atropine-receptor combination by itself produces no biologic response; atropine
merely decreases the number of receptors available for occupancy by acetylcholine.
Hence the response to a particular dose of acetylcholine is reduced. As the dose of
acetylcholine is increased, the agonist displaces atropine from the receptor until, at
a sufficiently large dose, all receptors are occupied by acetylcholine and a maximal
contractile response is obtained. Thus the log dose-effect curve for an agonist in the
presence of a competitive antagonist will be shifted to the right, indicating an alteration in the effective affinity of the agonist for its receptor; the shape of the curve and
the maximal response, however, are not altered by the competitive antagonist.

Competitive antagonism can also be demonstrated in the intact animal. In the
experiments illustrated in Figure 7-7, the response to the agonist — intravenously
administered histamine — was measured as a prompt but transient fall in blood pressure. Administration of the antagonist diphenhydramine (Benadryl) produced no
change in blood pressure. When diphenhydramine was administered prior to the
injections of histamine, the dose-effect curves for histamine were shifted farther and
farther to the right as the dose of the antagonist was increased. Since similarly shaped
curves with the same potential maximum were obtained, diphenhydramine is a com-

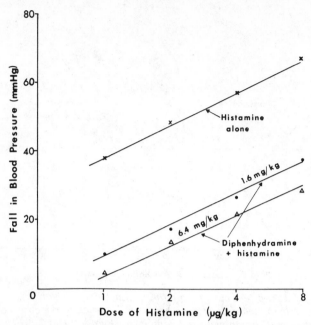

FIGURE 7-7. Log dose-effect curves depicting competitive antagonism in the intact animal. Abscissa: Dose of histamine (µg per kilogram) administered intravenously to an anesthetized dog. Ordinate: Fall in blood pressure (mm Hg) determined by difference in measurements just before and immediately after injections of histamine. The effect of increasing doses of histamine was first determined. The antagonist diphenhydramine was then given, followed by the same series of challenging doses of histamine. Two doses of diphenhydramine (1.6 and 6.4 mg per kilogram of body weight, respectively) were used. (Data from G. Chen and D. Russell, J. Pharmacol. Exp. Ther. 99:401, 1950. Copyright © 1950, The Williams & Wilkins Co., Baltimore.)

petitive antagonist of histamine — an *antihistaminic* whose antagonism can be completely overcome by the administration of sufficient histamine.

We would anticipate that a noncompetitive antagonist influences the log dose-response curve very differently from a competitive antagonist. First, there is a decrease in the maximal height of the response curve. This follows from the fact that even a large excess of agonist cannot displace the antagonist from all the receptor sites and, therefore, cannot achieve 100 per cent receptor occupancy in the presence of the antagonist. The agonist-antagonist curve will still be shifted to the right, however, since the response to a particular dose of agonist will be reduced as a result of the decreased availability of receptors. The slope of the curve is also reduced in proportion to the degree of noncompetitive antagonism produced. All these characteristics of noncompetitive antagonism are illustrated in Figure 7-8 for the effect of two

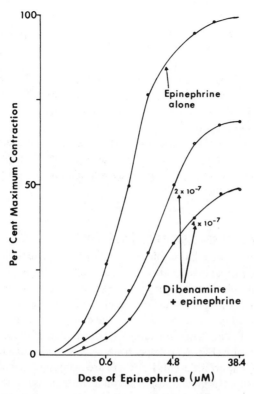

FIGURE 7-8. Log dose-effect curves depicting noncompetitive antagonism. The effect of epinephrine on the isolated cat spleen preparation is shown in the absence and presence of the noncompetitive antagonist dibenamine. The ordinate shows the response as percentage of the maximum contraction obtainable under the conditions of the experiment. The abscissa shows the dose of epinephrine as micromolar concentrations. The curve on the left is for epinephrine alone, and the middle and right-hand curves are for epinephrine in the presence of 2 and 4 x 10⁻⁷ molar concentrations of dibenamine, respectively. (Modified from R. K. Bickerton, J. Pharmacol. Exp. Ther. 142:99, 1963. Copyright © 1963, The Williams & Wilkins Co., Baltimore.)

concentrations of the antagonist dibenamine[1] on the contraction of an isolated animal spleen in response to the agonist epinephrine.

The noncompetitive antagonism exemplified by dibenamine may be considered reversible. As dibenamine is eliminated from the body or from the biologic system, the response of the receptor to the agonist is slowly restored. The pharmacologic effect produced by an organic phosphate insecticide, such as parathion, is an example

[1] Dibenamine is an experimental drug, the forerunner of a group of agents that have limited clinical use in the treatment of certain types of shock.

of irreversible, noncompetitive antagonism. Parathion produces its effect by inhibiting the enzyme cholinesterase. The product formed by the interaction of the insecticide and the enzyme is so stable that the restoration of enzyme activity depends on the synthesis of new enzyme.

The type of drug antagonism we have been discussing is termed *pharmacologic antagonism* since the antagonism interferes with the mechanism by which most pharmacologic effects are produced — it interferes with the formation of an agonist-receptor complex. There are, however, other ways in which one drug may decrease the observed response to another without directly interfering with receptor occupancy. We shall discuss these other types of drug antagonism in Chapter 10 together with the many ways in which the prior or concurrent administration of one drug modifies the effects of another drug.

THE QUANTAL DOSE-RESPONSE RELATIONSHIP

So far, we have examined the relationship between dose and effect only in the system of a single biologic unit capable of graded response, i.e., capable of showing a progressively increasing magnitude of effect with progressively increasing concentration of a drug. We saw that graded dose-effect curves could be obtained in a simple system, such as the isolated small intestine, as well as in the complex system of the intact animal. The response elicited — in our examples, contraction of muscle (Fig. 7-2) and lowering of blood pressure (Fig. 7-7), respectively — was measurable on a *continuous scale* — and this is the important point. For there are many pharmacologic effects which cannot be measured as graded responses on a continuous scale; they either occur or do not occur. For example, if one were determining the relationship between the dose of a barbiturate and its propensity to induce sleep, the effect could be measured only as an all-or-none response — either sleep was induced by a particular dose, or the individual was still awake. Another, yet obvious, example is the determination of the relationship between dose and the ultimate toxicity of a drug; here the criterion of response is whether the experimental animal is dead or alive after a particular dose is administered. The all-or-none response is known as the *quantal* response.

In the graded type of dose-effect relationship, it is assumed that the response of an individual biologic unit increases measurably with increasing concentration of drug. In the quantal type the assumption is made that the individual units of the system respond to their maximum capability or not at all. To examine the graded dose-effect relationship, we obtain quantitative data of response at each of several doses administered to a single biologic system. To explore the relationship between dose and quantal response, however, we must use many individuals and obtain *enumerative* data of the *number* either responding or not responding to each given dose. The quantal dose-response curve, then, does not relate dose to an expression of intensity of effect, but rather to an expression of the *frequency* with which any dose of a drug produces an all-or-none pharmacologic effect. In toxicity tests in animals the quantal response may be death or the appearance of a particular adverse effect, such as convulsions. In clinical trials the quantal response may be the abrupt disappearance of a symptom, such as pain or irregular heartbeat, or the appearance of an unwanted effect, e.g., nausea or vomiting.

The Normal Distribution Curve

Let us examine a quantal dose-response curve for a group of animals when the observed response is death, as measured by cessation of respiration. We will use a large group composed of members of a single species. To ensure uniformity within the group, all members will be of the same strain, sex, age and approximate weight, and will have been bred and kept in the same environmental conditions. Each animal will receive drug X in progressively larger doses (calculated on the basis of body weight) until a dose is reached that is just sufficient to cause death. Such a minimally effective dose of any drug that evokes a stated all-or-none pharmacologic response is called the *threshold* dose.

One of the first observations we would make in our experiment is that not all the animals died at the same threshold dose. In fact, even though we chose an apparently uniform group of animals, we find that it is necessary to use a wide range of doses in order to affect all the individuals. If we tally the number of animals for which any given dose is lethal and plot these numbers in order of uniformly increasing threshold doses, we obtain a bar gram, or histogram, of the distribution of frequencies of response. This is illustrated in Figure 7-9, not for our hypothetical drug X, but for ethyl

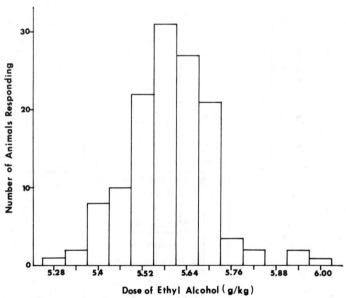

FIGURE 7-9. Frequency histogram showing relationship between dose and effect. Progressively larger amounts of ethyl alcohol were injected into each of 130 rats until respiratory failure occurred. The dose (in grams per kilogram of body weight) that killed each particular animal was recorded. All animals dying following a dose increment of 0.06 g per kilogram of body weight were grouped together.

alcohol administered in a carefully controlled experiment to a group of rats. Now we can clearly see that only a few animals respond at the lowest doses and another small number at the highest doses. Larger numbers of animals respond to any given threshold dose lying between these extremes. But the maximum frequency of response occurs in the middle portion of the dose range.

The larger the number of subjects studied, the greater the likely range of doses between the extremes. With an infinitely large number of animals we arrive at the smooth, symmetrical, bell-shaped curve known as the *normal frequency distribution* (Fig. 7-10). The curve is called *normal* because it is a very common or natural distribution found almost everywhere. We could obtain normal distribution curves for data of such items as the IQ's of thousands of people, or the variations in a dimension of a part which is manufactured in large quantities, or even the probability of possible outcomes on the throws of two dice. And in pharmacology the quantal curve describing the distribution of minimal doses of a drug that produce a given effect in a group of biologic subjects fits the normal curve reasonably well, whether the effect observed is therapeutic, adverse or even lethal. In other words, the drug doses required to produce a quantitatively identical response in a large number of test subjects are distributed in the normal pattern.

Since the normal distribution expresses the frequency of occurrence of random values of different magnitude, we may well ask, "Why does the quantal dose-effect

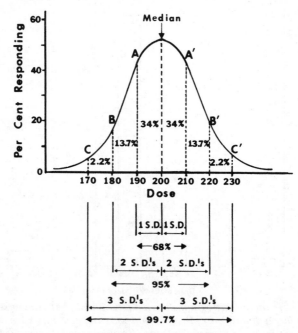

FIGURE 7-10. Normal curve representing the theoretical distribution of quantitatively identical responses of individual animals following administration of drug X to a uniform population.

curve obtained in an apparently homogeneous group of animals so closely resemble the normal distribution curve?" The only answer is that our initial assumption of homogeneity was incorrect. Differences *do* exist among individuals, even when we minimize errors of measurement and eliminate the variables of species, strain, age, sex, weight and other factors under our control. But the nature of these differences becomes apparent only when a *group* of individuals is challenged, as by the administration of a drug. The graded dose-effect curve, constructed from data relating intensity of response to drug dosage in a single or average individual, obscures the biologic variation. The quantal curve, made up of the all-or-none responses of single individuals, readily discloses the variability that normally exists within a seemingly uniform group.

It is not surprising that there is wide variation in the quantity of a drug required to produce a given response in a group of test subjects. Rather, it is to be expected in view of the innate complexity of the biologic system and the many intercoupled processes involved in getting a drug to and from its site(s) of action. In Chapter 9 we shall discuss in some detail the more important factors known to contribute to and account for biologic variation. For the variables that may affect drug response in individuals must be taken into account if drugs are to be used successfully as therapeutic agents. But even though individuals are not alike in their response to drugs and may require personalized adjustment of dosage, general guidelines for the intelligent use of any drug are still needed. The methods devised to quantitate the phenomenon of pharmacologic variation provide these guidelines and help to minimize errors of prediction.

Concepts Statistically Derived from the Quantal Dose-Effect Curve

It is never possible to examine an infinitely large group of subjects experimentally. To obtain the desired information, we must resort to studying samples taken from the population — the collection of items defined by a common characteristic. Then, with the use of appropriate statistics, we can reach general conclusions from the fragmentary data. Since the doses for quantal responses to drugs are so often distributed normally, the statistical procedures applicable to the normal curve can also be applied to the quantal dose-response curve.

The normal distribution curve (see Fig. 7-10) extends to infinity in both directions, never quite reaching zero. Theoretically, this means that a few individuals will respond to infinitely low doses, whereas a few others will have infinitely high thresholds. In actual experiments, finite minimal and maximal threshold doses are determined. But the true shape of the normal curve warns that wide extremes of responsiveness, or lack of responsiveness, may be encountered when a drug is administered to many individuals. Important as this point is, neither the minimally nor the maximally effective dose is a characteristic which can be used to distinguish different populations from each other. These extremes in response are not representative of the group of values but depend on the size of the population measured. Inspection of the normal distribution curve shows, however, that most responses tend to cluster around a central value. This measure, or parameter, of central tendency is the *median*, the value on the abscissa which bisects the area of the curve so that 50 per cent of the population lies on either side of the midpoint. The median is an average, a representative and distinguishing characteristic of a frequency distribution which is unaffected by the few values at the extremes of the curve. For the quantal dose-effect curve this average is the *median effective dose,* abbreviated ED50; it is the smallest dose required to produce a stated effect in 50 per cent of the population. For the distribution shown in Figure 7-10, the ED50 is 200 units. When death is the response, the ED50 is termed the *median lethal dose,* or LD50. The median effective dose can also be designated as the median analgesic dose, AD50, or the median convulsive dose, CD50, or as the median of any other stated response.

Even though the great majority of responses do not differ very much from the median, it is obvious that a number of responses are markedly different from this average value. So, to characterize a frequency distribution curve fully, we need more than the median; we also need a measure of the range of variability about this average value so that we can determine the spread of the population on either side. The most useful measure of variability, or dispersion, of the normal distribution curve is the **standard deviation** (or *root-mean-square deviation*). Unlike the median, which is calculated only from the *number* of individuals in the sample, the standard deviation takes into account all the individual values, even those at the extremes, since its calculation is based on the difference of each observation from the mean value. The standard deviation and the median are the only two parameters needed to describe completely any normal distribution curve. Although the standard deviation is a little difficult to calculate, it is readily visualized: it is the distance along the abscissa from the median to the steepest point of the curve, the point of inflection. In Figure 7-10 the vertical dotted lines A and A' correspond to 1 standard deviation (SD) on either side of the median.

What is the significance of the standard deviation and how can it be used to determine the dispersion of the population about the median? The standard deviation tells us what fraction of all the measurements will be found within this specified distance. The area under the curve enclosed by one standard deviation on either side of the median represents about 68 per cent of the total area enclosed by the whole distribution curve. Therefore, we would find that we make little error in assuming for drug X on Figure 7-10 that about two-thirds of the total number of individuals tested would respond to doses no lower than 190 and no higher than 210 units, i.e., the ED50 ± 1 SD.[2]

If we mark off along the abscissa a distance equivalent to 2 standard deviations on either side of the median (dashed lines B and B'), we find that about 95 per cent of the total distribution lies within these limits; less than 1 per cent of the distribution lies more than 3 standard deviations away from the median (dashed lines C and C'). Thus, for the data in Figure 7-10, almost all measurements lie between 170 and 230.

This is a rough rule, of course. But if the distribution is a reasonably symmetric

[2] Obviously, the number of individuals capable of responding to doses lower than 190 units would also be capable of responding to doses lying between 190 and 210 units.

bell-shaped curve, these measures of central tendency and dispersion have great practicality. Even when the distribution is not normally spread on an arithmetic, abscissal scale, it frequently can be changed mathematically to units that are normally distributed — by using a logarithmic scale on the abscissa, for instance. Hence, knowing merely the median and the standard deviation, we have a broad picture of the whole distribution; we know the dose which would be expected to produce the stated effect in 50 per cent of the individuals tested, and we know the range of doses which may be needed to ensure a response in two-thirds of the individuals or in almost all the individuals.

Although the bell-shaped curve provides adequate information concerning the average response to a drug and the individual variation within a group of subjects, the data are more conveniently handled when other graphic representations are employed. A conventional method of doing this is to plot the data in the form of a curve relating the dose of the drug to the cumulative percentage of subjects showing the response. To represent the data of Figure 7-9 in this way, we first take the number of individuals responding to any given dose and convert this figure to a percentage of the total number tested. We then plot at each dose level the total percentage of animals responding to that dose and to *all lower doses*. By repeating this summation for every dose level studied, we arrive at the S-shaped, or sigmoid, curve shown in

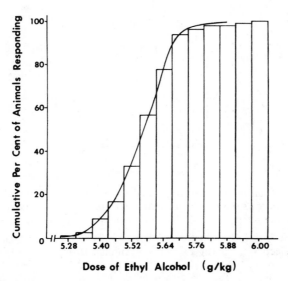

Dose of Ethyl Alcohol (g/kg)

FIGURE 7-11. Quantal dose-response curve (summation of the frequency histogram, Fig. 7-9). Every bar of Figure 7-9 is added to all preceding bars as dose is increased. The total number of animals responding at each dose and to those below is converted to per cent of total animals (130). The curve is drawn through the midpoints of the summated bars. For example, a total of 21 rats, or 16.2 per cent of the total, died by the time the fourth dose was administered. At the fifth dose — 5.52 g per kilogram — 22 more died, giving a total of 43 rats, or 33.1 per cent of the total number.

Figure 7-11.[3] This curve resembles the graded dose-effect curve shown in Figure 7-2. But it should be remembered that the graded curve expresses the relationship between change in effect and change in dose, whereas the quantal curve provides a measure of the variation in threshold dose needed to produce a stated effect in a group of subjects.

When drugs are being tested in the laboratory for their effectiveness and propensity to produce toxic or undesirable effects, it is too costly and inefficient to determine the individual minimally effective dose for each animal. In practice the test animals are divided into a number of groups of equal size, and each member of a single group is given the same preselected dose, but different groups receive different doses. The animals responding to a given dose will be those of the group for which the dose is threshold or *above* threshold; the number of animals responding in each

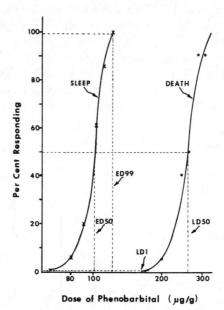

Dose of Phenobarbital (µg/g)

FIGURE 7-12. Quantal dose-response curves representing the cumulative number of animals responding as the dose is increased. Groups of 20 mice were injected with different doses of phenobarbital. The following results were obtained:

% Animals Asleep	Dose (µg/g)	% Animals Dead	Dose (µg/g)
5	80	5	200
20	90	15	220
60	103	40	240
85	110	50	260
100	120	90	280
		90	300

[3]Methods of transforming the quantal dose-response curves to straight lines are given in the Glossary under the heading **normal equivalent deviation.**

group will increase with increasing size of dose. For example, the data in Figure 7-12 were obtained by administering phenobarbital to eleven groups of twenty mice, each group receiving a different dose. Loss of the righting reflex was taken as the indication that an animal was asleep, and cessation of respiration, that an animal was dead. The number of animals responding at each dose level was recorded. When the percentage of animals responding was plotted against the corresponding dose level, S-shaped curves were obtained just like those for the distribution of the threshold doses of individual animals in the groups. The reason for this, of course, is that in both methods, any dose along the curve gives the percentage of animals responding to that dose and to all lower doses.

The statistical methods applicable to the quantal dose-effect curve can also be applied to the graded type of response if the measured response is made all-or-none. To do this, an arbitrary intensity of effect is selected and the response is called positive whenever the threshold or level is either reached or exceeded. For example, a 40 to 50 per cent reduction in heart rate might be used as the criterion of therapeutic response to a drug which slows the heart beat (Fig. 7-13). In the same manner, any effect of a drug may be treated as a quantal response.

Evaluation of Drug Safety

The data in Figure 7-12 are for a single agent administered in various doses to groups of animals of the same species. As dose was increased, two separate curves were obtained, one for the hypnotic effect of the barbiturate and one for its lethal effect. These curves illustrate an important principle of pharmacology: there is no *single* dose-response relationship that can adequately characterize a drug in terms of its full spectrum of activity. The ideal drug would produce its desired effect — its therapeutically useful effect — in all biologic systems without inducing any side-effect, i.e., an effect other than that for which the drug is administered. But there is no ideal drug. Most drugs produce many effects, and *all* drugs produce at least two effects. And it is also a truism that no chemical agent can be considered entirely safe. For any drug, there is some dose that will produce a *toxic effect* — one deleterious to the subject or even life-threatening.

Given the fact that any chemical can be expected to produce toxic effects, the risks entailed in its use must be weighed against its effectiveness before it can be considered a salutary agent. In Chapter 11 we will discuss the specific ways in which the use of drugs may be harmful. At this point, we shall consider only the general principles involved in the quantitative evaluation of drug safety.

The safety of a drug depends on the degree of separation between the doses producing a desirable effect and the doses at which adverse effects are elicited. Since both the therapeutic and undesirable effects of a drug can be characterized by quantal dose-response curves, we can use these curves to obtain a statement of the margin of safety of the drug. For example, we can calculate the median lethal dose and the median therapeutic dose and express these as a fraction. Such an expression is known as a *therapeutic ratio*. The LD50/ED50 for the data in Figure 7-12 is about 2.6. This ratio tells us that about two and one-half times as much barbiturate is required to

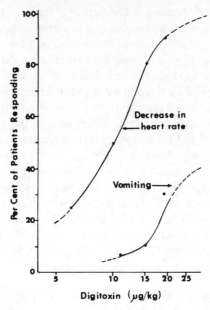

FIGURE 7-13. Quantal dose-response curve of a graded response. Ten patients with cardiac irregularities were given a single oral dose of digitoxin at intervals of one week. The desired response was made quantal by determining the dose that produced a 40 to 50 per cent decrease in heart rate. The undesired effects were nausea and vomiting. The curve at the left shows the per cent of patients responding with the desired effect, and that at the right, with the undesired effect (dashed curves indicate theoretical responses to doses above and below those actually used). The overlap of the curves is so great that even at ED50, a few patients would be expected to show an adverse effect. For individual patients this type of relationship may be even more critical. For example, one patient required 15 mg per kilogram of body weight for the desired effect and vomited at a dose of 18 mg per kilogram, an increase in dose of only 20 per cent. (Redrawn from D. F. Marsh,
Outline of Fundamental Pharmacology, *1951. Courtesy of Charles C. Thomas, Publisher, Springfield, Illinois.)*

produce a lethal effect in 50 per cent of the animals as is needed to induce sleep in the same proportion of animals.

The aim of drug therapy, however, is *to achieve the desired therapeutic effect in all individuals without the risk of producing a hazardous effect in any.* Obviously, a measure of drug safety based on the doses at the lowest toxic and highest therapeutic levels of response, such as LD1/ED99, is more realistic and more consistent with this aim than is the ratio LD50/ED50. Even the term applied to the therapeutic ratio LD1/ED99 connotes this idea of relative safety; it is called the *certain safety factor* (CSF). The CSF for phenobarbital is about 1.34 (Fig. 7-12). A CSF greater than 1.0 indicates that the dose effective in 99 per cent of the population is less than that which would be lethal in 1 per cent of the population. A CSF less than unity is indicative of overlap between the maximally effective and minimally toxic doses.

An alternate expression of drug safety, the *standard safety margin,* is also calculated from the extremes of the quantal dose-response curves. The standard safety
margin has the dimension of per cent; it is the percentage by which the ED99 has to
be increased before the LD1 is reached:

$$\text{Standard safety margin} = \frac{\text{LD1} - \text{ED99}}{\text{ED99}} \times 100$$

Thus the dose of phenobarbital which is predicted to be effective in all but 1 per cent
of individuals needs to be increased by 34 per cent before the drug would be lethal
to 1 per cent of the population.

We saw earlier that the values at the ends of the dose-effect curve depend on the
size of the population being measured. These values are less precise than the median
dose, which is derived independently of the number of observations and is unaffected
by the extremes. However, the advantages of using measures of drug safety based on
the LD1/ED99 far outweigh the imprecision of this ratio. This can be more fully
appreciated when we examine how the interpretation of therapeutic indices is affected
by the slopes of the dose-response curves.

Let us first consider the case in which the curves for desirable and undesirable effects
parallel each other, as illustrated in Figure 7-14 for phenobarbital (Ph) and drug A.

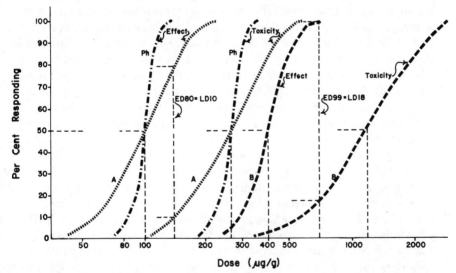

*FIGURE 7-14. Quantal dose-response curves for effect and toxicity of pheno-
barbital (Ph), drug A and drug B. The ordinate represents the per cent of animals
responding and the abscissa shows dose (μg per gram of body weight) on a logarithmic scale. Groups of 20 mice were injected with different doses of each of the three
drugs. The responses observed were loss of righting reflex (effect) and cessation of
respiration (toxicity). The LD50/ED50 of phenobarbital and drug A is 2.6; the
LD50/ED50 of drug B is 3.0.*

Theoretically, this would be the relationship whenever the lethal or toxic effects are a continuation, or the result of a continuation, of the therapeutic effect. If the therapeutic ratio LD50/ED50 were the criterion of drug safety, drug A and pheno-barbital would be judged equally safe since this ratio is numerically the same for both drugs. An entirely different evaluation of relative safety is reached, however, if we compare these agents on the basis of their respective CSF's. The slopes of the curves for phenobarbital are sufficiently steep that there is a separation between the maximally effective dose and the minimally toxic dose. This margin of safety of phenobarbital is denoted by a CSF greater than 1.0. The slopes of the dose-response curves for drug A are much flatter than those for the barbiturate. As a consequence, the efficacy of drug A overlaps its toxicity. For example, the dose of Drug A effective in 99 per cent of the population corresponds to the dose at which toxicity may be anticipated in 30 per cent of the individuals. Even at a dose effective in 80 per cent of the population, 10 per cent may show toxicity. When the CSF for drug A is calculated, it is found to be far less than unity, and its standard safety margin has a negative value. Thus, when the safety of drug A is measured by methods utilizing the extremes of the dose-response curves, drug A is shown to be not at all safe.

Death or toxicity may result from any of several mechanisms unrelated to that producing the desired effect. In this event the dose-response curves usually do not parallel each other, and the ratio between efficacy and toxicity is different at different levels of responses. The curves for drug B in Figure 7-14 illustrate the situation when the slope of the toxicity curve is flatter than that for the therapeutic effect. Again, whereas the ratio derived from the median doses is rather large, this index is misleading and gives a false assessment of the relative safety of the drug. Thus, for considerations of drug safety it is not enough to know only how the median doses are related. What must be known as well is how the *slopes* of the curves are related, and this is reflected by the ratio LD1/ED99. Whether or not the curve for toxicity parallels that for efficacy, the flatter the curves, the greater the likelihood of undesirable effects occurring within the therapeutic range of doses, and the smaller the value of the CSF.

It was previously pointed out that whereas all drugs are capable of eliciting at least two responses, most drugs can and do produce many more effects. Since almost all drug effects are dose-dependent, the methods used to relate mortality and efficacy can also be employed in assessing the relationship between the desired effect and any other effect. Thus a drug may have as many therapeutic indices as it has side-effects.

Some side-effects, such as nausea or dizziness, although therapeutically useless, may be merely unpleasant and uncomfortable. Even when the dose-response curves for such nontoxic effects fall well within the range of therapeutic doses, this does not ordinarily become a deterrent to the use of the drug. For example, the use of digi-toxin or other digitalis preparations is frequently associated with nausea and vomiting, as would be anticipated from the large overlap in the curves for desired and undesired effects (Fig. 7-13). The appearance of these unpleasant effects is taken as the criterion of the beginning of toxicity when digitoxin dosage is being adjusted for a particular patient. However, the great therapeutic value of digitalis and its con-

geners, and the lack of any other drug with a wider margin of safety, amply justify
their continued use. But there are other side-effects of drugs which, though not
necessarily lethal, may nevertheless seriously impair normal function. The gastrointestinal bleeding sometimes associated with the use of aspirin in the treatment of
rheumatic fever and the hearing deficit occasionally induced by the antibiotic streptomycin are cases in point. Whether a drug with unavoidable toxic effects is safe
enough to be used under any conditions depends on the availability of safer drugs
and the prognosis were the drug to be withheld. Judgments of therapeutic usefulness can be made only when the severity of the illness and the potential benefit of
the drug are weighed against the risks of serious toxicity. For example, most anticancer drugs are highly toxic since they affect rapidly growing normal cells as well
as cancer cells; but the nature of the disease warrants drug treatment despite the
many adverse effects the drug may cause.

THE SELECTIVITY OF DRUG ACTION
In our discussions of drug-receptor interactions we indicated that the majority of
drugs show a remarkable degree of selectivity. They act at some sites to produce
their characteristic effect, whereas their presence at other cells, tissues or organs does
not lead to any measurable response. How can this be reconciled with the statement
that most drugs produce many effects? The fact that a drug may produce a multiplicity of effects does not contradict the earlier statement about selectivity. Nor does
this fact challenge the receptor concept of the specificity of drug action, i.e., that
interactions occur only when the chemical structure and configuration of drug and
receptor are complementary. On the contrary, the dose-effect relationships help to
clarify what is meant by selectivity and specificity of drug action.

First of all, let us consider how, within the framework of receptor theory, a drug
can produce more than one effect and still be a special key fitting only a specific,
preexisting lock. The answer is actually very simple: a specific receptor may be
located at more than one site in the intact organism. At each site, the response trig-
gered by the combination of the drug with the specific biologic entity is observed as
an alteration in the physiologic function of that particular anatomic region. Let us
take the acetylcholine receptor, for example. Earlier in this chapter we saw that the
muscles of the isolated small intestine contract in response to acetylcholine. Atropine
inhibits this contractile response by competing with acetylcholine for receptor sites.
The acetylcholine receptor, however, is widely distributed and is present in many
tissues and organs in addition to the intestinal muscle (cf. Chap. 13, Drugs Affecting
the Autonomic Nervous System). Thus, when atropine is administered orally or parenterally so that it can be distributed throughout the body, many other effects of
its inhibitory activity at the acetylcholine receptor become evident. In the stomach,
the effect of atropine is to decrease the hydrochloric acid secreted in response to
acetylcholine. In the oral mucosa, the action of atropine leads to the production of
"dry mouth" by interfering with the flow of saliva stimulated by acetylcholine. In
the eye the antagonistic effect of atropine is observed as an increase in the diameter
of the pupil. Yet atropine is a very *specific* drug — it antagonizes only the actions

of acetylcholine or drugs that closely resemble acetylcholine. The several effects produced by atropine are the consequence of a *single mechanism of action* but a multiplicity of sites where this action is manifest.

The spectrum of effects produced by the antihistaminic drug diphenhydramine contrasts sharply with that of atropine. As Figure 7-7 indicates, diphenhydramine can competitively antagonize the effects of histamine by vying with the agonist for binding sites on the receptor. Histamine receptors, like those for acetylcholine, are widely distributed, so that many effects result from the antihistaminic action of diphenhydramine, e.g., prevention of the vasodilator activity of histamine on small blood vessels or antagonism of the constrictor action of histamine on smooth muscles of the respiratory tract. The action of diphenhydramine is not limited, however, to histamine receptors. Because of structural similarities to atropine, diphenhydramine can also antagonize the actions of acetylcholine and produce many of the effects of atropine. Diphenhydramine also exhibits local anesthetic activity like that of procaine and, by other actions in the central nervous system, produces a state of somnolence. Diphenhydramine is a *nonspecific* drug — not because it produces many effects, but because the effects it produces are the consequence of *more than one mechanism of action.*

We may well ask, then, why is diphenhydramine called an antihistaminic drug? The answer to this question clarifies what we mean by selectivity of drug action. A drug is usually described by its most characteristic effect or by the action thought to be responsible for the effect. From a consideration of the dose-effect relationship, the most characteristic or prominent effect is the one produced at doses *lower* than those required to elicit other responses. A drug is considered *selective* when the effect for which it is being administered can be produced in nearly all individuals at doses which produce its other effects in only a few individuals. Thus, selectivity of drug action is measured by the therapeutic indices — certain safety factor or standard safety margin. Since diphenhydramine is called an antihistaminic drug, we anticipate that the curve for its antihistaminic activity would lie to the left of curves for all its other effects. This is indeed the case. But diphenhydramine is not an especially selective drug: there is a great deal of overlap between the curve for histamine antagonism and those for other effects. In particular, the overlap of the curve for the desired effect and that for drowsiness is so great that this side-effect would be expected to occur in large segment of the population receiving the drug; calculation of the standard safety margin with respect to inhibition of salivation also yields a relatively large negative value.

Clinically, diphenhydramine causes somnolence in about half of those who take the drug, and about one in four persons also experiences other side-effects like dry mouth. Whereas the occurrence of dry mouth would be a nuisance, the drowsiness so often encountered might be a desirable, adjunctive effect in patients about to retire for the night. If an individual had to remain alert in order to operate an automobile, however, sleepiness would be an undesirable accompaniment of therapy. In any case, although diphenhydramine is a very useful antihistaminic agent, it is neither a specific nor a selective drug.

Although atropine is a specific drug, it too is not selective; inhibition of the action of acetylcholine at a number of different sites is produced by about the same dose of the antagonist. For example, if atropine were administered to decrease gastric acidity, dry mouth would be expected to occur almost routinely as a side-effect of therapy. In contrast, the pharmacologic effects of heparin are almost entirely confined to the blood and, as such, are both specific and selective. We have mentioned previously that heparin prevents the coagulation of blood by combining with macromolecules essential to this process. Its toxic effect is the result of a continuation of its therapeutic effect — too much anticoagulant activity leading to spontaneous bleeding. The limitation in the number of effects heparin may produce is related to the fact that the biologic entity with which heparin combines has a limited physiologic role and anatomic distribution.

The choice of the route of drug administration may sometimes confer selectivity of action on a drug that is ordinarily nonselective. For example, if the ophthalmologist applies atropine directly to the surface of the eye in order to dilate the pupil, the other pharmacologic effects of atropine may be largely averted. The quantity administered to achieve the local effect on the pupil is usually too small to yield a concentration, after absorption, that would be sufficient to elicit responses at sites other than the eye.

Differences in distribution of drug within the intact organism can also make one drug more selective than another acting by the same mechanism. This type of selectivity usually results from differences in an agent's ability to traverse certain biologic barriers. Drugs with structures similar to atropine (some of the quaternary ammonium compounds referred to previously) are examples of chemicals with selectivity of action through selective biologic permeability. These atropine-like compounds may decrease gastric acidity or salivary secretions or have effects similar to atropine on the eye and the small intestine. However, the water-soluble quaternary ammonium compounds do not traverse the so-called blood-brain barrier as readily as does lipid-soluble atropine. Consequently, when administered at sites outside the central nervous system, the quaternary ammonium compounds, unlike atropine, do not have activity within the brain. Atropine and the atropine-like quaternary ammonium compounds combine specifically with the acetylcholine receptor, but the latter drugs show fewer effects than atropine because they cannot reach as many receptor sites.

Very few drugs are as selective as heparin. And not all drugs that produce multiple effects are as specific as atropine — more than one mechanism of action may be involved. But it is clear that selectivity and specificity are the most important characteristics of a drug in determining its therapeutic usefulness. The greater the selectivity and specificity, the less the likelihood of undesirable effects and the greater the margin of safety.

SYNOPSIS

One of the most fundamental principles of pharmacology states that the intensity of response elicited by a drug is a function of the dose administered. In one sense we can take this to mean simply that as the dose of a drug is increased, the magnitude of effect is also increased. Or we can say that as the dose of a drug is increased, the number or proportion of individuals exhibiting a particular, stated response is also increased. These two fundamental relationships between dose and response have been termed *graded* and *quantal,* respectively. The graded and quantal dose-response relationships are examined by different techniques, and each type provides different information about the quantitative aspects of drug action. Both types can be clearly and precisely defined with the use of special descriptive forms called *dose-effect* or *dose-response* curves, which are graphic representations of mathematical expressions.

The graded response is examined by administering increasing amounts of drug to a single subject, or to a specific organ or tissue. As dose is increased, the pharmacologic response increases in a continuous fashion, first in large and then in progressively smaller increments, until additional increases in dose elicit no further increase in effect.

The graphic representation of the typical relationship between graded response and dose takes the form of a hyperbola with concavity downward when effect (the dependent variable) and dose (the independent variable) are expressed in arithmetic units. When the units of measure of either the dose or the response, or both, are transformed mathematically from arithmetic units to other units, the form of the curve is also altered. In the transformation most frequently used, the dose is changed to the logarithm of the dose or, alternatively, the abscissal scale is made logarithmic. Such a transformation converts the hyperbola into an S-shaped curve with a central segment that is practically linear. The midpoint of the log dose-effect curve is identified with the dose at which 50 per cent of the maximum response is elicited. Drugs that produce similar effects by acting at the same receptor generally have similarly shaped log dose-effect curves with the same maximum. Their linear middle segments also are usually parallel.

The receptor concept and the reversibility of drug-receptor interaction permit us to explain the graded type of dose-effect relationship on the basis of the laws governing chemical equilibrium. In the drug-receptor reaction, the reacting substances are the drug and the unoccupied receptors and the product is the drug-receptor complex. However, in order to apply the law of mass action to the dose-response phenomenon, two important assumptions are made. First, the drug response is directly proportional to the percentage of the total receptors occupied by the drug, so that the latter is estimated in terms of the response observed. Second, the amount of drug combined with receptors is negligible, and thus the concentration of free drug remains essentially unchanged during the reaction. At equilibrium (the point at which the response to a given concentration of drug has attained its full level), the percentage of total occupied receptors is proportional to the product of the drug concentration times the percentage of unoccupied receptors. The drug concentration does not change during the reaction; only the proportion of free and occupied receptors changes. This means, then, that the ratio of the percentage of occupied receptors to that of unoccupied receptors is proportional to the dose of drug administered. The mathematical expression of this statement is the equation for a hyperbola. It is thus possible to explain the graded dose-response relationship in terms of the percentage of total receptors occupied; a maximum response would be equivalent to 100 per cent occupancy of receptors.

From the mass action interpretation of dose-effect curves, it follows that when several drugs acting at the same receptor produce effects of equal magnitude, the percentage of total receptors occupied must be the same for each drug. It does not follow, however, that equal concentrations of each drug at the receptor lead to effects of equal intensity. The intensity of effect produced is *directly* proportional to the percentage of total receptors occupied by a drug. But the percentage of the total receptors occupied by a drug is a function of drug concentration as well as of the drug's ability to combine with its receptor. The ability of a given drug to combine with a particular receptor is a constant; it is known as the *affinity* constant. Different drugs have different affinities for the same receptor site. The concentration of drug needed to produce a stated intensity of effect at a given receptor varies inversely with its affinity. Therefore, to produce effects of equal intensity requires a lower concentration of a drug with a higher affinity than of a drug with a lesser affinity. And it follows that the position of the log dose-effect curve on the abscissa reflects the affinity of a drug for its receptor, i.e., the greater the affinity, the closer the curve to the ordinate.

The positions of the dose-effect curves of several drugs along the abscissa also provide an expression of the relative potencies of the drugs — potency being the dose of a drug required to produce a standard effect. The closer the dose-effect curve to the ordinate, the smaller the dose required to produce a given effect and the more potent the drug. Only drugs that act at the same group of receptors and that are capable of eliciting the same maximal response can be compared with respect to potency. However, potency is determined only in part by a drug's affinity for the receptor; it is also influenced by absorption, distribution, biotransformation and excretion, the factors that determine how much drug will reach the receptor. The potency of a drug tells us nothing about its effectiveness or safety and is, therefore, a relatively unimportant characteristic.

Drugs are called antagonists when they interact with a receptor and produce no response of their own but impair the receptor's capacity to combine with an active drug — an agonist. The effect is a reduction in the apparent affinity of the agonist for its receptor. An antagonist is said to be competitive when its inhibitory effects can be surmounted by excess agonist. In this type of antagonism there is parallel displacement of the log dose-effect curve to the right but no change in the maximum. An antagonist is said to be noncompetitive when it does not compete with the agonist for the same sites on the receptor but inactivates the receptor in such a way as to prevent its effective combination with an agonist. Noncompetitive antagonists cannot be displaced by excess agonist. As a consequence the log dose-effect curve will still be shifted to the right, but the maximum response will be lower, reflecting the inability of agonist to attain 100 per cent receptor occupancy in the presence of the antagonist.

The graded curve gives us information about the dose required to produce a specified intensity of effect in an individual. But individuals are not alike; each is the product of his inheritance and the environmental conditions to which he has been exposed from conception. Since the general principles of pharmacology are formulated for the "average" but hypothetical person, we need some means of evaluating the "average" dose-response relationship that will be representative of a group of individual values. We also need to know the variability about this average, so that we can get a broad picture of the relationship between dose and effect among all individuals. The quantal dose-response relationship provides this information.

The concept of averageness indicates a tendency for a group or "sample" of items to distribute themselves equally on both sides of a dividing line. To determine this central value dividing the sample into two groups of equal numbers requires the enumeration of all the individual values of the sample and then the calculation of the point of equal division – the *median*. Thus the quantal dose-response relationship is determined by noting the *frequency* with which any dose of a drug evokes a stated, fixed (all-or-none) pharmacologic effect. The quantal curve describes the distribution of minimal (or threshold) doses that produce a predetermined effect in a population of individual organisms. The median of the quantal curve is the dose at which 50 per cent of the population manifests the given effect and 50 per cent does not. Hence the term *median effective dose,* ED50, or *median lethal dose,* LD50, is used to express the smallest dose required to produce the stated or lethal effect, respectively, in 50 per cent of the population.

The quantal dose-effect curve takes on a bell shape like that of the normal distribution when the frequency of occurrence of threshold doses is plotted against the actual doses needed to elicit the stated quantal response. This means that, whereas the great majority of individual effective doses differ relatively little from the median, very marked departures from the median dose are not at all infrequent. In order to measure this variability about the average value in the most meaningful way, we use the parameter *standard deviation.* We find, with very little error, that about two-thirds of the population responds to doses lying no lower than 1 standard deviation below and no higher than 1 standard deviation above the median. About 95 per cent of the distribution lies less than 2 standard deviations away from the median, and less than 1 per cent of the total population lies beyond 3 standard deviations from the median.

The quantal dose-response curve takes on an S shape when the number of individuals responding at each dose level is integrated from the lowest to the highest doses. This cumulative curve can be more conveniently used for the analysis of data, such as in the assessment of drug safety or drug selectivity.

Every drug has at least two quantal dose-response curves, one for the desired therapeutic effect and one for a toxic effect. It is imperative, then, to assess the relative safety of a drug in terms of its potential danger relative to its potential usefulness. An approximate statement of relative safety may be obtained by comparing the LD50 with the ED50. The larger the ratio of this therapeutic index, the greater the relative safety. However, this index alone is not sufficient for a true assessment of drug safety, since median doses tell nothing about the slopes of the dose-response curves for therapeutic and toxic effects. If the slopes are flat, there may be a great deal of overlap between the curves even when the median doses are widely separated. Since the aim in therapy is to achieve a salutary response in 100 per cent of the patients and a toxic effect in none, drug safety can be better assessed by using a ratio derived from the extremes of the respective quantal curves, such as LD1/ED99. This ratio is known as the certain safety factor (CSF). Another useful measure of safety is the standard safety margin: the percentage increase in the ED99 (the dose effective in 99 per cent of the population) needed to produce a lethal or toxic effect in 1 per cent of the population.

Few drugs are so specific that they manifest only two effects. Most drugs have many effects and thus many dose-effect curves. If all the effects produced by a single drug are due to a single mechanism of action, then the drug is still said to be specific. If the effects are due to several mechanisms of action, the drug is nonspecific. However, a drug's selectivity depends on its capacity to produce one particular effect in preference to others — to act in lower doses at one site than those required to produce effects at other sites. Thus the relationship of the curves for different effects of a single drug determines its selectivity. Selectivity can be measured by the same ratios used to assess drug safety, and these indices may express selectivity of drug action with respect to two potentially beneficial or two potentially toxic effects. Certainly, selectivity of action is one of the more important characteristics of a drug.

GUIDES FOR STUDY AND REVIEW

What factors determine how much of the quantity of drug administered reaches a site of action? How does one go about studying the relationship between the dose of drug administered and the magnitude of effect produced?

What are dose-response curves? In dose-response curves what is the independent variable? the dependent variable? By convention, on which scale is each of these variables plotted? What is the typical form of the curve representing the relationship between graded response and dose when both variables are plotted on an arithmetic scale? What is the typical shape of the curve when the dose is expressed on a logarithmic scale? What are the advantages of using semilogarithmic graphic representations of dose-effect relationships?

How does the graded dose-effect relationship differ from the quantal dose-response relationship? How is each type of dose-response relationship examined? What information does the graded dose-effect relationship give us? the quantal dose-response relationship?

How can you explain the graded type of dose-effect relationship in terms of the laws governing chemical equilibrium? In the drug-receptor interaction what are the reacting substances? what is the product? What assumptions must be made about a drug-receptor interaction in order to apply the law of mass action?

How are the dose-effect curves of two drugs related to one another when the two drugs produce the same pharmacologic response by acting at the same receptor? What can you infer about the mechanisms of action of two drugs that elicit qualitatively similar pharmacologic responses but which have nonparallel log dose-effect curves?

What is the magnitude of the effect produced by a drug when it occupies 100 per cent of its receptor? According to the mass action interpretation, when two drugs acting at the same receptor produce effects of equal magnitude, what must be true about the total receptors occupied by each drug?

When two drugs produce the same response by the same mechanism, what determines the concentration of each drug that is required to produce effects of equal intensity? What is the relationship between affinity and concentration of drug needed to produce a stated intensity of effect at a given receptor? How can apparent and relative affinities be determined from log dose-effect curves?

How is potency defined? How does potency differ from affinity? How can the relative potencies of several drugs be determined from their log dose-effect curves?

What is an antagonist? an agonist? How can a competitive antagonist be distinguished from a noncompetitive antagonist? How does the log dose-effect curve of an agonist in the absence of an antagonist compare with its log dose-effect curve in the presence of a competitive antagonist? in the presence of a noncompetitive antagonist? How is the maximum response of an agonist affected by a competitive antagonist? a noncompetitive antagonist?

How do you define median? What is a median effective dose? an ED50? an LD50? What is a threshold dose?

What is the shape of the quantal dose-response curve when the frequency of occurrence of threshold doses is plotted against the actual dose needed to elicit the stated quantal response? when the number of individuals responding at each dose level is integrated from the lowest to the highest doses?

How do you define standard deviation? What does the standard deviation tell you about the variability of a population? What percentage of a population is included within 1 standard deviation on either side of the median? within 2 standard deviations on either side of the median? 3?

What is the term given to the ratio LD50/ED50? What does this ratio tell you about the relative safety of a drug? Does this ratio given any indication of the relative slopes of the dose-response curves for therapeutic and toxic effects? Why is knowledge of the relative slopes of the curves for therapeutic and toxic effects important for the assessment of the safety of a drug? What expressions of drug safety are more realistic and consistent with the aim of drug therapy? How do you calculate the certain safety factor (CSF)? the standard safety margin? How are these measures useful in evaluating the relationship between therapeutic effect and any other effect of a drug?

What is meant by "specificity" of drug action? by "selectivity" of drug action? How is selectivity of drug action assessed? How does selectivity determine the therapeutic use and usefulness of a drug?

SUGGESTED READING

Ariens, A.J. *Molecular Pharmacology: The Mode of Action of Biologically Active Compounds,* Vol. 1. New York: Academic, 1964.

Clark, A.J.   *The Mode of Action of Drugs on Cells.* London: Arnold, 1933.

Finney, D.J.   *Statistical Methods in Biological Assay,* 2d ed. London: Griffin, 1964.

Gaddum, J.H.   Methods of biological assay depending on a quantal response. *Spec. Rep. Ser. Med. Res. Council* (Lond.) 183:5, 1933.

Gaddum, J.H.   Quantitative and Human Pharmacology. In A.S.V. Burgen and J.F. Mitchell (eds.), *Pharmacology,* 6th ed. London: Oxford University Press, 1968. P. 195.

Goldstein, A. *Biostatistics: An Introductory Text.* New York: Macmillan, 1964.

Litchfield, J.T., Jr., and Wilcoxon, F.   A simplified method of evaluating dose-effect experiments. *J. Pharmacol. Exp. Ther.* 96:99, 1949.

Marsh, D.F.   *Outline of Fundamental Pharmacology.* Springfield, Ill.: Charles C. Thomas, 1951.

Moroney, M.J.   *Facts from Figures.* Harmondsworth, Eng.: Penguin, 1956.

Riggs, D.S.   *The Mathematical Approach to Physiological Problems: A Critical Primer.* Baltimore: Williams & Wilkins, 1963.

8. GENERAL PRINCIPLES OF THE QUANTITATIVE ASPECTS OF DRUG ACTION
II. Time-Response Relationships

It bears repeating that one of the most important principles of pharmacology is that the magnitude of drug effect is a function of the concentration of drug at the site where the action-effect sequence is initiated. As we have seen, the dose administered is a critical factor in determining the intensity of response produced. But the quantity of drug put into the system only delineates the ultimate concentration that can be attained at the site of action. The proportion of the dose actually contributing to the concentration at an active site is the net result of many processes going on simultaneously: (1) the rate and extent of absorption from the site of application; (2) the rate and extent of tissue distribution; (3) the rate of biotransformation to active or inactive metabolites; and (4) the rate of excretion (Fig. 8-1). If we set aside the differences that exist among individuals, it follows that the variability in the intensity of the biologic effects elicited in response to a single dose of an agent must result from variability in absorption, distribution and elimination (biotransformation and excretion).

In order to establish the relationship between the dose administered and the magnitude of drug effect, we had to exclude the other variables which influence concentration at the site of action. We did this by measuring the effect at a particular time — at a point when the concentration at the site was sufficient to produce a minimum, maximum or other preselected level of response. Now we want to determine how factors other than dose are related to the amplitude of drug effect. Since the other factors operating to affect the concentration at a site of action are all rate functions, we can obtain an overall picture of their influence by following the magnitude of drug effect as it changes with time after the administration of a single dose. *Pharmacokinetics* is the term applied to the branch of pharmacology that deals with the factors influencing the magnitude of drug effect by determining the amount of drug at various sites in the body as a function of time.

The time course of drug action can be divided into three distinct phases: (1) the time for onset of action, or latency; (2) the time to peak effect; and (3) the duration of action (Fig. 8-2).

Latency is the time between the administration of a drug and the first measurable

205

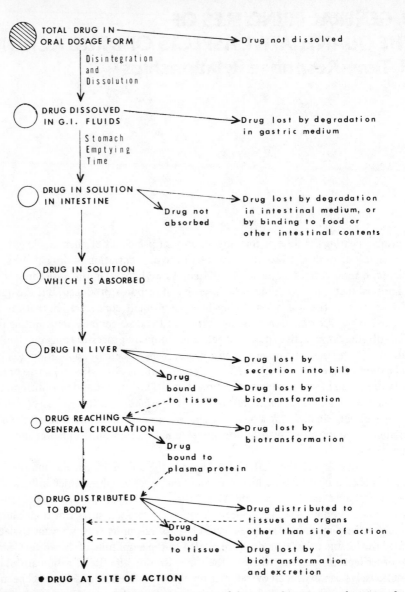

FIGURE 8-1. Factors modifying the quantity of drug reaching a site of action after a single oral dose.

signs of response. Although modified indirectly by the processes of elimination, it is determined largely by the rate of accessibility of the drug to its site of action. This includes the rates of absorption, distribution and localization within the target organ or tissue. The time for onset of action may in some cases include the delay occasioned by the need for biotransformation of the drug from an inactive to an active form.

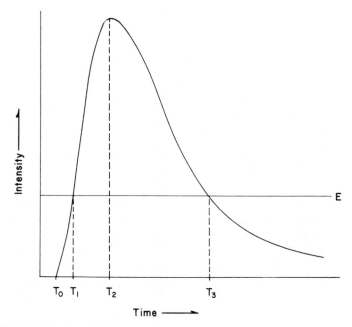

FIGURE 8-2. Intensity of effect as a function of time. Drug administered at Time 0 (T_0). E = minimum level of measurable response; T_0 to T_1 = time for onset of drug effect; T_0 to T_2 = time to peak effect; T_1 to T_3 = duration of action.

The peak effect for most drugs occurs when the drug concentration at a site of action has reached its maximum level. The time needed to reach this point is determined by the balance between the rate processes operating to get the drug to its site of action and those responsible for removing the agent from the site and from the body.

The duration of action of a drug extends from the time of onset of an effect to the time when the response is no longer perceptible. This phase of the temporal course of drug action is affected primarily by the rates of the elimination processes but is also modified by continuing absorption from the site of administration. In addition, compensating physiologic reflexes set in motion by the response to the drug itself may contribute to the termination of drug effect. (For example, nitroglycerin used in the treatment of coronary artery disease produces a fall in blood pressure. This fall induces compensatory reflexes which attempt to correct the disturbance and return the blood pressure to normal levels.)

The time course of drug action is frequently studied by correlating the amplitude of effect with the concentration of drug present in the blood at various times after administration. We have seen that the blood circulation occupies a central position with regard to absorption, distribution and excretion. A drug is absorbed from its site of administration (or administered directly) into the blood before it is distributed to the organs and tissues; and in the process of excretion, the movement of drug occurs in the reverse direction. The conventional use of blood levels as the correlates of intensity of drug effect is based on the assumption that the concentration of a drug in the blood is a faithful indicator of its concentration at the site of action. This is indeed the case when the equilibrium between blood and tissues occurs at a rapid rate. But when the movement of a drug from the blood to its site of action is slow, the intensity and duration of effect may not be synchronous with the changes in blood levels. For example, when an anesthetic dose of the poorly lipid-soluble drug phenobarbital is administered intravenously, 10 to 15 minutes elapse before any effects are seen, and anesthesia takes about 30 minutes to appear. During this latency period, the blood level falls rapidly while the concentration of phenobarbital within the brain slowly rises (Fig. 8-3). The time course of the changes in brain concentration coincides with the onset of action, but there is a lack of correspondence between changes in blood levels of phenobarbital and the time course of effects produced. However, for many drugs the changes in concentration in blood *do* mirror the changes in concentration at the effector site, as illustration in Figure 8-4 for the analgesic pentazocine. It is obvious that blood levels of drugs can be conveniently measured in man as well as in experimental animals, whereas drug concentration at sites of action can be determined only in animals, and even then only with much difficulty. We shall use these blood level data, therefore, in some of our considerations of the time course of drug action.

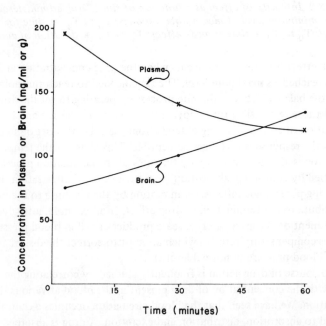

FIGURE 8-3. Plasma and brain concentrations of phenobarbital after intravenous administration to animals. The dose was 100 mg per kilogram. Onset of anesthesia was at 30 minutes after administration. (Data from L. C. Mark et al., J. Pharmacol. Exp. Ther. *123:70, 1958. Copyright © 1958, The Williams & Wilkins Co., Baltimore.)*

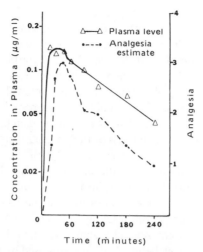

Time (minutes)

FIGURE 8-4. Plasma concentrations of pentazocine and its effect on relief of pain in humans at various times after intramuscular administration of 45 mg per 70 kg of body weight. Pain evaluation or analgesia: 0 = no pain relief; 1 = some relief; 2 = moderate relief; 3 = high degree of relief; 4 = complete relief, or no pain. The results represent the average of eight patients. (Redrawn from A. B. Berkowitz, J. H. Asling, S. M. Shnider and E. L. Way, Relationship of pentazocine plasma levels to pharmacological activity in man. Clin. Pharmacol. Ther. 10:320, 1969.)

We shall begin by examining separately (1) the rate of entry of a drug into the blood circulation, i.e., its rate of absorption into the body; and (2) its rate of elimination from the blood and from the body. We shall then see how the kinetics of the rise and fall in blood levels of a drug affects the duration of action of a single dose of the drug and delineates the frequency with which multiple doses may be given.

RATE OF DRUG ABSORPTION

Most drugs move across biologic barriers in accordance with the principles of passive diffusion and at a rate proportional to the concentration gradient. This means, of course, that as absorption proceeds, the total amount of drug available at the site of administration diminishes and the concentration gradient becomes progressively smaller. Since the rate of diffusion is always proportional to the gradient produced by the amount of drug still to be absorbed, the rate of absorption also decreases with time. The rate of absorption is constant and independent of the amount of drug available for absorption only when facilitated diffusion or active transport is involved, and then only at drug concentrations which saturate the carrier mechanism. At concentrations below saturation, the rates of the specialized transport processes and passive diffusion can be similarly characterized, i.e., *a constant fraction of the total amount of drug present is transported in equal units of time* (cf. pp. 63-67). Thus, most drug absorption follows the kinetics of a *first-order* reaction, a reaction whose velocity is proportional to the concentration of a single reactant (cf. pp. 143-144).

The time course of absorption of phenobarbital (Fig. 8-5) is typical of drugs showing first-order absorption kinetics. These data were obtained by determining the amount of drug remaining in the intestine at various times after administration. If no biotransformation takes place at the site of administration, then the amount of drug which has disappeared from the depot directly represents the amount of drug absorbed. Such techniques of obtaining information about the isolated process of absorption are, by and large, applicable only to experimental animals. However, very good approximations of the rate of drug absorption in man have been made indirectly by mathematical analyses of blood levels of the drug, corrected for the portion lost through elimination.

Although constant-rate absorption is the exception rather than the rule for most drugs, the rate of entry into blood can be made independent of the amount of drug available for absorption. Constant-rate absorption can be achieved whenever the conditions of administration provide a supply or reservoir of drug to replenish the quantity removed from the site. A good example is seen in the special case of the administration of gaseous anesthetics. The apparatus used by the anesthetist con-

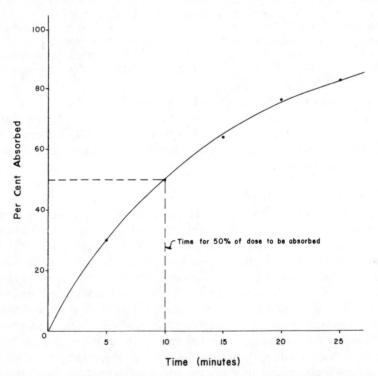

FIGURE 8-5. Absorption of phenobarbital from the small intestine of the rat. Each point on the curve represents the mean absorption in 4 to 6 rats calculated from the amount of drug remaining in the intestine at the end of the particular interval.

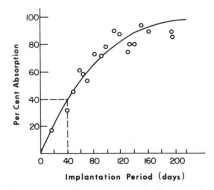

FIGURE 8-6. Rate of absorption of testosterone pellets in the human. Pellets were accurately weighed and then implanted subcutaneously and allowed to remain in these depots for varying intervals. After removal, each pellet was reweighed. Each point represents the per cent absorbed from a single pellet in a single subject. (From P.M.F. Bishop and S.J. Folley, Lancet *1:434,1944.)*

stantly supplies drug to be mixed with the air that the patient inhales and, thus, replaces the quantity of drug removed during each breath the patient takes. However, the more usual way of making drug absorption proceed at a rate that approaches a constant is through the preparation of special dosage forms (cf. pp. 88–89, 96-97). Compressed pellets of hormones for subcutaneous implantation provide a remarkable example of such sustained-release preparations. As Figure 8-6 shows, about 1 per cent of the total amount of administered testosterone is absorbed each day for at least forty days. After this time, the absorption rate ceases to be practically constant and gradually diminishes. Other types of sustained-release medications, such as oral preparations of antihistaminics (cf. p. 88) or special solutions of insulin for subcutaneous injection (cf. p. 96), are also designed to achieve a nearly constant rate of absorption, but obviously for shorter periods. In all these instances, the relatively constant rate of drug entry into blood is accomplished by making the disintegration or dissolution of drug from the dosage form the rate-limiting process for absorption.

RATE OF DRUG ELIMINATION
The rate at which a drug disappears from the body is dependent on the rate of its biotransformation to inactive products and on the rates of its excretion by one or more routes. Collectively, these processes are called *elimination.* We stated previously that, for many drugs, the changes in concentration in blood reflect the changes in the amount of drug in the body. Thus the net rate of all the processes involved in terminating the presence of a drug in the organism may be determined by following the rate of decrease of blood levels of the agent. And when the drug is administered intravenously, the rate of decline directly represents the overall rate of drug elimination uncomplicated by the kinetics of drug absorption. The rate of elimination of a given agent determined after its intravenous administration is a property characteristic of

the drug. It is a constant for a particular individual, provided other agents or conditions do not change the rate of biotransformation or excretion.

As a general rule, elimination, like absorption, follows first-order kinetics. Most drugs disappear from the body and the blood at a rate which is dependent upon the blood concentration at any given moment. When the concentration is high, the rate of disappearance (amount of drug per unit time) is rapid; when the blood level is low, the rate of elimination is slow. Ideally, the concentration of drug in the body will decline with time in the form of the typical "decay" curve shown in Figure 8-7A for the elimination of ethanol in the dog following administration of a small dose. Since it is a constant fraction of the alcohol present in the body that is eliminated in each equal time interval, conversion of concentration to the logarithmic scale yields a straight line, as in Figure 8-7B.

When the elimination of a drug follows first-order kinetics, the rate of elimination can be described by a single, simple index. This index is called the *biologic half-life*, or half-time for elimination, $t_{1/2}$. It is the time required to eliminate one-half of the quantity of drug that was present in the system at the point when the measurement was begun. The biologic half-life of ethanol, for example, is found by measuring the time needed for a given blood level to decline to one-half this value. From Figure 8-7 this is seen to be about twenty minutes whether we use the blood level obtained immediately after administration or an intermediate one as our point of reference. The information conveyed by a knowledge of the half-time for elimination is useful, first of all, because it permits comparison of the elimination rates of several drugs, provided they all follow first-order kinetics. But from the practical standpoint, as we shall see below, its greatest utility is in calculating the frequency with which multiple doses of a drug can be safely administered.

When the rates of biotransformation and excretion are proportional to the amount of drug remaining in the body, the overall rate of elimination will also be first order. We would anticipate an exception to the rule of first-order elimination, however, if either of these processes proceeds at a constant rate, i.e., follows zero-order kinetics. The effect on the overall rate of elimination will depend on which process — biotransformation or excretion — plays the major role in elimination and which is the zero-order process. A few examples in which one of the processes involved in elimination is governed by zero-order kinetics will illustrate the general phenomenon.

Rate of Biotransformation

Since all drug biotransformation is mediated by enzymes, the factors determining the kinetics of biotransformation are, of course, those that determine the velocity of an enzymic reaction (cf. pp. 142–144). When the substrate concentration is low and active sites on the enzyme are available for occupancy, the rate of biotransformation will be first order. However, zero-order kinetics obtain at substrate concentrations that are high enough to saturate the enzyme or overtax the supply of a cofactor. As the substrate or drug concentration falls below saturation levels, the rate of reaction ceases to be constant and reverts to first order. While it is theoretically possible for *any* drug to be biotransformed at a constant rate, most drugs are administered in

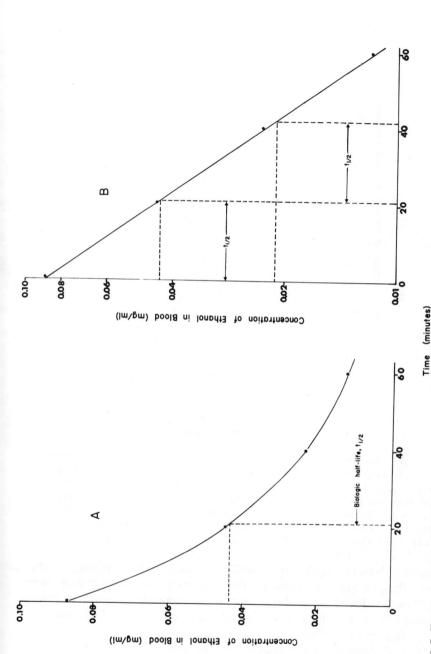

FIGURE 8-7. First-order rate of elimination: decline of ethanol content in blood following intravenous administration of a small dose to a dog. The abscissa represents time after the first point. In A, the ordinate is concentration in blood (mg per milliliter) on an arithmetic scale; in B, on a logarithmic scale. Biologic half-time, $t_{1/2}$, is about 20 minutes. (Modified from E. K. Marshall, Jr., and W. F. Fritz, J. Pharmacol. Exp. Ther. 109:431, 1953. Copyright © 1953, The Williams & Wilkins Co., Baltimore.)

213

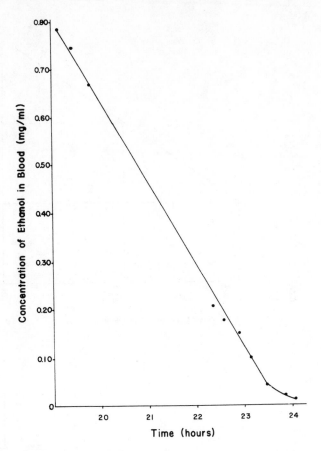

FIGURE 8-8. Zero-order rate of elimination; curve illustrating decline of ethanol content in blood following intravenous administration of a large dose to the same dog as in Figure 8-7. The abscissa represents the time beginning 19 hours after administration. The plotted data show the change from zero-order to first-order kinetics when low concentrations are reached between 23 and 24 hours after administration. (From E. K. Marshall, Jr., and W. F. Fritz, J. Pharmacol. Exp. Ther. *109:431, 1953. Copyright © 1953, The Williams & Wilkins Co., Baltimore.)*

amounts which lead to concentrations well below the saturation levels of their enzyme systems. Thus, zero-order biotransformation is generally not a factor in drug elimination. However, there are a number of drugs whose elimination is known to depend on a metabolic reaction that can be saturated at drug concentrations commonly reached after ordinary doses.

The fate of ethanol in humans and other animals provides a good example of how a zero-order mechanism of biotransformation affects the overall rate of drug elimination. It is of practical as well as theoretical importance, since this biotransformation process exhibits zero-order kinetics at a drug concentration produced by

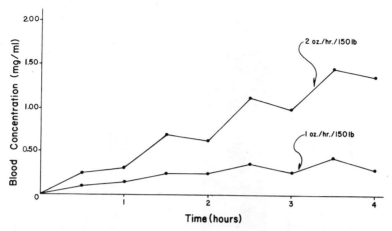

FIGURE 8-9. Accumulation of ethanol in blood of human subjects following in-gestion of 1 or 2 ounces of 100-proof whiskey (50 per cent ethanol) every hour. First drink at time 0 and one drink each hour thereafter. Lower curve: Dose, 1 oz per hour; each point is the mean of samples from 25 males. Upper curve: Dose, 2 oz per hour; each point is the mean of samples from 10 males. (Redrawn from R. B. Forney and F. W. Hughes, Alcohol accumulation in humans after prolonged drinking. Clin. Pharmacol. Ther. *4:619,1963.)*

the ingestion of a very small quantity of alcohol – about one average-sized drink of whiskey.

Ethanol undergoes a series of oxidative reactions whose end products are carbon dioxide and water:

$$C_2H_5OH \longrightarrow CH_3CHO \longrightarrow CH_3COOH \longrightarrow CO_2 + H_2O$$

The enzyme system responsible for the conversion of alcohol to acetaldehyde is saturable at extremely low concentrations of substrate. Hence, the rate of metabolism of ethanol in humans is essentially constant irrespective of the quantity of alcohol present in the body.

The rate of elimination of ethanol also is almost constant, since biotransformation is the primary pathway for its removal from the body. Normally less than 2 per cent of the total alcohol administered or ingested is excreted in the urine, exhaled through the lungs or lost in perspiration. Consequently, the decline in blood levels after intravenous administration of alcohol closely follows zero-order kinetics until very low blood concentrations are reached. This is clearly evident from a comparison of the data in Figure 8-8 with those in Figure 8-7A. (Note that the data in both figures are for the same animal.) Even twenty hours after the administration of a very large dose, the blood alcohol level is seen to decrease linearly, indicating that the rate of disappearance is constant and independent of the substrate concentration (Fig. 8-8). For example, the blood level declines from 0.62 to 0.46 mg per milliliter between

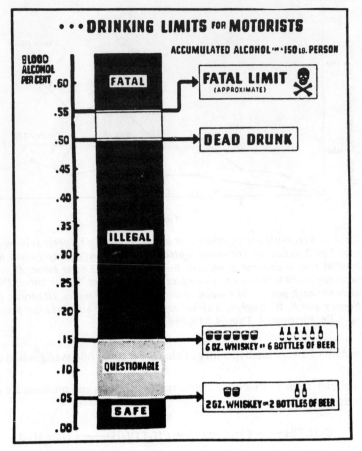

FIGURE 8-10. Relationships between ingestion of various alcoholic beverages, alcohol levels in the blood and the ability of an individual to drive an automobile after consuming alcohol. (N.B. Blood alcohol per cent equals the number of grams of ethanol per 100 ml of blood; e.g., 0.1 alcohol per cent = 0.1g per 100 ml blood, or 100 mg per 100 ml blood, or 100 mg per cent.) (From R. N. Harger, in J. P. Economos and F. M. Kreml [eds.], Judge and Prosecutor in Traffic Court. Chicago: American Bar Association and the Traffic Institute, Northwestern University, 1951.)

twenty and twenty-one hours, and in the next hour the decrease is also 0.16 mg per milliliter. Only when the blood level has fallen below 0.1 mg per milliliter does the rate become first order. Elimination starts out as a first-order process when the dose administered is small and the initial blood concentration does not exceed saturation levels (Fig. 8-7).

The average human adult metabolizes about 8 g (10 ml) of pure ethanol per hour although there is considerable biologic variation in the rate of ethanol elimination (cf. Fig. 7-9). This quantity is equivalent to about 20 to 25 ml of liquor (40 to 50 per cent ethanol), less than 1 ounce of whiskey or one 12-ounce bottle of beer. The slow rate of ethanol elimination and its independence of the quantity present in the body are, obviously, the cause of the well-known effects associated with a too-rapid rate of multiple dosing (Fig. 8-9). Alcohol is distributed throughout the total body water, which in a 70-kg person is about 40 liters. If the body contained 1 fluid ounce of whiskey, the calculated blood level of alcohol would be about 0.25 mg per milliliter (or 0.025 per cent); at 2 fluid ounces the blood would contain 0.5 mg per milliliter (or 0.05 per cent).[1] To arrive at these figures, the assumption has to be made that all of the dose was instantly available for distribution. In actuality it would take the ingestion of more than 1 ounce to produce this level because absorption is not instantaneous, and some elimination takes place before absorption is complete. Objectively measurable effects of alcohol, such as impairment of visual acuity, have their onset at blood levels between 0.15 and 0.55 mg per milliliter, whereas mild intoxication is associated with blood levels of 1 mg per milliliter (or 0.1 per cent), a body content of about 4 oz of whiskey (Fig. 8-10). In the mildly intoxicated individual, the duration of effective blood concentrations would be about three hours, and about five hours would be needed to eliminate the dose taken at the outset.

Aspirin is another commonly used drug which shows unusual characteristics of elimination. This is again of practical importance since the effects of enzyme saturation become evident at blood levels attained with the ordinary analgesic dose of aspirin: two tablets, or 600 mg. As a consequence of zero-order kinetics, the relative rate of elimination of aspirin diminishes as the dose increases. From Figure 8-11

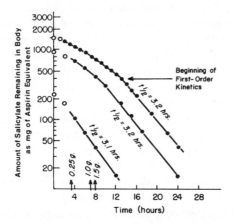

FIGURE 8-11. Elimination of salicylate by a normal 22-year-old male as a function of dose. Doses taken were 0.25, 1.0 and 1.5 g aspirin, respectively. Vertical arrows on the time axis indicate the time necessary to eliminate 50 per cent of the dose. Half-times ($t_{1/2}$) are for straight-line portion of curves where rate is first order. (Modified from G. Levy, J. Pharm. Sci. 54:959, 1965. Reproduced with permission of the copyright owner.)

[1] The blood alcohol per cent is defined as the number of grams per milliliter, multiplied by 100. Concentrations of ethanol in blood are also frequently expressed in terms of mg%; milligram per cent is defined as the number of milligrams per 100 milliliters.

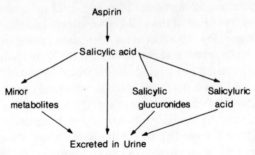

FIGURE 8-12. Biotransformation of aspirin in man.

it can be seen that it takes longer to eliminate 50 per cent of the quantity administered as the dose increases from 0.25 to 1.5 g. (Note that in Figure 8-11 the rate of
aspirin elimination is depicted in terms of the amount remaining in the body, instead
of the blood concentration of aspirin. This is in accordance with the assumption that
the concentration of drug in blood is indicative of drug concentration in the body, and
vice versa.)

   A number of processes are involved in the biotransformation of aspirin, two of
which are saturable under the conditions of its clinical use. Aspirin is first hydrolyzed
to salicylic acid, a rapid reaction with a half-time of one-quarter hour. Salicylic acid,
in turn, is conjugated partly with glucuronic acid and partly with glycine. These
conjugates, together with some minor metabolites and free salicylic acid, are excreted
almost exclusively in the urine (Fig. 8-12). All the processes of biotransformation
and excretion are first order with the exception of the conjugation of salicylic acid
with glycine to form salicyluric acid and with glucuronic acid to form the ether glucuronide (cf. p. 147). Salicyluric acid formation has been found to change from
first-order to near zero-order kinetics when the amount of salicylic acid in the
body exceeds the quantity derived from the biotransformation of less than 1 g of
aspirin; the glucuronide conjugating system is saturated at somewhat higher levels of
salicylic acid. When conventional dosage forms are administered and the aspirin is
absorbed normally, it would take only two tablets to reach the level at which salicyluric
acid formation ceases to be a first-order phenomenon.

   When the salicylic acid derived from aspirin in the body is below saturation levels,
the overall rate of elimination of salicylate follows first-order kinetics because all the
elimination processes are first order, as shown in Figure 8-11 for the elimination of
the 0.25 g dose of aspirin. The half-time of elimination under first-order conditions
is about 3.1 hours. At these low doses the major process responsible for salicylate
elimination is its conjugation with glycine, since the first-order rate of salicyluric
acid formation is much faster than the rates of the glucuronide syntheses. When
doses of aspirin of 1 g or more are administered, the glycine conjugation reaction
becomes practically zero order and the glucuronide conjugation with the phenolic
group of salicylate also approaches the limit of its capacity. As a consequence, the

overall rate of elimination of the salicylate derived from large doses of aspirin displays complex kinetics, indicative of a mixture of apparent zero-order and first-order processes. As Figure 8-11 shows, the curves for the 1.0 and 1.5 g doses of aspirin do not become linear until the salicylic acid remaining in the body drops to the quantity equivalent to about 300 mg of aspirin. This indicates a lack of conformity with first-order kinetics. Below 300 mg the curves for all three doses are linear and first order. Moreover, the time required to eliminate 50 per cent of the salicylate in the body lengthens as the dose of aspirin increases, because less of the more rapidly formed salicyluric acid is contributing to the overall elimination process.

Rate of Excretion

The kidney plays the major role in excretion of drugs, and, as has been seen, urinary excretion begins with glomerular filtration of any drug that is not bound to plasma proteins. The rate of appearance of drug in the glomerular filtrate is dependent on the rate at which the drug is presented to the kidney. This rate is always proportional to the levels of drug in plasma, since a constant fraction, one-fifth, of the volume of blood coming to the glomerulus is filtered per unit of time. Thus, glomerular filtration is a first-order rate process with respect to the free (non-protein-bound) drug. The final concentration of drug in voided urine is determined by how much of the filtrate is passively reabsorbed after filtration as the urine travels through the tubule. The rate of passive reabsorption is also first order because it is proportional to the concentration gradient established between the tubular urine and blood. Since glomerular filtration and passive reabsorption represent the mechanisms by which most drugs are excreted, it follows that the excretion of most drugs is usually first order.

Active tubular secretion is an important mechanism of urinary elimination only for certain organic acids and bases (cf. pp. 134–135, 137). Since the rate of active transport is limited by availability of carrier, secretion becomes zero order at blood levels of drug which saturate the carrier mechanism. Here the overall rate of excretion is partly first order due to glomerular filtration and partly zero order. However, below saturation levels the rate of urinary excretion is always proportional to the concentration of drug in the blood. (The same principle applies to those drugs which are actively secreted by the liver into bile.) Although the potential exists for the establishment of zero-order kinetics for those drugs actively secreted by the tubules, their maximal secretory capacity appears rarely, if ever, to be exceeded in drug therapy. Penicillin is a case in point. The secretory capacity for penicillin in a person with normal kidneys is so high that even massive doses — greater than those ordinarily needed even in intensive therapy — do not yield blood levels which saturate the process. Indeed, this rapid elimination is one of the drawbacks of penicillin therapy. If it were possible to saturate the renal secretory process with extremely large doses of penicillin, it would perhaps be unnecessary to use special dosage forms to prolong its sojourn in the body.

In using blood concentration data to evaluate the kinetics of drug elimination, the assumption is made that the rate of decline of blood levels after intravenous injection reflects the rate at which drug is leaving the entire body. This means that the rate of decrease in blood levels is also a reflection of changes in the *amount of drug remaining in the body.* We have just said that the rate of urinary excretion of drug is predictably proportional to blood levels under most conditions, i.e., the rate of urinary excretion is usually first order. Consequently, the rate of appearance of drug in the urine also represents the rate at which the amount of drug remaining in the body changes with time (Fig. 8-13). Urinary excretion data can serve, then, as another means of determining kinetics of drug elimination. All we need to know is the amount of drug *unexcreted* at any time after administration. When the drug is not metabolized and is excreted only in the urine, the amount of drug remaining in the body can be calculated directly from the total dose administered and the quantity of drug excreted in the given interval. Thus:

Total dose administered − Amount excreted = Quantity of drug remaining in the body

When urinary excretion represents the mechanism by which most of a drug is removed from the body, the overall rate of elimination generally follows first-order kinetics. A constant fraction of the drug still in the body will be excreted per unit time. Therefore, a straight line is obtained when the amount of drug unexcreted is plotted on a logarithmic scale against time on an arithmetic scale. This is illustrated in Figure 8-13 for penicillin, whose elimination is primarily the result of urinary excretion. Under these conditions, the half-time for excretion, about twenty-five minutes,

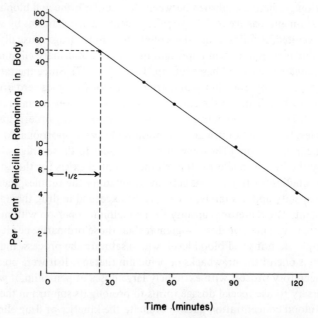

FIGURE 8-13. *First-order elimination of penicillin. Penicillin G (50,000 units, 30 mg) was injected intravenously in a dog at 0 time. (Modified from H. K. Beyer et al.,* Am. J. Physiol. *166:625, 1951.)*

is almost identical to the half-time for elimination and can be read directly from the graph.

When a drug is biotransformed as well as excreted, the kinetics of its elimination can also be interpolated from urinary excretion data, provided the products of bio-transformation appear in the urine. In this situation, the amount of drug unexcreted is calculated from the difference between the total urinary content of unchanged drug plus its metabolites and the quantity of drug originally administered. This is how the data of Figure 8-14 for "amphetamine remaining to be excreted" were obtained. The total quantity of unchanged amphetamine plus its metabolites (expressed as amphetamine) was determined in the urine for each given interval. The amount of amphetamine remaining in the body was then calculated for each point of the graph by subtracting from the dose administered the cumulative sum of amphetamine plus its metabolites excreted up to that point. As Figure 8-14 indicates, the kinetics of amphetamine elimination is shown to be first order whether evaluated from blood level or urinary excretion data.

The data in Figure 8-11 for aspirin were also obtained by determining the rate of urinary excretion of its metabolites. The urinary output of unchanged salicylic acid (there is almost no unchanged aspirin excreted), salicyluric acid and the glucuronide conjugates was measured at various times after aspirin administration. The total amount of aspirin eliminated in the given interval is then equal to the quantity that

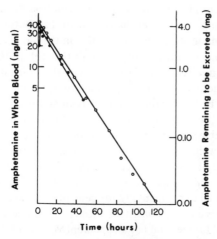

FIGURE 8-14. Elimination of amphetamine following administration of 10 mg to a human subject. Total urinary content of unchanged amphetamine plus its metabolites (expressed as amphetamine) was determined for each given interval. The amount of amphetamine remaining in the body was then calculated for each point of the graph by subtracting the cumulative urinary content of amphetamine and its metabolites from the dose administered. (● = concentration in whole blood in nanograms per milliliter [1 ng = 0.001 μg]; ○ = amphetamine, in milligrams, remaining to be excreted.) (From M. Rowland, J. Pharm. Sci. 58:508, 1969. Reproduced with permission of the copyright owner.)

has to be biotransformed to yield the sum of the voided metabolites. In turn, the amount of unexcreted aspirin can easily be determined from the difference. Thus the ordinate of Figure 8-11 represents the amount of aspirin remaining in the body, calculated from the total excretion of its metabolites at various times after administration. That the elimination of aspirin in doses of 1 g or more does not conform to first-order kinetics is readily ascertained from this semilogarithmic plot of amount remaining in the body versus time. Under appropriate conditions, then, the rate of excretion of a drug can be used to determine not only its overall rate of elimination, but also the type of kinetics this elimination follows.

The half-lives of chemical agents may vary widely when urinary excretion is the primary mechanism of elimination, e.g., about one-half hour for penicillin to one week for digitoxin to more than nine years for the metal strontium. Since the rate of passage into urine is generally proportional to the blood level, these enormous differences in half-lives of elimination can arise only from differences in the rates at which free drug is presented to the kidney and in the extent of tubular reabsorption. If glomerular filtration is the only mechanism by which a drug enters the urine, then the availability of drug for excretion will be strictly dependent on the amount of unbound drug arriving at the glomerulus (cf. p. 135). The greater the degree of protein binding, the slower the overall rate of elimination. Protein binding will, of course, have little influence on the overall rate of excretion for those drugs actively secreted by the tubules. For the most part, however, the variability in the half-life of urinary excretion of drugs arises from differences in distribution within the body and not in plasma protein binding. The greater the volume of distribution of a drug, the smaller the amount of the administered dose remaining in the blood and the lower the concentration of drug presented to the kidney per unit time (cf. p. 103). For agents not biotransformed and not bound to plasma protein, the shortest half-lives are associated with drugs distributed only within the plasma-water, the intermediate ones with those distributed to the extracellular fluid compartment and the longest with those distributed in the entire content of body water. Drugs belonging to the last category are usually lipid soluble, and this property is conducive to extensive reabsorption from the tubular urine as well. The theoretical relationships between elimination half-time and apparent volume of distribution are shown in Table 8-1 for drugs cleared by glomerular filtration and tubular secretion (cf. pp. 135–137). The actual half-life of elimination determined experimentally for penicillin, between twenty-five and thirty minutes (Fig. 8-13), is entirely consistent with the theoretical value. Penicillin is secreted by the renal tubules and has an apparent volume of distribution greater than that of extracellular fluid but less than that of total body water. As would be predicted from Table 8-1, its half-life should lie between thirteen and forty-four minutes, as it does.

The theoretical half-lives in Table 8-1 were calculated by assuming that the movement of drug into the fluid compartments of the body is readily reversible. That is to say, when the concentration gradient within extravascular fluid compartments favors movement in the opposite direction, drug moves back into the blood. However, no limits can be set for how long a drug may remain in the body when it is

Table 8-1. Theoretical Relationship Between Elimination Half-Time and Volume of Distribution in the Human Being

Mechanisms of Urinary Excretion	Drug Distributed in[a]		
	Plasma Water (3,000 ml)	Extracellular Fluid (12,000 ml)	Body Water (41,000 ml)
Glomerular filtration — 130 ml/min	16 min	64 min	219 min
Tubular secretion — 650 ml/min	3 min	13 min	44 min

[a]Entries in each column are values of the fastest possible elimination half-time. Elimination half-times have no upper limit; renal clearance may be extremely low (near zero) if a drug is extensively reabsorbed or protein-bound, or has an apparent volume of distribution greater than total body water due to extensive tissue binding.
Source: Modified from A. Goldstein, L. Aronow and S. M. Kalman, *Principles of Drug Action.* New York: Hoeber Med. Div., Harper & Row, 1968. P. 197.

strongly bound to tissue components and, thus, restricted in its outward movement. The long half-lives of digitoxin and strontium, as well as many other agents, are due to sequestration within tissues or organs. Drugs that undergo extensive reabsorption also have longer half-lives than are indicated by the rates at which they are filtered or secreted into the proximal tubule.

Although the biologic half-time is the index of how long a drug will remain in the body, it does not always indicate the duration of drug action. There are some instances when the duration of action of a drug outlasts its presence in the organism. These are usually cases in which the mechanism of action of a drug involves the destruction or depletion of a body constituent necessary for normal function. The responsible agent may have disappeared from the scene before the body can adequately compensate for the functional loss through replenishment. For example, the action of the organic phosphate insecticides persists beyond their residence in the body and until the enzymes which they have destroyed are resynthesized.

With the exception already noted, the duration of action of a drug is the time during which effective concentrations are present in the body. For drugs with comparatively short half-lives, there is a relatively close correspondence between duration of action and rate of elimination. But for drugs with comparatively long half-lives, the concentration of drug may fall to ineffective levels long before the drug has disappeared from the body. This is certainly true for agents which are highly bound to various tissue components and only slowly released from these stores. For example, the bright yellow antimalarial drug quinacrine (Atabrine) has a biologic half-life of about ten days. All patients receiving the drug for more than a week develop a yellow discoloration of the skin as a result of drug-binding. After the drug is discontinued, the altered pigmentation (which causes no ill effects) persists from several weeks to months, depending on the dosage and length of therapy.

Another important principle concerning the duration of effective concentration may be derived from the fact that most drug elimination is first order. This principle

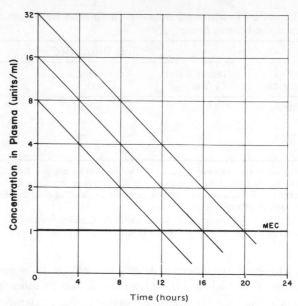

FIGURE 8-15. Relation between duration of action and dose for a drug eliminated by first-order kinetics. Biologic half-life is 4 hours. If action lasts until the drug remaining in the body is reduced to the minimal effective concentration (MEC, shown in graph as 1 unit), then the duration of action increases as the logarithm of the dose increases. (Note that the units along the ordinate are on a geometric scale.)

states that if the duration of action lasts until the drug concentration falls to a certain point, then the *duration of action increases as the logarithm of the dose increases.* The reason for this relationship can be easily deduced from the following example. Suppose that drug X has a biologic half-life of four hours and that its just-effective concentration in the body corresponds to 1 unit per milliliter of plasma. A dose is given which will establish a plasma concentration of 8 units per milliliter. The duration of action will then be twelve hours, or three half-lives (Fig. 8-15). When the dose is doubled, i.e., sufficient to yield 16 units per milliliter of plasma, the duration of action is extended only four hours, or one biologic half-life, since in the first four hours the plasma level will fall to 8 units per milliliter. Redoubling the dose so that the initial plasma level is 32 units per milliliter again increases the duration of action by only four hours. Thus, geometric increases in dose produce linear increases in duration of action. This relationship implies that, for a drug which is eliminated rapidly, it is in practice almost impossible to produce a prolonged action by giving massive doses. Moreover, the quantity of drug that can be safely administered at one time is limited by the dose-related toxicity of the drug.

THE TIME COURSE OF DRUG ACTION AFTER SINGLE DOSES
So far, we have considered the temporal course of drug action only in a piecemeal fashion. We have examined the factors that influence the ascending portion of the

time-response curve separately from those that determine its descending portion. Now we shall consider how all these factors acting in concert affect the overall time course as well as the separate phases of drug action.

To understand how the rate of drug accessibility influences the time-response relationship, we need only recall how the properties of drugs and the characteristics of the biologic barrier influence the rate of drug movement within the body (cf. Chaps. 4 and 5). The faster an agent moves across membranes, the faster it attains an effective concentration at its site of action; the slower the transfer, the longer the latent period between administration and onset of effect. Thus, differences in lipid solubility, state of ionization and molecular size are responsible for differences among agents with respect to time of onset of action. This is well illustrated by comparing the onset of anesthesia following administration of thiopental (Fig. 8-16) with that following phenobarbital administration (see Fig. 8-3). Thiopental is about one hundred times more lipid soluble than phenobarbital and is also less completely ionized in body fluids. As a consequence, thiopental penetrates into the brain so rapidly that the onset of anesthesia is almost instantaneous. Phenobarbital penetrates so slowly that it has no usefulness as an anesthetic agent in man, since it takes about thirty minutes for anesthesia to begin.

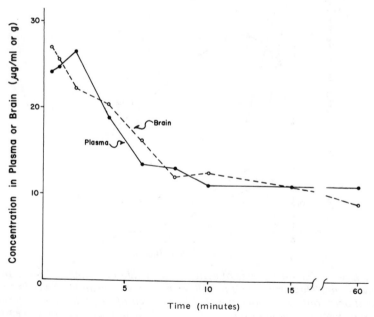

FIGURE 8-16. Plasma and brain concentration of thiopental after intravenous administration (15 mg per kilogram of body weight) to rats. Onset of anesthesia was between 1 and 2 minutes. (•——• = plasma; ○----○ = brain.) (Modified from A. Goldstein and L. Aronow, J. Pharmacol. Exp. Ther. 128: 1, 1960. Copyright © 1960, The Williams & Wilkins Co., Baltimore.)

The ways in which the characteristics of the biologic barrier influence the time course of drug action can best be seen when a single agent is administered in equal doses by several routes to the same individual. Under these conditions, most of the variables are reduced to a minimum. The administration of equal doses by all routes ensures that the same quantity of drug is potentially available to its sites of action. Carrying out the experiment in a single individual eliminates biologic variation in rates of drug distribution and excretion. Thus the differences in drug levels attained following administration by the several routes can be directly attributed to differences in rates of absorption. Figure 8-17 shows such data for penicillin. It is evident that the time needed to reach a just-effective blood concentration becomes longer as the barriers interposed between the site of application and the circulation increase in number. Since transfer of drug across the gastrointestinal epithelium is slower than movement from interstitial space into the circulation, the delay in onset of action is longest by the oral route.

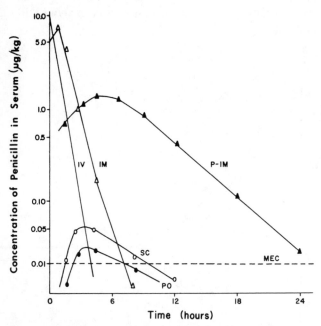

FIGURE 8-17. The time course of action of penicillin following various routes of administration. Three milligrams per kilogram of body weight were administered on different occasions to the same subject. Blood levels of penicillin were determined at various times after administration. The antibiotic was dissolved in water for administration intravenously (IV), intramuscularly (IM), subcutaneously (SC) and orally (PO), Procaine-penicillin in oil was given intramuscularly (P−IM). MEC represent the minimal effective serum concentration. (Modified from D. F. Marsh, Outline of Fundamental Pharmacology, 1951. Charles C Thomas, Publisher, Springfield, Illinois.)

The penicillin data (Fig. 8-17) also point out rather forcefully how the route of administration can alter the duration of action, the amplitude of the peak concentration and the time to this maximum level. Our points of reference for comparison are the data obtained following intravenous administration of penicillin. This route yields the highest and most rapidly attainable blood concentrations because the entire dose is placed directly into the bloodstream. The duration of action of an intravenous dose also measures the rate of elimination unmodified by absorption. Figure 8-17 shows that, even though the dose is sufficient to establish an initial concentration one-hundred-fold greater than the minimum effective level, the action of intravenously administered penicillin lasts only five hours.

When an aqueous solution of penicillin is given intramuscularly, the amplitude of the peak concentration attained is not much lower, and the duration of action not much longer, than after intravenous injection. Moreover, the peak blood level is reached soon after the drug is deposited in the muscle. Together, these facts signify that the rate of absorption from the intramuscular site is extremely rapid; so rapid, in fact, that the major portion of the dose reaches the blood before very much elimination has taken place. The rate of decline of blood levels then approaches that following intravenous injection, since little influence is exerted by continued absorption. In contrast, after subcutaneous administration, a much lower peak is reached at a later time, yet the duration of effective concentrations is somewhat longer. The lower and later peak indicates that the rate of absorption is insufficient to keep up with the rate at which penicillin is being eliminated. But continued absorption even at a rate slower than elimination is sufficient to compensate partially for the drug that is being lost. As a result, the duration of action of the subcutaneous dose is longer than that given intramuscularly. The lowest and latest peak is associated with oral administration, the route with the slowest rate of absorption. Again, continued entry of drug into the body provides for a duration of action of orally administered penicillin longer than that given intravenously. We would anticipate that this should be equally true for the comparison between the oral and subcutaneous routes. That it is not true for penicillin is due to the fact that only about one-third of an oral dose is absorbed, whereas nearly the entire dose is available to the system following subcutaneous administration.

The ways in which routes of administration influence the time course of drug action permit us to draw some important conclusions about the relationship between the rates of absorption and elimination when both are first order. If the rates of biotransformation and excretion are not changed by the existence of some abnormal condition, then the absolute rate of elimination of any given agent remains the same, regardless of its route of administration. The index of rate of elimination is, of course, the biologic half-life determined after intravenous injection, in which situation it is independent of absorption. Thus, for equal doses of a given drug, it is a change in the rate of absorption which produces a change in its time course of action. And for any agent, the slower the rate of absorption relative to elimination, the later are the minimally effective and peak concentrations attained and the lower is the value of the latter. The duration of action will also become longer with a slower rate of absorption provided that (1) the rate of absorption is sufficiently rapid relative to elimination to yield levels above the minimal effective concentration, and (2) the entire dose at a site of application is absorbed.

The duration of action of a drug, such as penicillin, which is rapidly eliminated is not altered very much, as we have just seen, by changing its rate of absorption *as long as absorption remains first order.* The duration of action, however, can be markedly prolonged when the kinetics of absorption approaches zero order. The administration of special dosage forms may approach this end because the drug is released at a rate slower than its rate of absorption. For example, penicillin combines with procaine to form a salt that goes into aqueous solution very slowly compared with the potassium salt of penicillin. The rate of dissolution of procaine-penicillin in body fluids is even further reduced when it is administered in oil. As a result, absorption proceeds at a nearly constant rate for a considerable period. A single intramuscular injection of procaine-penicillin in oil provides therapeutic drug levels for more than twenty-four hours (curve labeled *P–IM* in Fig. 8-17), whereas the same dose of penicillin in water is effective for little more than five or six hours.

THE KINETICS OF DRUG ACCUMULATION FOLLOWING MULTIPLE DOSES

Multiple Dose Schedules

The aim in most therapeutic situations is to produce an alteration in a particular function of an organism and to maintain this change for an adequate period. This calls initially for attaining an effective concentration of drug in the body and then for keeping this level relatively constant. Achieving an initial effective concentration is a simple matter if an appropriate route and dose are used. It is the maintenance of this effective level which poses problems. We have seen that increasing the size of the dose is not only ineffective in prolonging drug action but also limited by considerations of dose-related toxicity. However, the duration of drug action can be safely prolonged by continually putting drug into the system to counterbalance that which is lost through biotransformation or excretion or both. Sustained-release preparations, if available, represent one way of doing this, but the more usual procedure is to give repeated doses of drug at regular intervals.

It is obvious, since the rates at which different drugs are eliminated from the body vary widely, that no single schedule for repeated dosage would suffice for each and every drug. But the development of a rational dosage schedule for any drug is governed by principles applicable to all agents and is a relatively simple procedure for drugs that are eliminated by first-order kinetics. For any given agent we need to know: (1) what concentration will produce the desired effect; (2) what dose will yield this concentration; and (3) how long the level of drug in the body will remain effective after the selected dose is administered. What constitutes an effective concentration of drug in the body is determined by the dose-response relationships of the therapeutic agent. The magnitude of the dose required to produce this particular drug level depends on the route of administration and the volume of distribution of the given drug. And the biologic half-life of the drug tells us how long an effective level of drug will remain in the body.

Let us suppose that drug X, with a biologic half-life of four hours, produces its desired effect when the total quantity of drug in the body is at least 1 g but not greater than 2 g. If we administer an initial dose of 2 g, we would immediately achieve this goal (assuming instantaneous absorption and distribution). After four hours, ·however, the level in the body would have fallen to half this amount, or 1 g. We could then replace the quantity of drug lost by giving an additional 1 g dose. If we continued giving 1 g every four hours, the drug level in the body would never exceed 2 g since the quantity lost between doses equals the quantity replaced at the next dosing interval. The rate of drug administration which just establishes, but does not exceed, the desired drug concentration in the body is the *maintenance dose rate.* In our example, if a body content of between 1 and 2 g represents the required effective drug concentration, then 1 g every four hours is the maintenance dose rate, and 1 g is the *maintenance dose* of drug X. The larger initial dose of 2 g, which was used to achieve the desired drug level quickly, is called a loading dose or *priming dose.*

What would happen if we began therapy with drug X by administering the maintenance dose of 1 g from the start? Or, alternatively, if we continued administering the priming dose of 2 g every four hours? If we administer the maintenance dose from the outset, the amount of drug X in the body would rise until a maximum of 2 g were present. This is so because more drug is being given than is being eliminated in the dosing intervals up to the point at which the body content is 2 g. At a body content of 2 g, however, the rate of elimination — 1 g every four hours — would equal the rate of drug entry into the body, and no further accumulation would occur. Simple arithmetic shows that it takes 7 doses to just about reach this point (Table 8-2). If we administer the priming dose every four hours, the amount of drug in the body will also increase until the rate of elimination equals the rate of drug entry into the body, and it would again take about 7 doses to approximate this point (Table 8-2). But since the rate of administration is 2 g every four hours, the level of drug in the body has to be 4 g before the rate of elimination will be 2 g every four hours. Thus, if a drug is given at regular intervals and if a constant fraction of what is present in the body is eliminated in the interval, *the amount of drug in the body will accumulate until the quantity cleared in the interval between doses is equal to a single dose.*

If the assumption is made that each single dose is absorbed instantaneously, marked fluctuations in the level of drug in the body will occur due to elimination during the intervals between doses. In the example cited, just before the second 1 g dose is administered, only 0.5 g would be present. Just after the instantaneous absorption of the second dose, the body content would be 1.5 g. There would be ever greater fluctuation when 2 g were administered every four hours. It can be readily appreciated that after oral administration the fluctuation in the body content of drug would be less severe, provided that the entire oral dose were absorbed well within the dosing interval. Continued absorption of drug tends to flatten out the fluctuations due to drug elimination in the intervals between doses. When the rate of drug entry into the body becomes constant, i.e., when it is near zero order, there will no longer be fluctuations. The extent to which the drug content in the body rises and falls can also be minimized

Table 8-2. Accumulation of Drug X in the Body[a]

	Dosing Interval												
	1		2	3		4		5		6		7	
	A[b]	B[c]	A	B	A	B	A	B	A	B	A	B	A
Administration of 1 g of drug X: Body content (g)	1.0	0.5	1.5	0.75	1.75	0.88	1.88	0.94	1.94	0.97	1.97	0.99	1.99
Administration of 2 g of drug X: Body content (g)	2.0	1.0	3.0	1.5	3.5	1.75	3.75	1.88	3.88	1.94	3.94	1.97	3.97

[a]Half-life of drug X = 4 hours. Dosing interval = 4 hours.
[b]Figures in columns headed "A" represent the amount of drug X in body immediately after a dose is given.
[c]Figures in columns headed "B" represent amount of drug X in body just before dose is given.

by shortening the interval between doses. However, the amount of drug administered per dose must also be adjusted to match the amount eliminated in the new interval. For example, if drug X were given every two instead of every four hours, less than one-half of the amount present in the body would be eliminated in the two-hour interval. Were the maintenance dose to remain 1 g, drug X would continue to accumulate beyond the desired level, since more drug was being put into the system than was being eliminated in the interval between doses. To avoid this accumulation, the maintenance dose must also be adjusted to correspond to the decreased amount being eliminated in the shorter dosing interval.

For any given interval between doses, the slower the rate of elimination, the smaller the degree of fluctuation in drug levels, since a smaller fraction of drug is lost from the body during the interval. By the same token, the maintenance dose will represent a progressively smaller fraction of drug present in the body as the rate of elimination becomes slower. Take, for example, drug Y with a biologic half-life of twenty-four hours. In a four-hour interval only about one-tenth of the drug in the body is cleared, whereas one-half of drug X, with a biologic half-life of four hours, is eliminated in an equal period. Thus, if we wished to maintain drug Y at a body content of 2 g, we would require a maintenance dose of only one-tenth this amount, or 0.2 g, once the desired level had been established. As in the case of drug X, we could establish this 2-g level quickly by administering a priming dose of 2 g and then continuing at four-hour intervals with the small maintenance dose. But if we started with the maintenance dose rate of 0.2 g every four hours, how long would it take to reach the 2-g level for drug Y in the body? The lower curve of Figure 8-18 indicates that even after three days, only about 90 per cent of the desired body content could be reached on this schedule. To obtain the full 2-g level would require almost six days. The upper curve of Figure 8-18 shows that when a dose of 0.4 g of drug Y is given every four hours, it requires only twenty-four hours to attain a level greater than 90 per cent of the desired body content. If administration at this higher dose rate were continued beyond twenty-four hours, the body content of drug Y would climb until a 4-g level was reached (dashed line in Fig. 8-18). Once the desired body content of 2 g was reached with the higher dose, however, institution of the maintenance dose rate would prevent further accumulation. We may conclude from these data that when administration starts with the maintenance dose (the quantity of drug lost in the interval between doses), the slower the rate of elimination, the longer it takes to establish a desired level of drug; thus, drugs which are slowly eliminated from the body also accumulate slowly compared with drugs having short half-lives.

When circumstances call for drug therapy, it is almost always imperative to produce an effective concentration in the body as quickly as possible, certainly within a few hours. For drugs with slow rates of elimination, which preclude the rapid buildup of effective drug concentrations through administration of the maintenance dose, the obvious solution is to increase the magnitude of the initial doses. Thus, the initial use of priming doses followed by maintenance doses to establish an effective drug concentration quickly and maintain it indefinitely is the usual procedure for drugs with excessively long half-lives. The dosage schedule for digitoxin used in the treat-

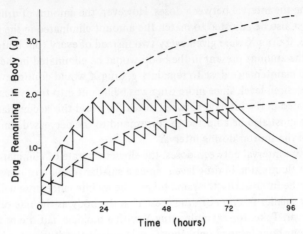

FIGURE 8-18. Accumulation of drug with repeated dosage at regular intervals. Biologic half-life = 24 hours. Dosage intervals = 4 hours. In lower curve, dose is 0.2 g; in upper curve, dose is 0.4 g for the first six doses, then 0.2 g. Zig-zag solid lines represent fluctuations in blood level in intervals between doses. Dosage was stopped at 72 hours. Dashed lines indicate course of continued accumulation if dosage were continued at original dosage level. (After J. H. Gaddum, Nature [Lond.] 153:494, 1944.)

ment of patients with congestive heart failure is a case in point. The biologic half-life of digitoxin is about seven days; about 10 per cent of the drug present in the body is eliminated daily. It would take weeks to establish a therapeutic drug concentration if the maintenance dose were administered from the start. Clearly, this would constitute improper therapy for a patient whose life may depend on how rapidly the abnormal condition can be brought under control. Ordinarily, in *digitalization,* the entire quantity of drug needed to produce an effective drug concentration is given, in divided doses, during a single day. This is followed by much smaller daily maintenance doses — doses just sufficient to replace what is lost during the dosing interval. The priming dose of digitoxin needed to establish appropriate therapeutic drug levels is not given as a single dose because this drug has a very narrow margin of safety (cf. Fig. 7-13). By giving divided doses, the physician can stop further administration if the patient manifests toxic reactions at doses corresponding to the lower end of the dose-toxicity curve.

Ideally, the laws governing the accumulation of drugs in the body should be applied to the administration of every agent, since no single fixed schedule is appropriate for all drugs. Although the method of administration of many drugs is soundly based, convenience and patient comfort frequently dictate less rational procedures. Adherence to principles is of particular importance, however, for drugs that are rapidly eliminated as well as for those that are slowly removed from the body. In the former case, it is easy to produce an effective concentration quickly but difficult to maintain this level without marked fluctuations. For drugs that are slowly eliminated, it is difficult to attain effective levels rapidly without priming doses, but toxic amounts can accumulate easily unless attention is paid to this possibility.

Cumulative Toxicity

Any chemical agent that gains access to the body has the potential for producing a toxic or deleterious effect. Cumulative toxicity, however, is associated only with agents whose residence time in the body far outlasts their duration of effective concentrations, i.e., agents whose time course of action *does not* correspond to the temporal course of their elimination. Obviously, this category includes agents with biologic half-lives measured in days, weeks or months instead of hours, where concentrations may fall to ineffective levels long before the drugs disappear from the body. Such agents also have the exceptional propensity for slowly accumulating upon repeated exposures even to small quantities until the total amount in the body is sufficient to produce toxicity. However, cumulative toxicity may also be associated with certain agents whose half-lives are relatively short. The agents in this category are highly lipid soluble and have their sites of action within tissues that are rapidly perfused with blood. Redistribution from these sites to tissues receiving lower rates of blood flow leads to the termination of action, even though considerable quantities of drug still remain in the body.

The cumulative toxicity of slowly eliminated chemicals is well exemplified by certain metals like lead which become tightly bound to various components of tissues. This binding is responsible for the very long half-life of lead, in excess of two months. In turn, the slow rate of elimination results in a slow rate of accumulation upon chronic exposure to relatively low levels of the metal. For example, individuals living in industrialized countries are exposed to lead in air and food as an ordinary, rather than as an exceptional, event. The sources of the lead are primarily leaded gasoline and industrial contaminants from the manufacture of items such as paint, insecticides or batteries. An additional source of exposure in children is through the ingestion of chips of lead-containing paint and of soil or household dust containing precipitates of airborne lead. Whereas only 5 to 10 per cent of ingested lead is absorbed from the gastrointestinal tract, 30 to 50 per cent of the lead inspired with air finds its way into the bloodstream. When the rate of lead entry into the body exceeds its rate of elimination, the excess lead is stored in various tissues, such as the kidney, liver and bone. The toxicity of lead arises from its ability to interfere with many cellular functions by inhibiting essential enzyme processes. What is so insidious is that toxic symptoms may appear before there is any awareness that chronic exposure to a dangerous environmental pollutant has occurred.[2]

Accumulation resulting in toxicity may also be seen with an agent like bromide ion, which was once widely utilized as a sedative and in the treatment of epilepsy. It has been supplanted in modern therapeutics by agents that are safer and more effi-

[2] The United States Environmental Protection Agency, by establishing air quality standards for lead and by decreasing the use of leaded gasoline, has taken major steps to eliminate this source of environmental pollution.

cacious. However, it is still used by the general public for a variety of ailments, and preparations containing bromides are freely available without prescription. The bromide ion has a volume of distribution somewhat greater than extracellular fluid. Since it is not bound to tissue components, one might anticipate that its sojourn in the body would be relatively short. Nevertheless, it has a half-life of about twelve days. Its rate of excretion is slow because it is handled by the kidney in much the same way as chloride ion, i.e., it is filtered at the glomerulus and largely reabsorbed in the tubules. The maintenance dose of bromide ion, about 0.9 g per day, if taken from the start, would produce no ill effects, because almost six weeks would elapse before effective concentrations would be attained in the body fluids. This rate of accumulation, inevitable as it is, is much too slow, since no one taking the drug on his own volition would wait so long for an effect. Thus, large doses are taken to produce an effect rapidly. And, if dosage were continued at the same priming dose rate (a common practice), cumulative poisoning would soon occur. Table 8-3 shows how bromide accumulates when what appears to be a moderate dose, 1 g three times a day, is taken for a prolonged period. The minimal effective blood concentration is about 50 mg per 100 ml, and this level is only attained after a week. After three weeks of continuous administration at the same rate, the blood level rises to 110 mg per 100 ml a blood concentration that may well produce toxic effects. Rashes and mental disturbances consisting of impaired thought and memory, dizziness and irritability are the most common manifestations of chronic bromide intoxication. Although bromides are still one of the nonprescription drugs that cause self-induced poisoning, the trend in recent years has been to omit them from over-the-counter formulations. Drug manufacturers in the United States have apparently heeded the conclusions published in the *AMA Drug Evaluations* (cf. p. 24) that bromides are "useless as hypnotics" and that "their use is deemed inadvisable."

The role which tissue redistribution plays in cumulative toxicity is clearly seen in the case of an agent like thiopental. Thiopental is extremely lipid soluble and diffuses rapidly across biologic barriers. Thus the rate at which it reaches various parts of the body is directly dependent on the rate of blood flow through the particular organ or tissue. The brain, liver, kidney and heart are perfused by blood more rapidly in proportion to their mass than are other body masses (cf. Table 5-5). Together, these organs, which constitute only about 6.5 per cent of body weight, receive more than 70 per cent of the cardiac ouptut, or about 4 liters of blood per minute in the aver-

Table 8-3. Accumulation of Bromide when 1 g Potassium Bromide Is Taken 3 Times a Day by an Adult[a]

Bromide Content	Duration of Administration (wk.)					
	3 days	1	2	3	4	5
In body (g)	5.6	11	19	22	24	25
In plasma (mg/100 ml)	28	55	95	110	120	125

[a] Body weight 60 kg.

age 70-kg individual. It is for these reasons that thiopental reaches its maximum concentration at its site of action in the brain within 1 to 2 minutes after intravenous administration (see Fig. 8-16). At this time the concentration in brain is similar to that in the plasma. The more slowly perfused areas of the body, such as muscle and skin, acquire the drug at a much slower rate; it takes 15 to 30 minutes for thiopental to reach its maximum level in these lean tissues (Fig. 8-19). Several hours may be required before thiopental reaches its peak concentration in fat, an even more poorly perfused tissue. But as the lean tissues first and then the fat take up the drug, its plasma concentration declines and thiopental diffuses back out of the brain as well as out of the other rapidly perfused organs. Within 15 to 30 minutes after a single intravenous dose, the amount of thiopental within the brain falls below an effective concentration, and the action of the drug is terminated — the patient awakens.

Because of its high lipid solubility, thiopental is readily reabsorbed from the glomerular filtrate and is eliminated from the body almost entirely by biotransformation. However, its rate of biotransformation is slow, only 10 to 15 per cent being metabolized in one hour. This means that a large fraction of the dose administered is still present in the body at a time when its pharmacologic effect is no longer apparent. Thus the brief action of a single dose of thiopental is the result not of elimination but of redistribution initially to muscle and to other lean tissues. The long sojourn of thiopental in the body is due to its subsequent redistribution from lean tissues to

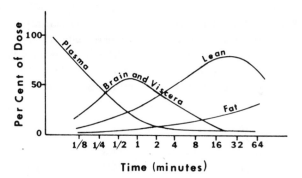

FIGURE 8-19. Theoretical distribution of thiopental in different tissues and organs at intervals after its intravenous administration, as predicted mathematically and compared with direct measurements in human blood and fat. The brain and viscera (liver, kidney and heart) are the rapidly perfused areas of the body. The curve labeled Lean represents the per cent of thiopental in the more slowly perfused areas of the body, such as muscle and skin. One minute after administration the plasma contains only 12 per cent of the original dose; the rapidly perfused brain and viscera, 55 per cent; the poorly perfused lean tissues, 28 per cent; and the fat, 5 per cent. Thirty minutes after injection the plasma contains about 2 per cent of the original dose; the rapidly perfused organs, only 5 per cent; the fat, 18 per cent; whereas the poorly perfused lean tissue contains about 75 per cent. (Modified from H. L. Price, P. J. Kovnat, J. N. Safer, E. H. Conner and M. L. Price, The uptake of thiopental by body tissues and its relation to the duration of narcosis. Clin. Pharmacol. Ther. 1:16, 1960.)

fat depots. The same factors which limit the rate of entry of thiopental into the poorly perfused tissues also account for its relatively slow egress from these tissues as drug is eliminated by biotransformation. If thiopental is readministered before the large fraction of a previous dose has been removed from lean tissues and fat, the effect of the second dose is to prolong the duration of action of thiopental. The concentration gradients between plasma and lean tissues, and between these tissues and fat, would be decreased by the concentrations of drug still present in the less rapidly perfused areas. As a result, the initial plasma concentration falls more slowly. And in turn, the rate of outflow of thiopental from the brain to plasma is slowed and the duration of drug action becomes longer. The persistence of thiopental in tissues unrelated to its pharmacologic effect explains its cumulative effects upon repeated administration.

Under the usual circumstances of its administration, the accumulation of thiopental in adipose tissue presents a problem only to the anesthetist. However, the same principles that account for rapid redistribution of this highly lipid-soluble drug also account for the slow accumulation of other lipid-soluble drugs and poisons in the fat depots of the body. Among such chemicals is the insecticide DDT (chlorophenothane); its former wide use afforded many opportunities for humans and animals to come in contact with it over an extended period.[3] The quantity necessary to produce even minimal signs of toxicity is large. With judicious use, this quantity would almost never be ingested by animals or by human beings eating plants or the flesh of animals exposed to the environmental contaminant. But once in the body, DDT is very slowly eliminated, primarily by biotransformation. Thus, DDT would accumulate in the fat depots if the rate of elimination were slower than the rate of ingestion. While the drug remains in the adipose tissue, it is harmless. It is only when it is mobilized from these fat stores (as in food deprivation or marked weight loss) that the released drug may be harmful if the quantities stored and then released are large.

SYNOPSIS

The time course of drug action is delineated in terms of the effective drug concentration that is attained in the body following drug administration. The time to a minimally effective concentration denotes the onset of drug action, the first measurable response; the total time an effective concentration is present in the body defines the duration of drug action.

The time course of drug action is determined by the rates of absorption, distribution and elimination of the drug and is dependent on the dose administered. The concentration of a drug in the blood at various times after administration may be used to describe the temporal course of drug action if the assumption is made that there is a correlation between the pharmacologic response and the concentration of the drug in blood. For many drugs this assumption is sufficiently valid to yield approxima-

---

[3] The use of DDT is now restricted by law.

tions of their time course of action. This relationship does not hold for drugs which act irreversibly, since their effects may persist long after the drugs have left the body.

Most drugs are absorbed at a rate proportional to the amount present at the site of application at any given moment, i.e., the rate of absorption usually follows first-order kinetics. When a supply of drug is available to replace that removed by absorption, a constant amount of drug rather than a constant fraction of the quantity present, is absorbed per unit time. This zero-order rate of absorption is usually approached through the use of sustained-release medications which make dissolution or disintegration of the preparation the rate-limiting factor in the drug's absorption. The faster the rate of absorption, the sooner the onset of action. (This is true even for agents which are inactive until they are biotransformed.) The faster the rate of absorption relative to elimination, the sooner the maximum drug concentration is attained and the higher is the actual value of this peak. And for any given rate of absorption, the larger the dose administered, the faster the onset of action, the higher the peak concentration and the longer the duration of action.

The rate of absorption of a given agent is determined by its physiocochemical properties and by the number and kind of biologic barriers which it must traverse to reach the bloodstream. Thus different drugs may have different rates of absorption from the same site of application, but a single agent will have different rates of absorption only when administered by different routes or in different dosage forms. Ordinarily, absorption of drugs given orally is slower than by the other common routes of administration. However, this slower rate of absorption leads to less fluctuation in the levels of drug present in the body as they change with time after administration. When a completely absorbable drug is absorbed at a rate relative to elimination which provides for effective drug levels, the duration of action tends to be longer after oral than after other routes of administration.

The overall rate of elimination of most drugs is also proportional to the amount of drug present or remaining in the body, since each of the elimination processes (biotransformation, excretion and tissue redistribution) usually follows first-order kinetics. The excretion of drugs by glomerular filtration, and their tissue redistribution in accordance with rates of passive diffusion and blood flow, are usually first order. Renal tubular secretion and biotransformation are the only processes with the potential for proceeding at constant rates, independent of the amount of drug remaining to be eliminated. The organic anionic and cationic drugs that are secreted by the renal tubule are rarely given in doses large enough to saturate the carrier mechanisms. Therefore apparent zero-order kinetics of excretion is the exception rather than the rule. Any drug biotransformation can become zero order at levels which saturate the enzyme system. This does not occur frequently. However, it is a factor in the rates of elimination of some drugs, including the common agents ethyl alcohol and aspirin, even when these are taken in small quantities.

The rate of urinary excretion is dependent on the rate at which drug is presented to the kidney. The rate of filtration is further dependent on the amount of unbound drug coming to the glomerulus. The greater the volume of distribution, the smaller the concentration of free drug in blood. Therefore the greater the volume of distribution, the slower the rate of excretion. Also, the more extensive the reabsorption of drug from the tubular urine, the slower the rate of excretion. Moreover, since urinary excretion is usually first order, the time course and overall rate of drug elimination may be determined by following the rate of appearance in urine of unchanged drug and its metabolites (provided the kidney is the organ of drug excretion).

Information concerning the rate of elimination of a drug can be summarized in a useful number called the biologic half-life. This index is the time needed to reduce the amount of unchanged drug in the body to one-half its value. It is measured under postabsorption and postdistribution conditions, i.e., when the amount of drug in the body is not modified by continuing absorption. Therefore, the biologic half-life is most conveniently determined from the rate of decline of blood levels following intravenous administration. The biologic half-lives of different agents vary over a wide range from minutes to years.

If all the elimination processes are first order, the biologic half-life of the drug does not change with dose; it will always take the same amount of time to eliminate one-half of the drug present in the body. This means that doubling the dose does not double the duration of action of a drug but increases it only by one biologic half-life. Thus, for drugs eliminated by first-order kinetics, increasing the dose is not an effective way of increasing duration of action and, furthermore, is limited by dose-related toxicity. When a zero-order process is involved in the elimination of a drug, the time to eliminate 50 per cent of the drug becomes progressively longer as the dose increases; the amount of drug eliminated per unit time ceases to be a constant fraction of that remaining in the body and approaches a constant amount of drug.

Most therapeutic situations call for the administration of more than one dose of a drug. Decisions concerning the frequency with which multiple doses should be administered are particularly important for two classes of drugs: (1) those which are so rapidly eliminated that effective concentrations are difficult to maintain, and (2) those which are so slowly eliminated that accumulation to toxic levels may easily occur. The principles governing the selection of appropriate dosing schedules apply equally to both classes. These principles involve (1) giving an initial dose that will establish but not exceed the desired drug concentration in the body, and (2) continuing to administer drug in an amount equal to that lost from the system. If a drug is given at regular intervals and if the dose given at the beginning of an interval equals the amount of drug eliminated during the previous interval, the drug will not accumulate in the body. In other words, when the quantity of drug put into the body equals the quantity of drug removed from the body in the interval between doses, no accumulation will occur. This quantity of drug is called the maintenance dose. If the maintenance dose is administered at regular intervals from the outset of therapy, the amount of drug in the body will rise until the amount eliminated in the interval between doses is equal to the maintenance dose. Thus, for a given dosing interval, the shorter the half-life of a drug, the more rapidly will the desired level of the drug be attained; the longer the half-life, the more slowly will the content of drug in the body rise when the maintenance dose is given from the start. Since in most cases it is necessary to produce an effective drug concentration rapidly, large doses, called priming doses, are given initially. When the desired level of drug in the body has been achieved, therapy is continued with the smaller maintenance dose.

Knowledge of the time course of drug action is important in determining how rapidly and for how long a drug may be expected to act, as well as in determining the relative dosage by different routes of administration. Knowledge of the relationship between rates of drug entry into and elimination from the body is fundamental to understanding the rationale of dosage schedules and of drug accumulation in the body.

GUIDES FOR STUDY AND REVIEW

What do we mean by latency or time for onset of action? by duration of drug action? When can changes in concentration of a drug in the blood be used to describe the time course of drug action?

How does the rate of absorption change with time for a drug that is absorbed by a process of passive diffusion? What does this mean in terms of the amount absorbed in equal units of time? How is the amount absorbed per unit time related to the amount remaining to be absorbed?

How does the rate of absorption change with time when the kinetics of absorption approaches zero order? How can the rate of absorption be made to approach zero order? How and when do rates of disintegration and dissolution affect the kinetics of absorption? When would it be desirable to have absorption governed by zero-order kinetics?

Does a change in the rate of drug absorption influence the onset of drug action? the duration of drug action? the maximum effect produced by a given dose? How does an increase in the rate of absorption affect the time course of drug action? How does the route of drug administration affect the time course of drug action? Does a decrease in the rate of absorption always lead to an increase in duration of drug action? Under what circumstances may a decrease in the rate of absorption lead to a decrease in duration of action?

What processes determine the rate of drug elimination? If the overall rate of drug elimination is proportional to the amount of drug remaining in the body, what does this tell you about the kinetics of biotransformation and excretion?

When is the rate of drug biotransformation zero order? What is the relationship between the rate of biotransformation and the amount of drug remaining in the body when biotransformation is zero order? when biotransformation is first order? What common drugs are biotransformed by metabolic reactions that are zero order following the administration of ordinary or small doses? How does this zero-order biotransformation affect the duration of action of the drug after a single small dose? a single large dose? multiple doses?

What is the only process of urinary excretion that can display zero-order kinetics? Is this an important factor in the urinary excretion of any drug? What is usually true concerning the kinetics of excretion for drugs that are eliminated primarily by the urinary route?

What does the index *biologic half-life,* $t_{1/2}$, describe? How is this index measured? Does the biologic half-life change with the dose of drug administered? Under what conditions is the $t_{1/2}$ the same as the time required to eliminate 50 per cent of an administered dose? when is it different?

When urinary excretion is the primary mechanism of elimination, how does volume of drug distribution, protein-binding or lipid solubility influence the biologic half-lives of drugs?

Drug X is eliminated by first-order kinetics. If the dose of drug X is doubled, how much will its duration of action be extended? Why? For a drug rapidly eliminated, is it practical to try to produce a prolonged action by giving massive doses?

How is the biologic half-life of a drug useful in calculating the frequency with which multiple doses of a drug can be safely administered? Will there be drug accumulation in the body if a drug is given in a dose equal to the amount of drug eliminated during the interval between doses?

What is meant by maintenance dose? by priming dose? When is the use of priming doses essential for effective drug therapy?

Why is cumulative toxicity upon repeated drug exposure associated with agents whose residence time in the body far outlasts their duration of effective concentration? How do small doses of lead compounds (which in themselves are pharmacologically ineffective) produce cumulative toxicity with chronic exposure? How does tissue redistribution explain the cumulative toxicity of drugs such as thiopental or chlorphenothane (DDT)?

SUGGESTED READING
Gaddum, J.H.   Repeated doses of drugs. *Nature* (Lond.) 153:994, 1949.

Levy, G.   Relationship between elimination rate of drugs and rate of decline of their pharmacologic effects. *J. Pharm. Sci.* 53:342, 1964.

Levy, G.   Dose-dependent Effects in Pharmacokinetics. In D.H. Tedeschi and R.E. Tedeschi (eds.), *Importance of Fundamental Principles in Drug Evaluation.* New York: Raven, 1968.

Levy, G., and Tsuchiya, T.   Salicylate accumulation kinetics in man. *N. Engl. J. Med.* 287:430, 1972.

Nelson, E.   Kinetics of drug absorption, distribution, metabolism and excretion. *J. Pharm. Sci.* 50:181, 1961.

Taylor, J.D., and Wiegand, R.G.   The analog computer and plasma drug kinetics. *Clin. Pharmacol. Ther.* 3:464, 1962.

Wagner, J.G.   Drug accumulation. *J. Clin. Pharmacol.* 7:84, 1967.

Wagner, J.G.   Pharmacokinetics. *Annu. Rev. Pharmacol.* 8:67, 1968.

9. FACTORS MODIFYING THE EFFECTS OF DRUGS IN INDIVIDUALS
Variability in Response Attributable to the Biologic System

Our considerations thus far have made it obvious that many factors play a role in determining the biologic effects observed when a chemical agent interacts with a living organism. The more complex the biologic system, the greater the number of variables that may affect the ultimate response. Some factors influence the *nature*, or *pharmacodynamics*, of the drug response; these result in effects such as allergic responses that are qualitatively different from those for which the drug is usually administered. Most factors that modify the effects of drugs, however, do so by altering their *pharmacokinetics* and, thereby, the *intensity* of the response. Once recognized, these quantitative changes in the usual effects of drugs can be corrected by appropriate dosage adjustment. We have already discussed the most important factor in determining the intensity of a biologic effect in any individual — the dose of drug administered. But the intensity of drug effect is also dependent on how much of a dose reaches a site of action at any one time and how long the drug remains there in effective concentrations. Thus it follows that even for a single dose of a single agent, the variability in the intensity of response among different individuals must result from irregularities in absorption, distribution, biotransformation or excretion.

Most of the factors known to influence the nature or intensity of the response to drugs can be conveniently categorized on the basis of the source of the variability. The variables attributable to the biologic system account for differences in response to drugs among individuals of the same species as well as different species. This category includes such items as body weight and size, age, sex and other inherited characteristics, and the general state of health. The second category includes the variables attributable to the conditions of administration, such as the dose, dosage form, route and previous administration of the same or a different drug. These factors largely account for the differences in response observed in a single individual on different occasions. In this chapter we shall identify the major biologic sources of variability which make an individual respond to a drug in an unusual manner — unusual in the sense that the response is different from that anticipated in the "average" subject or in the majority of a population. In Chapter 10 we shall deal with the ways in which the repeated administration of a single drug and the interactions of concurrently administered drugs modify the effects produced.

BODY WEIGHT AND SIZE

The magnitude of drug response is a function of the concentration of drug attained at a site of action, and this concentration is related to the volume of distribution of the drug. For a given dose, the greater the volume of distribution, the lower the concentration of drug reached in the various fluid compartments of the body. Since the volume of interstitial and intracellular water is related to body mass, weight has a marked influence on the quantitative effects produced by drugs. One would antici-pate that a particular quantity of drug might be more effective in lighter subjects than in heavier ones, and in general, small persons require lower amounts of drugs than large persons in order to produce effects of equal intensity.

The average adult dose of a drug is calculated on the basis of the quantity that will produce a particular effect in 50 per cent of a population between 18 and 65 years of age and weighing about 70 kg (150 lb). Since the dose required is roughly propor-tional to body size, the variation in effects produced by a drug can be reduced when the dose is determined on the basis of a certain amount per kilogram of body weight. Thus:

$$\text{Dose required} = \frac{\text{Average dose}}{70\ \text{kg}} \times \text{Weight of individual (kg)}$$

This method of adjusting dosage to eliminate a source of biologic variation may be quite suitable for those persons whose weights are within the limits considered normal for their height and age. But for abnormally lean or obese individuals, dosage adjust-ments must also take into account the changes in ratios of body water to body mass. In the obese subject the total volume of body water is about 50 per cent of the body weight, whereas the value is closer to 70 per cent for the lean individual (Table 9-1). It is for this reason that body surface area, which is based on both height and weight,

Table 9-1. Effect of Age, Sex and Body Type on Body Composition

	Age (yr.)	Mean Body Weight (kg)	Total Body Water (% body weight)	Fat (% body weight)
Infant	Less than 3 mo.	3.5–8.3	70	
Infant	1	10	57	
Male	20–30	72	58	19
	40–50	77	56	25
	60–70	77	54	25
Female	16–30	58	52	29
	40–50	62	49	35
	60–70	64	42	45
Obese male	31	100	49	33
Lean male	26	69	70	7

is often a more discriminative index than weight alone for adjustment of drug dosage over a wide range of body sizes.[1]

AGE

Some effects of age on the quantitative aspects of drug activity are inseparable from those attributable to size, since the two variables are directly related during the early part of life. However, age, not size, is the more dominant factor in the variability of drug action in the infant and young child. And the elderly also frequently respond to drugs in a manner that cannot be imputed merely to differences in body weight. These individuals at the extremes of the life-span are often unusually sensitive to drugs; their responses occur at the far left of the normal distribution and quantal dose-response curves. This apparent increase in sensitivity is associated with changes in rates of absorption, distribution, biotransformation or excretion.

In the elderly, there is a normal decline with aging in the integrity of the various organs and systems involved in the absorption and elimination of drugs. There may be decreased responsiveness to drugs administered orally due to a lowered efficiency of absorption. But what is observed most often is an increased sensitivity because of impaired ability to biotransform and excrete drugs. Since the elderly are likely to respond to drugs in a manner quantitatively different from the average adult, cautious estimates of drug dosage are always indicated.

At the other end of the age scale, in newborn infants, particularly premature infants, many of the enzyme systems responsible for normal metabolic conversions and drug biotransformations are underdeveloped. For example, many of the important microsomal enzymes concerned with oxidation and glucuronide conjugation are either lacking or present in very low quantities. As a consequence, natural metabolites such as bilirubin (cf. p. 146) or drugs such as acetanilid, aminopyrine (Pyramidon) and hexobarbital are biotransformed very slowly (or not at all) in the young of humans and other animals (Table 9-2). These enzyme systems develop quickly, however. Most

Table 9-2. Effect of Age on Biotransformation

Drug	Drug Biotransformed[a] (μM/g) at Age:		
	2 Weeks	3 Weeks	Adult
Hexobarbital	4.2	10.3	16.6
Aminopyrine	0.34	1.41	5.2
l-Amphetamine	1.9	15.1	21.1
Acetanilid	2.9	5.2	7.8
Chlorpromazine	11.4	31.5	32.3
p-Nitrobenzoic acid	1.76	5.28	8.1

[a]Micromoles of drug metabolized or metabolite formed per gram of protein of liver.
Data from J. F. Fouts and R. H. Adamson, *Science* 129:897, 1959.

[1]Nomograms for determination of body surface area from height and weight are available, e.g., D. DuBois and E. F. DuBois, *Arch, Intern. Med.* 17:865, 1916.

of them increase to adult levels within one to eight weeks after birth, and within the first year of life all are probably as active as they will ever be.

The renal excretion of drugs is also depressed in the very young, primarily as a result of a decreased rate of presentation of drug to the kidney. As Table 9-1 indicates, water constitutes a greater percentage of the total body weight of the infant than of individuals in other age groups. The greater volume available for distribution lowers the concentration of drug in the blood coming to the kidneys. In addition, the volume of blood flowing through the kidney per unit time is smaller in the infant in proportion to this total body water content. Because of the greater volume of distribution and the lower rate of blood flow, the rate at which drugs are filtered by the infantile glomerulus is relatively slow. For example, the half-time of elimination of inulun is three times longer in the average infant than in the average adult, despite the corrections that are made for differences in relative body water content. Drugs that are secreted by the renal tubular cells, such as para-aminohippuric acid (PAH), are also eliminated more slowly in infants than in adults (cf. p. 137). This deficiency in all likelihood is traceable to the incomplete development of the active transport processes.

The existence of these defective mechanisms for drug elimination in the infant has important therapeutic implications. Depending on the route and frequency of administration, drug action tends to be either heightened or prolonged, or both, even when dosage is adjusted according to body size. If the appropriate dose is given by a route in which absorption is rapid, the concentration attainable at a site of action — and therefore the intensity of response — is likely to be no different from usual. Effective drug levels, however, will persist for longer periods (Fig. 9-1A). An increase in the duration of action of a single dose of a drug is not in itself harmful and may even be salutary. Rather, the danger lies in the accumulation to toxic levels if the spacing

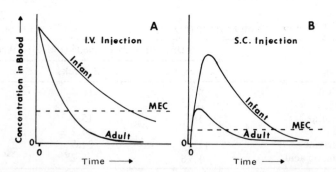

FIGURE 9-1. Effect of age on the maximum blood concentration and duration of action of a drug. (A) Drug A given by intravenous route to an adult and a 3-month-old infant in equivalent doses based on milligrams of drug per kilogram of body weight. (B) Drug B given by subcutaneous injection to an adult and a 3-month-old infant in equivalent doses based on milligrams of drug per kilogram of body weight. (MEC = minimum effective concentration in blood.)

between doses does not take into account the higher residual drug level in the infant's body prior to each successive dose (cf. pp. 228–233).

Ordinarily, the rate of passive diffusion is unaltered in the infant. If anything, it may be increased because of incomplete development of the anatomic barrier. This is certainly true for the blood-brain barrier, which is unusually permeable in the newborn. The newborn can also absorb large molecules, such as proteins, from the gastrointestinal tract, and this increased permeability may extend to still other chemical entities. A decreased rate of absorption is likely only for those few agents that are actively transported; these transport mechanisms may be deficient at other barriers as they are in the renal tubular epithelium. Since most drugs are absorbed by passive diffusion, it follows that the rate of absorption of drugs is, for the most part, the same in the very young as in the adult. Nevertheless, when drugs are administered by slow-absorption routes, the ensuing changes in the time course of action may be more deleterious to the infant than if administration were by fast-absorption routes. When a dose of a drug is rapidly absorbed, the rate of elimination has little effect on the maximum concentration reached in the body (cf. Fig. 8-17). But when the rate of absorption is slow, the peak drug concentration attained is determined by the rate of absorption *relative* to elimination. For a given rate of absorption, the slower the rate of elimination, the higher the peak drug level and the greater the magnitude of drug effect following equivalent dosage. Thus a drug given by a slow-absorption route in a dosage calculated by weight will yield higher peak levels in the infant than in the adult because of the reduced elimination rate in the infant (Fig. 9-1B). Under these circumstances of administration, the likelihood of cumulative toxicity with repeated administration is also greater than by fast-absorption routes; not only does a single dose yield a higher drug level in the infant compared with the adult, but the higher level also prevails for a longer period (Fig. 9-1B).

The combination of depressed renal function and decreased rates of drug biotransformation can now adequately account for many drug toxicities in the newborn infant that previously were inexplicable. For example, the antibiotic chloramphenicol (Chloromycetin) is conjugated with glucuronic acid to the extent of about 90 per cent in the adult. The conjugated antibiotic is excreted rapidly by renal tubular secretion as well as by glomerular filtration. The important hepatic enzymes which are involved in glucuronide conjugation are not fully developed until after three or four weeks of extrauterine life. Consequently, in the newborn child, when chloramphenicol is administered, most of it remains as the free, unconjugated drug. Not only is the free drug poorly eliminated in the urine due to reabsorption from the glomerular filtrate, but glomerular filtration in the neonate is itself relatively inefficient. Therefore, a normal therapeutic dose calculated on the basis of body weight leads to high and prolonged levels of free chloramphenicol in the newborn. And it is the unconjugated drug which is pharmacologically active. Successive dosage on the usual schedules only aggravates the situation and produces free drug levels associated with severe toxicity. A number of deaths resulted from this routine adaptation of adult dosage to use in infants before it was recognized that the newborn baby is different from the adult in more than just size. Once the reasons for the neonate's vulnerability to chloramphenicol-induced toxicity were disclosed, the potential adverse effects were avoided.

The deficiency of enzymes in infants as well as other factors involved in their growth and development also render them more susceptible than older children to nontherapeutic chemicals in their environment. For example, infants less than 6 months old are extraordinarily sensitive to agents that convert hemoglobin, the oxygen-carrying protein of red blood cells, to methemoglobin, which cannot carry oxygen. Two factors are responsible. First, fetal hemoglobin is oxidized to methemoglobin more readily than is the adult form of the protein; fetal hemoglobin is only slowly replaced by adult hemoglobin during the first five or six months of life. Second, the young infant — but not the older child — is deficient in the enzyme necessary to reduce methemoglobin to hemoglobin. Consequently, it takes only very small quantities of a chemical, such as an aniline dye, to produce methemoglobinemia in an infant. Even the amount of aniline dye used in inks for marking diapers has proved at times sufficient to cause this toxicity.

These two factors plus a third developmental variable also account for the severe, sometimes fatal, methemoglobinemia seen when formulas for infants are prepared with water that contains inorganic nitrates. (Water from wells is a particularly insidious source of this potentially toxic chemical in rural communities because of the extensive use of nitrate-containing fertilizers.) This represents a qualitatively differ-

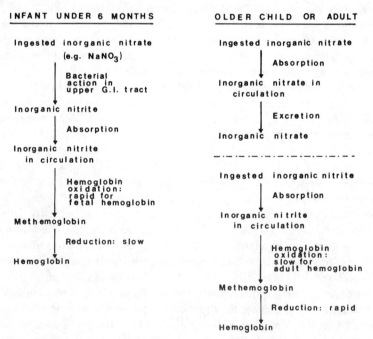

FIGURE 9-2. Effect of age on the potential toxicity of inorganic nitrates and nitrates.

ent effect in very young infants, since inorganic nitrate does not lead to methemoglobin formation in older children and adults. Hemoglobin is not oxidized to methemoglobin by inorganic nitrate; the nitrate must first be reduced to inorganic nitrite. In infants, but not in older individuals, ingested inorganic nitrate is converted to nitrite by the enzymic activity of bacteria present in the upper gastrointestinal tract. It is the nitrite that is absorbed and that interacts with hemoglobin which causes the toxicity in infants. Nitrate-reducing bacteria require a near-neutral or only slightly acidic environment to grow. In older individuals, bacteria do not normally invade or multiply in the upper intestine since the entering stomach contents produce an unfavorable acidic environment. Consequently, in older subjects, the ingested nitrate is not chemically altered within the intestine; it is absorbed as such before it reaches an area where bacterial action can affect it. In contrast, the less acidic stomach contents of infants provide conditions of pH conducive to bacterial growth within the upper small intestine. Thus it is the decreased acidity of the upper intestinal tract of infants compared with that of older individuals which is the factor responsible for the qualitatively different response to ingested nitrate (Fig. 9-2).

SEX

Simply on the basis of weight, women may require smaller doses of drugs than men to manifest the same magnitude of response. For drugs with a narrow margin of safety, these differences may necessitate a dosage reduction for women. There also may be sex differences in response to drugs because of the unequal ratios of lean body mass to fat mass. In the adult female, adipose tissue represents a greater and water a smaller percentage of total body weight than in the adult male (see Table 9-1).

Whereas differences in drug effects attributable to sex appear to be of only minor consequence, in pregnant women the use of all drugs except those essential to maintain pregnancy should be approached with caution. As was mentioned earlier (Chapter 5, Distribution from Mother to Fetus) almost any agent in maternal blood may cross the placental barrier, and drugs with little potential for producing adverse effects in the mother may prove most harmful to the developing embryo or fetus. Drugs given to the mother at parturition may also have long-lasting effects in the newborn; the latter not only may lack the mechanisms necessary for terminating the action of many drugs, but also loses those of the mother as soon as contact with the maternal circulation is severed.

GENETIC FACTORS

A few members of a supposedly homogeneous population respond to drugs in an entirely unusual and highly unpredictable fashion. These responses may take the form of extreme sensitivity to small doses or insensitivity to high doses of a drug whose administration normally produces qualitatively similar effects only at much higher or lower doses. Or the drug reactions may be qualitatively different from the effects usually observed in the majority of subjects. The term *idiosyncrasy* (Gr. *idios,* "one's own," "peculiar," "distinct"; *synkrasis,* "a mixing together") has long been used to denote both quantitatively and qualitatively abnormal drug response. Although this terminology recognized that the peculiar responses were not explicable in the same terms as other commonly encountered biologic variations, the reasons for their occurrence remained obscure. Relatively recent advances in biochemical genetics provided the knowledge necessary to seek plausible explanations for these phenomena. The mechanisms underlying the unusual responses to several drugs have now been elucidated and shown to be of genetic origin; it is quite likely that all drug idiosyncrasies will turn out to be genetically conditioned abnormalities. Thus the term *idiosyncrasy*, as it applies to drug reactivity, has taken on a more satisfactory meaning; it may now be more precisely defined as a *genetically determined*, abnormal response to a drug. And the relatively new, increasingly important branch of pharmacology that deals with the study of genetic modifications of drug response is known as *pharmacogenetics*. Before considering the abnormal drug responses that have been shown to be idiosyncratic, we shall discuss briefly the basic genetic mechanism involved and how idiosyncrasies can be recognized.

The Genetic Basis of Abnormal Drug Responses

The structure, function and development of each entity of a biologic system are determined by heredity. All the genetic information transmitted from generation to generation is contained in genes, the submicroscopic, chemical entities located at various areas on chromosomes. Chromosomes always exist in pairs, each species having its own characteristic number. There are 23 pairs of chromosomes in humans, only one pair of which carries the X or *sex-determining gene*. In the female, each of the two sex chromosomes has the X gene. In the male, only one of the sex chromosomes carries the sex-determining gene; the chromosome lacking the X gene is represented by Y. The term *sex-linked* describes any inherited trait carried on the X chromosomes; a trait located on any of the other 22 pairs of chromosomes (in humans) is referred to as an *autosomal* trait.

An inherited trait is controlled by either a single gene, a pair of genes or many genes. If many genes are involved in the transmission of a specific trait, the inherited characteristic shows continuous variation within the species. In other words, if multigenetic or multifactorial inheritance is involved, the specific trait shows a normal distribution within a population, i.e., it follows a normal, bell-shaped distribution curve (cf. Fig. 7-10). The distribution of height in humans is a typical example of an inherited trait whose magnitude is continuously variable (Fig. 9-3A). In contrast, if an inherited trait is determined by a single gene, there can be no continuous variation; the individual either possesses the characteristic or lacks it. Maleness or femaleness is a good example of such *discontinuous* variation.

The biotransformation of atropine in rabbits furnishes a model of discontinuous variation that is more pertinent to our discussion. Certain members of this species possess an enzyme called atropine esterase which hydrolyzes atropine, whereas the enzyme is completely lacking in other rabbits. A single gene or pair of genes controls the production of atropine esterase, and the enzyme appears to be completely absent in animals that have not inherited this autosomal trait. The enzyme is also absent in most mammalian species, including the human. Rabbits capable of hydrolyzing

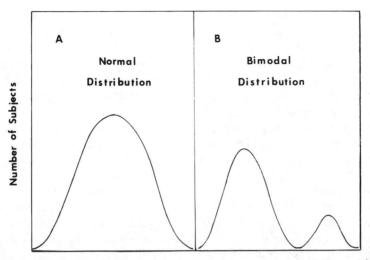

FIGURE 9-3. Continuous and discontinuous biologic variation. (A) Normal frequency distribution, schematically representative of an inherited trait that is continuously variable, such as the distribution of height in human beings. This type of distribution is also representative of the rate of biotransformation of a drug like salicylic acid or the effect of a drug like ethanol in a population. Such normal frequency curves are characteristic of multigenetic inheritance. (B) Bimodal frequency distribution, schematically representative of an inherited trait that is controlled by a single gene or pair of genes. This type of discontinuous variation may indicate a genetically determined abnormality in drug biotransformation or drug effect. The response of rabbits to atropine may be depicted by B, the curve at the left representing the frequency of response to increasing doses of atropine in animals lacking atropine esterase and the curve at the right, the response in animals possessing the enzyme.

atropine are much more resistant to the drug's effects than those which lack this mechanism for eliminating the drug. If progressively larger doses of atropine were administered to a substantial number of rabbits and the frequency with which a certain dose produced death were determined, the frequency could not be expressed as a normal distribution. Rather, the studied population would be found to be divided into two distinct groups — there would be discontinuous variation, such as illustrated by the bimodal distribution in Figure 9-3B. The bell-shaped curve at the left in B may be considered representative of the group lacking atropine esterase and responding to lower doses of atropine. The curve on the right would represent the response of rabbits possessing the gene for the hydrolyzing enzyme which renders them able to tolerate higher doses of the drug. The spread of values within the two groups indicates that other factors — multigenetic factors, which are responsible for the commonly observed biologic variations — are also influencing the responsiveness of all rabbits to atropine.

The discontinuity of a frequency-response curve is characteristic of the idiosyncratic reaction and distinguishes this type of reactivity from the normal resistance to high doses of a drug or sensitivity to low doses. The few individuals responding to very low or very high doses of alcohol, for example, as shown in Figure 7-9 (and schematically by Fig. 9-3A), do not represent a population separate from the normal. The continuous biologic variation observed in this and all dose-response relationships may have a genetic basis, but this is probably of multigenetic origin, unlike the single genetic determinant of drug idiosyncrasy. Thus, when the response to a drug indicates a discontinuous variation, it is highly suggestive of the existence of genetically abnormal responders within the group being studied. Subsequent investigation often reveals the particular hereditary defect responsible for the unusual reaction to the drug. And such defects are almost always found to involve the alteration of a protein.

But how do such abnormalities occur in the first place? Information for the synthesis of all cell proteins is encoded in the gene. Every protein in the cell is assembled from individual amino acids in accordance with the specifications of its genetic code. The correct assembly depends upon the fidelity with which the genetic message is transcribed and translated. And the normal replication process is remarkable in this respect. Errors rarely occur more often than once in one hundred thousand replications. But unless these errors, or *spontaneous mutations,* can be recognized as such and either rejected or repaired, they will persist. For if the alteration is not incompatible with life, the mutation will not only be replicated in the normal manner but will itself become permanently encoded in the gene. A mutation which affects the ability of the progeny to carry on a vital function will not be perpetuated since the progeny will not survive. A mutation which alters the specifications of the genetic code for a nonvital function may become a permanent, heritable change in a germ cell. The progeny of the union of that altered germ cell with another will appear as genetically abnormal individuals. Thus, abnormalities that manifest themselves as the altered ability to direct the synthesis of nonvital proteins originate as mutations.

These mutations may be expressed as the complete absence of a given protein or as variously altered proteins in which the modification is usually only the substitution of a single amino acid. Such replacement of a single amino acid by another in the normal hemoglobin structure produces a number of different abnormal hemoglobins. For example, substituting valine for glutamic acid at a particular location in the hemoglobin protein causes sickle cell anemia. The red blood cells possessing this genetically modified hemoglobin tend to aggregate in the capillaries, and this clumping together renders them more susceptible to lysis. The substitution of glutamic acid for valine at a different position in the hemoglobin structure makes the protein more readily oxidizable to methemoglobin. Even though individuals with this hereditary defect, unlike the newborn infant (cf. p. 246), have the enzyme to reduce the methemoglobin to hemoglobin, the former tends to accumulate. The life-span of the affected erythrocytes is shortened by this methemoglobin accumulation, since in this case the presence of an altered protein makes the cells more susceptible to rupture. Individuals with this genetic defect are exceedingly sensitive to nitrites and other drugs that cause methemoglobinemia.

Mechanisms of Drug Idiosyncrasies

Proteins occupy a singularly dominant position with respect to pharmacologic activity. As structural components of receptors and as enzymes, proteins play an essential part in the initiation and termination of the action of most drugs. And the interaction of some proteins with drugs influences distribution by mediating or inhibiting drug transfer across biologic membranes. It is not surprising, then, that the mechanisms responsible for idiosyncratic drug reactions, in the instances in which they have been elucidated, have been traced to genetic modification of specific proteins. In fact, such genetic alterations may go undetected until the abnormal system is suitably challenged by a drug. Some of the important discoveries of inheritable abnormalities have been made when the responses to some drug, or the biotransformation of a drug, indicated a discontinuous variation.

Hence, the various mechanisms involved in idiosyncratic responses may be categorized according to the role which the altered protein usually plays in drug activity. The alteration of an enzyme normally responsible for drug biotransformation may prolong or shorten the duration of action if this reaction is the principal mechanism for the drug's elimination. Abnormalities of proteins of other systems may either result in a prolonged effect of a drug, or be manifest as a novel drug response. Modifications that change the combining capacity of nonreceptor proteins may lead either to decreased responsiveness if an agent is unable to reach its target site or to unusual responses if a chemical reaches extraordinary sites of distribution. Finally, alteration of a receptor protein may lead to increased or decreased intensity of drug effect. Examples of each type of idosyncrasy are listed in Table 9-3 and briefly discussed below.

Abnormalities in Biotransformation Processes

An excellent example of how genetic abnormalities of drug-inactivating enzymes affect duration of action is provided by the muscle-relaxing drug succinylcholine. This drug is widely used in surgical procedures in which relaxation of muscles is desirable for a short period. Normally, succinylcholine is so rapidly hydrolyzed by the cholinesterases of plasma and liver that its action persists for only a few minutes after its administration is completed. In a few patients, however, the drug has been found to produce muscular relaxation and apnea (partial or complete suspension of respiration) of several hours' duration. Subsequent investigations of cholinesterase activity in the affected patients and their families revealed the presence of atypical cholinesterase as a genetically determined trait. The frequency of occurrence of this genetic abnormality in the population as a whole is about 1 in 3,000.

Another well-documented case of genetic variation in the biotransformation of drugs in humans is that of isoniazid, an agent useful in the treatment of tuberculosis. Here, it is an enzyme of a conjugation process, acetylation, which is affected. Figure 9-4 shows the frequency distribution of the rate of biotransformation of isoniazid (as measured by the plasma concentration of free drug six hours after administration) in 267 individuals belonging to 53 families. The discontinuous variation is clearly

Table 9-3. Drug Idiosyncrasies Classified According to the Role of the Genetically Altered Protein in Drug Activity

Genetic Abnormality of Protein of	Type of Alteration	Chemicals Whose Activity Is Affected	Manifestation of Abnormality
Drug Biotransformation Processes			
Plasma cholinesterase	Decreased activity	Succinylcholine	Prolonged drug effect
Plasma cholinesterase	Increased activity	Succinylcholine	Decreased responsiveness to drug
Acetylation	Reduced quantity of enzyme	Isoniazid	Increased toxicity due to accumulation
Microsomal oxidation	Decreased activity	Phenytoin (Dilantin)	Increased toxicity due to accumulation
Atropine esterase	Presence in <u>some</u> rabbits	Atropine	Decreased responsiveness to drug
Normal Enzymes or Functional Proteins			
Methemoglobin-reducing enzyme	Markedly decreased activity in erythrocytes	Nitrites, phenacetin, sulfa drugs and other drugs that oxidize hemoglobin	Prolonged methemoglobinemia; decreased oxygen-carrying capacity of hemoglobin
Enzymes involved in synthesis of blood-clotting factors	Decreased affinity for drug	Coumarin anticoagulants	Marked decrease in response to drug
Hemoglobin	More easily oxidized to methemoglobin	Nitrites and other drugs that oxidize hemoglobin	Propensity to develop methemoglobinemia; erythrocytes rupture due to methemoglobin accumulation
Enzyme involved in glucose metabolism	Reduced quantity of enzyme in erythrocytes	Primaquine, quinine, sulfa drugs, aspirin and phenacetin	Novel drug effect; hemolytic anemia; decreased number of circulating red blood cells due to lysis

Distribution			
Specific plasma protein: ceruloplasmin	Deficient synthesis	Copper in diet	Novel drug effect; excessive free, ionized copper distributed to and accumulated in various organs and tissues
Intrinsic factor	Deficiency leading to poor absorption	Vitamin B_{12} in diet	Depressed formation of new erythrocytes
Receptors			
Taste receptors	Altered combining capacity	Phenylthiourea	Inability to taste bitterness

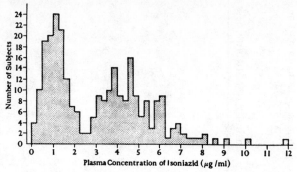

FIGURE 9-4. Plasma concentration of isoniazid determined 6 hours after its oral administration (9.8 mg per kilogram of body weight) to 267 members of 53 families. The frequency distribution shows a bimodality, with the mean plasma concentration for one subpopulation at about 1 μg per milliliter and for the other subpopulation, between 4 and 5 μg per milliliter. The subpopulations were designated "rapid inactivators" and "slow inactivators." (From D. A. P. Evans, K. A. Manley and V. C. McKusick, Br. Med. J. 2:485, 1960.)

seen: one group of individuals may be classified as "rapid inactivators," the other as "slow inactivators." Acetylation is the major pathway of elimination of isoniazid; slow inactivators have been found to possess a reduced quantity of the enzyme which acetylates the drug. In this case, then, the genetic abnormality is a difference in the amount of available enzyme rather than an alteration in the enzyme protein itself. The individuals with the enzyme deficiency are more prone than normal persons to develop serious toxic effects on the usual dosage schedule. This has practical significance, since the incidence of slow inactivators is very high among certain geographic groups: 44 to 54 per cent in American Caucasians and Negroes; 60 per cent in Europeans and only 5 per cent in Eskimos.

Abnormalities in Functional Proteins and Enzyme Systems Other than Those of Biotransformation

We have already discussed how the low level of an enzyme system that is essential for reducing methemoglobin to hemoglobin partially accounts for the infant's sensitivity to chemical agents producing methemoglobinemia (cf. p. 246). Fortunately, in normal infants the deficiency is usually corrected within a few months after birth. There are, however, individuals who, at any age, show an abnormally prolonged duration of methemoglobinemia following exposure to nitrites, phenacetin, sulfa drugs or other agents capable of oxidizing hemoglobin to methemoglobin. This prolonged drug action is due to a genetic defect, the absence of the methemoglobin-reducing enzyme. In the normal person, a small amount of methemoglobin (about 1 per cent of the total hemoglobin) is always present in the circulating blood as a result of the spontaneous oxidation of hemoglobin. Physiologically, the amount of methemoglobin is held in check primarily by the normal activity of the reducing enzyme. In individuals afflicted with hereditary methemoglobinemia and lacking the normal defense mechanism, the quantity of methemoglobin may rise to as much as 30 to 50 per cent of the total hemoglobin. Such a decrease in available hemoglobin seriously impairs the capacity of erythrocytes to carry oxygen to the cells. But this level of methemoglobin is not incompatible with life. A decrease in the oxygen-carrying capacity of red blood cells does not become lethal until methemoglobin concentration reaches about 70 per cent of the total hemoglobin. It can be readily appreciated, however, that in individuals with hereditary methemoglobinemia, the use of drugs which form additional methemoglobin may be extremely hazardous.

Another genetic defect in an enzyme system of the red blood cell is manifest as a novel drug effect in some individuals, particularly Negro, Near Eastern and Mediterranean males. In these genetically abnormal subjects the administration of the usual daily doses of the antimalarial drug primaquine produces a profound, acute reduction in the number of circulating red blood cells. The novelty of this effect is evidenced by the fact that no comparable hemolytic anemia can be provoked in nonsusceptible individuals even at doses many times greater than the usual dose. The susceptible individuals differ from normal subjects in having red blood cells that are deficient in an important enzyme involved in glucose metabolism.[2] The activity of this enzyme system is essential for maintenance of cellular integrity. The trait is carried on the X chromosome and is, therefore, sex-linked. Persons with this trait can also develop hemolytic anemia in response to many other agents, e.g., quinine, sulfanilamide, aspirin, phenacetin and unidentified compounds present in fava beans.[3] The sensitive individuals appear to be adversely affected, however, only when challenged by these drugs.

Abnormalities in Drug Absorption and Distribution

Another type of anemia, juvenile pernicious anemia, also has its origin in the inherited lack of a protein. In this instance the protein is one essential for the intestinal absorption of vitamin B_{12}, a nutrient indispensable for the normal formation of red blood cells. In the absence of sufficient quantities of the vitamin, the number of circulating red blood cells is reduced as a result of a decreased rate of formation. The protein needed for vitamin B_{12} absorption, called *intrinsic factor,* is synthesized in the gastric mucosa and secreted into the stomach. When intrinsic factor is present, vitamin B_{12} combines with it and is carried to the ileum, where the complex attaches to the ileal surface. The vitamin is then transported across the intestinal mucosal cells and absorbed directly into the bloodstream. In the absence of intrinsic factor, the small quantities of vitamin B_{12} present in the normal diet escape absorption. Vitamin B_{12}

---

[2] The deficient enzyme is glucose-6-phosphate dehydrogenase (G6PD), just one of many enzymes involved in the complicated process by which glucose is metabolized ultimately to carbon dioxide and water. Cells deficient in G6PD are unable to maintain normal levels of another compound, glutathione. Glutathione is a reducing agent which, by combining with oxidizing agents in the cell, prevents the oxidizing agents from damaging cellular components. In the absence of sufficient glutathione, these oxidizing agents in the red blood cells can produce hemolysis.

[3] A popular vegetable among Europeans.

absorption not mediated by intrinsic factor occurs only in the presence of quantities of the vitamin much greater than those made available from the usual dietary intake. Pernicious anemia also develops in adults, but unlike the juvenile form of the disease, a genetic basis has not yet been clearly established.

According to the definition of a drug, the effects produced by the absence of intrinsic factor cannot truly be considered a *drug* idiosyncrasy. Even though vitamin B_{12} is administered as a drug to correct the abnormality, it is ordinarily regarded as a food constituent vital to normal development and nutrition. Antithetically, the genetically determined deficiency of a specific plasma protein, ceruloplasmin, converts a normal dietary constituent into a toxic chemical agent. The abnormality is known as Wilson's disease, and the dietary constituent is copper. Only a small quantity of copper is absorbed from the total amount ingested in the daily diet. Normally, almost all of the absorbed metal is incorporated into ceruloplasmin at the time this specific plasma protein is being newly synthesized. As a result, about 98 per cent of the copper in plasma is present as a firmly bound part of the protein structure. And in the normal state, the amount of copper incorporated into ceruloplasmin each day is counterbalanced by an equal daily elimination (by the intestine) of the copper-containing protein. Thus, in normal individuals, plasma-water and tissues contain negligible amounts of copper in the free, ionic state, since there is little free metal left in plasma to be distributed. In Wilson's disease, however, the plasma-water contains a greater than normal quantity of free copper ions; there is insufficient synthesis of the copper-containing protein for the adequate removal of the copper absorbed into the circulation each day. As a result, free copper ions are distributed to the tissues, where they become bound to various components. It is the slow accumulation and deposition of copper, particularly in liver and brain, that produces the toxicity and clinical manifestations of the disease.

Abnormalities in Drug Receptor Proteins

Almost all the known genetically determined abnormalities in drug responses fall into the first three categories discussed, since drug receptors and their protein components do not lend themselves readily to study in isolation. Indeed, drug idiosyncrasies that can be directly linked to genetic alteration of receptors are known only for those receptors that mediate the senses of taste and smell. For example, some few persons are unable to taste the compound phenylthiourea, even in concentrations one hundred times greater than those at which most people find it an extremely bitter substance. When various populations were studied to determine their taste thresholds for phenylthiourea, the frequency of response was found to have a bimodal distribution, i.e., the subjects could be divided into two distinct groups, one of "tasters," the other of "nontasters." The results of one such investigation are shown in Figure 9-5.

The interactions of chemicals with taste or smell receptors show the same types of specificity that are characteristic of the interaction of drugs with other receptors. Thus, when we are able to identify the receptor macromolecules responsible for the biologic effect of drugs, we may anticipate that some drug idiosyncrasies will also be traced to genetic alterations in these systems.

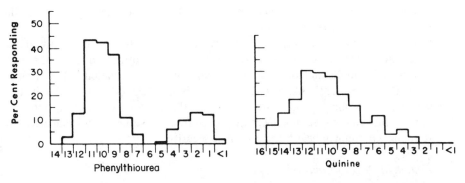

FIGURE 9-5. Distribution of taste thresholds for phenylthiourea and quinine. Tests were performed in 200 Belgian women. Values on the abscissa are for increasing concentrations, left to right; each concentration differed by a factor of 2 from the one before. Subjects unable to taste even the most concentrated solutions are included in the category labeled 1. The normal distribution of the ability to taste quinine indicates that subjects unable to taste phenylthiourea were not deficient in the ability to taste all bitter substances. (Modified from A. Leguebe, Bull. Inst. R. Sci. Nat. Belg. 36:1, 1960.)

The Importance of Pharmacogenetics

The objectives of pharmacogenetics are twofold: (1) the investigation and identification of the genetic basis for unusual drug responses, and (2) the development of methods for predicting those individuals who will react abnormally to drugs. Although routine investigations of large populations may not be justified considering the rarity of some idiosyncratic responses, thorough investigations are warranted in relatives of individuals in whom the diagnosis of a drug idiosyncrasy has been made. Thus the practical value of pharmacogenetic studies lies in their use to predict a potentially deleterious response to a drug before the drug is administered.

Interspecies Variation

So far we have considered genetically controlled differences in drug responses only as observed among individuals of the same species, primarily human. However, genetic factors that influence the pharmacologic action of drugs are even more apparent when comparisons of drug responses are made between species. These interspecies differences in reactions to drugs, often remarkable, also have a direct bearing on the use of drugs in the human. The initial investigations of the pharmacologic properties of a drug are carried out in a variety of laboratory animals. Because of interspecies variations, however, neither the efficacy nor toxicity of a compound in the human can be predicted solely from results obtained in other species. Thus, on the one hand, interspecies differences preclude the automatic transfer to human subjects of knowledge gained in animal experimentation. This means that the value of a drug can be ultimately ascertained only in the species in which it is to be used. (We shall deal more fully with this topic in Chapter 14.) On the other hand, without species variation in the response to drugs, there could be no drug therapy of organisms causing disease;

the very success of the drug depends on its ability to cause selective injury to invading organisms, such as bacteria, without injuring the host.

Interspecies variations in response to drugs, both quantitative and qualitative, have their origins in differences in absorption, distribution or biotransformation of the drugs, as well as in dissimilarities in integral functions or organization of the living matter. There are countless known examples of these species differences. We shall cite only a few to illustrate how they complicate the development of therapeutic agents for human use, yet implement the search for agents to destroy living matter interfering with human health and economic security.

Variation in Drug Biotransformation

Variation in drug biotransformation among species, even among closely related species such as mammals, is the rule rather than the exception. Thus the most probable cause of species differences in the response to drugs is the variability in the proportion of an administered dose of a drug that remains available to sites of drug action. These variations in drug biotransformation may be expressed qualitatively, as species differences in the pathways of metabolism, or quantitatively, as differences in the rate of biotransformation by reactions which are common to several species.

Differences in the pathway of biotransformation may appear as an inability of a particular species to carry out a given reaction due to the absence of an enzyme system generally found in other species. For example, glucuronide conjugation does not occur to any great extent in cats, although the reaction is a very common pathway of biotransformation for many drugs in dogs, rats and rabbits as well as humans. Again, dogs are unable to carry out some acetic acid conjugations which represent the principal routes of biotransformation in humans, rats and rabbits of agents such as the sulfa drugs. But even when there are no species differences in the occurrence of one or more enzyme systems, a single drug may be biotransformed by different reactions or at entirely different rates in various species. Amphetamine, for example, is biotransformed in humans, dogs and mice by similar mechanisms. In mice, however, the degree of biotransformation is more extensive than in the other two species. Amphetamine is biotransformed in the rat by processes different not only from those in the mouse but also from those in yet another species, the guinea pig. The pathway of biotransformation of ephedrine, a drug closely resembling amphetamine in structure and pharmacologic activity, is entirely different in rabbits from that in rats, dogs and humans. But, in the case of ephedrine, almost no biotransformation takes place in the human, whereas the dog converts most of the drug into an equally active agent. Yet the microsomal enzyme systems responsible for the metabolism of amphetamine or ephedrine in any one of these species are present in all the species examined, as evidenced by their activity in the biotransformation of other drugs. Thus, even though a particular reaction occurs in many species, there appears to be no rationale for predicting the extent of the reaction with different compounds in the same species or with a given drug in different species. The data in Table 9-4 emphasize not only how great may be the species differences in rates of biotransformation of a single drug, but also that these differences display no consistent pattern.

Table 9-4. Comparative Half-Lives[a] of Biotransformation of Drugs in Various Species

Drug	Human Being	Rhesus Monkey	Dog	Mouse	Rat	Rabbit	Cat
Hexobarbital	6		4.3	0.3	2.3	1	
Meperidine (Demerol)	5.5	1.2	0.9				
Phenylbutazone (Butazolidin)	72	8	6		6	3	
Ethyl biscoumacetate (Tromexan)	2		21			2	
Antipyrine	12	1.8	1.7				
Digitoxin	216		14		18		60
Digoxin	44		27		9		27

[a]Values in hours required to biotransform 50 per cent of a dose of drug.

This vast species variation in drug biotransformation largely account for the equally wide species differences in the therapeutic or toxic effects of chemical substances. This is what poses such great problems in the testing and development of new drugs. The evaluation of new agents for their efficacy and safety in humans begins with studies in laboratory animals such as mice, rats, rabbits, dogs and cats, and the decision to test or use an agent in human subjects is largely determined by the data obtained from these initial studies. For example, in a developmental program seeking an anticoagulant drug with a short duration of action in humans, the therapeutically useful agent ethyl biscoumacetate (Tromexan) would have been discarded on the basis of its prolonged action in dogs (Table 9-4). On the other hand, studies in rabbits would have given a good indication of the drug's short duration of action in humans, since in both these species the biologic half-life is about two hours. These same studies, however, illustrate the complexities involved in projecting animal data directly to humans. Ethyl biscoumacetate is biotransformed in both the human and the dog by the same metabolic reactions, despite the differences in rate. The rabbit utilizes an entirely different pathway for the inactivation of the anticoagulant, even though the rate of biotransformation is the same as in humans.

The projection to humans of data obtained in animals can have more serious consequences when a chemical produces toxic effects in the human that were unanticipated from the initial studies in animals. This may occur when biotransformation in humans is much slower than in other species or yields a toxic metabolite that is not formed by the species originally studied. Although the quest continues for an animal species that closely resembles the human in its handling of all drugs, the hope of finding the ideal specimen appears remote. Even studies in primates, the species closest to humans on the evolutionary scale, appear to have no better predictive value in man than have studies carried out in the dog (see Table 9-4). Since animal studies must always serve as a guide, and since the vast species differences in drug response is well recognized, how can the dilemma be resolved so that translation of results to humans is less uncertain? No simple answers to this question are available, but present knowledge — or the lack of it — certainly suggests that drug testing should be conducted on a wide variety of species, including those with close phylogenetic relationship to man.

Other Sources of Species Variation in Response to Drugs

So far we have considered only how the inescapable fact of species variation in response to drugs handicaps the development of agents to be used for their direct pharmacodynamic effects in humans. Here, the most important factor appears to be variations in rate and pattern of drug biotransformation. But differences in renal or biliary excretion, binding to plasma proteins, tissue distribution or other factors may also contribute to the phenomenon. Species variation takes on an entirely different perspective, however, when it is a question of developing chemicals to eliminate organisms that threaten human economic security, comfort or health. Now the greater the dissimilarity between species, the greater the likelihood of achieving the therapeutic goal: producing irreversible damage to the undesirable species, the *uneconomic* species, while leaving the desirable species, the *economic* species, unaffected. And under these circumstances, species variation in structure or organization of the living matter or in metabolic reactions supplying energy for growth and survival becomes more pertinent than differences in drug biotransformation or availability to receptor sites.

The classic example of the destruction of an uneconomic species without harm to the economic species is that of the action of sulfanilamide (or sulfonamides in general) on various bacterial infections of humans or other mammals. Many microorganisms require the vitamin folic acid (pteroylglutamic acid) for growth and use para-aminobenzoic acid (PABA) for the synthesis of this essential metabolite. Sulfanilamide is closely related to PABA in structure (Fig. 9-6) and interferes with the incorporation of PABA into the vitamin. The drug acts as a competitive inhibitor of the enzyme involved in the first step of folic acid synthesis. In the absence of sufficient quantities of folic acid, the bacteria are unable to sustain growth. Folic acid is also an essential metabolite for cells of mammals, but these species cannot synthesize the vitamin and must acquire it as a preformed constituent of the diet. Hence, since PABA is not an essential metabolite for animals, sulfanilamide can selectively affect bacteria which require PABA without equivalent injury to host tissues.

A difference in structure readily explains why penicillin is relatively inert toward

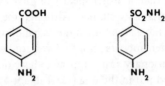

Para-aminobenzoic acid   Sulfanilamide

FIGURE 9-6. Structure of para-aminobenzoic acid (PABA) and sulfanilamide.

mammalian cells but lethal to bacteria. The actively multiplying bacterium must be able to assimilate certain soluble substances from its environment and to maintain these at intracellular concentrations higher than those in its external surroundings. A rigid cell wall surrounding a cellular membrane affords the bacteria the needed protection to remain intact despite the pressure gradients established between the inside and outside of the cell. Penicillin suppresses the formation of the bacterial cell wall. Thus, microorganisms growing in the presence of the antibiotic fail to synthesize the rigid structure which will protect them from their usual hypotonic environment. As a result, the cell-wall-deficient bacteria are unable to withstand the differences between the internal and external osmotic pressures; the cell membrane ruptures, and complete lysis occurs. Human or animal cells lack a cell wall, and their intracellular contents are isotonic with their extracellular environment. The selective toxicity of penicillin for bacteria arises, then, from inhibition of the synthesis of a structure vital but unique to the microorganism.

The dramatic effectiveness of antibacterial drugs arises from the fact that they act on target systems which are indispensable for either bacterial reproduction or survival but are either nonessential or nonexistent in mammals. When the differences between the economic and uneconomic species are less qualitatively distinctive or merely quantitative in nature, the selectivity of drug action is also less spectacular. For example, certain organic compounds which contain the metal antimony are effective in the treatment of schistosomiasis, a disease caused by various parasitic worms commonly known as *blood flukes*. The metabolism of glucose proceeds at a very rapid rate in the schistosomes, and their survival is largely dependent on this metabolic process. The antimonial drugs inhibit the activity of one of the enzymes essential for the metabolism of glucose. This enzyme is present in mammals as well, but is much less sensitive to inhibition by the drugs containing antimony. Therefore, the usefulness of antimonials in schistosomiasis is due, in part at least, to species differences in the nature of an enzyme and to the greater dependence of the parasite on energy supplied by glucose metabolism. The species difference is not great enough, however, to preclude all adverse effects on the host. Hopefully, continued investigations will disclose in other uneconomic species the true qualitative differences that exist between microorganisms and mammals. Then these uneconomic species will also be subject to attack by selectively toxic chemicals.

GENERAL CONDITIONS OF HEALTH

Almost all the principles of pharmacokinetics have been developed from data collected in normal, healthy subjects. Drugs, however, are usually administered to people in whom a physiologic or biochemical process is functioning at other than normal levels. It is to be expected, then, that a disease-induced or drug-induced abnormality may modify a drug effect, just as an inherited abnormality may produce an altered drug response in the individual afflicted. The multitude of diseases makes it impossible to summarize briefly the effects of all the potential variables involved, but a few examples will help to point up the varying susceptibility to drugs that may be encountered when they are administered to patients.

Physiologic variables such as changes in body temperature, in the water content of various body compartments or in the pH of body fluids may understandably modify the effects of drugs. For example, we have seen that differences between infants and adults, or between men and women, with respect to their content of body water, may influence the volume of distribution of a drug. By analogy, the volume of drug distribution will be affected by states of dehydration or overhydration (edema). The degree of ionization of drugs that are weak acids or bases is dependent on the pH of the medium in which they are dissolved. Therefore, changes in the pH of body fluids, as in acidosis or alkalosis, may alter the rate of distribution or excretion of some drugs by changing their rate of passage across biologic membranes (cf. pp. 133–134).

The occurrence of serious toxic effects in some patients being treated with various antidepressant drugs provides a bizarre example of how *some foods* can alter the anticipated response to drugs. Toxic symptoms appeared after the patients ate certain cheeses, such as Camembert, cheddar, Stilton and Roquefort. These cheeses and other foods like pickled herring, red wine and chicken liver are rich in tyramine, a naturally occurring amine that is normally metabolized rapidly by the enzyme monoamine oxidase. The affected patients, however, were being treated with drugs that are effective monoamine oxidase inhibitors. The inability of these patients to metabolize the ingested tyramine turned an ordinarily harmless food component into a toxic substance capable of producing sharp rises in blood pressure and, in a few cases, fatal cerebral hemorrhage. Appropriate warnings are now carried on the labels and inserts of all such drugs so that future incidents of toxic reactions may be avoided.

A drug-induced abnormality in body function precipitated the unexpected results of the interaction of monoamine oxidase inhibitors with normal foodstuffs. The effects of some drugs can also be considerably modified by disease-induced abnormalities in the physiology or biochemistry of the body. However, the underlying disturbance does not always offer a reasonable explanation for the altered response observed. In severe renal or liver disease, drugs that depend on these organs for their elimination must, understandably, be used with caution. A decreased rate of biotransformation or excretion may lead to cumulative toxicity if the usual dosage schedule is maintained. Abnormal susceptibility to drugs in some other diseases is also well recognized, as, for example, in individuals with an excess secretion of thyroid hormone. The hyperthyroid patient can tolerate larger doses of morphine than the individual with normal thyroid function, but responds to doses of epinephrine that barely affect the latter. The exact relationship between the thyroid hormone and the drugs is unknown, however. And in many other diseases, a modified drug response, although frequently observed, is not consistently correlated with the impaired function, so that the explanation remains obscure.

PSYCHOLOGIC FACTORS: THE PLACEBO EFFECT
It is astonishing how many therapeutic successes primitive doctors effected despite their ignorance of the causes of disease. Although some of these successes may have been realized through the use of agents that are still part of our therapeutic armamentarium, possibly the majority were based on the healing powers of suggestion.

For even with our present-day knowledge of normal bodily functions and the manner in which these functions are deranged by disease, it is frequently difficult to separate the pharmacologic effects of drugs from effects of psychologic origin or, for that matter, to distinguish between truly organic symptoms of illness and the equally real symptomatology arising from psychic and emotional factors. Experimental evidence indicates that many of the component changes in disease, including fever, headache, nausea and even more serious symptoms, can be brought about by impulses originating in the cerebral cortex. In the same way, the mere act of administering a drug may produce effects of varying severity which are totally unrelated to the drug's pharmacologic action. When the effects of a drug are temporally correlated with its administration and cannot be attributed to its chemical properties — its pharmacodynamic activity — they are known as *placebo effects.* An inert substance disguised as a drug, such as the sugar lactose, is called a *placebo* (L., "I shall please").

Placebo responses result, in part, from the strong motivation of the patient and the physician that the drug have its desired effects. How the impressions created at the time of drug administration may influence the therapeutic result is well illustrated by a study in two groups of patients with ulcers. All patients received a placebo. The patients in the first group were given the dummy drug by their physician, who told them that it was a new medication which would undoubtedly produce relief. A nurse administered the placebo to the second group with the statement that it was an experimental drug, the effects of which were not yet fully established. Excellent relief of symptoms was obtained in 70 per cent of the patients in the first group, whereas only 25 per cent of the second group showed a favorable response.

The effects of many drugs, particularly effects on mood and behavior, may also be modified by environmental conditions. For example, drugs used in the treatment of the anxiety and tension in psychiatric disorders appear to be more effective in relatively neglected and economically disadvantaged patients confined in large state hospitals than in patients residing in expensive, small, highly staffed hospitals. The influence of environmental factors is not limited, however, to the subjective effects of drugs, as the following study illustrates. A group of normal subjects were placed on controlled food and water intake, and their physical activity was regulated. The response measured was the urinary output induced by the drinking of a large quantity of water in a short period. Here, water was being used as the drug. For the two weeks of the study, the daily administration of water and the collection of urine always took place in the same laboratory room and under identical conditions. At the end of the conditioning period, a single swallow of water — about 1 ounce — was given to the subjects in the same laboratory. This small quantity induced a urinary output similar to that in response to the large quantities that had been ingested during the conditioning period. On the other hand, in an entirely different setting under otherwise similar conditions, the ingestion of 5 ounces of water (an amount smaller than that used in conditioning) produced a volume of urine directly proportional to intake. The results suggested that a particular therapeutic environment had a deep significance for the subjects and that the response of a vital regulatory mechanism was influenced by a situation that was meaningful to the individuals.

The administration of placebos also may produce effects that involve complex mechanisms, as for instance a significant reduction in the lipoprotein content of plasma or changes in the number of certain circulating blood cells (eosinophils). Thus it bears emphasizing that placebo effects are not imaginary. And just because they are real phenomena, they must be taken into account in pharmacology. First, the placebo may, under appropriate but limited circumstances, be used as a therapeutic aid. This is indicated, however, only when a physician, after a considered diagnosis, decides that there is no better form of drug or other therapy and that the administration of a placebo may elicit some beneficial results. But the more justifiable and important place of placebos in pharmacology is in evaluating the true pharmacologic efficacy of drugs. The results of many investigations indicate that the administration of a placebo produces a variety of positive responses in about 30 to 35 per cent of the population. Studies also show that there is no specific group of individuals who can be classified as "placebo responders"; at one time or another, all subjects may respond to placebos. Moreover, there is a lack of consistency not only in the frequency of placebo responses from study to study, but also in the kind of response observed. Since all drugs may produce placebo effects, the placebo response obviously represents a complicating factor in the study of drugs, particularly in human subjects. In Chapter 14, in discussing the development of a new drug, we shall see how the placebo response is evaluated within each experiment to ensure that the information obtained about drug action is meaningful.

REMARKS

We shall postpone summarizing the contents of this chapter until we have discussed the factors modifying drug response that are associated with the conditions of drug administration. Then at the conclusion of Chapter 10, having viewed modification in drug response from the perspective of the variability attributable both to the biologic system and to the conditions of drug administration, we can summarize the many contributory factors from another point of view.

GUIDES FOR STUDY AND REVIEW

How may differences in body weight and size affect the intensity of response to a given dose of drug? On what basis is the average adult dose of a drug calculated? Why would body surface area be a more discriminative index than body weight for adjustment of drug dosage?

In which population groups would age be most likely to influence the response to a given drug dosage? What factors are responsible for variability in drug response in the elderly? in the very young?

In the very young, what factors account for changes in rates of drug absorption? for changes in rates of drug elimination? How do changes in the rate of drug absorption or rate of elimination affect the quantitative response to a drug in the very young? How does a decrease in the rate of elimination affect the *maximum concentration* in the body of a drug that is rapidly absorbed? slowly absorbed? How does a decrease in the rate of elimination affect the duration of action of a drug that is rapidly absorbed? slowly absorbed? When is it necessary to adjust the size of a single dose of a drug? the frequency of administration of a drug?

How do we now define the term *idiosyncrasy* with respect to response to a drug? How does the quantal (frequency) dose-response relationship distinguish between the normal variability in response to a drug and the variability due to an idiosyncratic response? The normal frequency distribution (continuous variability) is associated with which type of inheritance? The bimodal (discontinuous) biologic variation is associated with which type of inheritance?

Why are idiosyncratic responses to drugs usually attributable to genetic modifications of specific proteins? What is an example of an abnormal drug response that is brought about by a genetic modification in an enzyme of biotransformation? by a genetic modification in hemoglobin?

How does interspecies variation in drug response complicate the development and testing of therapeutic agents to be used in humans? What are the most important factors (or sources) of species variation in response to drugs? For what general types of drugs is a marked difference between species a desirable and indeed an essential circumstance?

What are some of the physiologic variables other than age, body weight and size that may modify the response of an individual to a given dose of drug? How can diet affect drug response? How can severe liver or kidney disease influence the maximum effect and duration of action of a single dose of a drug? of multiple doses of a single drug? In the presence of liver disease, what dosage adjustments are necessary with respect to a drug eliminated primarily by biotransformation? In the presence of kidney disease, what dosage adjustments are necessary with respect to a drug eliminated primarily by urinary excretion?

How do psychologic factors influence the response to a drug? What is a placebo effect? What is a placebo?

What percentage of a population may be expected to display a "placebo response"? What form may a placebo response take? Are "placebo responders" always the same group of individuals or may anyone at some time respond to a placebo? How does the placebo response affect the determination of a drug's efficacy? In the development of a new drug, how is the placebo response evaluated to ensure accurate information about a drug's potential efficacy?

SUGGESTED READING

Bonner, D.M. *Heredity.* Englewood Cliffs, N.J.: Prentice-Hall, 1961.

Bourne, H.R. The placebo — a poorly understood and neglected therapeutic agent. *Ration. Drug Therap.* 5(11):1, 1971.

Clarke, C.A., Price-Evans, D.A., Harris, R., McConnell, R.B., and Woodrow, J.C. Genetics in medicine, a review: Part II. Pharmacogenetics. *Q.J. Med.* 37:183, 1968.

Done, A.K.   Perinatal pharmacology. *Annu. Rev. Pharmacol.* 6:189, 1966.

Jacob, F., and Monod, J.   Genetic regulatory mechanisms in the synthesis of proteins. *J. Mol. Biol.* 3:318, 1961.

Kalow, W.   *Pharmacogenetics, Heredity and the Response to Drugs.* Philadelphia: Saunders, 1962.

Koch-Weser, J.   Serum drug concentrations as therapeutic guides. *N. Engl. J. Med.* 287:227, 1972.

La Du, B.N.   Genetic Factors Modifying Drug Metabolism and Drug Response. In B.N. La Du, H.G. Mandel, and E.L. Way (eds.), *Fundamentals of Drug Metabolism and Drug Disposition.* Baltimore: Williams & Wilkins, 1971. P. 308

La Du, B.N., and Kalow, W. (eds.).   Pharmacogenetics. *Ann. N.Y. Acad. Sci.* 151:691, 1968.

Lasagna, L., Laties, V.G., and Doban, J.L.   Further studies on the "pharmacology" of placebo administration. *J. Clin. Invest.* 37:533, 1958.

Peters, J.H.   Genetic factors in relation to drugs. *Annu. Rev. Pharmacol.* 8:427, 1968.

Proceedings of an international symposium on comparative pharmacology. *Fed. Proc.* 26:963, 1967.

Stanbury, J.B., Wyngaarden, J.B., and Frederickson, D.S.   *The Metabolic Basis of Inherited Disease* (3d ed.). New York: McGraw-Hill, 1972.

Watson, J.D.   *Molecular Biology of the Gene.* New York: Benjamin, 1965.

10. FACTORS MODIFYING THE EFFECTS OF DRUGS IN INDIVIDUALS
Variability in Response Attributable to the Conditions of Administration

We have already discussed in detail how the size of the dose administered, the pharmaceutical formulation and the route and frequency of administration modify the effects produced by a drug. Although these four factors are the most important variables attributable to the conditions of administration, several others may also profoundly affect the response to a drug. All these other factors have one condition in common: the effects they produce are dependent on the previous administration of the same or a different drug. We shall discuss first the modified drug effects that may be seen following the repeated administration of a single agent, and then how the sequential or concurrent administration of two different drugs may enhance or diminish the effects of either or both drugs.

MODIFIED DRUG EFFECTS AFTER REPEATED ADMINISTRATION OF A SINGLE DRUG

Drug Resistance

The term *drug resistance* describes a state of decreased responsiveness, or complete lack of responsiveness, to drugs that ordinarily inhibit growth or cause cell death. Drug resistance is therefore a phenomenon which, by definition, may be associated only with drugs used to eliminate (1) an uneconomic species such as insects, bacteria or other parasites; or (2) rapidly growing cells such as cancer cells in higher organisms.

Origin of Drug Resistance

The sequence of events leading to the emergence of a strain of bacteria with altered drug response is typical of the general phenomenon of the development of drug resistance. When a strain of bacteria is exposed for the first time to an antibacterial agent, the effect produced is what is anticipated: retardation of the normal growth rate or reduction in the size of the bacterial population. As drug therapy continues, however, bacterial growth resumes, indicating that the organisms now present are unaffected by the same concentration of drug that was inhibitory or lethal to the original population. Thus a bacterial population that was initially sensitive to a drug has become insensitive; it has *acquired* resistance. The clinical consequences of this acquired resistance in a patient under treatment for an infection can readily be appreciated. If the pathogenic organism is one which would normally respond to the drug being used, the patient would at first show improvement. Then when resistance developed, the patient would suffer a relapse as the infecting organism became refractory to the previously used drug.

How do organisms such as bacteria acquire this resistance to the toxic effects of drugs? The answer lies in the fact that some species of microorganisms undergo spontaneous mutation. Populations of many bacteria do not consist solely of genetically identical cells; they are normally composed of individuals with different degrees of inherited susceptibility to an antibacterial drug, including some genetically altered cells that are completely drug-resistant. The number of spontaneous mutants that are drug-resistant may be as few as one in ten billion cells. In the presence of an antibacterial agent, the mutants that are insensitive to the drug survive and multiply, giving rise eventually to an entirely new drug-resistant population. Thus the drug permits survival of the least susceptible organisms. And the appearance of drug resistance during therapy merely represents selective multiplication of those insensitive mutants that were present *from the beginning of the infection.* The only role that the drug plays is to select out the resistant cells at the expense of the sensitive strain.

The fact that it is the microorganism, and not the patient, that becomes resistant to the drug also accounts for the increase and spread of drug-resistant strains of bacteria within a human or animal population. Extensive and prolonged use of a particular antibacterial agent provides the opportunity for eliminating the bulk of sensitive microorganisms while sparing the resistant mutants. The latter become the predominant strain and spread from infected patients to uninfected individuals and from them to the community. For example, in the United States in 1940 to 1941, over 70 per cent of patients with gonorrhea were rapidly cured by the use of various sulfa drugs. Four years later these same drugs failed in 70 per cent of the patients, since many strains of the gonococcus had become resistant to sulfonamides. Fortunately, penicillin became available for use at this time and proved to be successful in treating the sulfonamide-refractory gonococcal infections. As a rule, microorganisms resistant to a particular drug like sulfanilamide tend to be equally insensitive to other chemically related agents, such as other sulfonamides. However, they remain sensitive to chemically dissimilar agents such as penicillin.

The genetic determinant of drug resistance may also be transferred from insensitive organisms to other organisms that are not direct offspring of the resistant cells. Cell-to-cell contact is necessary for this phenomenon, called *infectious drug resistance* (Fig. 10-1.) Drug resistance may be acquired by a sensitive organism in contact with an insensitive organism of the same or a different strain of the same species, or even of a different species. This has considerable clinical significance since it means that the genetic determinants of drug resistance may be transferred from a nonpathogenic to a pathogenic bacterial species. Reports from many areas of the world indicate that an increasing number of diseases are caused by microorganisms that have acquired resistance to several drugs by infectious transferral. The widespread use of antibacterial agents not only in medicine but in agriculture (livestock feed) is undoubtedly a contributory factor. Again, by preventing the growth of drug-sensitive organisms, the

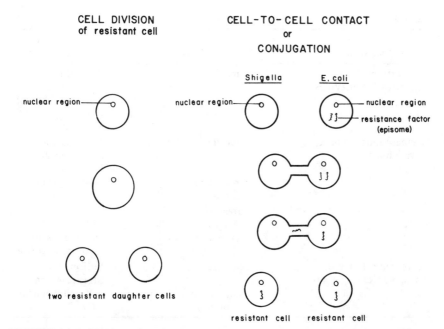

FIGURE 10-1. The transfer of drug resistance. In cell division, drug resistance is transferred from the parent cell to daughter cells together with all the other genetic information contained on the chromosomes of the parent cell. This type of transfer retains the resistance to a drug within the particular strain and species of bacteria. In conjugation, the carrier of the genetic determinant for drug resistance, the episome, is independent of the chromosomes of the host bacterium. This extrachromosomal fragment, found in the cytoplasm and not in the nucleus, is self-replicating. When a resistant cell conjugates with (or contacts) a nonresistant cell of the same or different strain or species, the resistance factor is passed to the nonresistant cell. In the figure this is shown as the transfer of drug resistance from the usually harmless, nonpathogenic Escherichia coli to Shigella, a pathogenic bacterium which causes dysentery.

drug promotes the survival of those bacteria which can spread the infectious drug resistance.

The best means of overcoming drug resistance is to prevent its emergence in the first place. This can be accomplished most effectively by avoiding unnecessary, promiscuous use of antibacterial agents. Once it has been established that a particular agent can reasonably be expected to have a salutary effect, adequate doses should be given to stop the multiplication of microorganisms as quickly as possible. Drug treatment should begin early and continue for a sufficiently long period to ensure that all the infectious organisms are eradicated before treatment is discontinued.

Mechanisms of Drug Resistance

There are a number of mechanisms that can account for the drug resistance of the genetically altered organisms, but we shall consider only those which have been shown to be most frequently responsible for the phenomenon (Table 10-1).

Table 10-1. Mechanisms and Examples of Drug Resistance

Mechanism	Resistant Species	Drug to Which Resistance Acquired
Elaboration of specific inactivating enzymes	Bacteria	Penicillin Kanamycin Chloramphenicol
	Insects	DDT Malathion
Decreased intracellular availability	Bacteria	Tetracycline Sulfonamides Isoniazid
	Cancer cells (animal)	6-Mercaptopurine Methotrexate
	Parasites: malarial trypanosomes	Chloroquine Organic arsenic-containing drugs
Decreased affinity of drug for its target site	Bacteria	Sulfonamides Streptomycin
	Cancer cells (animal)	6-Mercaptopurine

ELABORATION OF SPECIFIC INACTIVATING ENZYMES. This is one of the best-documented mechanisms by which mutants resists the activity of antibacterial agents. For example, the main basis for the bacterial resistance to penicillin is the production of the enzyme penicillinase, which hydrolyzes the antibiotic to inactive metabolites. The production of this enzyme (as well as that of all enzymes) is genetically controlled; a microbial cell must possess the necessary genetic information in order to synthesize the active penicillinase molecule. Entire populations of some species of bacteria are natural producers of penicillinase and have always been penicillin-resistant because of the presence of large amounts of the enzyme. In such normally resistant bacteria, penicillinase is a *constitutive* enzyme, i.e., an enzyme that is an integral part of the normal organization of the cell.

Organisms which are initially sensitive may acquire resistance to penicillin in one of two ways. Some bacterial species have the genetic potential to synthesize penicillinase but produce it only in amounts too meager to protect the cells even against low concentrations of penicillin. However, penicillinase is also an *inducible* enzyme, and in the presence of an inducer (usually one of the penicillins), the enzyme is elaborated by capable cells in increasingly greater quantitites. Whereas trace amounts of penicillinase in an entire population, or large amounts in a few cells, are insufficient to protect the bacteria, an entire population producing penicillinase can cooperatively provide the means for survival. This is the type of penicillin resistance that can best be prevented by early use of large enough doses of penicillin to eradicate the organism before the emergence of increased enzyme activity.

The second way that mutants of normally sensitive bacteria can acquire resistance to penicillin is by penicillinase becoming a constitutive rather than an inducible enzyme. These mutants become the dominant forms by the mechanisms previously described: (1) selective multiplication in the presence of the drug of those insensitive variants arising from random mutations; and (2) infectious transfer of drug resistance. Mutants possessing constitutive enzymes produce large quantities of penicillinase even in the absence of the drug. Individuals infected by these insensitive organisms manifest an immediate rather than a delayed resistance at first exposure to penicillin.

Insect populations may also acquire resistance to various insecticides by producing specific inactivating enzymes. For example, insects that have become insensitive to malathion have been found to possess a greatly increased capacity to convert the insecticide to a nontoxic metabolite before its conversion to the toxic metabolite malaoxon (cf. Fig. 6-21 and p. 163).

DECREASED INTRACELLULAR AVAILABILITY. When a drug acts intracellularly, any change that significantly decreases its rate of entry renders the cell resistant to the action of the drug. Changes in the permeability characteristics of the cell membrane may decrease the rate of passive diffusion, whereas changes in a carrier system may diminish the rate of facilitated diffusion or active transport. In either case the result is a lowered concentration of drug within the cell.

Malarial parasites that have become resistant to the antimalarial drug chloroquine have been found to take up less drug than sensitive plasmodia. The drug resistance to arsenic-containing organic compounds acquired by trypanosomes (the organisms causing sleeping sickness) has also been attributed to decreased intracellular concentrations of drug. And the resistance developed in certain animal malignancies to a number of drugs has been shown to involve a decrease in their rate of penetration into the cancer cells. However, little is known about the mechanisms whereby human cancer cells develop resistance to these same anticancer drugs.

DECREASED AFFINITY OF DRUG FOR ITS TARGET SITE. We have seen that genetic modifications of specific proteins are responsible for idiosyncratic drug responses. The altered protein or enzyme, originating as an error in the normal replication process, becomes permanently encoded in the gene if the alteration is compatible with life. Analogously, genetic modification may be responsible for drug resistance when an alteration occurs in a protein which is the specific target of the drug causing growth inhibition or cell death. If the drug cannot interact with the altered protein as readily as with the normal protein, the cells containing the former will survive at the expense of those containing the latter. For example, sulfa drugs inhibit the growth of sensitive bacteria by competing with PABA for binding sites on the enzyme catalyzing the first step in the synthesis of folic acid (cf. p. 260). In resistant bacteria the sulfa drugs can no longer interact effectively with this enzyme and, consequently, do not inhibit the incorporation of PABA into the essential vitamin. The enzyme is altered only with respect to the drug and can still combine effectively with its normal substrate. Thus, genetically determined alterations in an enzyme of some bacteria are responsible for their resistance to the action of sulfa drugs.

Drug Allergy

Allergy is an adverse response to a foreign chemical resulting from a previous exposure to the substance; it is manifested only after a second or subsequent exposure and then as a reaction *different from the usual pharmacologic effects of the chemical.* Since drug allergy occurs in susceptible individuals who usually comprise only a small fraction of all people receiving the particular drug, it could be classified as a variability in drug response attributable to the biologic system. It is discussed here, however, to emphasize the fact that a drug can produce an allergic reaction only after a previous *sensitizing* contact with the agent or with one closely related in chemical structure. Since a minute amount of an otherwise safe drug may elicit the allergic response, the term *hypersensitivity* frequently is improperly used to describe the sensitization reaction. And since the allergic response is unusual, it is also often confused with the idiosyncratic response. The inappropriateness of both these terms is readily revealed by considering the mechanism involved in the production of the allergic response and the characteristics of the reaction itself.

The Mechanism of the Allergic Reaction

Drug allergies are produced by essentially the same mechanisms as other allergies such as hay fever or food allergy. As far back as 1913, the Englishman Sir Henry H. Dale, who won the Nobel Prize in Medicine in 1936 for research in other areas, suggested that an allergic response involves a typical immunologic reaction.

The immune response is a normal defense mechanism that is set in motion when a foreign agent like bacteria is introduced into the body for the first time. The invasive organism stimulates the formation of specific proteins called *antibodies.* By definition, any substance which induces the synthesis of antibodies is an *antigen.* After the period required for their production, usually from several days to more than a week, the newly formed antibodies, or *immunoglobulins*, are found in blood plasma and other body fluids as well as in various tissues. The appearance of the antibodies signals the development of immunity to the particular antigenic bacteria (or other antigen), i.e., the antibodies react with the antigen which stimulated their production to form antigen-antibody complexes. It is the formation of such complexes that normally confers protection against the further development of disease by nullifying the otherwise damaging invading agents. Thus the immune system is the body's conventional way of safeguarding itself from harmful foreign substances such as bacteria or viruses.

These antigen-antibody interactions show a remarkable degree of physicochemical specificity. It is the antigen itself which is responsible for this; antigens are also macromolecules, usually proteins, with a large number of determinant chemical groups, or "antigenic sites." Indeed, the action of an antibody upon the antigen that stimulated its production is usually compared to that of a lock and its key. However, the lock-and-key concept of the antigen-antibody reaction is somewhat different from the analogous interpretation of the interaction of a drug and its receptor. In the latter the drug is the key which must fit the preexisting lock, the receptor, in order to open the way for the events that follow. In the antigen-antibody reaction there is a prefabricated key, the antigen, for which a specific lock, the antibody, must be fashioned. After the specific lock (antibody) has been installed, only the original key (antigen), or one very similar, can release what lies behind the locked door.

Allergic reactions, like the immune responses to bacteria, also begin with the formation of rather specific antibody proteins capable of complexing with their corresponding antigens. Since the substances responsible for hay fever or food allergy are either proteins or complex macromolecules, it is understandable in the classic immunologic context how these materials may act as antigens. But if antigens must be proteins or other big molecules with specific regions which can act as antigenic determinants, how can simple compounds like aspirin take part in the allergic reac-

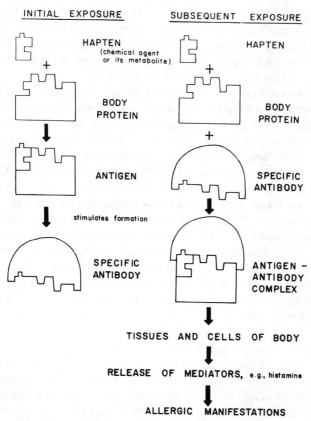

FIGURE 10-2. Mechanism of the allergic response. In the initial exposure, the drug (hapten) combines with a body protein to form the antigen, which then stimulates the formation of specific antibodies. The present concept of the immunopathogenesis of histamine release from most cells upon subsequent exposure to the hapten involves the following sequence of events: (1) the specific antibodies bind at one end to most cells, leaving antigen-binding sites free to react; (2) the antigen binds to antibody at antigen-binding sites; and (3) the antigen-antibody complex triggers the release of histamine.

tion? Drugs which are small molecules and which are relatively simple in structure do not become antigenic until they combine with body proteins. It is the relatively stable complex formed between a drug and a conjugate protein which is the active antigen. Simple chemicals capable of binding rather firmly with a protein to form a product that has antigenic properties are termed *haptens;* the structure of the hapten in the hapten-protein complex determines the specificity of the induced antibody.

The initial contact of an individual with a foregin material having potentially antigenic properties, and the ensuing formation of a specific antibody, comprise the sensitizing portion of the immune mechanism. The reaction part of the total phenomenon is seen only when the sensitized individual is reexposed to the antigen or hapten. The problem in allergy is that the formation of the antigen-antibody complex triggers a series of events that can be highly damaging. Thus, in the allergic individual, a normally protective and essential mechanism goes awry. The antibodies induced by bacteria or viruses act to neutralize these organisms on subsequent invasions. But the antibodies produced in response to haptens convert drugs which are harmless, if used properly, into noxious substances.

It is important to stress that the manifestations of drug allergy are the consequences of antigen-antibody actions and are unrelated to the pharmacologic activity of the eliciting drug. In some cases, the allergic response may be manifest as tissue damage or cell destruction resulting from attachment of the antigen-antibody complex to the tissue or cell. However, in the majority of allergic reactions, the antigen-antibody complex is not directly responsible for the manifestations of allergy. Rather, the complex reacts with various tissues and cells of the body by processes not clearly understood and causes them to release certain substances which then provoke the symptoms (Fig. 10-2). These *mediators* are present in the body in inactive form and become pharmacologically active only when liberated. One of the chief mediators of allergy in humans is histamine, a natural amine widely distributed throughout the body and stored in especially high concentrations in cells called mast cells. It is because the allergic response is due to the release of one or more of these mediators[1] that various *allergic manifestations are effects characteristic of the mediators* and not of the allergenic drugs.

Manifestations of the Allergic Reaction

Allergic reactions to drugs manifest themselves as a variety of symptoms involving various organ systems and ranging from minor skin rashes to an often fatal collapse of blood pressure (Table 10-2). Reactions may be localized or widespread, and the symptoms may appear immediately or within hours to days following administration of the eliciting drug to the sensitized individual.

The immediate response is probably due to the release of histamine by the antigen-antibody complex. The reaction may involve the respiratory and gastrointestinal tracts, the blood vessels, the skin, or all of these. Characteristic symptoms include

---

[1] Serotonin (5-hydroxytryptamine) and bradykinin are also known mediators; most likely there are many other mediators not yet identified.

Table 10-2. Common Manifestations of Allergic Reactions in the Human

Tissue or Organ	Symptom	Hapten Commonly Involved
Skin	Hives (urticaria) and generalized itching	Penicillin, aspirin
	Rashes	Barbiturates, sulfonamides, streptomycin
	Exfoliative dermatitis (loss of superficial skin layers)	Tetracycline, streptomycin, phenobarbital
Mucous membranes (particularly of nose and eye)	Inflammation, swelling and excessive secretions	Sulfonamides, barbiturates
Respiratory tract	Difficulty in breathing	Penicillin, local anesthetics, aspirin, heroin
Vascular system	Fall in blood pressure	Penicillin, aspirin
Blood and blood-forming tissues[a]	Reduction in the number of one or more types of circulating blood cells	Aminopyrine (Pyramidon) Quinidine

[a]The presence of an antibody that reacts specifically with the sensitizing drug has been demonstrated in the case of each of the drugs cited as well as for a number of other drugs. Such demonstrations provide proof that drug allergy can account for some disorders of blood and the blood-forming tissues.

difficulty in breathing due to constriction of the airways of the upper respiratory tract (bronchial asthma); swelling of the mucous membranes; and a fall in blood pressure. *Anaphylaxis* is the most serious immediate type of allergic response. In its severest form — anaphylactic shock — death may occur within a few minutes as a result of complete obstruction of respiratory passages and the precipitous lowering of blood pressure.

Inflammation and excessive secretions of the nose and eyes (as in hay fever) and generalized hives and itching may also be manifest as immediate allergic responses. But they are not typical of the immediate response, since their appearance is sometimes delayed. The severity of the delayed allergic responses may vary from trivial skin eruptions to disorders of the blood and blood-forming tissues and even to fatal loss of superficial layers of skin (*exfoliative dermatitis*).

The pattern of allergic response to an agent is not entirely predictable in different individuals or in the same individual at different times. On the other hand, one or more allergic symptoms may be more commonly associated with a particular drug than are others from among the entire gamut of possible responses. For example, hives and generalized itching are the symptoms most frequently seen when individuals sensitized to penicillin are reexposed to the antibiotic. However, fatal anaphylactic reactions have followed the administration of as little as 1 μg of penicillin. The important point is that the pattern of allergic response is dependent on the kind and amount of mediator(s) liberated, or the tissue or cell damage caused by the antigen-antibody reaction; it is independent of the chemical structure or pharmacologic effects of the eliciting drug.

Incidence of Allergic Reactions to Drugs

So many different drugs have haptenic qualities that allergic responses represent the largest single group of adverse drug reactions. The frequency of allergic reactions to most drugs appears to be low, however. For example, one of the most common offenders is penicillin. Yet the incidence of allergic responses may be not greater than 5 to 10 per cent among the patients receiving the antibiotic. The overall incidence of allergy to aspirin, a more widely used drug, is probably in the order of 0.2 per cent. On the other hand, some drugs, such as caffeine, have no known incidence of allergic response; and some, such as phenylethylhydantoin (Nirvanol), lead to allergic manifestations in virtually everyone. The latter agent, designed for use in epilepsy, was withdrawn after a brief trial because of its allergenic propensity.

These estimates of the frequency of allergic drug responses are based, of course, on the number of such occurrences that have been reported and recorded. They do not ordinarily include the frequency of occurrence of mild allergic reactions. Nor do they take into account all those individuals who have received a particular drug and have not manifested adverse effects. Moreover, it is often difficult to prove that the response is indeed the result of an antigen-antibody reaction. The only unequivocal evidence that a drug has produced an allergic reaction is the presence of specific antibodies in plasma or tissues. Thus the best available estimates of potential allergenicity do not really assess the attendant risk to the patient using a particular drug. Even if valid estimates of the frequency of allergic responses to a given drug were available, they could be used only to predict the fraction of a population that might be expected to be allergic. They would have no predictive value for the response in a single individual, and at present there are no generally reliable and safe procedures by which sensitization to a drug in an individual can be ascertained before drug administration.[2] It is for these reasons that drugs which are known haptens, such as many of the antibiotics, should be reserved for use only in those illnesses in which they may be lifesaving.

In some instances, the hapten is not the drug administered but is a product of its biotransformation. For example, the allergic response to the local anesthetic procaine is caused by the antigenicity of one of its metabolites, para-aminobenzoic acid (PABA). Occasionally, too, the antigen-antibody reaction is not entirely specific for the hapten which induced the formation of the antibody. Thus, individuals sensitized to procaine may show an allergic response to other local anesthetics whose biotransformation yields either PABA or a compound closely related to PABA in structure. We

---

[2]Skin patch tests or skin injection tests may themselves be hazardous, since the small quantity of drug used in these diagnostic procedures may be sufficient to induce an allergic response.

saw earlier that sulfanilamide is sufficiently similar in structure to PABA to be able to inhibit its enzymic incorporation into folic acid. This structural similarity is also characteristic of other antibacterial sulfa drugs. And in some individuals allergic to procaine, the first administration of a sulfonamide will also elicit the antigen-antibody reaction. The term *cross-sensitization* denotes this lack of absolute antibody specificity for the hapten which induced its formation. It is not possible to predict whether an individual will manifest cross-sensitization to agents other than the original eliciting hapten. Thus in patients with a known history of allergic responses to a drug, it is safest to avoid using any agent that may substitute for that drug in the antigen-antibody reaction.

The Distinguishing Characteristics of Drug Allergy

Drug allergy, toxicity and idiosyncrasy are adverse effects which, fortunately, may be considered unusual in that they occur infrequently. It is important to distinguish these three effects from each other, however, since the differences among them influence the subsequent use of a drug which produces any one of them. A sharp differentiation can be made on the basis of occurrence, dose-response relationships, the mechanism by which they are produced and the particular manifestations of the adverse effects (Table 10-3).

The occurrence of toxicity as an adverse effect can be considered unusual only in the context of quantal dose-response curves and therapeutic indices. First, toxic responses to any drug may be produced in every individual exposed to the agent simply by increasing the size of the dose. Also, if considerable overlap exists between the curves for desirable and undesirable effects (cf. Fig. 7-13), the toxic effects would not be regarded as unusual since a sizable fraction of the total population may show adverse effects at doses that are well within the therapeutic range. On the other hand, given a drug with a certain safety factor of 1.0 or greater (cf. Fig. 7-12), the appearance of toxicity would be infrequent. Toxicity would be evident only in the few individuals who require a maximum dose to elicit the desired effect and who also show adverse effects at doses lying at the lowest extreme of the toxicity curve. (Individuals showing such extreme sensitivity to an action of a drug could be called hypersensitive; hence the confusion in using the term *hypersensitivity* in referring to the allergic state.) A simple reduction in the dose may be sufficient to eliminate this type of adverse effect of any drug.

The size of the dose, however, does not determine whether an individual will have an idiosyncratic or allergic response to a drug. Idiosyncratic responses occur infrequently and only in genetically abnormal subjects. Heredity may also play a role in determining whether an individual is susceptible to one or more antigenic substances. But only in allergy is prior exposure to the offending drug an absolute essential for the subsequent development of the adverse response. That prior exposure has occurred may not always be known. It may occur inadvertently through environmental contact or dietary intake. For example, moldy foods, such as bread or certain cheeses, or milk from penicillin-treated cows may be the sources of sensitization to this antibiotic.

Table 10-3. Distinguishing Characteristics of Toxic, Idiosyncratic and Allergic Responses to Drugs

	Toxic Response	Idiosyncratic Response	Allergic Response
Occurrence			
Incidence in population	In all subjects, if dose high enough	Only in genetically abnormal subjects	From a few per cent to 100 per cent, depending on drug
Incidence among drugs	All drugs	Few drugs	Many drugs
Circumstance	Prior exposure unnecessary	Prior exposure unnecessary	Prior exposure essential
Dose-response relationship	Dose-related	Dose-related	Independent of dose; erratic relationship
Mechanism	Drug-receptor interaction	Drug-receptor interaction	Through antigen-antibody reaction; specific antibody formed in response to first dose of antigen
Effect produced	Determined by drug-receptor interaction; depends on eliciting drug	Determined by drug-receptor interaction; depends on eliciting drug	Independent of eliciting drug; determined by mediators released by or direct action of antigen-antibody complex
Effect antagonized	By specific antagonists	By specific antagonists	By antihistaminics, epinephrine or anti-inflammatory steroids like cortisone

Both toxic and idiosyncratic effects are the result of drug-receptor interactions and consequently show the usual dose-response relationships. Thus the pharmacologic effects observed are determined by both the physicochemical properties of the drugs and their ability to combine with specific receptor sites. In contrast, the manifestations of the allergic reaction are unrelated to the structure or pharmacologic activity of the particular eliciting drug; they are mediated through endogenous substances released by the antigen-antibody complex. There is, therefore, no predictable dose-response relationship between the hapten and the allergic effects. A minute amount of an otherwise safe drug may not only sensitize an individual but also elicit a severe allergic reaction. Conversely, an ordinary therapeutic dose may elicit only mild allergic symptoms in the sensitized patient. Moreover, since the effects seen in allergy do not result from the interaction of the antigenic drug and its normal receptor, the allergic response cannot be overcome by agents antagonizing the actions of the eliciting drug. Indeed, drugs which antagonize the allergic responses to one drug may be useful against similar effects of any antigenic drug. For example, nalorphine can abolish the toxic effects of an overdose of morphine or counteract the rare idiosyncratic response to the narcotic analgesic. Nalorphine is useless, however, in treating allergic responses to morphine, whereas an antihistaminic drug may have ameliorative effects.

Drug Tolerance

Tolerance is a condition of *decreased responsiveness* which is acquired after prior or repeated exposure to a given drug or to one closely allied to it in pharmacologic activity. Tolerance is characterized by the necessity of increasing the size of successive doses in order to produce effects of equal magnitude or duration. Alternatively, it is an inability of the subsequent administration of the same dose of a drug to be as effective as the preceding dose.

Tolerance may be acquired to various effects of many drugs, especially those of narcotic analgesics or **opioids**, barbiturates, alcohol and other agents depressing the central nervous system; nitrites; atropine; and central nervous system stimulants like lysergic acid diethylamide (LSD), amphetamine, nicotine and caffeine (Table 10-4). The tolerance developed to drugs that profoundly affect mood, thought and behavior is frequently associated with either physical or psychologic dependence, or both. The interrelationship of tolerance and these other factors is discussed separately in Chapter 12. Here we are concerned only with the general aspects of the phenomenon of drug tolerance and the mechanisms responsible for its development.

Given that the quantitative effect of a drug is determined by its concentration and extent of chemical reaction at an effector site, there are only two ways whereby an individual can become tolerant to a drug. Tolerance may be the consequence of conditions which produce (1) a decrease in the effective concentration of the agonist at the site of action, or (2) a reduction in the normal reactivity of the receptor. Tolerance developed by the first mechanism is called *drug-disposition tolerance*; that by the second is *cellular* or *pharmacodynamic tolerance.*

Drug-disposition tolerance may occur when a drug reduces its own absorption or its rate of transfer across any biologic barrier, or when it increases its own rate of

Table 10-4. Mechanisms and Examples of Drug Tolerance

Drug Disposition Tolerance	Pharmacodynamic Tolerance
Barbiturates	Barbiturates
Glutethimide (Doriden)	Glutethimide
Alcohol	Alcohol
Meprobamate	Meprobamate
Phenylbutazone	Morphine and other
Benzpyrene	narcotic analgesics
	Nalorphine (antagonist
	of narcotic analgesics)
	Amphetamine
	Methamphetamine
Tachyphylaxis	Methylphenidate
Ephedrine	Lysergic acid diethylamide
Tyramine	Caffeine
Morphine	Nicotine
	Tachyphylaxis
	Nitrites
	Atropine

elimination. The best examples of tolerance produced by this mechanism are provided by drugs like phenobarbital, glutethimide (Doriden) and meprobamate, which are capable of increasing their own rates of biotransformation through stimulation of microsomal enzyme systems (cf. Table 6-7 and Fig. 6-19). However, drug-disposition tolerance accounts for only a small part of the total tolerance developed to these and other agents acting on the central nervous system; a reduction in the normal reactivity of receptors plays the principal role (see below).

Whether drug-disposition tolerance is exhibited as a decrease in peak effect and duration of action, or only as the latter, strongly depends on the route of drug administration. When a drug is given intravenously, the initial concentration at the target site — and hence the magnitude of effect observed — will be the same in tolerant and nontolerant subjects. In both, the entire dose will be distributed before differences in rates of biotransformation can significantly influence drug availability. However, as a result of the increased rate of drug elimination, the duration of action will be shorter in the tolerant state than it was before tolerance was developed. This means, of course, that the intravenous dose producing a toxic or lethal effect is essentially the same for both the nontolerant individual and the subject made tolerant to the drug by this mechanism. In contrast, when a drug is given to the tolerant subject by a slow-absorption route, both the duration of action and the peak effect observed will be reduced. This is so because, for any given drug, the faster the rate of elimination relative to absorption, the lower the peak concentration attained and the shorter the duration of action. Whereas the rate of absorption remains the same in the tolerant and intolerant state, the rate of elimination is increased in the tolerant individual.

Tolerance is sometimes the indirect effect of the administered drug, even though it develops as the consequence of a reduced effective concentration of an agonist at its target site. For a number of drugs do not produce all their effects by direct combination with a receptor. Instead, they act at other cellular sites to release endogenous, physiologically active substances like histamine, which are inactive in their bound form (see Chap. 13 for full discussion). Once released from their storage sites, these endogenous substances become agonists and combine with receptors to initiate an action-effects sequence (Fig. 10-3). (This is analagous to the antigen-antibody complex giving rise to the symptoms of allergy.) These stores of endogenous, active substances may be gradually depleted if the interval between doses of the drug which releases them is too short to permit their replenishment. As the stored quantity of the physiologic agonist is diminished, the effect elicited on repeated administration of the same or larger doses of the releasing agent is correspondingly reduced. For example, the histamine stored in various cells and tissues can be set free by morphine. One of the effects produced by the released histamine is a dilation of cutaneous blood vessels, readily observed in humans as flushing of the face, neck and upper thorax. If small doses of morphine are given to an animal over a period of several weeks, there is little attenuation of this peripheral vasodilatation. However, with large doses, tolerance develops rapidly, due mainly to the unavailability of adequate stores of histamine. The term (cf. Table 10-4) *tachyphylaxis* is used to describe the acute development of tolerance to the rapid, repeated administration of a drug.

Tachyphylaxis may also occur as a result of a change in the sensitivity of the target cells. A case in point is the tolerance to nitroglycerin observed among workers exposed to this drug in the manufacture of explosives. During the first few days of their exposure, new employees frequently suffer severe headaches, dizziness and nausea. These symptoms quickly disappear as pharmacodynamic tolerance develops. But they may reappear if the worker returns to his job after a few days' absence; hence the term *Monday disease* to describe the return of symptoms after a weekend away from work. When nitroglycerin is used to treat angina pectoris, tolerance is rarely seen, since continuous exposure to the drug is not customary. Although the mechanism of tolerance to nitrites is unknown, it does not result from more rapid elimination of drug or decreased availability of drug to sites of action.

Pharmacodynamic or cellular tolerance is usually observed as a slowly developed phenomenon rather than as acute tolerance or tachyphylaxis. This is the type that accounts for much of the tolerance that is seen with various drugs acting on the central nervous system to produce changes in mood and behavior. The mechanisms of this tolerance, however, have not been elucidated for any of the drugs. Generally speaking, it must be attributed to some kind of adaptation of the cells within the brain which renders them insensitive to the action of the drugs. This altered reactivity of target sites within the brain is the primary mechanism for the development of tolerance, even for the central nervous system depressants which can increase their own rate of biotransformation. The tolerance developed to barbital provides an example of the evidence available to support this view. Barbital, unlike most other barbiturates, is biotransformed very slowly, if at all, in laboratory animals and humans; its actions are terminated by excretion. Consequently, repeated administration of barbital

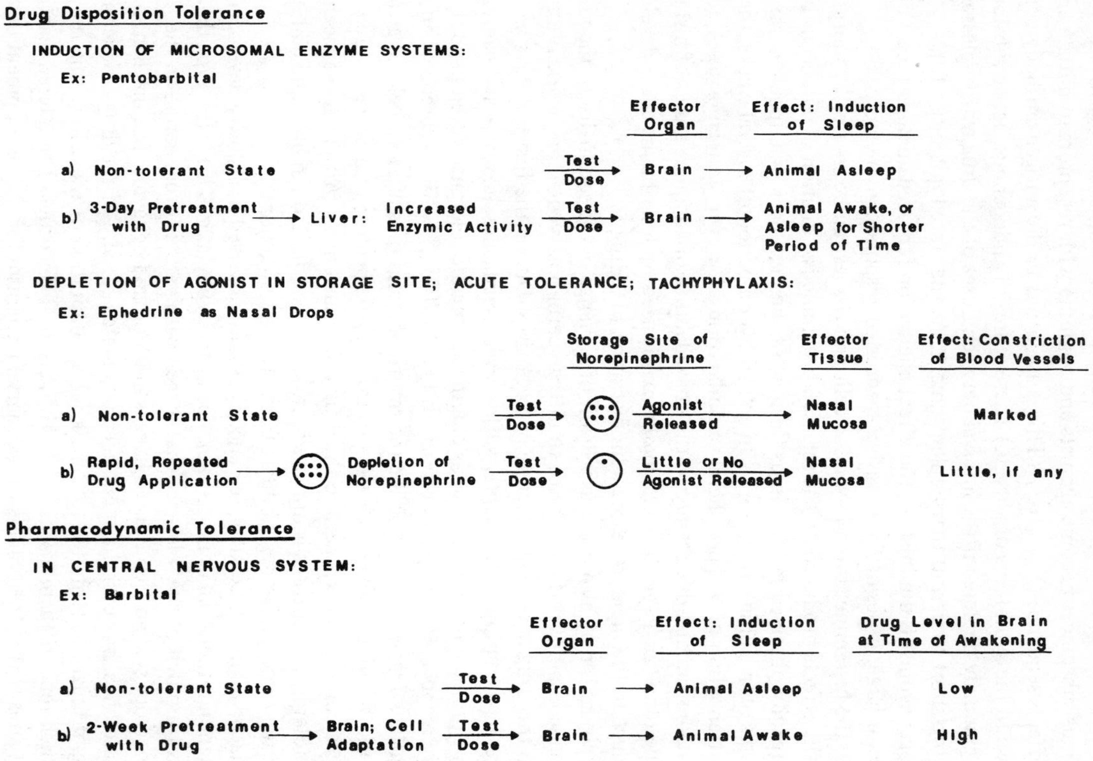

Drug Disposition Tolerance

INDUCTION OF MICROSOMAL ENZYME SYSTEMS:

Ex: Pentobarbital

	Effector Organ	Effect: Induction of Sleep

a) Non-tolerant State

Test Dose → Brain → Animal Asleep

b) 3-Day Pretreatment with Drug → Liver: Increased Enzymic Activity

Test Dose → Brain → Animal Awake, or Asleep for Shorter Period of Time

DEPLETION OF AGONIST IN STORAGE SITE; ACUTE TOLERANCE; TACHYPHYLAXIS:

Ex: Ephedrine as Nasal Drops

Storage Site of Norepinephrine		Effector Tissue	Effect: Constriction of Blood Vessels

a) Non-tolerant State

⊙ Test Dose → Agonist Released → Nasal Mucosa → Marked

b) Rapid, Repeated Drug Application → ⊙ Depletion of Norepinephrine

○ Test Dose → Little or No Agonist Released → Nasal Mucosa → Little, if any

Pharmacodynamic Tolerance

IN CENTRAL NERVOUS SYSTEM:

Ex: Barbital

Effector Organ	Effect: Induction of Sleep	Drug Level in Brain at Time of Awakening

a) Non-tolerant State

Test Dose → Brain → Animal Asleep — Low

b) 2-Week Pretreatment with Drug → Brain; Cell Adaptation

Test Dose → Brain → Animal Awake — High

FIGURE 10-3. Mechanisms of development of drug tolerance.

282

does not increase its own rate of elimination from the body. Thus, when tolerance is developed to barbital, it cannot be attributed, even in part, to a decrease in the effective concentration of drug at the site of action. When the relationship between sleeping time and drug concentrations within the brain is determined, animals made tolerant to barbital are found to awaken at brain levels of barbital significantly higher than those at which nontolerant animals are still asleep. It is well to point out, however, that this adaptation of cells within the brain is not akin to the development of drug resistance. In drug resistance, sensitive cells are destroyed at the expense of insensitive mutants which then become the dominant population. Within the brain, however, the cells which become tolerant are the same cells which were originally sensitive to the drug, since little or no cell renewal takes place in the brain.

It is apparent from what has been said that the development of tolerance may proceed by a number of mechanisms and that more than one of these may be operative in any given case. Tolerance to morphine, for example, may involve a decreased sensitivity of target cells within the brain as well as tachyphylaxis due to depletion of a physiologically active substance. And stimulation of microsomal enzyme systems in addition to a change in the reactivity of brain cells may account for the development of tolerance to barbiturates. The degree of tolerance produced also varies widely from one group of drugs to another. For example, the habitual user of morphine may tolerate doses many times greater than the dose that would be lethal for a nontolerant person. In contrast, whereas individuals tolerant to alcohol or barbiturates have fewer and less marked effects from moderate doses of these agents than do abstainers, both tolerant and nontolerant subjects are affected almost equally by high or near-lethal doses of these depressants. Tolerance also does not develop uniformly to all the pharmacologic effects of a drug. In the case of morphine, for example, the highly tolerant individual exhibits tolerance to the central nervous system effects of the drug but continues to have "pinpoint" pupils and constipation.

Another characteristic of the tolerant state is that of cross-tolerance among drugs belonging to the same group of agents. For instance, individuals made tolerant to morphine are also tolerant to heroin, methadone and other narcotic agents, but not to alcohol or barbiturates. On the other hand, the alcoholic may have some degree of tolerance to barbiturates but has none to the opioids. Tolerance disappears when administration of the drug that produced the phenomenon is discontinued. The rate of disappearance may be rapid, as in the case of nitrites, or prolonged, as for morphine. The special features associated with discontinuance of the use of drugs that act on the central nervous system are discussed in Chapter 12.

DRUG INTERACTIONS

It has been estimated that the average hospitalized patient may receive as many as six to ten different drugs during his confinement. In chronic disease states such as epilepsy, diabetes and heart disease, when the patient contracts another illness, the conjoint administration of several drugs may be mandatory. There are also other therapeutic situations in which multiple-drug therapy may constitute good practice. But there are many occasions when more than one drug is given to an individual, regardless of whether this is warranted. Whatever the rationale for administering several drugs concurrently, the question arises of how these drugs may affect each other's actions.

Two drugs administered at the same time may act wholly independently. For example, aspirin may lower the body temperature of the fevered patient while an appropriate antibacterial agent is eliminating the organism responsible for the disease as well as the fever. The effect of aspirin is apparently unaltered by the presence of the antibacterial agent, and vice versa. On the other hand, there are many known instances — and more come to light continually — of the concurrent use of two drugs changing the effects of one or both. The results may be a response greater than was anticipated, a decrease in effectiveness of one or both drugs, or an unanticipated toxicity. Many of the adverse effects are dose-dependent and occur only when sufficiently large doses of the interacting drugs are used. Some of the interactions may be trivial in nature, while others have proved disastrous. For example, the combination of a monoamine oxidase inhibitor, such as tranylcypromine, with another antidepressant agent like imipramine may produce convulsions, delirium and death. Thus it is the consequence of a given interaction that is significant, rather than the fact that two drugs may interact. But to ensure the effectiveness and safety of multiple-drug therapy, the potential for drug interaction must be evaluated.

We are not concerned here with the ways in which the prior administration of one drug may influence the subsequent administration of another in connection with the development of drug resistance, allergy or tolerance. We shall limit our discussion to the interactions that occur when one agent alters the absorption, distribution, biotransformation or excretion — or enhances or opposes the action or effects — of another drug.

Some of these interactions, such as the inhibition or induction by one drug of enzymes required for the biotransformation of other drugs, have already been discussed (cf. pp. 158–165) and will be mentioned again only briefly. To avoid ambiguity, however, we will begin by defining the terms used to describe the combined effects of drugs.

Terminology

Summation, Additive Effect and Synergism

Summation, additive effect and synergism refer to different situations in which the combined effect of two (or more) drugs acting simultaneously is either equal to or greater than the effect of each agent given alone (Fig. 10-4). When two drugs elicit the same overt response, regardless of the mechanism of action, and the combined effect is the algebraic sum of their individual effects, the drugs are said to exhibit *summation*. The term *additive effect* is usually used in those cases in which the combined effect of two drugs acting by the *same* mechanism is equal to that expected by simple addition. (Of course the magnitude of the combined effect must be within the capacity of the system to respond.) Thus, when small doses of codeine and aspirin are concurrently administered for the relief of pain, the combined effect is called summation since the two drugs act by different mechanisms. However, aspirin

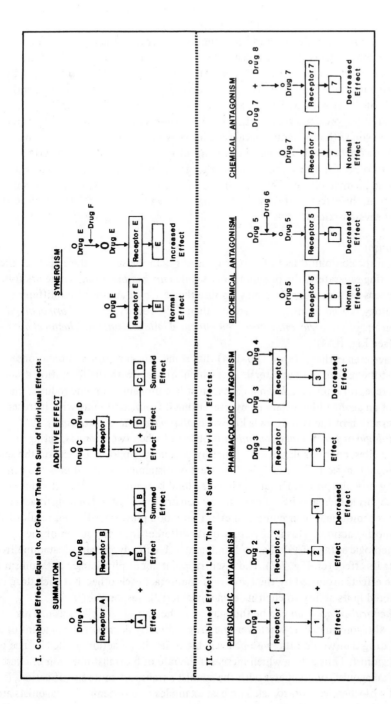

FIGURE 10-4. Classification of drug interactions.

285

and phenacetin, which also exhibit summation, apparently act on the same receptors, and their combined effect is an additive effect.

In *synergism,* the joint effect of two drugs is greater than the algebraic sum of their individual effects. The term is usually reserved for cases in which two drugs act at different sites and one drug, the synergist, increases the effect of the second drug by altering its biotransformation, distribution or excretion. Thus in synergism the intensity of the effect may be potentiated or the duration of action prolonged. The exaggerated response to tyramine that has been observed in patients being treated for depression with monoamine oxidase inhibitors is an example of synergism (cf. p. 262). As previously indicated, the amount of tyramine ingested with certain cheeses or other foodstuffs, such as herring, ordinarily is too small to produce a detectable pharmacologic effect. But in the presence of a drug which prevents its destruction, the effect of this small quantity of tyramine is potentiated, even to the point of severe toxicity.

Antagonism

Any time the conjoint effect of two drugs is *less* than the sum of the effects of the drugs acting separately, the phenomenon is called *drug antagonism.* There are four mechanisms by which one drug may oppose the action of another, and different terminology is used to distinguish among them. The four types are *pharmacologic antagonism; physiologic antagonism; biochemical antagonism;* and *chemical antagonism* (see Fig. 10-4).

We have seen earlier (cf. pp. 180–184) that some drug-receptor combinations manifest themselves only as interactions which interfere with the formation of an agonist-receptor complex. When an antagonist like diphenhydramine reduces the effect of an agonist like histamine by preventing it from combining with its receptor, the interaction of the two drugs is known as *pharmacologic antagonism.*

Physiologic or *functional antagonism* is observed when two agonists, acting at different sites, counterbalance each other by producing opposite effects on the same physiologic function. For example, the effect of histamine on blood pressure can be offset by norepinephrine. Histamine lowers blood pressure by dilating blood vessels; norepinephrine increases blood pressure by constricting vessels. Each agent acts at its own receptor, and their combined effect on blood pressure is the net result of the two opposing actions. This is obviously quite different from the action of the pharmacologic antagonist diphenhydramine, which actually prevents histamine from exerting its effect (cf. Fig. 7-7). The essential point about physiologic antagonism is that the effects produced by the two drugs counteract each other, but each drug is unhindered in its ability to elicit its own characteristic response.

Biochemical antagonism can be thought of as the opposite of synergism. This type of antagonism occurs whenever one drug indirectly decreases the amount of a second drug that would otherwise be available to its site of action in the absence of the antagonist. Thus a drug which increases the rate of biotransformation or excretion of an agonist, or competes with the agonist's transport to its site of action, is termed a biochemical antagonist. The best examples of biochemical antagonists are the many agents, such as phenobarbital, which induce the microsomal enzyme activity responsible for the biotransformation of other drugs (cf. Table 6-7).

The fourth kind of antagonism, *chemical antagonism,* is simply the reaction between an agonist and an antagonist to form an inactive product. The agonist is inactivated in direct proportion to the extent of chemical interaction with the antagonist. For instance, the anticoagulant effect of the strong, negatively charged macromolecule heparin is antagonized when the drug combines with strongly basic dyes (toluidine blue) or basic proteins (protamine). This is analogous to the neutralization of excess gastric acid by any of the antacid drugs such as aluminum hydroxide or sodium bicarbonate.

Mechanisms Responsible for Adverse Effects Resulting From Drug Interaction

The word *adverse* applies not only to drug interactions that lead to a toxic manifestation, but also to those in which the combined drug action results in less than desired effectiveness. Examples of the major adverse interactions of commonly used drugs are listed in Table 10-5. Ordinarily, such adverse responses do not emanate from the additive effects of drugs acting at the same receptor site or from pharmacologic or physiologic antagonisms. The combined effects produced by such drug interactions may be readily predicted from the known pharmacology of the agents involved and can be taken into account before multiple-drug administration. Generally, drugs exhibiting summation do not cause problems when used concomitantly, since their combined effects also may be anticipated on the basis of available pharmacologic knowledge. Adverse reactions of combined medication are commonly associated with drugs that act synergistically or are chemically or biochemically antagonistic. Thus the mechanisms usually responsible for the adverse effects associated with drug interactions are those in which one drug affects the absorption, distribution, biotransformation or excretion of another.

Intestinal Absorption

Since the oral route is the one most frequently used for drug administration, drug interactions influencing absorption are most likely to occur within the gastrointestinal tract. One drug affects the absorption of another primarily by altering the amount of drug available for absorption, rather than by influencing the absorptive mechanism per se. A good example of such interaction is provided by cholestyramine, a drug used to lower plasma levels of cholesterol, high levels of which are considered to be a risk factor in predisposing individuals to coronary heart disease. Cholestyramine, a nonabsorbable resin, indirectly lowers plasma cholesterol levels by binding bile acids and preventing their reabsorption from the intestine and their enterohepatic cycling (cf. pp. 138–139). Plasma cholesterol levels fall in response to decreased enterohepatic cycling of bile acids since there is increased hepatic conversion of cholesterol to bile acids and since bile acids are required for the intestinal absorption of cholesterol itself. The same binding characteristics that make cholestyramine useful in the treatment of hypercholesterolemia also account for the resin's interference in the

Table 10-5. Major Adverse Interactions of Commonly Used Drugs

Interacting Drugs		Type of Interaction of Mechanism	Adverse Effects
A	with B		
Alcohol (acute intoxication)	Antihistaminics	Additive	Increased depression of central nervous system
	Barbiturates Meprobamate Anticoagulants	} Synergistic; biotransformation of B inhibited by A	Increased bleeding tendency
Alcohol (chronic abuse)	Barbiturates Anticoagulants Antidiabetic agents like tolbutamide	} Biochemical antagonism of B by A through enzyme induction	Decreased effect of B
Anticoagulants, like dicumarol	Salicylates (high doses) Quinidine Quinine	} Additive	Increased bleeding tendency
	Tolbutamide	Synergistic; displacement of B by A from plasma protein	Excessive lowering of blood sugar
Antidepressant drugs; monoamine oxidase inhibitors like pargyline or tranylcypromine	Barbiturates Meperidine Alcohol	} Synergistic; biotransformation of B inhibited by A	Increased depression of central nervous system
	Tolbutamide	?	Excessive lowering of blood sugar
	Antidepressant drugs like imipramine	?	Excitement, delirium and convulsions

Drug A	Drug B	Mechanism	Result
Phenylbutazone / Sulfonamides / Salicylates	Tolbutamide	Synergistic; displacement of B by A from plasma proteins	Excessive lowering of blood sugar
Phenylbutazone / Sulfonamides	Dicumarol	Synergistic; displacement of B by A from plasma proteins	Increased bleeding tendency
Phenobarbital / Glutethimide / Meprobamate	Dicumarol	Biochemical antagonism of B by A through enzyme induction	Decreased effect of B
Laxatives (prolonged use) / Diuretics, like chlorothiazide (Diuril)	Digitalis	Excessive loss of potassium ion from body produced by A	Increased toxicity of B
Antacids	Tetracycline / Isoniazid	Chemical antagonism; decreased absorption of B	Decreased effect of B
Cholestyramine	Dicumarol / Digitalis / Thyroxine	Chemical antagonism; decreased absorption of B	Decreased effect of B
Salicylates (small doses)	Probenecid	?	Decreased activity of B; decreased excretion of uric acid
Probenecid	Cephaloridine	Synergistic; inhibition of urinary excretion of B	Increased toxicity of B

absorption of a variety of drugs such as chlorothiazide, phenobarbital, thyroxine, anticoagulants and various digitalis preparations.

Reduced absorption of drugs may also result from interactions with preparations used to neutralize excess gastric acid. For example, antacids containing calcium or magnesium form nonabsorbable complexes with tetracycline, thereby decreasing the amount of the antibiotic absorbed. This example of chemical antagonism also illustrates how a patient, through self-medication with antacids to relieve gastrointestinal distress, may inadvertently decrease the effectiveness of an agent prescribed by a physician. Antacids may enhance the absorption of a basic drug like quinine by increasing the fraction of drug present in the nonionized and more absorbable form. Although changes in the alkalinity or acidity of the gastrointestinal tract affect the rate of absorption of ionizable drugs, this usually does not produce significant alterations in drug effectiveness or safety. However, drugs that decrease the rate at which the stomach empties its contents into the small intestine may markedly affect the absorption of drugs concomitantly administered. For example, codeine, morphine, atropine and chloroquine are known to delay gastric emptying and to depress the rate of absorption of other drugs as well as of foodstuffs. And on the whole, there is more evidence for drug interactions resulting in decreased effectiveness through diminished absorption than for increased toxicity due to enhanced absorption.

Distribution

We have seen that many drugs bind to nonreceptor tissue components, such as plasma proteins (cf. pp. 105–107). Since the drug that is bound to nonreceptor macromolecules is free neither to move to its site of action nor to produce a biologic effect, the binding sites represent sites of drug loss. These secondary binding sites also represent a reservoir of drug which may be made available to exert its pharmacologic effect. Certain drugs compete for binding sites on plasma or other proteins; a drug which binds more strongly may displace the drug forming weaker bonds. In this way one drug may have a synergistic effect on another. For example, phenylbutazone can displace a number of other agents from proteins, including salicylates, penicillin, sulfonamides, anticoagulants like dicumarol and warfarin, and some of the drugs other than insulin used in the treatment of diabetes. In most instances the increased effectiveness of the displaced drug is not very significant. However, this type of interaction may have serious consequences for anticoagulants and antidiabetic agents whose dosage has been very carefully adjusted for individual patients. Excessive amounts of anticoagulants can produce an increased bleeding tendency, and increased amounts of antidiabetic agents may lower blood sugar to undesirable levels.

Biotransformation

There are many examples of enhanced drug activity brought about by the inhibition of the biotransformation of one drug by another. This phenomenon is so well recognized that it rarely results in unanticipated events following prescribed, combined medication with well-established drugs. The problems encountered with the monoamine oxidase inhibitors, of course, were due to the unknown presence of tyramine in the various foods. But this adverse reaction might have occurred just as readily if the patients, during self-treatment for a cold, had used one of the popular non-prescription cough or cold remedies containing other reactive amines.

There are also many examples of decreased drug activity brought about by the acceleration of the biotransformation of one drug by another; this type of biochemical antagonism results from the induction of drug-metabolizing enzymes (cf. Table 6-7). Since the data obtained in laboratory animals are not always applicable to humans (cf. pp. 258–260), drug interactions involving enzyme induction are not always predictable. Indeed, some cases in which the effectiveness of one agent was unexpectedly reduced by concomitant administration of a second drug remained unexplained until subsequent investigation revealed the second drug to be an enzyme inducer.

Some drugs such as ethanol can either inhibit or enhance microsomal enzyme activity depending on the circumstances of drug administration. For instance, during acute ingestion of an intoxicating amount of alcohol, microsomal enzyme activity may be inhibited, but after chronic ingestion of alcohol for a prolonged period, there may be enzyme induction. These effects of ethanol on microsomal enzymes are of little consequence in the metabolism of ethanol itself, since nonmicrosomal enzymes account for most of the conversion of ethanol to acetaldehyde. However, the opposing effects of ethanol on microsomal enzymes help explain why interactions of alcohol with other drugs biotransformed by these enzymes vary with the amount of alcohol consumed and with the duration of alcohol use (see Table 10-5). It is well known, for example, that the usual hypnotic dose of barbiturates is relatively ineffective in the sober alcoholic but produces a greater than expected effect in the inebriated alcoholic. Enzyme induction and an increased rate of biotransformation can account for the diminished effect of barbiturates in the sober alcoholic and inhibition of barbiturate biotransformation for the increased response in the intoxicated.

Renal Excretion

The quantity of a drug excreted in the urine depends in the first place on how much is presented to the kidney. This, in turn, is determined by extrarenal factors: the amount of drug remaining in the body; the degree of protein binding; and the volume of drug distribution. Once a drug reaches the glomerular filtrate, only reabsorption from or active tubular secretion into the urine will affect the amount ultimately voided. For ionizable drugs the rate of reabsorption can be markedly influenced by changes in the pH of the glomerular filtrate (cf. pp. 133–134). Thus, any drug that produces an alkaline urine enhances the excretion of weakly acidic drugs, whereas an agent that leads to an acidic urine increases the urinary elimination of a weakly basic drug. Many of the drugs given specifically to increase the volume of voided urine — diuretics — affect the excretion of other drugs by altering urinary pH. And we cited earlier how the administration of sodium bicarbonate can hasten the excretion and shorten the duration of action of phenobarbital, a procedure useful in the treatment of poisoning by this agent.

We have seen that a number of drugs which are organic acids or bases are actively secreted by the renal epithelial cells, and it is the availability of carrier which limits the rate of active transport (cf. p. 137). Hence a drug that uses the same transport system as another agent will reduce the secretion of the second agent when the system is saturated by the simultaneous presence of the two substances. This type of biochemical interaction has greater theoretical than practical significance as far as multiple-drug therapy is concerned; there are only a few therapeutic situations which call for the concurrent administration of two drugs known to share the same renal tubular secretory process. Such combined therapy may be important, for example, in the treatment of resistant infections which require the administration of enormous doses of penicillin. Here, probenecid may be coadministered to decrease the rate of elimination of the antibiotic. On the other hand, administration of probenecid concurrently with the antibiotic cephaloridine may lead to increased cephaloridine toxicity as a consequence of the inhibition of its tubular secretion.

The fact that organic anionic drugs are secreted by the same transport process as uric acid, a normal waste product of the body, is of practical significance. For example, blood levels of uric acid may be increased above normal as a side-effect of therapy with some diuretic agents like chlorothiazide (Diuril) which are also actively secreted by the renal tubule. In some susceptible individuals this inhibition of uric acid secretion contributes to the appearance of gout, a disease associated with excessive uric acid content of the body.

A change in the rate of drug elimination is, of course, reflected as a change in duration of action: an increase in the rate of excretion will shorten the duration of action, and vice versa. Whether a change in the rate of urinary excretion also alters the intensity of drug effect depends on the rate of absorption. For drugs rapidly absorbed, there will be little change in the maximum drug level attained in the body, since most of the drug is available for distribution before much excretion occurs. When a drug is slowly absorbed, however, changes in rates of elimination may have considerable influence on the levels of drug in the body. A decreased rate of excretion may permit drug concentrations to rise to toxic levels, whereas an increased rate may prevent the attainment of effective drug concentrations.

Drug Mixtures

The type of muliple-drug therapy we have been discussing involves the concurrent but separate administration of more than one drug. This is quite different from the simultaneous administration of several drugs mixed in a single pharmaceutical preparation. Conjoint but separate administration permits manipulation of the dosage of individual drugs so that the greatest benefit can be attained with the least possibility of undesirable effects. The timing of the administration can also be adjusted as required. Neither individual dosage nor timing is possible in the case of the single multiple-drug preparation. The fixed-dose drug mixture has another disadvantage when toxic effects occur; it is frequently impossible to ascertain which drug was responsible. Because of the disadvantages and possible risks associated with fixed-dose mixtures, there are only a few occasions when their use is justified.

SYNOPSIS

Drug effects are never identical in all individuals, or even in the same individual at different times. Yet the majority of people respond to most drugs in a fashion similar enough to permit the calculation of a standard therapeutic dose for a drug. However, this "average" dose merely represents a starting point from which to estimate the appropriate dose for a given subject. The many variables contributing to the individuality of a complex living organism, or associated with the conditions present at the time of drug administration, must also be considered as factors potentially capable of modifying the usually observed drug effect.

We have considered the many factors contributing to individual variability in drug response from the perspective of the origin of the variability. Now we can summarize their influence on drug effects from the point of view of whether they produce quantitative or qualitative changes as a result of modifications in (1) absorption, (2) distribution, (3) biotransformation, (4) excretion, (5) receptors or target sites or (6) interactions unrelated to the normal pharmacodynamics of the drug.

Absorption. Differences in the rate and extent of absorption account in large part for the quantitative differences in an individual's response to drugs after administration by different routes. It is likely that differences in absorption, particularly after oral administration, also account for much of the commonly observed biologic variation in the responsiveness to drugs.

The rate of stomach emptying is one of the principal factors influencing rate of absorption, since the largest portion of the oral dose of most drugs is absorbed in the upper part of the small intestine. The rate at which the stomach empties its contents into the intestine is influenced by many factors, including the presence of food or of drugs which alter gastric motility. Occasionally, the interaction of the drug with certain food components or chemical agents results in a large fraction of the dose becoming unavailable for absorption. The more usual event is a decrease in the rate of drug absorption with but little change in the total amount of drug absorbed over a longer period.

There may be decreased efficiency of drug absorption in both the very young and the elderly individual, but this factor is of lesser consequence in their altered quantitative response to drugs than are other pharmacokinetic factors. However, qualitative differences in response to chemicals in the very young infant have been associated with differences in intestinal absorption.

Genetic abnormalities in drug absorption are relatively rare. The best documented example is the inherited lack of intrinsic factor, a biologic entity secreted by the gastric mucosa and essential for the normal absorption of vitamin B_{12}.

Distribution. Changes in the response to drugs attributable to modifications in drug distribution may be brought about by differences in (1) the ratios of total body water or fat to body mass, (2) the binding capacity of nonreceptor proteins or (3) the permeability of a biologic barrier.

The average dose of a drug is calculated for the individual whose total content of body water is about 58 per cent of body mass. Even after dosage is adjusted according to body weight, very young infants or very lean individuals may be less responsive to drugs distributed in body water than the average adult man, since their body water content is a larger percentage of their body weight. Conversely, the average woman or the obese individual might show a greater response. Pathologic conditions in which the normal body content of water is depleted (dehydration) or excessive (edema) may also alter the drug response. For drugs that are highly lipid soluble, the differences in body content of fat between males and females, and between lean and obese individuals, may influence the intensity of drug effect.

Many drugs bind to plasma or other proteins to varying degrees, and the fraction bound does not exert a pharmacologic effect until it is dissociated from the protein complex. Because many drugs compete for the same binding sites on plasma proteins, one drug may displace another when both are administered concurrently. The displaced drug is then free to leave the plasma and to act in concentrations higher than are ordinarily attained after the same dose given in the absence of the second drug. Whether the displaced drug will produce a large enough change in drug concentration at receptors to result in significant increases in response depends on its volume of distribution; the smaller the volume of distribution, the greater the increase in concentration.

A decrease in the quantity of available plasma proteins as the result of disease, malnutrition or genetic abnormality may also lead to an increased intensity of drug effect. In a few cases the inherited lack of a plasma protein may result in a novel effect, if the chemical is ordinarily bound and thus confined to plasma. In the genetically deficient individual, the unbound chemical is free to leave plasma and exert effects at sites to which it is normally not distributed.

Genetic alterations in the permeability or transport characteristics of parasitic and cancer cells can alter the ability of these cells to take up drugs that cause growth inhibition or cell death. This is one of the mechanisms by which resistance develops to antibacterial, antimalarial or anticancer drugs.

Biotransformation. Changes in the rate of drug biotransformation play a major role in variability in drug response because so many factors can affect the activity as well as the quantity of enzymes participating in these chemical reactions. Differences in pathways of biotransformation as well as in rates also account in large part for the differences in drug response between individuals of different species.

A decrease in the rate of biotransformation results in an increased duration of action or a greater magnitude of drug effect, or both. Conversely, an increase in the rate of enzymic activity leads to a decreased responsiveness or to a shorter duration of effective drug levels in the body, or both. When biotransformation converts an inactive agent to an active metabolite, an increased rate of biotransformation produces more rapid onset of drug effect.

The inhibition of the biotransformation of one drug by another is the most common mechanism of enhancing drug effect. But other factors such as age, genetic abnormalities and pathologic conditions may also make some individuals more sensitive than others to low doses of drugs. In the very young infant, the immaturity of the enzyme systems for drug inactivation is responsible. In the elderly, it is a generally impaired ability to carry out enzymic reactions effectively. In genetically abnormal individuals, the altered enzyme may be unable to combine effectively with its drug substrate, or there may be an altered ability to synthesize the enzymes that catalyze specific drug biotransformations. Drug biotransformation also may be depressed in certain types of liver disease which affect the microsomal enzyme systems.

Many drugs increase the activity of the microsomal enzymes involved in drug biotransformation by stimulating their synthesis. The concurrent use of a drug which enhances the rate of biotransformation of a second drug necessitates an increase in dosage of the latter to produce effects equal to those in the absence of the inducer. If the enzyme-inducing drug is suddenly withdrawn, severe toxic effects may occur unless the dosage of the second drug is suitably lowered. The decreased responsiveness to subsequent doses of a drug such as phenobarbital, which increases its own biotransformation, is one of the mechanisms for the development of tolerance to the particular drug.

The elaboration and induction of specific inactivating enzymes are also important mechanisms for the development of drug resistance in certain uneconomic species, such as bacteria and insects. The strains which have acquired specific enzymes or increased the quantity of these enzymes are capable of inactivating drugs that are lethal or inhibitory in the strains not possessing the enzyme activity.

Excretion. Modifications which influence the excretion of a drug or its metabolites ordinarily produce only quantitative changes in the effects of drugs, since it is only the rate of removal from the body which is affected. The kidney, as the principal organ for drug excretion, is also the site where most of these changes in rate of drug removal take place. And almost all the factors which modify the rate of urinary excretion produce a decrease in rate which, in turn, leads to an increased duration of drug action. However, factors that increase the rate of drug presentation to the kidney usually produce an increase in the rate of drug excretion and the consequent decrease in duration of drug action.

Alterations in the rate of urinary excretion of drug may be the result of changes in the rate of either glomerular filtration, tubular reabsorption or tubular secretion. In infants (as in the elderly), the decrease in rates of both glomerular filtration and tubular secretion is primarily responsible for the impaired ability to excrete drugs. In infants the filtration rate is decreased because there is less blood flowing through the immature kidney and the volume of distribution of drug is greater than in the adult. Incomplete development of active transport processes accounts for the decrease in rate of tubular secretion in the infant.

For drugs not extensively reabsorbed, any pathologic condition that decreases the rate of drug presentation to the glomerulus decreases the rate of drug removal from the body. A decreased rate of glomerular filtration may result from decreased glomerular blood flow, a diseased glomerulus or an increased volume of drug distribution (as in edema). Conversely, an increased rate of glomerular filtration may result from increased glomerular blood flow, a decreased volume of drug distribution or a decrease in the amount of drug normally bound to plasma proteins.

Changes in the pH of the tubular urine will affect the rate of reabsorption of ionizable drugs. The rate of reabsorption will be decreased by a pH which favors the ionization of a drug, since the passive reabsorption of ions is so much slower than that of nonionized substances. The converse is equally true. Changes in urinary pH may be brought about by disease, by drugs which influence the normal formation of urine, as well as by the intake of large quantities of acids or bases, or by foods which give rise to acidic or alkaline excretory products.

Alterations in the rate of the renal tubular secretory mechanisms affect the excretion of only those organic acids or bases, either normal metabolic products or drugs, which are transported by these processes. Decreased tubular secretion may be the consequence of interaction of drugs competing for the same secretory mechanism or of pathologic conditions which decrease renal blood flow or impair the function of the secretory processes themselves.

Drug Receptors or Target Sites. Alterations in a receptor or a target site of a drug may be manifested as either an idiosyncratic response, drug resistance or drug tolerance. In the genetically abnormal individual, the receptor for the drug may be entirely absent or altered to such a degree that even extremely high concentrations of drug cannot produce effective interaction.

In drug resistance an enzyme or protein of an uneconomic species is altered in such a way that the drug can no longer combine with it to produce its lethal or inhibitory effect. The altered enzyme retains its capacity to bind with its normal substrate, however. The strains which possess the normal enzyme or protein are not resistant to the action of the drug and are inhibited or destroyed. As a consequence, the mutant strains, possessing the altered protein, survive and multiply and eventually become the predominant strains. This mechanism has been shown to account, in part, for the resistance developed to some antibacterial and anticancer drugs.

The development of tolerance is characterized by decreased responsiveness to a drug upon repeated administration. Tolerance is developed to many drugs which act in the central nervous system to produce changes in mood and behavior. Although the mechanisms of this tolerance remain a mystery, there is ample evidence to indicate that it must be attributed to cells within the nervous system having become adapted in some way to the action of the drugs. This kind of development of tolerance through cellular adaptation also occurs outside the central nervous system with respect to the action of drugs such as the nitrites.

Interactions Unrelated to the Normal Pharmacodynamics of the Drug. Factors which modify the pharmacokinetics of a drug, with few exceptions, produce an alteration only in the intensity of an anticipated pharmacologic effect. Although such factors make it difficult to predict whether a given individual will manifest extreme sensitivity or unusual resistance to the average dose of a drug, the character of the response will be as expected. Qualitatively different responses as a result of modified pharmacokinetics occur only when drug biotransformation yields unusual products or when altered patterns of distribution permit a chemical to reach extraordinary sites of action. But when the administration of a drug elicits effects unrelated to its normal pharmacodynamic activity, then neither the intensity, the nature nor the occurrence of the response can be predicted beforehand. This certainly is true for allergic or psychologic (placebo) responses to drugs. It is also true for most idiosyncratic responses unless the mechanisms of the specific genetic defect and its patterns of inheritance are known and the patient's family history is available.

The allergic response has a number of important characteristics which distinguish it from a toxic or idiosyncratic effect. The allergic response (1) requires prior exposure to the chemical and a primary sensitizing period before the individual manifests the response to subsequent exposures; (2) is a consequence of antigen-antibody interaction; (3) is unrelated to the usual pharmacologic effects of the eliciting drug; (4) is determined by the activity of the mediators released or the tissues or cells damaged by the antigen-antibody complex; (5) shows no consistent relationship between the severity of symptoms elicited and the size of the dose of eliciting drug; and (6) is antagonized by drugs like antihistaminics, epinephrine or hydrocortisone, but not by specific antagonists of the drug which produces the allergy.

Since many drugs may produce allergic responses, allergy is one of the most frequent side-effects of drug therapy. The incidence within the population of an allergic response to a given drug, however, is usually very low. Unfortunately, one cannot predict which patient will manifest an allergic reaction to what drug, or which of the many possible allergic symptoms will constitute the response.

The placebo response is not a pharmacologic effect of a drug, since it is unrelated to the physicochemical properties of the eliciting drug. It is a psychologic response to drug administration induced by the circumstances of the administration and by the wish of patient and physician for a successful outcome. The intensity and nature of a placebo response following the administration of either an active drug or a material masquerading as an active drug vary widely and are completely unpredictable. All drugs may produce placebo effects, and any individual at some time may be a "placebo responder."

Idiosyncratic reactions are seen as novel drug effects when an inborn error affects the constitution of cells in such a way that they become susceptible to unusual interactions with certain drugs. Under ordinary circumstances the cell can compensate for the inherited abnormality. Indeed, the abnormality frequently is first revealed when an affected individual is exposed to a drug and has an unexpected response.

GUIDES FOR STUDY AND REVIEW
What are the general types of altered drug response that can occur only after repeated administration of a single drug (or of a drug closely related in structure)?

How is the phenomenon of drug resistance distinguished from that of drug tolerance? With what types of drugs is the phenomenon of drug resistance associated? What do we mean by "economic species"? "uneconomic species"?

What are the origins of drug resistance? What is infectious drug resistance? Why is infectious drug resistance of such great clinical significance? What is one of the most common mechanisms by which an uneconomic species acquires drug resistance, for example, the bacterial resistance developed to penicillin?

What is drug allergy? Why does an allergic response to a particular drug require prior exposure to that drug or to one very similar in structure? Does the allergic response show the usual dose-response relationship? How does this differ from the relationship between the dose and a toxic response to a drug? between the dose and an idiosyncrati response to a drug? What is the incidence of the allergic response in a population? the toxic response? the idiosyncratic response?

How is the allergic response related to the structure or pharmacologic activity of the drug eliciting the allergic response? What are some mediators of the allergic response? What types of drugs can be used to counteract the allergic response? How is this different from the way in which toxic or idiosyncratic responses to drugs are antagonized?

What is drug tolerance? Experimentally how would you determine whether an individual has acquired tolerance to a particular drug? To what types of drugs is tolerance usually acquired?

What do we mean by "drug-disposition tolerance"? What is the mechanism by which drug-disposition tolerance is produced to a drug such as phenobarbital? How does drug-disposition tolerance affect the duration of action of a given dose of a drug compared to the duration of action of the same dose in the nontolerant state? Why is the intravenous dose producing a toxic or lethal effect essentially the same for both the nontolerant individual and the subject made tolerant to the drug by the mechanism of increased rate of drug elimination? Why is the peak effect of a drug reduced in the latter tolerant individual when the drug is given by a slow-absorption route?

What is tachyphylaxis? What is an example of a drug that produces tachyphylaxis?

What do we mean by pharmacodynamic or cellular tolerance? The repeated use of what types of drugs usually produces pharmacodynamic tolerance? What do we mean by cross-tolerance among drugs? What kinds of drugs exhibit cross-tolerance?

How does the tolerance developed to narcotic analgesics like morphine differ from that developed to alcohol or barbiturates? Does tolerance develop uniformly to all the pharmacologic effects of a drug? To which of the characteristic pharmacologic effects of morphine does tolerance develop? not develop?

What are the terms that are used to describe the combined effect of two or more drugs acting simultaneously? What is the term used to refer to the situation in which two drugs elicit the same pharmacologic response and the combined effect is the algebraic sum of these individual effects? What is the special term used when both drugs act by the same mechanism? What do we mean by synergism? How does a synergist increase the effect of another drug?

What do we mean by the term *drug antagonism*? What are the four types of drug antagonism and how are they distinguished from one another? What is an example of each type of drug antagonism?

The decreased bioavailability of orally administered tetracycline in the presence of a magnesium-containing antacid is an example of what type of drug interaction?

The increased bleeding tendency produced when an anticoagulant drug is displaced from protein-binding sites by another drug is an example of what type of drug interaction?

The decreased effectiveness of an anticoagulant drug in a patient who starts taking phenobarbital is an example of what type of drug interaction?

The action of an antihistaminic drug to alleviate some of the symptoms of an allergic response is an example of what type of drug interaction?

The use of epinephrine in preparations of local anesthetics is an example of what type of drug interaction?

SUGGESTED READING

Azarnoff, D.L., and Hurwitz, A. Drug interactions. *Pharmacol. Physicians* 4:1, 1970.

Davis, B.D., and Maas, W.K. Analysis of the biochemical mechanisms of drug resistance in certain bacterial mutants. *Proc. Natl. Acad. Sci. U.S.A.* 38:775, 1952.

Eddy, N.B. The Phenomena of Tolerance. In M.G. Sevay, R.D. Reid, and O.E. Reynolds (eds.), *Origins of Resistance to Toxic Agents.* New York: Academic, 1955.

Gaddum, J.H., and Schield, H.O. Drug antagonism. *Pharmacol. Rev.* 9:211, 1957.

Garb, S. *Undesirable Drug Interactions and Interferences.* New York: Springer, 1971.

Hamburger, R.N. Allergy and the immune system. *Am. Sci.* 64:157, 1976.

Levine, B.B. Immunochemical mechanisms of drug allergy. *Annu. Rev. Med.* 17: 23, 1966.

Medical Letter. Adverse Interactions of Drugs. In *Reference Handbook.* New York: Drug and Therapeutic Information, Inc., 1975. Pp. 3–10.

Moyed, H.S. Biochemical mechanisms of drug resistance. *Ann. Rev. Microbiol.* 18:347, 1964.

Parker, W.C. The biochemical basis of allergic drug response. *Ann. N.Y. Acad. Sci.* 123:55, 1965.

Seevers, M.H., and Deneau, G.A. Physiological Aspects of Tolerance and Physical Dependence. In W.S. Root and F.G. Hofmann (eds.), *Physiological Pharmacology.* New York: Academic, 1963. P. 565.

Swedler, G. *Handbook of Drug Interactions.* New York: Wiley, 1971.

Wolf, S. The pharmacology of placebos. *Pharmacol. Rev.* 11:689, 1959.

11. DRUG TOXICITY

Desired effect and *toxic effect*, when used to describe the end-results of the interaction of a drug and a biologic system, are relative terms. They take on real meaning only within the context of the circumstances under which the chemical-biologic reaction occurs. Certainly, *desired effect* indicates that the purpose for which a drug is being used has been achieved. And *toxic effect* always means that a harmful effect has been produced on some biologic mechanism. Yet the two terms are occasionally synonymous, as for example when the action of a pesticide like malathion saves a farmer's crop by eliminating a plant-destroying insect. This same effect would be considered very undesirable from another standpoint were the farmer accidentally exposed to quantities sufficient to make him ill or cause his death.

Drug safety and drug toxicity are also relative concepts. Phenobarbital, for example, is considered a relatively safe drug since the dose producing the desired effect in most individuals is appreciably lower than that producing toxicity in even a small percentage of the same population (cf. pp. 191–195 and Fig. 7-12). Penicillin also is relatively nontoxic, since it can effectively eliminate the microorganisms responsible for certain diseases without harming the great majority of human or animal hosts. But malathion is not regarded as a safe drug despite the fact that it is a useful insecticide. For even though, on the basis of dose per unit of body weight, it is much less toxic to humans, other mammals and birds than it is to many insects (cf. p. 163), its administration to these higher animals produces no salutary effects. Its usefulness as an insecticide presupposes that it can be administered by mechanical means in a manner and in amounts that will harm only the uneconomic or undesirable species.

We can also evaluate the relative safety and toxicity of a drug by comparing it with other drugs having similar actions and used for similar purposes. These comparisons can be made on the basis of the relative margins of safety (the difference between the dose producing a lethal effect and that producing the desired effect), or the relative severity or incidence of any undesirable effects. Penicillin, for example, elicits a much higher incidence of allergic responses than does the antibacterial agent neomycin. Yet in nonallergic individuals, penicillin is the safer drug by far since it is virtually nontoxic to host tissues and cells.

What do these examples tell us about drug safety and harmfulness as relative phenomena? First, they tell us that the relative safety of a drug is judged in terms of its effects on a species considered desirable or economic[1]; relative drug toxicity can be evaluated in terms of both the economic and the uneconomic species. Second, when the sites of action for the desired and toxic effects occur within the same organism, the *dose* is the single factor that determines the degree of harmfulness of the compound (except when the harmful effect is the result of an immune response). But when an economic species uses a chemical to eliminate an undesirable species, it is the degree of *species specificity* or *selective toxicity* that determines the margin of safety for the species which it is desirable to maintain.

When a drug is intended for use in an economic species, it is implicitly understood that dosage can be regulated to produce the desired effect in most individuals without causing significant harmful effects to members of the economic species. This is true whether the purpose of administering the drug is to effect a change in the physiologic function of the economic species itself or to eliminate an uneconomic species. In contrast, if a chemical is not intended for use in an economic species there is no dose that can be introduced into the species that will be both effective and noninjurious. If the dose is sufficiently small there may be no effects, untoward or otherwise; but a dose large enough to produce an effect will produce only an undesirable effect. A substance that acts in a noxious manner and by physicochemical means to cause harmful or lethal effects when introduced into a biologic system is, by definition, a *poison*. Thus a chemical is considered a poison when it exerts an injurious action in the majority of cases in which it reacts with a living organism. There is no sharp line of demarcation, however, between a poison and a drug intended for introduction into an economic species; in large enough doses, *any* chemical agent, even food and water, can cause harmful effects. As Paracelsus recognized so long ago, "All things are poisons, for there is nothing without poisonous properties. It is only the dose which makes a thing a poison."

The study of the harmful actions of chemicals on living organisms is the particular province of that branch of pharmacology known as toxicology (cf. pp. 18–19). Since any chemical agent has the potential to cause injurious effects in some biologic mechanism, the subject matter of toxicology is, understandably, vast. We need formulate no new principles, however, to understand the essentials of toxicology; the principles of pharmacology are applicable to the study of both the beneficial and the toxic effects of chemicals that interact with living organisms. Thus the magnitude of the toxic response, like the intensity of any response (except an allergic one), is a function of the concentration of the chemical at the site(s) of action. And this in turn depends on many factors we have already discussed: (1) the physicochemical properties of the agent; (2) the route and rate of its introduction into the organism; (3) the rate of its absorption, distribution, biotransformation and excretion; and (4) the many other variables influencing the response of a biologic system. A separate

[1] What constitutes an "economic" species is also relative; it may be interpreted very differently by the public health official, the marine biologist, the agriculturist, the ecologist, and others concerned with the adverse effects of chemical compounds on biologic systems.

discussion of the adverse effects of chemicals is warranted nevertheless, since toxicity has become a crucial aspect of the use of therapeutic agents and a major societal problem in the form of exposure to chemicals contaminating the atmosphere, food or water.

We shall limit our discussion to considerations of the types of toxic reactions and the means by which they occur, the incidence of untoward effects of chemicals and the general principles underlying the treatment of drug toxicity. We shall simplify our task by dividing the many biologically reactive chemicals into two distinct categories based on whether or not they are intended for use in humans. All the drugs used in the treatment, cure, prevention or diagnosis of disease; for population control; as food additives (sweeteners, flavoring agents and preservatives); or as cosmetics will fall into one category. For convenience, we shall refer to this category as *therapeutic agents* or *medicinals,* even though the purpose of administering food additives and cosmetics is not to produce biologic effects. The second category comprises those chemicals which are not intended for introduction into humans, but which are potentially capable of producing biologic effects upon incidental, accidental or (maliciously) intentional exposure. This group includes agents produced for use by humans, such as cleaning and polishing agents, paints, petroleum products and pesticides, as well as industrial waste materials, noxious gases and nonfood plants. We shall refer to chemicals in this second category as *poisons.*

CLASSIFICATIONS OF TOXIC REACTIONS

In textbooks of toxicology, toxic agents are usually grouped by chemical classes, e.g., heavy metals, oxidizing agents, acids. Or the various chemicals may be grouped according to the locale of exposure to the source of toxicity — household poisons, industrial poisons and so forth. From the standpoint of pharmacology, classification based on the types of toxic effects produced or the sites in the body where they occur is more appropriate.

Types of Toxic Effects Produced

Toxic reactions may be classified as *acute, subacute* or *chronic* on the basis of the rate of onset of symptoms and the rate and duration of exposure to the offending agent. Toxicity is said to be acute when symptoms which imperil the individual develop shortly after introduction of the drug into the body. Acute toxicity is usually produced by the single or sudden intake of a drug in quantities large enough to cause severe depression of a vital physiologic function. For example, the ingestion of excessively large amounts of secobarbital (five to fifteen times the usual dose of 100 mg) quickly leads to a profound depresssion of respiration. Death from acute barbiturate poisoning may occur within one to two hours and is usually caused by a cessation of respiration resulting from inhibition of the center in the brain which controls involuntary breathing. Many of the deaths which occur in burning buildings are the consequence of sudden exposure to an atmosphere containing poisonous quantities of carbon monoxide. For example, death may occur within five to six minutes of exposure to air containing 1.5 per cent of the lethal gas. Death is not caused by a lack of oxygen in the air, but by a lack of oxygen in the victim's blood. Carbon monoxide's affinity for hemoglobin is nearly three hundred times that of oxygen's. The greater the concentration of carbon monoxide inhaled and the longer the exposure, the greater the decrease in the amount of oxygen that can be carried to the cells of the body. The ingestion of cyanides or inhalation of hydrogen cyanide gas may also produce a lethal effect in minutes. The cyanides interfere with cellular respiration but in a manner different from that of carbon monoxide; cyanides inhibit enzymes which promote the utilization of oxygen by the cell.

Subacute toxicity differs from acute toxicity only with respect to the conditions under which the subject is endangered by the drug. In subacute toxicity there is frequent, repeated exposure over several hours or days to a dose insufficient to produce deleterious effects when given as a single dose. This type of toxicity may develop in response to therapeutic agents when there is a malfunction of the mechanisms responsible for terminating the action of the agent. For example, tetracycline, which is eliminated primarily by urinary excretion, may accumulate to toxic levels within a few days in patients with impaired renal function. In the case of poisons, it is usually inadvertent and prolonged exposure that leads to toxicity. A farmer spraying his crops with malathion, for instance, if he is not adequately protected, might absorb enough insecticide through the skin or lungs over several hours to cause subacute toxicity.

Chronic toxicity usually occurs from repeated exposure over long periods to a chemical whose rate of entry into the body exceeds its rate of elimination. As we have seen (pp. 233–238), cumulative toxicity is usually associated with agents having biologic half-lives measured in days, weeks or months instead of hours. This is the type of poisoning that has occurred all too frequently in children living in old, dilapidated buildings painted with lead-containing preparations. Ingestion of flakes of chipped paint may continue over a period of many months before the signs of chronic lead poisoning emerge. Recognition of this source of poisoning in children living in slum housing provided the impetus for legislation banning the further use of lead-containing interior housepaints and for their removal from existing dwellings. Environmental lead, however, derived principally from automobile exhausts, still presents a clear health hazard to urban dwellers; infants and children remain the population at greatest risk because of the presence of precipitated airborne lead in playground soil and household dust. On the other hand, the rapid decline since 1965 in mortality due to lead poisoning among children under 5 years of age (see Fig. 11-2) is most encouraging. This decline is primarily attributable to the mass-screening programs established and currently in operation in many large urban centers; the early detection of hazardously high blood levels permits treatment to prevent death and, perhaps, serious toxicity. Workers in certain industries may also become accidental victims of environmental poisons upon repeated exposure to airborne chemicals in the form of fine particulate matter. Some of these particles, such as fibers of silica or asbestos, remain unabsorbed in the lungs and produce serious, irreversible lesions, but only after several years of constant impaction and deposition in alveolar tissue (cf. pp. 93–94).

Chronic toxicity can occur, however, upon continued exposure to an agent even when the causal agent is rapidly eliminated. It is as if the injury rather than the injurious agent accumulates; each dose of the offending agent produces some slight tissue damage that either is irreversible or is repaired at a rate slower than the rate of injury. For example, the separate ingredients in proprietary analgesic mixtures, e.g., aspirin, phenacetin and caffeine, are completely and rapidly eliminated from the body by biotransformation and excretion. Yet, there is presumptive evidence that constant and excessive self-medication with these proprietary analgesics over a period of years may be associated with irreversible kidney damage. This type of toxicity is not observed following frequent — but not continuous — use of these analgesic mixtures in recommended dosage. Benzene, a volatile liquid used in the manufacture of petroleum, explosives, plastics and pesticides, is also rapidly eliminated from the body. The toxicity that results from repeated inhalation of an atmosphere contaminated with low concentrations of benzene is insidious, however; depression of blood-cell forming elements in bone marrow may not develop until months or even years after chronic exposure to benzene vapors has stopped. In contrast, the symptoms of acute poisoning with benzene are related to depression of the central nervous system; death from acute overexposure is due to respiratory failure. Thus it is the circumstances under which an individual is exposed to a potentially toxic agent that determine the type of toxicity that ensues. And it is usually true that the symptoms of acute toxicity are different from those seen in chronic poisoning by the same agent.

Chemical carcinogenicity also may be considered a variant of chronic toxicity. Prolonged exposure of many years' duration to a variety of chemical agents, such as those contained in cigarette smoke, is associated with the development of destructive and characteristic cancers (see Toxic Substances Encountered in the Workplace, p. 313).

Sites of Toxic Actions

Local Actions

Certain chemicals not intended for use in humans, as well as some that are, may produce local injury at the site of initial contact with the body, usually on the skin or in the respiratory tract. A topical agent that causes destruction of tissue at the site of application is termed a *caustic* or *corrosive*. These caustic chemicals are called primary irritants; their action is nonselective and occurs in all cells in direct proportion to the concentration in contact with the tissue. Strong acids such as hydrochloric, sulfuric or nitric, and strong alkalis like sodium, potassium or ammonium hydroxide, are examples of agents that produce severe structural damage to tissues. A primary irritant effect may also be produced by gases which are converted to acids or bases when they react with water. High concentrations of ammonia gas, for example, can produce local injury to tissues when inhaled and converted to ammonium hydroxide on contact with the moist pulmonary surfaces. (Yet ammonium ion is a normal metabolite produced in the body by the catabolism of amino acids.) Gases such as sulfur dioxide and nitrogen dioxide, which are encountered as atmospheric pollutants (especially under smog conditions), also owe their toxic effects to conversion to acids within the lungs.

Primary irritants which are therapeutic agents are used topically for their **antiseptic** or **germicidal** properties. Many such agents are available in a variety of proprietary preparations, e.g., various derivatives of phenol (hexylresorcinol; hexachlorophene) or cresol (Lysol); compounds containing mercury (thimerosal, Merthiolate); inorganic compounds, such as iodine and silver nitrate, and acids, such as boric acid. When these agents are employed topically and for legitimate therapeutic purposes, they have some beneficial and few toxic effects. When one of these agents is taken into the body, its corrosive action is exerted on any tissue with which it comes in contact.

Systemic Actions

A chemical acts systemically only after absorption into the circulation and distribution by the blood to the cells and tissues capable of responding to it. Therapeutic agents administered for systemic effects are usually introduced into the body by the oral route or by subcutaneous, intramuscular or intravenous injections. The lungs, the alimentary canal and the skin represent the most important sites of absorption of chemicals not intended for use in human beings.

NONSELECTIVE TOXICITY. The systemic action of some chemicals, like the local action of primary irritants, may be nonselective in that the drugs may act by altering functions vital to cells in general. Thus a drug that modifies an enzymic reaction essential for energy production, growth or reproduction will affect this enzyme in any cell in the body to which the drug can gain access. Drugs with such actions are called *cytotoxic* or *protoplasmic poisons.* And when drugs modify cellular functions in this way, almost without exception they produce effects harmful to the cell. We have already noted that the toxic effect of cyanide in oxygen-dependent animals is mediated through its ability to inhibit cellular utilization of oxygen. Many heavy metals, such as arsenic and mercury, although markedly different in their physical and chemical characteristics, share the property of inhibiting various enzyme systems essential to normal cellular metabolism. As a result, the symptoms of poisoning by these heavy metals are referable to many tissues, organs and systems. The tissues and cells most easily disrupted are those with the greatest metabolic requirements or the lowest reserve capacity to carry on their overall function. Thus, rapidly proliferating tissues like the gastrointestinal mucosa and the blood-cell-forming elements of bone marrow, and the finely balanced cells of the renal tubules and nervous system, show early signs of toxicity.

It is noteworthy that the cytotoxic action of each of the agents cited is a *specific* action of the particular agent. The *nonselectivity* of the action of any one of these agents arises from the fact that it can exert its cytotoxic effect on many tissues and organs. When such drugs possess selectivity as well as specificity, the toxicity will be manifested in certain cells but not in others. The rationale for the use of cytotoxic agents in the treatment of cancer, for example, is based on the fact that these agents selectively attack rapidly proliferating cells. This selectivity is of limited usefulness, however, since the anticancer drugs do not discriminate between malignant and normal cells; thus they are also toxic to the rapidly multiplying cells of the bone marrow and gastrointestinal mucosa.

SELECTIVE TOXICITY OF THERAPEUTIC AGENTS. In contrast to the nonselective activity and toxicity of protoplasmic poisons, most therapeutic agents have a relatively high degree of selectivity or specificity of action, or both. As we have seen, selectivity and specificity are the most important characteristics of a drug in determining its therapeutic usefulness (cf. pp. 195–197). The greater the selectivity and specificity, the less likelihood of toxic effects occurring when therapeutic agents are used in recommended dosage. Toxic effects unrelated to idosyncrasy, allergy, concurrent drug therapy or pathology are unlikely in the majority of individuals given normal doses of drugs which have highly selective and specific sites and mechanisms of action. Excessive doses will produce toxic effects in all individuals. And obviously, except for the immune response, whenever a therapeutic agent produces a harmful effect, regardless of circumstantial or predisposing factors, the dose administered must be considered an overdose. The type of toxicity observed may be the result of a continuation of the therapeutic effect, as, for example, the occurrence of hemorrhage following overdosage with an anticoagulant. Or the toxicity may be produced by mechanisms unrelated to those responsible for the desired or intended effect of the drug, e.g., the excitement and convulsions associated, particularly in children, with acute poisoning by antihistaminic agents.

The frequency of unwanted effects associated with therapeutic agents depends on the circumstances of their use. However, even when we exclude accidental or voluntary overdosage and consider only the adverse effects of the correct drugs used in recommended dosage for the right indications, we find the incidence of untoward effects not insignificant. Although the true incidence is unknown for the general population, it is estimated that between 5 and 10 per cent of hospitalized patients experience some unwanted effects of drug therapy. Between 20 and 25 per cent of these are allergic manifestations. The remainder, in order of frequency, are referable to effects on the central nervous system, the gastrointestinal tract and the cardiovascular system. The most common effects include drowsiness, dizziness, nervousness, headache, insomnia, nausea, heartburn, abdominal distention, vomiting and diarrhea. Many of the effects that occur most often are not harmful and do not necessarily require withdrawal of the offending drug. Yet nonspecific changes in general well-being can be life-threatening when, for example, a drug induces suicidal tendencies. And excessive vomiting or diarrhea merits consideration as being serious in every instance.

The more serious aspects of the toxicity induced by therapeutic agents are those relating to pathologic changes in specific organs. The frequency with which these changes occur may be low (e.g., only a few tenths of 1 per cent of those using the drug), or even rare (e.g., less than 2 in 50,000 patients). Nevertheless, they represent the most hazardous and unpredictable complications of drug therapy. The sites most frequently attacked are the liver, kidney and blood-forming elements of bone marrow. For example, drugs like the phenothiazines (including chlorpromazine) and certain steroids may produce hepatotoxicity; renal tubular damage is a severe toxic effect of some antibiotics like tetracycline; and drugs like phenylbutazone and streptomycin may produce disorders of the blood. The liver and kidney are particularly vulnerable, since many drugs attain high concentrations in these organs. Some of the effects on the liver, kidney and bone marrow may be manifestations of drug allergy.

Chemicals that induce abnormal fetal development when administered to the pregnant animal are called *chemical teratogens.* That this type of toxic phenomenon could be induced by an ordinary, and supposedly harmless, therapeutic agent was dramatically and tragically demonstrated by what has since become known as the "thalidomide disaster of 1960–1962." In the aftermath of this tragedy, a wide range of medicinals, both old and new, have been tested and shown to have teratogenic effects in animals (Table 11-1). The potential teratogenicity of these agents in humans is unknown. But these investigations and the retrospective analysis of the effects of thalidomide indicate that there is a specific critical period during fetal development when malformations can be induced. The embryo is most susceptible to teratogenic effects during the period corresponding to organogenesis. In the human, this extends from about the twentieth day of gestation to the end of the first trimester. This means that part of the period of greatest vulnerability occurs in many instances before pregnancy is recognized or diagnosed. The uncertainty of the risk to the human embryo of drugs known to be teratogenic in animals obviously dictates their cautious use in any woman of child-bearing age. And until a drug is known to be reasonably safe by virtue of thorough investigation or long usage, it should be avoided altogether in women known to be pregnant.

Whereas the potential teratogenicity of some drugs has been recognized only recently, the tendency of some chemicals to produce cancer in animals and humans has been known for about half a century. Legally, except for one group of therapeutic agents, no chemical may be designated for use in humans which has been found to be capable of producing cancer in laboratory animals (cf. Chap. 14). The exception is the group of chemicals used to treat cancers in humans; many of these agents have been shown to be carcinogenic for laboratory animals. The unknown etiology of most spontaneous cancers, the long latent period involved in the chem-

Table 11-1. Chemicals Producing Teratogenicity in Various Laboratory Animals

Vitamin A
Nicotinic acid
Thiouracil (used in the treatment of hyperthyroidism)
Tetracycline
Streptomycin
Sulfanilamide
Tolbutamide (and other sulfonamide antidiabetic agents)
Heavy metals (inorganic mercury salts, lead, selenium, etc.)
Nicotine
Quinine
Chlorpromazine and derivatives
Salicylate
Caffeine

ical production of tumors and the low predictive power of animal tests for carcino-genicity make it impossible, however, to say that a compound will not be carcinogenic in man.

SELECTIVE TOXICITY OF POISONS. When *selectivity* is used in connection with the actions of poisons, the term has somewhat different connotations than when it is used to refer to the actions of therapeutic agents. Chemicals not intended for introduction into humans have selectivity only with regard to the types of toxic effects they may produce; they are not selectively capable of producing effects which are not harmful to humans. The selectivity of action of poisons may be mani-fested as an immediate harmful effect on a particular function or organ or as a delayed pathologic change in one or more specific organs. Many chemicals are capable of producing both immediate and delayed effects; the particular toxic symptoms that develop are determined by the conditions of exposure. For example, the initial effects of the ingestion of methyl alcohol (methanol or wood alcohol) are referable to the central nervous system and resemble those of intoxication with ethyl alcohol. The most serious toxic effect of methanol is the selective injury to retinal cells which results from the products of methanol biotransformation (probably formaldehyde; cf. p. 156). As little as $1/2$ ounce (15 ml) of methanol has caused blindness. The immediate effects of carbon tetracholoride (CCl_4), following either ingestion or inhala-tion of quantities sufficient to cause toxicity, are also initially on the central nervous system and consist of dizziness, headache, stupor, convulsions and coma. The delayed toxic effects of CCl_4 are on hepatic or renal tubular cells, or both. These delayed effects may either follow recovery from acute poisoning or occur as a result of chronic exposure in the absence of any marked effects on the central nervous system. The extent of tissue damage is a dose-related phenomenon, and the reversibility of the damage depends on the efficiency of the mechanisms of tissue repair. In chronic exposure to any chemical that produces tissue damage, the tissue will be able to per-form its functions only as long as the rate of repair keeps pace with the rate of injury.

That constant exposure to certain chemicals can induce cancer in humans was recognized as early as 1775, when soot was implicated as a causative factor in the high incidence of scrotal cancer among chimney sweeps. Many other examples of cancer as an occupational hazard came to light in the second half of the nineteenth century. These indicated that cancer-producing substances are also present in coal tar, crude paraffins, pitch, mineral oils and certain dyestuffs. But it was not until the early part of the twentieth century that cancer was produced by chemical means in experimental animals. Then the earlier clinical observations made in man were confirmed by laboratory demonstrations of the carcinogenic activity of the suspect chemicals. The responsible agents were subsequently isolated and identified and found to be polycyclic hydrocarbons, such as benzpyrene, and aromatic amines like naphthylamine. There are at present stringent laws to safeguard workers in those occupations in which a high incidence of cancer has been associated with particular chemicals (cf. pp. 314—315).

A great variety of compounds besides the polycyclic hydrocarbons and aromatic amines are now known to be capable of producing cancer in animals. Many of these occur in the environment and are derived from various sources, and some have been clearly incriminated in the production of cancer in humans. Since large segments of the population undoubtedly have contact with these agents, it becomes essential to determine how much of a hazard they constitute. However, establishing tolerance levels for potential environmental carcinogens and formulating measures to protect the general public pose serious practical problems which are as yet unresolved (cf. p. 316).

EVALUATION OF DRUG TOXICITY
The introduction of any new chemical into medicine, industry or everyday living carries with it certain potential hazards which must be assessed prior to its use. This potential toxicity is evaluated initially by measurements on experimental animals. The nature of the tests carried out is dictated by the intended use of the new chemical.

Chemicals Intended for Use in Humans
If the chemical is a potential therapeutic agent, the toxicity studies are conducted with a dual purpose in mind. First, since no active medicinal agent is without undesirable effects, it is essential to delineate the conditions under which these effects occur and to define the type(s) of toxicity which may be encountered. Second, the expected beneficial effects must be weighed against any possible harmful aspects of the agent's use, so that its margin of safety may be determined (cf. Chap. 7). These tests are carried out as acute, subacute and chronic studies in several species of laboratory animals in accordance with the guidelines established by regulatory agencies.[2]
In the United States this agency is the Food and Drug Administration. The rationale of these preclinical studies is based on the assumption that toxicity determinations in animals have predictive value for the harmful effects likely to occur in humans. This assumption is often valid, particularly when the toxic effect involves a physiologic function equally important to all species concerned, or when it is a continuum of the therapeutically desired effect. All too often, however, a newly introduced drug thought to be free of undue toxicity turns out to have serious toxic effects in humans of a nature unforeseen from the animal tests. In general, preclinical tests in animals fail to provide clues about human toxicity when the toxicity is a rare event or the toxic effect is detectable only in humans.

The number of animals that it is feasible to use in toxicity tests is very small compared with the large number of patients who will receive the drug once it is in widespread use. Therefore a toxic effect with a low incidence is unlikely to be picked up in preclinical animal testing, since the probability of detecting such an effect depends on the number of animals used. Effects with an incidence of less than 1 per cent are not apt to be disclosed in most animal studies. And toxic effects such as the blood disorders which occur in about 1 in 100,000 patients receiving chloramphenicol usually are not recognized as being caused by a drug until it has been in widespread clinical use for several years.

---

[2] This topic is discussed more fully in Chapter 14, in connection with the development of a new drug.

Table 11-2. Adverse Effects of Six Unrelated Drugs in Humans, Rats and Dogs[a]

Toxic effects observed in humans		53
Toxic effects observed in rats {	also found in humans	18
	not found in humans	19
Toxic effects observed in dogs {	also found in humans	29
	not found in humans	24
Toxic effects observed in humans and detected in neither rats nor dogs		23

[a]Each drug was used in at least 500 patients. Only those toxic symptoms were considered which could occur in all these species; subjective effects that could not be evaluated in animals (e.g., nausea and headache) and effects peculiar to humans (e.g., allergic reactions) were omitted.

Data from J. T. Litchfield, Jr., *Clin. Pharmacol. Ther.* 3:665, 1962.

Several toxic effects occur in humans that appear to have no counterpart in animals. The most serious among these are allergic reactions, skin lesions, some blood disorders and many central nervous system effects. Nausea, headache, dizziness, amnesia and mild depression are examples of minor effects not readily observable in animals which, nevertheless, frequently limit the use of a drug. But even when we exclude from consideration the effects that cannot be demonstrated in animals, toxicity tests in various species do not necessarily predict the kinds of effects that will be observed in humans. The magnitude of the problem of extrapolating data from animal experiments to humans is illustrated in Table 11-2. These data are a summary of a retrospective study of the effects of six drugs. The unwanted effects observed in humans during clinical use were compared with the toxic effects noted in experiments on rats and dogs. The 53 adverse effects reported in humans were of a nature that could have been detected in all three species. Yet, toxicity in the rat was a poor indicator of toxicity in humans. And results in the dog, while a good deal better, still indicated only about half the adverse effects encountered in patients. What is also noteworthy is that in both the rat and the dog, toxic effects were found that so far have not been observed with the use of these drugs in human patients. Thus, species differences in response to drugs may not only present problems in predicting toxicity in humans, but may also lead to discarding potentially valuable drugs on the basis of adverse effects that will never appear (cf. pp. 257–260). However, the results of this same study showed that effects which occurred in *both* rats and dogs provided correct predictions of human toxicity in 68 per cent of the cases. Such evidence suggests that toxicity testing in lower animals should include several species and that the results of all animal studies must be viewed in terms of the potential benefit of the new drug.

Chemicals Not Intended for Use in Humans

Pesticides

Studies of toxicity are also required for chemical compounds that are used by humans to eliminate insects, rodents, fungi, weeds and other organisms designated as pests. The regulations governing these studies are embodied in the Federal Insecticide, Fungicide and Rodenticide Act of 1975 which is administered by the Pesticide Regulation Divison of the Environmental Protection Agency (EPA). The purpose of this act is to ensure that quality products are available to the public, and that when properly used, these products will provide consumers with effective pest control without hazard to health or significant adverse effects upon the environment. Under the law as amended, all economic poisons must be registered prior to shipment intrastate as well as interstate. This applies to newly developed pesticides and also to those marketed prior to enactment of the new law. Since registration is effective for a period of only five years from the time of registration, products will also require reregistration at a later date.

Before a registration can be obtained, however, the manufacturer must submit data to the Registration Division of the EPA showing that the product *when used as directed*: (1) is effective against the pests listed on the label; (2) will not present an unacceptable risk to humans, animals or crops; (3) will not damage the environment and (4) will not result in illegal residues on food or feed.

The development of a pesticide includes preliminary studies conducted in the laboratory, greenhouse and small field plots in order to determine its inherent effectiveness against specific pests. Once this is established, additional evidence of its effectiveness and usefulness is obtained through advanced large-scale laboratory and field testing procedures that closely approach actual commercial use and that employ commercial application equipment. All tests consider factors of degree and duration of pest control and crop yield and quality.

The pesticide hazard to humans and domestic animals is assessed following administration by mouth, by application to the skin and in some cases, by inhalation. Acute toxicity by the oral route is determined in one mammalian species, preferably the rat, whereas the rabbit is the animal of choice for acute dermal LD50 studies. When the physical and chemical nature of the pesticide under conditions of use result in a respirable product, acute toxicity by the inhalation route is also evaluated. Subacute and chronic toxicity studies are designed to determine the adverse effects of multiple or continuous exposure for various periods; these may include assessment of oncogenic, mutagenic, teratogenic, reproductive and metabolic effects. If the pesticide is intended for outdoor use, data on acute and subacute toxicity to avian species and acute toxicity to fish are obtained. And if the pesticide may be expected to move readily from the application site by means of drift, volatilization or leaching in soil, then studies on toxic effects to susceptible nontarget plants are also undertaken.

The regulations governing research and development of an economic poison — a chemical that is intended to be used by, but not in humans — are now as stringent as are those for drugs that are intended for use in humans (cf. Chap. 14). No pesticide is registered by the EPA unless it has been shown to be effective for its intended use and to be safe when used as directed. To promote effective and safe use of economic poisons, the law also requires that products be properly labeled. The label on each package of pesticides must include: intended product use; composition, both active and inactive ingredients; directions for use; pests to be controlled; crops, animals or sites to be treated; dosage, time and method of application; and warnings

Table 11-3. Criteria for Cataloging Pesticides by Toxicity, and Label
Requirements Established by Federal Insecticide, Fungicide and Rodenticide Act

	Acute Oral LD Value	Signal Word and Antidote Statements
Highly toxic	0-50 mg/kg	"DANGER" "POISON" Skull and crossbones Antidote statement "Call physician immediately" "Keep out of reach of children"
Moderately toxic	50-500 mg/kg	"WARNING" No antidote statement "Keep out of reach of children"
Low-order toxicity	500-5,000 mg/kg	"CAUTION" No antidote statement "Keep out of reach of children"
Comparatively free from danger	5,000+ mg/kg	No warning. caution or antidote statement Unqualified claims of safety are not acceptable "Keep out of reach of children"

United States Department of Agriculture, Agricultural Research Service, Pesticides Regulation Division. March 9, 1962. Interpretation Number 18 of the Regulations for the Enforcement of Federal Insecticide, Fungicide and Rodenticide Act. 7 C.F.R. 362, Int. 18, Rev. 2.

to protect user, consumer of treated foods, and beneficial plants and animals. Antidotes and first-aid instructions are required only on products that have been judged "highly toxic"; the labels on such products must also bear the skull and crossbones and the word POISON in red on a contrasting background (Table 11-3). The signal words on the label such as "Danger," "Warning" and "Caution" are set by law and reflect the degree of toxicity of the pesticide as determined in the studies of its acute toxicity (Table 11-3).

Toxic Substances Encountered in the Workplace
There are 3,000,000 known chemicals! Although no one is certain exactly how many are in use today, this mind-boggling number includes the more than 100,000 different industrial chemicals that are incorporated into more than 300,000 consumer products marketed in the United States. Since every chemical has an inherent potential for producing toxicity, the average individual is exposed to an enormous number and variety of chemical hazards as an integral part of our industrial society. It is the workers who manufacture or handle these chemicals, however, who are the population at greatest risk. In 1970 alone the estimated new cases of occupational diseases in the United States totaled 300,000, many of which were due to exposure to toxic substances in the workplace. In consideration of annual figures such as this, Congress passed the Occupational Safety and Health Act of 1970 "to assure so far as possible every working man and woman in the nation safe and healthful working conditions

and to preserve our human resources." Under the provisions of the act, the Occupational Safety and Health Administration (OSHA) was created within the Department of Labor to (1) encourage employers and employees to reduce hazards in the workplace and to implement new, or improve existing safety and health programs, and (2) develop mandatory job safety and health standards and enforce them effectively.

Even prior to the establishment of OSHA, national consensus standards had been developed to serve as guides in assessing the health hazard of industrial environments. Among the most widely used were the lists of permissible concentrations — the limits of atmospheric contamination that would be considered safe — for about five hundred substances promulgated by the nationally recognized American Conference of Governmental Industrial Hygienists. Some of the standards established by OSHA since 1970 are based on those of the Conference as well as on those recommended by the American National Standards Institute. However, the older standards adopted by OSHA and those newly established are now mandatory and enforceable by law.

Some common environmental contaminants and their permissible limits are listed in Table 11-4. The values are estimations based on human experience, measurable physiologic responses and toxicologic data derived from animal studies; they represent levels of contamination to which it is believed nearly all humans may be repeatedly exposed day after day without adverse effects. (These are, of course, subject to change whenever they are found inadequate.) The standards are expressed as parts of gas or vapor per million parts of air (ppm), or approximate milligrams of particulate per cubic meter of air (mg/m^3). For some chemicals, e.g., ammonia, the standard only sets limits for exposure in any eight-hour shift of a forty-hour workweek; for other contaminants, e.g., benzene, the standard also includes a ceiling value that cannot be exceeded except under the conditions given. For example, an employee may never be exposed to a concentration of benzene above 5 ppm but may be exposed to one at 5 ppm only for a maximum period of ten minutes during an eight-hour work shift. Such exposure should be compensated by exposures to concentrations less than 1 ppm so that the cumulative exposure for the entire eight-hour shift does not exceed a weighted average of 1 ppm.

The current convention of expressing the toxicity of airborne chemicals in terms of parts per million parts of air, or milligrams per cubic meter, and of chemicals given or taken by other routes in terms of LD50 values has little meaning for the average individual. Even though dangerous or lethal doses of toxic agents are only tentatively established for humans, there is a need to express the relative toxicity of different chemicals in simple, understandable language. The American Industrial Hygiene Association has suggested the six categories given in Table 11-5 as a way of translating oral toxicity data obtained in animals into terms that are more meaningful to the general population.

Despite the great strides made in reducing gross occupational hazards and making both employers and employees more aware of the dangers associated with exposure to injurious chemicals in the workplace, occupational toxicity continues to present major problems. And the most serious, pervasive and insidious of these is occupational cancer (Table 11-6), the full impact of which is just beginning to be felt. The pervasive

Table 11-4 Standards Promulgated by the Occupational Safety and Health Administration (OSHA) for Common Environmental Industrial Contaminants

Substance	8-Hour Time Weighted Average[a]		Acceptable Ceiling Concentration[b]		Acceptable Maximum Peak Above the Acceptable Ceiling Concentration[b] for an 8-Hour Shift	
	ppm	mg/m³	ppm	mg/m³	Concentration (ppm)	Maximum Duration (min)
Ammonia	50.	35.	...		...	...
Carbon monoxide	50.	55.	...		...	...
Carbon dioxide	5,000.	9,000.	...		...	...
Ethyl alcohol	1,000.	1,900.	...		...	...
Liquid petroleum gas	1,000.	1,800.	...		...	...
Ozone	0.1	0.2	...		...	...
Sulfur dioxide	5.	0.3	...		...	...
Benzene	1.	...	5		5	10
Carbon tetrachloride	10.	...	25		200	5 in any 4 hours
Hydrogen sulfide	...	...	20		50	10 once only
Mercury	...	...	...	0.1 mg/m³	...	...

[a] 8-hour time weighted averages: An employee's exposure in any eight-hour work shift of a forty-hour workweek, shall not exceed the eight-hour time weighted average given for that material in the table.

[b] Acceptable ceiling concentrations: An employee's exposure shall not exceed at any time during an eight-hour shift the acceptable ceiling concentration limit given for the material in the table, except for a time period, and up to a concentration not exceeding the maximum duration and concentration allowed in the column under "acceptable maximum peak above the acceptable ceiling concentration for an eight-hour shift."

Table 11-5. Interpreting Animal Toxicity Data

LD50 of Single Oral Dose in Animals (dose/kg)	Degree of Toxicity	Probable Lethal Dose for 70-kg Man
0.1 mg	Extremely toxic	A taste
1–50 mg	Highly toxic	A teaspoonful
50–500 mg	Moderately toxic	An ounce
0.5–5.0 g	Slightly toxic	A pint
5–15 g	Practically nontoxic	A quart
15 g	Relatively harmless	More than a quart

Source: From H. C. Hodge and J. H. Sterner, *Am. Ind. Hyg. Assoc. Q.* 10:93, 1949.

and insidious nature of this occupational hazard can be appreciated by citing some gloomy figures and examples. The World Health Organization estimates that between 75 and 85 per cent of all cancers have environmental causes. To what degree occupational exposure contributes to these causes or how many workers are exposed to chemicals that may be carcinogens is not known. The National Institute for Occupational Safety and Health (NIOSH), which recommends standards for OSHA's adoption, has obtained evidence to indicate that more than 10 per cent of the 14,000 substances on its Toxic Substance List may be carcinogenic; which of these are important in workplace exposures, again, has not been evaluated. However, the first new health standard under the 1970 Occupational Safety and Health Act drastically curtailed workers' exposure to asbestos, a known carcinogen.[3] And all of the sixteen new health standards OSHA has set since 1970 involve cancer-causing substances. One of these is vinyl chloride, the basic ingredient in making polyvinyl chloride (PVC) which is used in about 55 per cent of today's convenience plastic products. OSHA acted very swiftly in response to the discovery that vinyl chloride causes a rare form of cancer and is a potent killer. Within three months of the first reports of cancer, an emergency temporary standard of 50 ppm was set. Six months later, a permanent standard of 1 ppm was promulgated when animal studies indicated that the temporary limit was too high. The fact that vinyl chloride was once considered so free of hazard that it was used as a general anesthetic agent illustrates the difficulties encountered in assessing the real carcinogenic potential of a chemical.

The latent period between first exposure and the development of cancer is much longer for most carcinogens than it is for vinyl chloride — usually ten to fifty years. Since the annual rate at which new chemicals enter the workplace is about 7 per cent, how can workers be protected from potential but unknown occupational carcinogens? The only answer can be to treat all chemicals as potential hazards until proven otherwise and to regulate exposures through enforcement of universal standards.

[3]The eight-hour time-weighted average airborne concentrations of asbestos fibers to which any employee may be exposed shall not exceed 2 fibers, longer than 5 micrometers, per cubic centimeter of air.

Table 11-6. Carcinogens Commonly Encountered in the Workplace

Agent	Organ Affected	Occupation
Wood	Nasal cavity and sinuses	Woodworkers
Leather	Nasal cavity and sinuses, urinary bladder	Leather and shoe workers
Iron oxide	Lung, larynx	Iron ore miners; metal grinders and polishers; silver finishers; iron foundry workers
Nickel	Nasal sinuses, lung	Nickel smelters, mixers and roasters; electrolysis workers
Arsenic	Skin, lung, liver	Miners; smelters; insecticide makers and sprayers; tanners; chemical workers; oil refiners; vintners
Chromium	Nasal cavity and sinuses, lung, larynx	Chromium producers, processers and users; acetylene and aniline workers; bleachers; glass, pottery and linoleum workers; battery makers
Asbestos	Lung (pleural and peritoneal mesothelioma)	Miners; millers; textile, insulation and shipyard workers
Petroleum, petroleum coke, wax, creosote, anthracene, paraffin, shale and mineral oils	Nasal cavity, larynx, lung, skin, scrotum	Contact with lubricating, cooling, paraffin of wax fuel oils or coke; rubber fillers; retort workers; textile weavers; diesel jet testers
Vinyl chloride	Liver, brain	Plastic workers
Coal soot, coal tar and other products of coal combustion	Lung, larynx, skin, scrotum, urinary bladder	Gashouse workers, stokers and producers; asphalt, coal tar and pitch workers; coke oven workers; miners; still cleaners
Benzene	Bone marrow	Explosives, benzene or rubber cement workers; distillers; dye users; painters; shoemakers
Benzidine	Urinary bladder	Dyestuffs manufacturers and users; rubber workers (pressmen, filtermen, laborers); textile dyers; paint manufacturers

From The National Cancer Institute, National Institutes of Health, Public Health Service, Department of Health, Education, and Welfare.

Environmental Toxicity

The hazards associated with the many chemical substances that are constantly being developed, produced and used in industry can reach well beyond the workplace, endangering the residents of a particular community or even the population as a whole. Poisoning of its water, air, land and food is the steep price society is paying for technologic advance. The year 1970 marked the beginning, however, of a comprehensive program and concerted effort to deal with the problems of widespread pollution of the biosphere when Congress established the United States Environmental Protection Agency (EPA). The creation of the EPA ended the piecemeal approach to our nation's environmental problems and filled the need for a single, strong agency to mount an integrated, coordinated attack on pollution.

The EPA is, first and foremost, a regulatory agency, having responsibilities for establishing and enforcing environmental standards. The process of setting standards, however, begins with a scientific research and monitoring program, since the nature of pollutants must be known before the environment can be treated. The EPA, therefore, carries out a diversified research program at the fifteen laboratories of its Office of Research and Development and also gathers information from scientific and technical advisory committees, from industry and from the scientific community as a whole. The aim is to obtain the basic knowledge needed to safeguard public health and to balance the benefits of a specific product against the hazards it might pose for the environment. Thus studies are designed to determine not only what a specific level of a specific pollutant does to human beings, but also what it does to crops and other vegetation; to domestic animals and wildlife; to marine plant and animal life; to concrete, steel and other building materials; to painted surfaces; and to fabrics.

Whereas research constitutes the essential scientific foundation for action to improve environmental quality, the EPA's authority to enforce the standards established subsequent to research is derived from the various laws passed by Congress since 1970. These include (1) the Clean Air Act as amended in 1974; (2) the Federal Water Pollution Control Act as amended in 1972; (3) the Marine Protection, Research and Sanctuaries Act of 1972, known as the "Ocean Dumping Act"; (4) the Safe Drinking Water Act of 1974; (5) the Federal Insecticide, Fungicide and Rodenticide Act of 1975; and (6) the Toxic Substances Control Act (TSCA) of 1976. The last of these is intended to provide additional regulatory authorities to deal with all hazardous chemicals that might lead to health and environmental damage. The TSCA mandates the EPA to obtain *from industry* data on the production, use and health effects of chemicals and to require testing of chemicals suspected of being harmful. If a new or existing chemical is determined to pose significant environmental or health hazards, its use may be banned or otherwise regulated by the EPA. Many cancer authorities believe that the TSCA will be a major step in controlling occupational cancer.

Although only a few years have elapsed since enactment of the laws creating the EPA and giving it the authority to implement and enforce regulations and standards, there have been significant areas of improvement in the quality of our environment. For example, in 1971 ambient (outside) air quality standards for five major air pollutants were set by EPA under the Clean Air Act[4]. As a result of this action, the national emission levels of four of the five major air pollutants declined between the years 1970 and 1975: total suspended particulates were reduced 33 per cent; sulfur dioxide, 4 per cent; hydrocarbons, 9 per cent; and carbon monoxide, 15 per cent from the 1970 level.

The changes in air quality which resulted from emission control plans indicate that fewer Americans are being exposed to unhealthy levels of air pollution. But since these are annual averages of air quality nationwide, these encouraging downward trends do not reflect conditions in a local area or short-term changes in degree of air pollution. The continuous monitoring and reporting of levels of air pollution by regional or local control stations are designed, however, to advise their respective communities of any possible adverse health effects resulting from extant air pollution. The Pollutants Standards Index (PSI) was developed by the Council on Environmental Quality and the EPA to achieve consistent and reliable reporting of the daily health effects associated with the quality of the air we breathe. The PSI values for five major pollutants are shown in Table 11-7. The data used to establish the descriptive categories ("good" through "hazardous") for varying degrees of air pollution are the criteria documents[5] used to set the National Air Quality Standards, the Federal Episode Criteria and Significant Harm levels. The PSI values can be used to report the daily status of air pollution in a local area in much the same way as the "burning index" is used to report the danger of forest fires. The guidelines for using the PSI advise reporting any index value that exceeds 100 in order to "alert" the public that the standard has been exceeded. For example, the air quality index for a particular day might be reported in a typical news broadcast as: "The PSI for today is 150, which falls into the 'unhealthful' category. The pollutant causing this condition is sulfur dioxide. Persons with existing heart or respiratory ailments should reduce physical exertion and outdoor activities. The forecast calls for no immediate change in conditions."

INCIDENCE OF POISONING

Awareness has been growing throughout the world of the increasing incidence of acute poisoning. It is estimated that in the United States alone the number of non-fatal poisonings exceeds one and a half million a year, although only about one-tenth of this figure is actually reported and tabulated. Chemicals are, however, documented as the direct cause of death in at least 10,000 persons annually. More than half of these chemically induced fatalities are the result of the use of chemical agents for suicidal purposes (about half of these by carbon monoxide, illuminating gas[6] and

[4] A sixth air quality standard, that for photochemical oxidants (ozone), was also set but data for this pollutant has been recorded for too short a time to be able to assess the effects of the regulations. New standards for lead will take effect in 1978.

[5] Air quality criteria are expressions of the scientific data of the relationships between various concentrations, averaged over a suitable time period, of pollutants in the atmosphere and their adverse effects upon public health and the environment.

[6] Gas manufactured from coal, still used in some areas of the United States and in many countries where natural gas is unavailable.

Table 11-7. Pollutants Standards Index for Reporting Possible Adverse Health Effects Resulting from Air Pollution

Index Value	Air Quality Level and Health Effect Descriptor	Pollutant Levels (mg/m³)					General Health Effects	Cautionary Statements
		Total Suspended Particulates (24 hour)	Sulfur Dioxide (24 hour)	Carbon Monoxide (8 hour) (mg/m³)	Oxidants (1 hour)	Nitrogen Dioxide (1 hour)		
500	Significant harm HAZARDOUS	1000	2,620	57.5	1,200	3,750	Premature death of ill and elderly; healthy people will experience adverse symptoms that affect their normal activity	All persons should remain indoors, keeping windows and doors closed. All persons should minimize physical exertion and avoid traffic
400	Emergency HAZARDOUS	875	2,100	46.0	1,000	3,000	Premature onset of certain diseases in addition to significant aggravation of symptoms and decreased exercise tolerance in healthy persons	The elderly and persons with existing diseases should stay indoors and avoid physical exertion. General population should avoid outdoor activity
300	Warning VERY UNHEALTHFUL	625	1,600	34.0	800	2,260	Significant aggravation of symptoms and decreased exercise tolerance in persons with heart or lung disease, with widespread symptoms in the healthy population	The elderly and persons with existing heart or lung disease should stay indoors and reduce physical activity

200	Alert	375	800	17.0	400	1,130	Persons with existing heart or respiratory ailments should reduce physical exertion and outdoor activity
	UNHEALTHFUL						
100	National Ambient Air Quality Standards	260	365	10.0	160		Mild aggravation of symptoms in susceptible persons with irritation symptoms in the healthy population
	MODERATE						
50	50% of National Ambient Air Quality Standards	75	80	5.0	80		
	GOOD						

From *EPA Journal.* 2:15, 1976.

automobile exhaust gases). Yet, even when we exclude the cases of poisoning by intentional self-administration, accidental poisoning due to therapeutic agents and other chemicals is still a major problem. The annual number of deaths caused by accidental exposure to carbon monoxide and other noxious gases (between 1,400 and 1,500) has remained relatively constant over the last twenty-five years. But the death toll due to ingestion of solids and liquids has more than doubled in the same period. And the percentage of these deaths attributable to poisoning by medicinal agents has risen from about 50 per cent to over 68 per cent (Fig. 11-1). The number of deaths due to accidental poisoning by therapeutic agents is not surprising, however, since more than half of all the reported poisonings are associated with this category of chemicals. Until a few years ago, one group of drugs — the barbiturates — accounted for more than one-third of all the fatalities caused by medicinal agents. Since 1970 the number of fatal poisonings with barbiturates has declined, but this has been offset by a continuing increase in poisoning by other types of sedatives, hypnotics and tranquilizers. The fashion in poisoning by nontherapeutic agents has also changed, as evidenced by the increase in deaths attributable to direct overdosage with alcohol. From 1961 to 1967, there was a sharp decline in the number of deaths due to ingested alcohol, but since then this number has more than doubled; the reasons for this are not apparent from the statistics available.

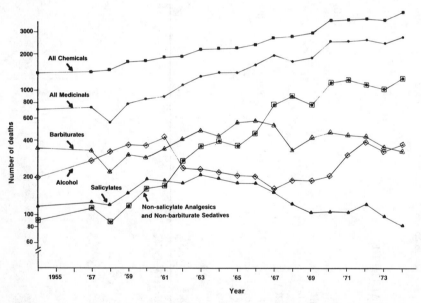

FIGURE 11-1. Deaths due to accidental poisoning by solid and liquid substances in all age groups, 1954–1974. Vital statistics are not available for years beyond 1974. (Data compiled from Vital Statistics — Special Reports, National Summaries. *Washington, D.C.: National Office of Vital Statistics, Years indicated. U.S. Department of Health, Education, and Welfare.)*

Table 11-8. Reports of Accidental Ingestions of Poisons in 1974 Classified by Age

Age (yr.)	Medicinals	All Substances
Under 1	482	2,109
1	8,285	29,106
2	16,431	36,577
3	10,476	19,125
4	3,915	7,658
5–9	2,837	7,163
10–14	2,371	4,621
15–24	12,939	17,395
25–44	10,126	13,084
45–64	2,666	3,785
>64	542	966
Unknown	6,991	19,968
Total for all ages	78,061	161,557

Source: Individual poison reports submitted to the National Clearinghouse for Poison Control Centers in 1974 by 479 centers in 45 states.

One of the most distressing sets of statistics on accidental poisoning is that for children under 5 years of age (Table 11-8). In 1965, accidental ingestion of potentially harmful chemicals by these young individuals accounted for 63,352, or 88.4 per cent, of all the reported cases. Fortunately, the mortality was proportionately much lower, since the 379 children under age 5 who died by poisoning that year represented only 18 per cent of the total deaths from poisons. In the period between 1965 and 1970 there was an encouraging decrease in the percentage of both non-fatal and fatal poisonings in children under 5 years of age (Fig. 11-2). Although the total number of cases of poisonings in the whole population rose 59 per cent in this five-year period, there was only a 12 per cent rise in the incidence of poisoning among the under-age-5 group. As the figures in Table 11-8 indicate, however, this decline in rate of poisoning was short-lived. Between 1970 and 1974, there was an increase of 54 per cent in the number of recorded poisonings by ingestion of chemical agents in children under 5 years of age. What is noteworthy and more reassuring is that this increased incidence of childhood poisoning was not paralleled by an increase in mortality. On the contrary, there has been a most gratifying decline recently in both the death rate and actual number of deaths due to accidental poisoning of the very young. In 1974, there were only 135 deaths from accidental poisoning among children under 5 years of age. This number is still tragically high, but it represents a 64 per cent drop in mortality within this age group over a nine-year period while the number of fatal poisonings for the entire population was steadily increasing.

This promising downward trend in deaths from accidental poisoning among children under 5 years of age can be accounted for largely by the sharp decline in the number of fatalities due to ingestion of medicines. Over the last decade or so, medicinal agents have been responsible for one-half to two-thirds of all deaths attributable to accidental ingestion of chemicals by individuals in the under-5-year age group (see Fig. 11-2). And, as can be clearly seen in Figure 11-2, the decline in

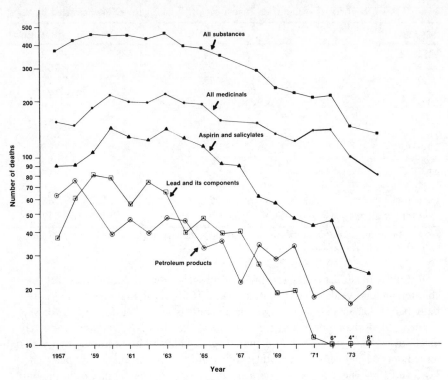

FIGURE 11-2. Deaths due to accidental poisoning by solid and liquid substances in children under 5 years of age, 1954–1974. Vital statistics are not available for years beyond 1974. (Data compiled from Vital Statistics – Special Reports, National Summaries. *Washington, D.C.: National Office of Vital Statistics, Years indicated. U.S. Department of Health, Education, and Welfare.)*

deaths due to medicinals is associated with a dramatic drop in the number of fatal poisonings due to aspirin – the number-one killer drug and poisoner in the very young (Table 11-9). From 1965 to 1974 there has been a decrease in fatal poisoning of 63 per cent for all medicines and 83 per cent for aspirin and its congeners.

The decrease in mortality due to poisoning by aspirin is a reflection of the lowered incidence of its ingestion among children under 5 years of age. In 1970 the percentage of poisoning by aspirin – 13.6 – was two-thirds of that in 1969. Compared to 1965, when aspirin ingestion represented 25.8 per cent of all reports of poisoning for this group, the 1970 percentage dropped by about one-half. A decrease in poisoning by baby aspirin (1 ¼ grains) was mainly responsible for the fall. The credit for this successful reduction in the ingestion of aspirin by children can be shared by (1) the pharmaceutical industry, which voluntarily set a limit of 36 baby aspirin tablets to a bottle; (2) the governmental and private organizations that campaigned intensively to make the public aware of the problem; and (3) the firms that instituted safety packaging on their own accord during 1970. Safety packaging for aspirin as well as

Table 11-9. Accidental Ingestion in 1974 by Type
of Substance among Children Under 5 Years of Age and in All Ages

Type of Substance	Under 5 Years		Total Cases All Ages	
	No.	%	No.	%
Medicines[a]	45,625	41.6	78,061	48.3
Internal	35,508	32.4	67,041	41.5
Aspirin	5,861	5.4	7,091	4.4
Other	29,647	27.0	59,950	39.1
External	10,117	9.2	11,020	6.8
Cleaning & polishing agents	17,871	16.3	20,571	12.7
Petroleum products	4,459	4.1	6,969	4.3
Cosmetics	10,968	10.0	10,610	6.6
Pesticides	6,193	5.6	9,678	6.0
Gases & vapors	131	0.1	1,024	1.0
Plants	8,245	7.5	11,097	6.9
Turpentine, paints, etc.	6,286	5.7	7,383	4.6
Miscellaneous	9,382	8.6	13,686	8.4
Not specified	585	0.5	1,878	1.2
Total	109,745	100.0	161,557	100.0

[a]Total of both internal and external medicines.

Source: Individual case reports submitted to the National Clearinghouse for Poison Control Centers in 1974 by 479 centers in 45 states.

other medicines became law in 1970 with the passage of the Poison Prevention Packaging Act, but the first safety packaging regulations only became effective in the latter part of 1972. That these packaging precautions are a powerful deterrent to poisoning by medicinals among children under 5 years of age is clearly evidenced by the mortality data for 1972 and 1974. Between 1972 and 1974 there was a 38 per cent drop in the number of deaths from accidental poisoning by all medicinals and an even more dramatic decline of 57 per cent for those attributable to aspirin. The incidence of nonfatal poisoning also appears to be declining.

The steady decline since 1963 in the number of fatal poisonings in very young children certainly must also be partly related to the widespread growth of poison control centers and the consequent increased accessibility of information about poisons. The concern about poisoning in young children and the need for information about the myriad chemicals which are potential poisons led to the inception of the first such center in Chicago in 1953. What began as a cooperative and integrated activity in one community quickly spread throughout the United States and Canada and to many other countries. There are at present almost six hundred poison control centers in the United States, coordinated and served by the Food and Drug Administration's National Clearinghouse for Poison Control in Washington, D.C.

Each poison control center is provided with an index, filed for rapid retrieval, which contains information on composition, toxicity, symptoms of poisoning and recommended treatment for most of the products sold and distributed within the

United States. In addition to therapeutic agents for human and veterinary use, the file contains references to household products, toiletries, cosmetics, pesticides, industrial chemicals, plants and fungi. Commercial firms whose products are included have cooperated willingly in providing the necessary data, despite the fact that trade secrets have had to be divulged. The centers are open to telephone inquiries 24 hours a day and provide information to anyone seeking help. Instant treatment information is also available at nine large regional centers through an electronic poison information network. Poison centers in Seattle, Boston, Detroit, Kansas City, Albuquerque, Atlanta, Baltimore, Salt Lake City and New Orleans are linked to a computer at the National Clearinghouse in Washington, D.C. At present the computer contains information on more than 10,000 household substances, and the FDA plans to expand the file to include 50,000 products. The National Clearinghouse also serves as a main center for the collection of data on all cases of poisoning reported at the cooperating centers. The data in Figures 11-1 and 11-2 and in Tables 11-8 and 11-9 were obtained from publications of the National Clearinghouse.

TREATMENT OF TOXICITY

From the earliest times to the not too distant past, the treatment of acute poisoning was based on the illusion that for each poison there was a specific antidote. But the physical law which states that for every action there is an equal and opposite reaction can be applied toxicologically in few instances. Only when the mechanism of action of a poison has been elucidated is it possible to develop effective measures to specifically antagonize the action of the offending agent. And this has been achieved for only a minority of the known poisons; a specific antidote is available in less than 2 per cent of all cases of poisoning. For the most part, treatment consists in applying basic pharmacologic principles to deal with the signs and symptoms of poisoning as they arise. Treatment of poisoning by either specific or nonspecific means is referred to as *antidotal therapy*. Any chemical agent used to counteract the action of the poison is termed an *antidote*.

The General Principles of Antidotal Treatment

It is axiomatic that prevention of poisoning is preferable to treatment and cure. But once poisoning has occurred, all antidotal treatment, both specific and nonspecific, is aimed at lessening the magnitude of the effect(s) produced by the chemical-biologic interaction. The intensity of any drug effect, whether toxic or salutary, is a function of the concentration of drug at the site where the action-effects sequence is initiated. And the concentration of drug at a site of action is a function both of dose — the quantity administered — and of time — the time involved in getting a drug to and from its site of action. Provided the effect is reversible, it will be produced only when and as long as there is an effective concentration of drug at the site. It follows that treatment of poisoning must be directed toward reducing the effective concentration at the site where the chemical interaction occurs. Thus to formulate the general principles of antidotal treatment, we need only apply what we already know about the relationship between time and drug effect.

Let us consider the case of a poison introduced into the body by the oral route at a dose sufficient to produce toxic but not lethal effects. The solid curve in Figure 11-3 represents the time course of action of such a poison. This curve is identical to that of Figure 8-2, except that we now consider E the minimum level of measurable toxic effect. The duration of the toxic effect extends from T_1 to T_3, and the intensity of the effect at any point in time is measured by the height of the curve above E. The faster the rate of absorption and distribution, the sooner the onset of toxic effects. The faster the rate of absorption relative to elimination, the sooner the maximum drug concentration is attained at a site of action and the greater is the intensity of effect. Or, from the standpoint of elimination, the slower the rate of elimination relative to absorption, the higher the maximum drug concentration (and the intensity of effect) and the longer the duration of action. Since the aim of antidotal treatment is to reduce the intensity and duration of the toxic effect (to decrease the area under the curve above E), there are two obvious ways in which this goal can be attained.

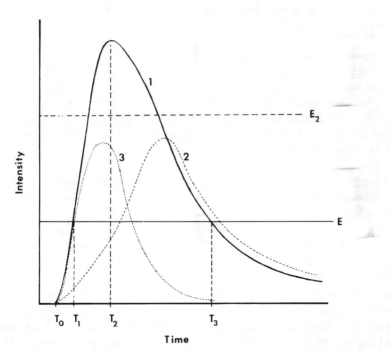

FIGURE 11-3. Intensity of toxicity as a function of time. Exposure to drug at time 0 (T_0). (T_0 to T_1 = time for onset of toxic effect; T_0 to T_2 = time to peak toxic effect; E = minimal level of measurable toxic response; T_1 to T_3 = duration of action; Curve 1 = time course of toxicity; Curve 2 = time course of toxicity when antidotal treatment decreases rate of absorption of toxic agent; Curve 3 = time course of toxicity when antidotal treatment increases rate of elimination of toxic agent; E_2 = minimal level of measurable toxic response when antidotal treatment raises threshold of toxicity.)

Either the rate of access of the drug to its site of action can be slowed (Curve 2), or its rate of removal from the body can be increased (Curve 3). By either procedure, the rate of elimination becomes faster *relative* to absorption and distribution; the maximum level of drug in the body and the intensity of effect are reduced. In practice, a reduction in the rate of access of drug to an effector site is achieved by removing the unabsorbed portion of the poison from the site of entry into the body, preventing further absorption or preventing distribution of the absorbed poison to its site of action. The rate of elimination is enhanced by mechanically or chemically increasing the rate of excretion, or by combining the poison with another chemical to form a less toxic, stable complex.

There is still a third procedure by which the aim of antidotal therapy can be achieved, and that is to elevate the minimal or threshold concentration at which the toxic effect occurs (E_2). This is accomplished either by administering a physiologic or pharmacologic antagonist or by employing mechanical procedures which compensate for the function(s) impaired by the poison. Now let us briefly examine the ways in which these principles are applied in both the nonspecific and the specific treatment of poisoning.

Nonspecific Therapy

The treatment of acute poisoning is always an emergency, but the judicious and rational use of therapeutic procedures is more effective than heroic measures which may do more damage than the poison itself. The Committee on Toxicology of the American Medical Association has published some excellent recommendations for first-aid measures to be used in poisoning emergencies, and these are presented in their entirety in Table 11-10.

The essentials of the nonspecific treatment of poisoning include (1) removal of the poison; (2) its identification; (3) administration of a suitable antidote; (4) promotion of elimination of the poison; and (5) supportive treatment of the patient. The order in which these actions are taken depends on the general condition of the victim, on the route of administration of the poison and on the poison itself.

The maintenance of respiration and circulation takes precedence over all other considerations. In essence, this is an application of the third procedure for accomplishing the goal of antidotal therapy. The maintenance of respiration by mechanical means or the administration of therapeutic agents to support the circulation are procedures for elevating the threshold of toxicity. The poison continues to exert its effect at its site of action, but the effect is overcome by measures which compensate for the physiologic functions impaired by the offending agent. There is also need to identify the poison as soon as possible so that rational and specific treatment may be instituted promptly. The immediate measures taken to prevent or retard absorption into the circulation depend on the route of drug entry into the body and on the general class of agent involved in the poisoning (Table 11-10). Copious washing with water is appropriate for the removal of any poison from the external surface of the body. But the procedures employed to remove unabsorbed poison from the gastrointestinal tract are dictated by the patient's condition and the type of poison ingested.

Vomiting is never induced as a means of removing ingested poisons in an unconscious patient or when the toxic agent is a petroleum product or a corrosive substance. There is too much danger of inhaling the poison into the lungs or of perforating a corroded esophagus or stomach. Gastric lavage may be used in the comatose patient, however, to remove a noncorrosive agent when appropriate precautions are taken to avoid the possibility of asphyxiation by inhalation of the stomach contents.

In the conscious patient, both gastric lavage and emetics can be employed to remove ingested poisons. Vomiting can be induced by the parenteral injection of apomorphine or by oral administration of syrup of ipecac. Apomorphine acts on the vomiting center of the brain and induces emesis within a few minutes after administration. Since it is given systemically, it is not eliminated with the vomitus and, therefore, has a great potential for exerting some of its other pharmacologic effects. Apomorphine is a derivative of morphine and has central nervous system depressant activity similar to that of its parent compound; its use and sale are no longer regulated in the same way as morphine (see Glossary under **Controlled Substances Act**), but a prescription is needed for its purchase. In contrast, ipecac induces emesis primarily by a direct action on the gastric mucosa and is eliminated with the vomitus, but takes 15 to 30 minutes to act. Yet despite this delayed onset of action, in the actual poisoning situation the removal of poison from the gastrointestinal tract can be accomplished with ipecac more quickly than with apomorphine. For ipecac can be readily available for immediate use in the home, where most poisonings occur; it can be purchased over the counter without prescription (in 1 fluid ounce quantities). With ipecac there need be no delay occasioned by getting the patient to a physician or hospital before administering an emetic. Since ipecac has a long shelf life, pediatric societies now advocate that it be kept on hand in the home in case of accidental poisoning in children. Recent studies indicate that syrup of ipecac is also preferable to gastric lavage as antidotal treatment in conscious patients: the emetic is more efficient in removing material from the gastrointestinal tract, and its use is less hazardous.

Once actual removal of an ingested poison has been attempted or accomplished, further absorption from the gastrointestinal tract may be retarded with large quantities of activated charcoal. If given within an hour of ingestion of a poison, it will effectively absorb a variety of agents, such as aspirin, chlorpheniramine (an antihistaminic agent), pentobarbital, propoxyphene (Darvon), strychnine, morphine, atropine, mercury and arsenic. The so-called universal antidote, a mixture of tannic acid, magnesium oxide and activated charcoal, is no longer recommended, since it is less effective than charcoal alone. Cathartics may also be used at times to hasten transit of the poison through the bowel, thus decreasing the opportunity for absorption of any material not removed by emesis.

In nonspecific antidotal therapy, an increase in the rate of drug elimination is usually the result of increasing the rate of urinary excretion of the poison. This is achieved by administering large amounts of water and a suitable diuretic agent in order to produce a copious flow of urine. The larger quantities of fluid entering the renal tubules may provide a less favorable concentration gradient for reabsorption of the poison and, in turn, the lower drug concentration may protect the renal tissue

Table 11-10.   First-aid Measures for Poisoning

The following recommendations on first-aid measures for poisoning have been adopted by the Committee on Toxicology of the American Medical Association. These recommendations are made in response to numerous requests to the American Medical Association for general instructions for poisoning emergencies. They are intended for use in educating the public in what to do when poisoning occurs.

Emergency telephone numbers:

Physician _____   Fire Dept. _____
Hospital _____ (resuscitator)
Pharmacist _____   Police _____
Rescue Squads _____

The aim of first-aid measures is to help prevent absorption of the poison. SPEED is essential. First-aid measures must be started at once. If possible, one person should begin treatment while another calls a physician. When this is not possible, the nature of the poison will determine whether to call a physician first or begin first-aid measures and then notify a physician. Save a poison container and material itself if any remain. If the poison is not known, save a sample of the vomitus.

Measures to Be Taken before Arrival of Physician

I. SWALLOWED POISONS

Many products used in and around the home, although not labeled "Poison," may be dangerous if taken internally. For example, some medications which are beneficial when used correctly may endanger life if used improperly or in excessive amounts.

In all cases, except those indicated below, REMOVE POISON FROM PATIENT'S STOMACH IMMEDIATELY by inducing vomiting. This cannot be overemphasized, for it is the essence of the treatment and is often a life saving procedure. Prevent chilling by wrapping patient in blankets if necessary. Do not give alcohol in any form.

A. Do not induce vomiting if:
1. Patient is in coma or unconscious.
2. Patient is in convulsions.
3. Patient has swallowed petroleum products (kerosene, gasoline, lighter fluid).
4. Patient has swallowed a corrosive poison (symptoms: severe pain, burning sensation in mouth and throat, vomiting).

CALL PHYSICIAN IMMEDIATELY.

(a) Acid and acid-like corrosives: sodium acid sulfate (toilet bowl cleaners), acetic acid (glacial), sulfuric acid, nitric acid, oxalic acid, hydrofluoric acid (rust removers), iodine, silver nitrate (styptic pencil).

(b) Alkali corrosives: sodium hydroxide (lye; drain cleaners), sodium carbonate (washing soda), ammonia water, sodium hypochlorite (household bleach).

If the patient can swallow after ingesting a corrosive poison, the following substances (and amounts) may be given:

For acids: milk, water, or milk of magnesia (1 tablespoon to 1 cup of water). For alkalies: milk, water, any fruit juice, or vinegar.

For patient 1–5 years old: 1 to 2 cups.
For patient 5 years or older: up to 1 quart.

B. Induce vomiting when noncorrosive substances have been swallowed:
1. Give milk or water (for patient 1–5 years old, 1 to 2 cups; for patient over 5 years, up to 1 quart).

330

2. Induce vomiting by placing the blunt end of a spoon or your finger at the back of the patient's throat, or by use of this emetic: 2 tablespoons of salt in a glass of warm water. When retching and vomiting begin, place patient face down with head lower than hips. This prevents vomitus from entering the lungs and causing further damage.

II. INHALED POISONS
1. Carry patient (do not let him walk) to fresh air immediately.
2. Open all doors and windows.
3. Loosen all tight clothing.
4. Apply artificial respiration if breathing has stopped or is irregular.
5. Prevent chilling (wrap patient in blankets).
6. Keep patient as quiet as possible.
7. If patient is convulsing, keep him in bed in a semidark room; avoid jarring or noise.
8. Do not give alcohol in any form.

III. SKIN CONTAMINATION
1. Drench skin with water (shower, hose, faucet).
2. Apply stream of water on skin while removing clothing.
3. Cleanse skin thoroughly with water; rapidity in washing is most important in reducing extent of injury.

IV. EYE CONTAMINATION
1. Hold eyelids open, wash eyes with gentle stream of running water immediately. Delay of a few seconds greatly increases extent of injury.
2. Continue washing until physician arrives.
3. Do not use chemicals; they may increase extent of injury.

V. INJECTED POISONS
(scorpion and snake bites)

1. Make patient lie down as soon as possible.
2. Do not give alcohol in any form.
3. Apply tourniquet above injection site (e.g., between arm or leg and heart). The pulse in vessels below the tourniquet should not disappear, nor should the tourniquet produce a throbbing sensation. Tourniquet should be loosened for 1 minute every 15 minutes.
4. Apply ice-pack to the site of the bite.
5. Carry patient to physician or hospital; DO NOT LET HIM WALK.

VI. CHEMICAL BURNS
1. Wash with large quantities of running water (except those burns caused by phosphorus).
2. Immediately cover with loosely applied clean cloth.
3. Avoid use of ointments, greases, powders and other drugs in first-aid treatment of burns.
4. Treat shock by keeping patient flat, keeping him warm, and reassuring him until arrival of physician.

Measures to Prevent Poisoning Accidents

A. Keep all drugs, poisonous substances and household chemicals out of the reach of children.
B. Do not store nonedible products on shelves used for storing food.
C. Keep all poisonous substances in their original containers; do not transfer to unlabeled containers.
D. When medicines are discarded, destroy them. Do not throw them where they might be reached by children or pets.
E. When giving flavored and/or brightly colored medicine to children, always refer to it as medicine – never as candy.
F. Do not take or give medicine in the dark.
G. READ LABELS before using chemical products.

Source: From Council on Drugs, *J.A.M.A.* 165:686, 1957.

from damage by the poison. When the poison is known to be a weak organic electrolyte, the urinary pH may be appropriately adjusted to favor ionization of the drug and, thereby, further inhibit reabsorption from the tubular urine (cf. pp. 133–134). Alkalinization of the urine by the administration of agents such as sodium bicarbonate and sodium lactate has been successfully used to treat poisoning by barbiturates. The urinary excretion of basic compounds, such as amphetamine, has been enhanced by acidification of the urine with ascorbic acid (vitamin C) given intravenously or arginine monohydrochloride given orally.

If a patient does not respond to forced diuresis or alteration in urinary pH, drug removal may be hastened by the use of chemical-mechanical dialyzing devices. The artificial kidney has been used successfully to remove salicylates, barbiturates and other drugs when the patient's condition was not correctable by more conventional means. Peritoneal dialysis may also prove effective in removing alcohols, such as methanol, and those drugs which are weak electrolytes. Although less efficient than the artificial kidney, it involves a much simpler procedure — normally, only the irrigation of the peritoneal cavity with an isotonic fluid.

Specific Therapy
Specific therapy for poisoning differs from nonspecific treatment only with regard to the availability of a specific antidote to counteract the toxic effect of a particular agent or group of agents. All the other measures used in the nonspecific treatment may still be required, even though a specific antidote is available. A specific antidote opposes the toxic effect(s) of another agent by acting as a chemical, pharmacologic or biochemical antagonist.

Prevention of Absorption or Distribution to Site of Action
The antidotes used to prevent further absorption of a toxic agent act locally as chemical antagonists (Table 11-11). They neutralize the offending agent either by a chemical reaction that leads to the formation of a new, harmless or nonabsorbable compound, or by complexing or binding the toxic agent. The use of weak bases, such as magnesium oxide or milk of magnesia, to neutralize ingested acids, or of weak acids like vinegar or lemon juice to neutralize alkalis, are examples of such chemical reactions. Detoxification by the mechanism of complex formation is exemplified by the use of deferoxamine in poisoning by therapeutic preparations of iron. This is an all-too-frequent occurrence in children. In 1975, 394 children under 5 years of age were poisoned following the ingestion of ferrous sulfate and other iron-containing tablets intended for adults being treated for iron-deficiency anemias. The oral administration of an antidotal agent, such as deferoxamine, can prevent the absorption of iron by the formation of a nonabsorbable complex which is eventually excreted in the feces.

The antidotal treatment of cyanide poisoning is an example of how chemical antagonism can prevent a poison from gaining access to its site of action. Once cyanide has combined with intracellular respiratory enzymes, no means are available to remove it from the enzyme protein. Thus, therapy is directed toward removing the cyanide *before* it can reach cells. The combination of cyanide with methemoglobin to form

Table 11-11. Toxic Agents, Specific Antidotes and Mechanisms of Antidotal Action

Toxic Agent	Specific Antidote	Mechanism of Action
Prevention of Absorption		
Iron	Sodium bicarbonate	Formation of relatively insoluble ferrous carbonate
Iron	Deferoxamine	Formation of nonabsorbable complex
Silver nitrate	Sodium chloride	Formation of insoluble silver chloride
Quinine, strychnine and nicotine	Potassium permanganate	Oxidation of poison
Fluoride ion	Calcium salt (milk, calcium lactate)	Formation of insoluble calcium fluoride
Prevention of Distribution to Site of Action		
Heparin	Protamine	Formation of complex that is removed by urinary excretion
Methanol	Ethanol	Prevents formation of poisonous metabolite
Enhancement of Rate of Elimination		
Bromide ion	Chloride ion	Accelerates excretion in urine
Strontium, radium	Calcium salts	Accelerates excretion in urine
Lead, nickel, cobalt and copper	Calcium disodium edetate (EDTA)	Removes metals from tissue binding sites by complex formation
Mercury, arsenic, gold and antimony	Dimercaprol (BAL)	
Copper	Penicillamine	Forms complex with toxin
Botulinus toxin and other toxins	Botulinus antitoxin and other antitoxins	
Organic phosphate insecticides (Parathion)	Pralidoxime	Removes poison from enzyme cholinesterase
Elevation of Threshold of Toxicity		
Morphine and other narcotic analgesics	Naloxone and related antagonists	Pharmacologic antagonism at site where toxic action is produced
Carbon monoxide	Oxygen	
Dicumarol	Vitamin K	
Organic phosphate insecticides	Atropine	

a nontoxic complex achieves this end. However, there is usually insufficient pre-formed methemoglobin in normal individuals to bind much cyanide. So to make sufficient methemoglobin available for this reaction, a nitrite, such as sodium nitrite, is administered. Methemoglobinemia itself does not present serious problems until more than half the available hemoglobin is converted to the non-oxygen-carrying form. Yet conversion of about 50 per cent of hemoglobin yields enough methemo-globin to combine with more than a fatal dose of cyanide. Cyanide may also be converted to the harmless thiocyanate ion by an enzyme that occurs normally in mammals. The reaction requires sulfate ion, however, and this is usually in short supply. When sulfate is supplied by the administration of thiosulfate, cyanide is rapidly biotransformed to the innocuous sulfur derivative. Thus the treatment of cyanide poisoning involves two mechanisms: (1) complexing with methemoglobin, whose formation is induced by nitrite; and (2) biotransformation to the nontoxic thiocyanate, which is accelerated by thiosulfate.

In contrast to cyanide poisoning, in which part of the treatment depends on the acceleration of its biotransformation, the specific antidotal treatment for methanol poisoning involves the inhibition of its biotransformation. Methyl alcohol is con-verted to formaldehyde and formic acid (cf. p. 156), both of which severely inhibit essential metabolic processes. The actions of these metabolites are potentially more toxic than the central nervous system depressant activity of the parent compound. The same enzyme that oxidizes methanol is responsible for the metabolism of ethanol, but conversion of the latter gives rise to harmless metabolites and proceeds at a rate five times faster than the corresponding reaction with methanol. This difference pro-vides the basis for the treatment of methanol intoxication. The administration of ethanol slows the rate of methanol biotransformation by competing for the oxidative enzyme, thereby slowing the rate of accumulation of the toxic metabolites of methanol.

Enhancement of Rate of Elimination

The termination of the action of a toxic agent may be hastened by specific antidotes in two ways: (1) by increasing the rate of the poison's excretion in the urine, or (2) by removing the poison from its site of action through complex formation. The treatment of bromide intoxication with sodium chloride is an example of the first mechanism. We have already discussed the insidious way in which bromide ion accu-mulates in the body; its rate of excretion is slow because it is handled by the kidney in much the same way as chloride ion (cf. p. 126). When chloride is administered in excess of the normal daily intake, the excess is excreted in the urine in order to maintain homeostasis. Increasing the amount of chloride in the tubular urine decreases the amount of bromide present relative to chloride, i.e., bromide now repre-sents a smaller fraction of the total chloride plus bromide. Thus in the presence of excess chloride ion, proportionately less bromide is reabsorbed. But just as bromide accumulates slowly, it is eliminated slowly, even in the presence of excess chloride ion.

The removal of a toxic agent from its site of action through the formation of a less toxic complex with a specific antidote is a very effective mechanism of detoxification. The action of the poison is terminated even before it is removed from the body. The agents dimercaprol (BAL, or British antilewisite) and calcium disodium edetate (EDTA) used in the treatment of poisoning by heavy metals are examples of such antidotal complexing agents. Additional examples are given in Table 11-11. The great value of compounds like BAL and EDTA lies in their ability to form tightly bound, nondissociable complexes with metal ions. This binding effectively removes the metal ions from circulation and promotes the continuing dissociation and complete removal of any metal which is reversibly bound to enzymes and other tissue components. The metal complexes are water soluble and are readily excreted in the urine. Thus the complexing agent not only terminates the action of the poison, but also serves to eliminate it from the body. For example, following the administration of EDTA to victims of lead poisoning, the urinary excretion of lead as the EDTA-lead complex may be as much as fifty times greater than in the untreated state.

Elevation of the Threshold of Toxicity

When the ability of an agonist to combine with its receptor is altered by the presence of a second drug which interacts with the same receptor, the phenomenon is known as pharmacologic antagonism. In the presence of a pharmacologic antagonist, the agonist acts as though it has become a less potent drug; much more agonist is required to produce responses equal in magnitude to those elicited before the addition of the antagonist. Thus in the presence of a pharmacologic antagonist, there is an increase in the minimal concentration of agonist required to produce a demonstrable effect; the dose-effect curve of the agonist is shifted to the right (cf. pp. 180–184).

All the specific antidotes acting to elevate the threshold of toxicity are pharmacologic antagonists (Table 11-11). They decrease the response to a given dose of a toxic agent by preventing the latter from exerting its full effect at the site where the toxic action is produced. For example, oxygen is a specific antidote for carbon monoxide poisoning, since oxygen competes with the noxious gas for hemoglobin and displaces the carbon monoxide bound to the protein. This is very different from the use of oxygen as a functional antagonist in the treatment of barbiturate poisoning, in which respiration is depressed by direct action of the poison on the respiratory center in the brain. The use of atropine in the treatment of poisoning by organic phosphate insecticides is another example of antidotal therapy utilizing the mechanism of pharmacologic antagonism. The toxicity of these insecticides is mediated through their inhibition of the enzyme cholinesterase. In the presence of the enzyme inhibitors, acetylcholine is not metabolized and is present in excessive amounts. Atropine, as an antagonist of acetylcholine at many receptor sites (cf. p. 195), diminishes some of the adverse effects produced by the inhibition of cholinesterase activity. The agent pralidoxime is another specific antidote used in the treatment of poisoning by organic phosphate insecticides (Table 11-11). But pralidoxime acts as a complexing agent and removes the offending drugs from combination with cholinesterase, thereby restoring the activity of the enzyme. The difference in the mechanisms by which atropine and pralidoxime act as specific antidotes in poisoning resulting from cholinesterase inhibition is an important distinction. In the presence of a pharmacologic antagonist, the toxic action of an offending chemical may be reduced, but the toxic agent is neither detoxified nor removed from the body by the specific antidote. This is in sharp contrast to the fate of a toxic agent in the presence of a complexing agent. Therefore, when pharmacologic antagonists are employed, the toxic effect of a poison may reappear if the rate of elimination of the antagonist is more rapid than that of the toxic agent. And it must always be borne in mind that the use of any chemical agent, even an antidote, carries its own potential for producing unwanted and toxic effects.

SYNOPSIS

A drug, in the broadest sense, is any chemical substance (except food) that affects a living organism. Even when we limit consideration of these chemical-biologic reactions to the species *Homo sapiens,* the number of substances which this broad definition embraces remains bewildering. And since any chemical agent, whether intended for use in humans or not, has some dose at which it will produce a harmful effect, the potential for chemicals to adversely affect the human organism is enormous.

The toxicity of agents intended for use in humans has become the most critical aspect of modern therapeutics. The introduction of more effective and more potent agents for therapeutic use has brought with it drug-induced adverse effects that are now called "diseases of medical progress." This is all the more reason for therapeutic agents to be used carefully and wisely, so that the expected benefits to be derived will outweigh the possible risks involved.

Whereas drug-induced diseases may be part of the price that has to be paid for more effective and better therapeutic agents, the toxicity associated with the non-therapeutic use of these chemicals can only be deplored. Poisoning by chemicals not intended for use in humans is also a major health problem. However, from the published morbidity and mortality statistics, it is apparent that the major incidence of poisoning is due to accidental as well as intentional use of therapeutic agents. And the vast majority of these accidental poisonings occur in children under 5 years of age. Increasing concern has led to many constructive measures to correct and reduce the hazards involved in the everyday exposure to potentially harmful chemicals of all types. But since exposure to many of these chemicals is unavoidable, more effort must be aimed at preventing the occurrence of toxicologic problems.

The best treatment for drug toxicity is prevention. But when poisoning occurs, nonspecific treatment is first aimed at supporting the vital physiologic functions, such as respiration and circulation, and at limiting further exposure to the offending agent. Removing the poison from the patient (or the patient from the toxic agent in the case of a contaminated atmosphere) and continuing adequate supportive measures as needed to antagonize and control the toxic effects may be all that is necessary. Given a little time, the normal mechanisms of drug elimination can be depended on to terminate the action of the offending agents.

Safe and effective specific antidotes are known for only a relatively few drugs. Yet because there are such specific agents, a positive identification of the cause of poisoning often facilitates therapy. Specific antidotes that prevent an agent from exerting its effects or that permanently remove it from its site of action are the most effective. Outstanding examples are the nitrites and thiosulfate used to treat cyanide poisoning, or the complexing agents used to treat heavy metal poisoning. The use of antidotal chemicals is not without hazard, however, and should be restricted to those situations in which irreparable damage or death may occur in the absence of their use. The objective of antidotal therapy, as with all therapy, is to achieve salutary effects without harm to the patient.

GUIDES FOR STUDY AND REVIEW

When is a chemical considered a poison? When does a chemical intended for use in humans become a poison? What is the single most important factor in determining the margin of safety of a chemical when the sites of action for the desired and toxic effects occur within the same organism? when an economic species uses a chemical to eliminate an undesirable species?

How do acute, subacute and chronic toxicities differ from each other? What is a primary irritant? How may primary irritants be used as therapeutic agents?

What do we mean by nonselective toxicity? selective toxicity?

What is the approximate incidence of adverse effects of therapeutic agents when these agents are correctly used in recommended dosage for the right indication? What kind of untoward effect is most common? What other untoward effects are commonly encountered? What effects represent the most hazardous and unpredictable complication of drug therapy? What is the one group of therapeutic agents that can be legally designated for use in humans even though they may have been found capable of producing cancers in laboratory animals?

In general, how is the toxicity of a chemical intended for use in humans evaluated? What regulatory agency in the United States sets the guidelines for this evaluation?

What types of toxic reactions are unlikely to be discovered in laboratory animal testing? What kinds of problems are encountered in extrapolating data from animal experiments to humans?

In general, how are chemicals that are used by humans to eliminate pests evaluated for their safety? for their efficacy? Is such assessment required by law? In layman's terms, when would a chemical be considered "extremely toxic"? "relatively harmless"? What information is required by law to appear on the label of a package of pesticide? How is the degree of toxicity of the product indicated on the label?

According to the published morbidity and mortality statistics, is the major incidence of poisoning (either accidental or intentional) due to use of therapeutic agents or nontherapeutic chemicals? What kinds of therapeutic agents are most responsible for fatal poisoning? What factors in recent years are responsible for the decline in the number of fatal poisonings in our young children? Do you know how to get professional help in a case of suspected poisoning?

What do we mean by antidotal therapy? What is an antidote?

What is the aim of all antidotal treatment? What are the three general procedures by which this aim can be achieved? What general procedures can be used to slow the rate of access of the drug to its site of action? What general procedures can be used to increase the rate of drug excretion? What procedures can be used to elevate the threshold concentration of drug needed to produce the toxic effect?

What are the essentials of the nonspecific treatment of poisoning? What measures take precedence over all other measures? Why is the maintenance of respiration or the administration of agents to support the circulation an example of procedures used to elevate the threshold of toxicity?

What first-aid measure should be taken immediately when a poison has been swallowed? How can vomiting be induced? For what types of poisons must vomiting *not* be induced?

What first-aid measures should be taken if poisoning is by inhalation? by skin contamination? by injection?

What first-aid measures should be taken in the case of chemical burns?

What measures should be taken to prevent poisoning accidents?

What do we mean by specific therapy of poisoning? What is a specific antidote for poisoning by therapeutic iron preparations that acts by preventing absorption of the drug from the gastrointestinal tract? What is the specific antidote for poisoning by methanol, and how does it act? What is the specific antidote for the treatment of lead poisoning, and how does it act? What are the specific antidotes for the treatment of poisoning by morphine and other narcotic analgesics, and how do they act to elevate the threshold of toxicity? What is the specific antidote for the treatment of poisoning by carbon monoxide?

SUGGESTED READING

Albert, A. *Selective Toxicity* (4th ed.). London: Methuen, 1968.

Brodie, B.B.   The Mechanisms of Adverse Reactions. In H. Rašková (ed.), *Mechanisms of Drug Toxicity* (Proceedings of the Third International Pharmacological Meeting, São Paulo, 1966), Vol. 4. New York: Pergamon, 1968. P. 23.

Burns, J.J.   Evaluation and mechanisms of drug toxicity. *Ann. N.Y. Acad. Sci.* 123:1, 1965.

D'Arcy, P.F., and Griffin, J.P. *Iatrogenic Diseases.* London: Oxford University Press, 1972.

Done, A.K.   Clinical pharmacology of systemic antidotes. *Clin. Pharmacol. Ther.* 2:750, 1961.

Done, A.K.   Pharmacologic principles in the treatment of poisoning. *Pharmacol. Physicians* 3:1, 1969.

Gosselin, R.E., Hodge, H.C., Smith, R.P., and Gleason, M.N. *Clinical Toxicology of Commercial Products: Acute Poisoning* (4th ed.). Baltimore: Williams & Wilkins, 1976.

Loomis, T.A.· *Essentials of Toxicology.* Philadelphia: Lea & Febiger, 1970.

Melmon, K.L.   Preventable drug reactions – causes and cures. *N. Engl. J. Med.*
284:1361, 1971.

Moser, R.H. (ed.).   *Diseases of Medical Progress – A Study of Iatrogenic Disease:
A Contemporary Analysis of Illness Produced by Drugs and Other Therapeutic
Procedures* (3d ed.). Springfield, Ill.: Thomas, 1969.

Zbinden, G.   Experimental and clinical aspects of drug toxicity. *Adv. Pharmacol.*
2:1, 1963.

12. THE PHARMACOLOGIC ASPECTS OF DRUG ABUSE AND DRUG DEPENDENCE

The earliest records of man's search for means to cope with the exigencies of his environment attest to his remarkable ingenuity in finding drugs that allay anxiety, elevate mood and, in general, furnish pleasure and satisfaction. Certainly, most ethnic groups had independently found methods of producing alcohol during a primitive stage in their development. Opium, the source of morphine, and solanaceous plants, the source of atropine and scopolamine, as well as the sources of hashish, nicotine, cocaine, caffeine and similar drugs, were also discoveries of primitive peoples. Among these agents known and used since antiquity are some that remain part of our modern therapeutic armamentarium. But these and many other ancient drugs are also among those which pose serious problems in our contemporary culture through their use for nonmedical purposes. Whether the ancients also recognized the social ills attendant on the use of drugs that provide the user with an escape from reality is clearly documented only in the case of alcohol. It wasn't until the late 1600s that descriptions of abuse appeared in the annals of medicine for other drugs (even opium, so widely used in ancient times for its soporific and analgesic properties). But surely there must have been individuals among ancient civilizations who used these drugs in a manner at odds with the society of their times. And in this context, drug abuse and drug dependence are equally as old as some of the drugs associated with these phenomena.

The term *drug abuse* refers to the excessive and persistent use, usually by self-administration, of any drug without due regard for accepted medical practice. The vast majority of drugs of abuse are agents that act on the central nervous system to produce profound effects on mood, feeling and behavior. This broad definition of drug abuse also includes the habitual use by laymen of drugs like laxatives, headache remedies, antacids and vitamins. However, inclusion of the word *persistent* excludes from classification as abusive the occasional nonmedical or inappropriate medical use of a drug, such as the indiscriminate use of penicillin to treat the common cold. This use of drugs for purposes or conditions for which they are unsuited (or even their appropriate use but in improper dosage) is better termed *drug misuse.*

The abuse of some drugs leads to *drug dependence,* a condition in which the user

341

has a compelling desire to continue taking the drug either to experience its effects or to avoid the discomfort of its absence. *Drug dependence* is a general term which is applicable to all types of drug abuse. It has been substituted for the terms *drug addiction* and *drug habituation*[1] on the recommendation of both the World Health Organization's Expert Committee on Addiction-Producing Drugs and the National (U.S.A.) Academy of Science's Committee on Problems of Drug Dependence. This was done in an effort to avoid confusion in classifying types of drug abuse under the older terminology, while calling attention to the fact that drug dependence is a feature common to all types of drug abuse. In addition, the use of the general term *drug dependence* carries no connotation of the degree of serious harm to the drug user or to society, or of the measures needed to solve the problems of drug abuse. Thus, within the context of drug dependence, we may discuss the interactions between the pharmacodynamic effects of the drug and the psychologic status of the individual separately from the larger aspects of the interactions between drug abuse and society. And we shall be concerned in this chapter only with drug dependence and not with the social, economic, psychologic, moral or legal issues which also enter into the complex phenomenon of drug abuse.

We shall confine our discussion to drugs of abuse that are agents acting on the central nervous system. As an aid to understanding these actions, we shall begin with an abbreviated account of the functional anatomy of the central nervous system.

THE FUNCTIONAL ORGANIZATION OF THE CENTRAL NERVOUS SYSTEM

The billions of cells of the body, each a unit in its own right, are transformed into interdependent and cooperatively functioning parts of a single entity — a human being — largely through the activities of the nervous system. The endocrine system and other chemical mechanisms also play important roles in the control and integration of the body functions. But it is the central nervous system that is the principal coordinator and director of all the activities of the tissues and organs of the body. By virtue of its capacity for rapid response, the central nervous system also provides the most effective mechanism by which the human can adjust to changes in his external environment. And it is the high degree of specialization of his brain that sets the human apart from all other animals in his ability to correlate and integrate information, to reason abstractly and to think creatively.

[1] The definitions of these two terms were proposed by the WHO Expert Committee on Addiction-Producing Drugs in its seventh report (1957):

Drug addiction is a state of periodic or chronic intoxication produced by the repeated consumption of a drug (natural or synthetic). Its characteristics include (1) an overpowering desire or need (compulsion) to continue taking the drug and to obtain it by any means; (2) a tendency to increase the dose; (3) a psychic (psychological) and generally physical dependence on the effects of the drug; (4) a detrimental effect on the individual and on society.

Drug habituation (habit) is a condition resulting from the repeated consumption of a drug. Its characteristics include (1) a desire (but not a compulsion) to continue taking the drug for the sense of improved well-being which it engenders; (2) little or no tendency to increase the dose; (3) some degree of psychic dependence on the effect of the drug, but absence of physical dependence and hence of an abstinence syndrome; (4) detrimental effects, if any, primarily, on the individual.

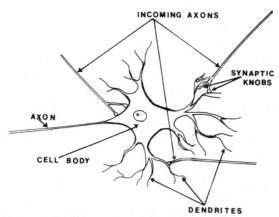

FIGURE 12-1. Nerve cell. A neuron may have many dendrites but has only one axon, which carries impulses away from the cell body. Nerve impulses from other nerve cells are transmitted from knobs of incoming axons to dendrites, or directly to the nerve cell body. A single neuron may receive impulses from many other neurons.

The central nervous system (CNS), enclosed by the vertebrae and the skull, is made up of the spinal cord, the brain and billions of nerve cells.

The *nerve cell* or *neuron,* the impulse-conducting unit, characteristically consists of a nucleated *cell body* (or soma), *dendrites* and a long process known as the *axon* or nerve fiber (Fig. 12-1). The dendrites, of which there may be many, receive impulses from other neurons or other types of cells and conduct them to the cell body. The axon, a single cytoplasmic extension of the cell body, conducts impulses away from the soma and stimulates other cells; there is usually only one axon, but this may have numerous branches or *collaterals.* Although neurons vary widely in shape and size and in the number, length and degree of branching of their processes, with respect to function they are divided into two main categories: *afferent* or *sensory* and *efferent* or *motor neurons.* Neurons which conduct impulses toward the CNS from the sense organs (e.g., eye or ear), or from receptors in tissues which are adapted to respond to different stimuli, are afferent neurons. Efferent neurons carry impulses outward from the CNS to the muscles, glands or other tissues and organs.

Neurons do not occur singly in vertebrates; the nerves that are visible on dissection are composed of bundles of both efferent and afferent nerve fibers. Outside the CNS these bundles are called *nerve trunks*; within the CNS they are usually referred to as a *tract*, or a *column.* [2] A cluster of cell bodies is known as a *ganglion,* but within the CNS the terms *nucleus, body* or *corpus* are also used to designate a group of associated nerve cell bodies.

The junction between two neurons at which impulses are transmitted from one to another is called a *synapse.* (The junction between an efferent fiber and a muscle or

[2]Within the CNS the bundle of nerve fibers is also referred to as a *fasciculus* (a little bundle), a *funiculus* (a little cord) or a *peduncle* (a little foot).

other tissue or organ which it innervates is known as a neuroeffector junction.) Transmission at the synapse is unidirectional, the impulse being conveyed from the axon of one neuron (the presynaptic cell) to the soma or dendrite, or both (or in some cases, the axon) of another neuron (the postsynaptic cell). The terminal branches of a single axon may impinge on a number of different cells, so that one axon may transmit impulses to hundreds of other neurons. Conversely, any one neuron may receive impulses from many different axons. In the CNS the impulses from the presynaptic fiber may excite or inhibit the postsynaptic neuron.

Transmission of impulses at the synapse is brought about chemically, not electrically as in the case of impulse conduction along the axon. At synapses the collaterals of the axon end in synaptic knobs or terminal buttons which contain numerous small vesicles. Nerve impulses arriving at the synaptic knobs cause these vesicles to liberate their contents, and the discharged chemical, rather than an electric current, affects the adjacent neuron. Outside the CNS the chemical transmitter, or neurohumors, released upon nerve stimulation have been identified as acetylcholine at all synapses and between nerves and skeletal muscles, and as acetylcholine or norepinephrine at other neuroeffector junctions. The transmitters at specific synapses in the CNS are not definitely known.[3] However, transmitter functions in the CNS have been proposed for acetylcholine and norepinephrine as well as for serotonin (5-hydroxytryptamine), dopamine, gamma-aminobutyric acid and some other amino acids which are present in the CNS. Undoubtedly, when the identities of the chemical transmitters within the CNS are disclosed, the precise mechanisms of action of the many drugs which act on the CNS will be elucidated in quick succession. For outside the CNS, many drugs are known to produce their effects either by mimicking, potentiating or inhibiting the actions of acetylcholine and norepinephrine or by altering the synthesis, storage, release or catabolism of these neurohumors (see Chap. 13). It seems quite likely that the drugs acting on the CNS will also be found to produce their characteristic effects directly or indirectly by altering the ability of neurons to transmit information to one another.

The *spinal cord* consists mainly of nerve fibers segregated into special functional groups, some transmitting sensory nerve impulses upward (the ascending tracts), others conveying efferent impulses downward to peripheral nerves and muscles (the descending tracts). The spinal nerves, thirty-one pairs in all, enter and emerge from each side of the spinal cord through spaces between the vertebrae. Each spinal nerve consists of a posterior (dorsal) root and an anterior (ventral) root. The posterior root contains the small bundles of afferent fibers that have united at each segment before entering the spinal cord, and the anterior root carries the efferent fibers that will divide after leaving the cord. Drugs may produce some of their effects by actions directly on the nerves within the spinal cord. Amphetamine, for example, enhances excitatory activities of some simple reflexes, such as the knee jerk elicited in response to a tap below the kneecap. This reflex involves only a single synapse between the afferent fibers carrying the sensory impulses and the efferent fibers to the leg muscles.

---

[3]There are some exceptions; for example, in the spinal cord, acetylcholine is known to be the transmitter at the synapse between the Renshaw cell and the motor neuron; in the cerebellum, norepinephrine is considered the transmitter at Purkinje cells.

The *medulla oblongata* is a direct extension of the spinal cord (Fig. 12-2). This region of the brain contains the so-called vital centers that regulate respiration, blood pressure (vasomotor center), heart rate and contractile force (cardiac center). The groups of synapses concerned with the reflex control of swallowing, coughing and vomiting also lie within the medulla. There are many drugs that produce their effects by stimulating or depressing one or another of these medullary centers. For example, respiration is depressed by alcohol, the barbiturates and narcotic analgesics through their actions on the respiratory center. Some drugs owe their therapeutic usefulness to their ability to affect a specific medullary center at doses usually below those which produce effects at other sites, e.g., cough suppression by codeine or the induction of vomiting by apomorphine.

The *pons* and *midbrain* along with the medulla constitute the *brainstem,* the part of the brain below the cerebrum. Ascending and descending tracts of fibers course through the pons, some of the descending fibers synapsing with neurons which enter the cerebellum. The midbrain also serves as a relay station for messages to and from the higher regions of the brain as well as for impulses concerned with vision and hearing.

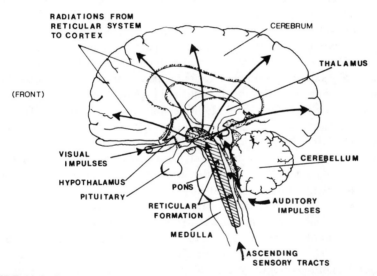

FIGURE 12-2. Structural and functional relationships of various parts of the central nervous system. The medulla contains control centers for respiration, blood pressure, heart rate and vomiting. The cerebellum is primarily concerned with the modulation and control of equilibrium, posture and movement. The hypothalamus is involved in the control and regulation of blood pressure, respiration, body temperature, body fluid volume, gastrointestinal activity and metabolism. Hypothalamic pathways also influence the emotional state, sleep and wakefulness. The thalamus is concerned primarily with sensory transmission and perception. The cerebrum is concerned with learning, memory, intelligence, reasoning, creative thought and imagination as well as with specific sensory and motor activities. The reticular formation influences the overall degree of activity of the CNS and is responsible for normal wakefulness and alertness.

The *cerebellum* lies close to and somewhat above the medulla and is connected to the brainstem by large tracts of fibers. Its primary functions are the modulation and control of equilibrium, posture and movements. Through feedback mechanisms to the periphery of the body and to other parts of the brain, the cerebellum coordinates and refines muscular activity and movement.

The *hypothalamus,* the area underlying the thalamus, is one of the central elements of systems concerned with control of the emotional state, of wakefulness and sleep and of alertness and excitement. The hypothalamus, as the principal locus of integration of the entire autonomic nervous system (see Chap. 13), is also involved in the subconscious control of many of the body's internal activities, including regulation of arterial blood pressure, respiration, body temperature, body fluid volume, gastrointestinal activity and fat and carbohydrate metabolism. The hormonal secretions of the endocrine glands, particularly those of the pituitary, are also influenced by the activities of the hypothalamus. Through its links with the thalamus and cerebrum, with various other regions of the brain and with organs involved in the basic life functions, the hypothalamus is in a most strategic position. It is not surprising that drugs which influence hypothalamic activity, either directly or indirectly, produce marked changes in an individual's behavior or in his ability to adapt to changes in his internal and external environments. For example, a drug such as the tranquilizer chlorpromazine is thought to act in part by suppressing the activity of many important behavioral areas of the hypothalamus and its associated regions of the brain.

The *limbic system,* intimately connected with the hypothalamus, is a collection of structurally and functionally interrelated brain centers lying deep inside the cerebral hemispheres and surrounding the thalamus and hypothalamus. The *amygdala* and *hippocampus* are two of the better studied components of the system. The limbic system is concerned with the complex emotions and instincts for survival — fear, feeding and mating. Thus it is involved with the integration of the emotional state with somatic and autonomic activities (cf. Chap. 13). Drugs such as the morphine-like opiates and antipsychotic agents that affect behavior may do so, in part, by altering the activity of the limbic system.

The *thalamus*, lying atop and to the right and left of the midbrain, is concerned primarily with sensory transmission and perception. All sensory impulses entering the spinal cord or brainstem synapse in the thalamus and are coordinated and interpreted before being relayed to the cerebral cortex. However, thalamic perception and interpretation of sensations of heat, cold, pain, touch or other types of sensory phenomena are rather gross and nondiscriminatory; the more refined, advanced sensations contributing to consciousness are interpreted through the cerebrum. Drugs that act on the thalamus may interfere with the orderly transmittal of sensory impulses such as pain, and this interference may be partially responsible for the action of some analgesic agents. But little is really known about the action of drugs on the thalamic region of the brain.

The *cerebrum*, by far the largest part of the human brain, is incompletely separated into right and left *hemispheres* by a median longitudinal fissure. At the base of this cleft, a band of fibers known as the *corpus callosum* connects the two cerebral hemi-

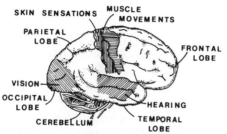

FIGURE 12-3. Lateral view of right cerebral hemisphere of the human brain, illustrating position of the four lobes and the areas concerned with special functions. The association areas (unshaded) contain fibers that form complex interconnections among all the impulses received in the cerebral cortex.

spheres. The *cerebral cortex* is the outer layer covering each hemisphere and the four large areas, or lobes, into which each half of the brain is divided (Fig. 12-3). The *frontal lobe* contains areas concerned with the control of muscular movements and speech as well as centers involved in coordinating muscular activity with the functions of the vital organs. The *parietal lobe* is responsible for the interpretation of sensations of heat, cold, touch and pressure with a specificity and fine discrimination not realized in the thalamus. The *occipital lobe* is the area for the perception and interpretation of visual stimuli, and a large part of the *temporal lobe* is involved with the process of hearing.

In lower mammals, almost the whole surface of the cortex is concerned with specific sensory or motor activities. In contrast, in humans the greatest bulk of the cerebral cortex is given over to associational fibers which form complex interconnections among all the impulses received in this region of the brain. These *association areas* make up almost all of the frontal and parietal lobes and much of the temporal and occipital lobes, and it is the size and degree of development of these association areas which place humans above other mammals. Learning and memory, intelligence and reasoning and those ideational processes unique to humans — creative thought and imagination — appear to be functions of the association areas.

Cortical activity may be depressed by drugs such as alcohol, phenobarbital or phenytoin, or stimulated by agents such as amphetamine and caffeine. The depressant activity may be manifested as a decrease in the acuity of sensory perception or as a decrease in muscular activity. Stimulation may be expressed as reduced fatigue, wakefulness, elation or increased mental or muscular activity. However, the basic actions of the drugs which produce either depression or stimulation are exerted on portions of the brain not directly concerned with motor activity.

Although it is possible to identify specific regions of the brain with particular functions, such as control of respiration, muscular activity, sensory perception and so forth, no one area of the CNS operates independently. Even though each part may have its own responsibilities, the various sections of the brain and spinal cord are interconnected and are constantly interacting with each other. This is perhaps best illustrated by considering how the *reticular formation* influences the overall degree of activity of the CNS.

The reticular formation, a complex network of cell bodies and interlacing fibers, begins in the medulla and extends upward through the midbrain to the thalamus (see Fig. 12-2). From the thalamus, fibers fan out to virtually all areas of the cerebral cortex. These upward projections of the reticular formation and thalamus are called the *ascending reticular activating system* (RAS). This system functions to control the overall degree of CNS activity and is basically responsible for normal wakefulness and alertness. The RAS has little intrinsic activity of its own, and in the absence of sensory impulses it is quiescent and the individual is relaxed, drowsy or asleep. Yet this system is instantly responsive to almost any type of sensory impulse, and stimulation of the RAS produces an arousal reaction and a state of wakefulness. By means of descending fibers the cortex is also able to increase the degree of activity of the RAS. Thus, once the RAS is stimulated, a "feedback" system from the excited cortex helps to maintain increased activity in the RAS.

The RAS also has an important descending component which can lead to increased or decreased activity of the peripheral muscles. When muscular activity is increased, this in turn feeds back to the RAS and promotes continued excitation. Many of the vital functions of the body are stimulated by the RAS, and this type of increased activity provides another feedback loop. Thus, once an individual has been awakened by the activation of the RAS, the feedback impulses from both the cerebral cortex and the periphery function to keep him awake. The neurons of the RAS are not capable of maintaining activity indefinitely, however, and after prolonged wakefulness they become fatigued or less excitable. The cycle then reverses itself, and the lessened activity of the RAS produces less and less activity in the feedback loops until most of the components of this complex system become inactivated and a state of sleep ensues. Drugs such as the barbiturates, which inhibit the RAS, can depress brain activity, induce sleep and, if the dose is large enough, may lead to unconsciousness and coma. Many other drugs, such as the general anesthetics and tranquilizers, also produce a decrease in the activity of the RAS.

During the wakeful state the RAS also controls the general level of attentiveness to external surroundings. But through its links with the thalamus, the RAS can excite or inhibit *specific* areas of the cortex. The latter may be one of the mechanisms whereby an individual can direct attention to certain aspects of his conscious mind while ignoring others. It would appear that the RAS plays a role in selecting the appropriate response to a given stimulus or condition and, in general, provides for integration of the activity of various parts of the CNS. Some of the effects of low doses of alcohol are the consequences of a depression of this integrating activity of the RAS (cf. p. 353).

GENERAL CHARACTERISTICS OF DRUG DEPENDENCE

The term *drug dependence* has two distinct and independent components: psychologic dependence and physical dependence.

Psychologic Dependence (psychic dependence; psychic craving; compulsive abuse): A condition characterized by an emotional or mental drive to continue taking a drug whose effects the user feels are necessary to maintain his sense of optimal well-being. The user's concept of optimal well-being may be considered abnormal or inappropriate, since judgment may be altered and there may be an incapacity to cope with and an indifference to life's problems. Psychologic dependence varies with the individual and with the drug and thus represents a complex interaction of personality factors and specific drug effects. When the desire to continue taking the drug becomes a "psychic craving" or "compulsion," the user may become preoccupied with drug-taking and drug-procurement. Such behavior is termed *drug-seeking behavior* or *compulsive drug use.* This represents the major problem of drug abuse, since it indicates that the user has lost control over the drug, and that the drug has acquired control over the user.

Physical Dependence: An altered or adaptive physiologic state produced in an individual by the repeated administration of a drug. That physical dependence has been induced during the prolonged use of a drug is revealed only when the drug is abruptly discontinued, or when its actions are diminished by the administration of a specific antagonist. Physical dependence manifests itself as intense physiologic disturbances called the *withdrawal* or *abstinence syndrome*; the specific symptoms and signs of a psychic and physical nature which make up the abstinence syndrome are characteristic for each drug type. The degree of physical dependence can be measured only by the severity of the withdrawal symptoms. For drugs like alcohol, the barbiturates and the narcotic analgesics, the withdrawal syndromes are so unpleasant and threatening that they are important factors motivating drug-seeking behavior and continued drug administration by the user to prevent their appearance.

The development of psychologic dependence is the *common denominator* in the abusive use of drugs that produce effects on the central nervous system. It may vary in intensity from the mild desire for the morning cup of coffee, to the more intense craving for a cigarette by the heavy smoker trying to give up the habit, to an overpowering obsession of the alcoholic to obtain a supply of drug such that he may knowingly drink unusual or poisonous mixtures. With certain types of drugs, such as cocaine and marihuana, psychologic dependence may be the only factor involved in their abuse. Thus, psychic dependence can and does develop to some drugs which do not induce physical dependence and which, therefore, do not give rise to an abstinence syndrome after discontinuance of drug use.

Physical dependence can also be induced by certain drugs and under some circumstances without any evidence of psychic dependence. For example, physical dependence can be developed to nalorphine, a drug which antagonizes the actions of morphine. The dependence manifests itself as a withdrawal syndrome when the drug is abruptly discontinued. However, no psychologic dependence develops to this agent, and it is not abused. Physical dependence also develops in patients receiving therapeutic doses of morphine or other narcotic agents for a period of several weeks. But the vast majority of these patients evince no desire to continue using the drug after the condition for which it was prescribed has been relieved — they develop no psychologic dependence. Hence, whereas psychologic dependence is the feature common to all drug abuse and may be the only factor involved in the abusive or compulsive use of some drugs, physical dependence alone does not lead to drug abuse. But physical dependence frequently accompanies the psychic dependence induced by drugs such as alcohol, barbiturates and the opiods (Table 12-1). Moreover, physical dependence occurring together with psychologic dependence is a powerful factor in reinforcing the compulsion to continue taking the drug.

The fact that some individuals do not develop psychic dependence to drugs which can induce this phenomenon in other subjects points to the presence of a predisposing factor in the person and not in the drug. The explanation that is widely accepted is that most drug abusers have deep-seated personality maladjustments and psychologic disturbances which would have surfaced even in the absence of drug use. This is particularly true of those who compulsively use drugs to which physical dependence also develops. Yet the number of emotionally disturbed individuals who are not drug abusers far exceeds the number who are. What we do not know, unfortunately, is why some individuals can occasionally use drugs like alcohol or experience other drugs of abuse and not be compelled to use the agents repeatedly, whereas others become drug abusers.

Many of the drugs that induce dependence also have the capacity to produce tolerance, the adaptive state characterized by diminished response to the same dose of a drug (cf. pp. 279–283). Yet tolerance and drug dependence are separate phenomena and may develop independently of each other. As we have seen, tolerance may be produced by many agents, such as nitrites, which have little or no potential for abusive use. On the other hand, drug abuse and drug dependence may occur in the absence of the development of any demonstrable tolerance. For example, no tolerance develops to cocaine despite the fact that it induces the highest degree of psychic dependence. Moreover, tolerance developed to drugs that are subject to abuse is not necessarily accompanied by physical dependence. The abusive use of lysergic acid diethylamide (LSD) is a case in point; marked tolerance develops to LSD, but withdrawal symptoms are not seen upon abrupt discontinuance of drug use. However, tolerance is almost invariably associated to some degree with the use of agents that do induce physical dependence (see Table 12-1).

Since the characteristics of the state of drug dependence are not the same for different drugs or groups of drugs, the nature of the dependence can be delineated only in terms of the agent(s) involved. For example, the dependent state may be designated as drug dependence of the barbiturate type, of the morphine type and so on. By using this explicit terminology a relationship among all drugs of abuse is indicated, but the specific pattern of the dependence is differentiated according to the causative agent(s). The drugs that are subject to abuse may also be classified on the basis of their characteristic pharmacologic effect on the central nervous system, i.e., general depressants, narcotic analgesics, stimulants and psychedelics (hallucinogens). Within any of these principal groups, agents may then be further classified into subgroups to clarify the particular type of drug dependence involved in specific cases.[4]

[4]This classification is quite different from that used to classify drugs of abuse under the Comprehensive Drug Abuse Prevention and Control Act, commonly referred to as the **Controlled Substances Act** (see Glossary for a fuller description of this act).

Table 12-1. Characteristics of Different Types of Drug Dependence

Agents	Psychologic Dependence	Physical Dependence	Withdrawal Syndrome	Tolerance
General Depressants Alcohol Sedative-hypnotics Barbiturates Glutethimide Methyprylon Chloral hydrate Paraldehyde Minor tranquilizers Meprobamate Chlordiazepoxide	Mild to strong; develops slowly	Develops slowly but to marked degree	Varies in intensity with duration and amount of drug intake; potentially severe and most dangerous; characterized by convulsions; deaths not uncommon	Irregular and incomplete; little tolerance to adverse effects of high doses; cross-tolerance among members of group
Narcotic Analgesics Natural opiates Synthetic derivatives of opiates Synthetic opiate-like drugs	Strong; develops rapidly	Early development which increases in intensity, paralleling increase in dosage	Severe symptoms but not life-threatening; may be precipitated by administration of narcotic antagonist	Striking degree of tolerance to all but effects on pupil and gastrointestinal tract; cross-tolerance with other opiates or opiate-like drugs
Stimulants Amphetamines	Mild to strong	Low degree	Mild	Marked but incomplete; cross-tolerance with amphetamine-like agents but not with cocaine
Cocaine	Strong	None	None	None
Psychedelics LSD Marihuana	Variable Mild to strong	None None	None None	Marked Low degree developed to high doses

GENERAL DEPRESSANTS OF THE CENTRAL NERVOUS SYSTEM

A variety of agents widely used for subjective purposes have in common the ability to produce a nonspecific but generalized depression of the central nervous system. Included in this category are ethyl alcohol; the sedative-hypnotics, principally the barbiturates but also nonbarbiturate agents; the so-called minor tranquilizers, and anesthetic agents (Table 12-2). These agents differ markedly in their physicochemical properties and in some of their pharmacologic actions; these differences account for their classification and therapeutic usefulness specifically as sedatives, hypnotics or anesthetics (cf. pp. 463–474, 477–478). But despite the differences that exist among the individual agents within the group, the pattern of dependence developed to the entire group is remarkably consistent.

All the general depressants of the CNS are abused to one degree or another for similar reasons: the drugs act to allay anxiety and decrease tension. All the agents in this group produce the same dose-related signs and symptoms characteristic of increasing depression of the central nervous system. The agents also resemble one another with respect to the pattern of development of psychologic dependence and the degree of tolerance acquired with continued use. Physical dependence also develops to all these agents, and the discontinuance of the use of any of them produces similar symptomatology. The drugs are essentially additive and inter-changeable; they show *cross-dependence,* the ability of one drug to suppress the manifestations of physical dependence induced by another and to substitute for the other in maintaining the physically dependent state. Such similarities among the general depressants of the central nervous system justify describing the dependence developed to any one of them under a single category. The barbiturates and alcohol are used as the standards of reference for the entire group, and the type of dependence is termed "drug dependence of the barbiturate-alcohol type"

Alcohol and the barbiturates, at all doses, produce a primary and continuous depression of the central nervous system. At low doses the effects are principally the result of depression of the reticular system, the more primitive part of the brain concerned with the maintenance of consciousness and the control of responsible behavior. Since the impulses ascending from the reticular activating system to the

Table 12-2. General Depressants of the CNS Used for Subjective Purposes

Ethyl alcohol	Minor tranquilizers
Sedative-hypnotics	Meprobamate (Miltown; Equanil)
Barbiturates	Chlordiazepoxide (Librium)
Secobarbital (Seconal)	General anesthetics
Pentobarbital (Nembutal)	Ether
Amobarbital (Amytal)	Nitrous oxide
Phenobarbital (Luminal)	Miscellaneous agents
Glutethimide (Doriden)	Glue
Methaqualone	Paint thinners
Methyprylon (Nodular)	Lacquer thinners
Chloral hydrate	
Paraldehyde	

cortex can be either excitatory or inhibitory, the behavioral responses that are observed will depend on which pathway is initially depressed. Thus the effects of low doses of alcohol and barbiturates are contingent on the degree of excitability of the central nervous system at the time of drug administration. This, in turn, depends on the environmental setting of drug use and on the personality of the user. In a quiet, nonsocial environment, the ascending excitatory influence may be impaired, and the sedation and drowsiness produced by the drugs are then readily equated with depression of the central nervous system. In a social setting, where there is a great deal of sensory input, the cortex may be freed from its integrating control by depression of the ascending reticular system. Under these circumstances the effects of low doses of drug are perceived as stimulation, whereas in fact they are the result of release from inhibition secondary to depression of those pathways of the reticular activating system that inhibit specific areas of the cortex. The paradoxical excitement — the talkativeness, the heightened vivacity, the increased self-confidence and the general loss of self-restraint — may be likened to the situation of an automobile parked on an incline being suddenly set in motion by releasing the brake. There is also loss of mental acuity and judgment and impaired motor coordination. As the dose is increased, and during chronic intoxication, these agents produce more of the same effects. There may be slurred speech; staggering; loss of balance and falling; loss of emotional control; stupor from which arousal is difficult; severe respiratory depression; and, finally, coma and death. Although low doses of alcohol and barbiturates impair mental and motor function to one degree or another, it is the untoward effects of high doses which produce the greatest harm to the individual and to society.

In the abusive use of alcohol there may be overt pathologic changes in tissues and organs, e.g., the liver, a factor not associated with dependence on other drugs of abuse. Alcohol, unlike other drugs, can be utilized by the body as a source of energy. This supply of calories often suppresses appetite, leading to dietary deficiencies which may be responsible in part for the pathologic conditions seen in chronic alcoholism.

Drug abuse and drug dependence occur in all degrees with the alcohol-barbiturate class of drugs. Abusive use ranges from occasional sprees of gross intoxication to prolonged, daily use and chronic intoxication. Ethyl alcohol is the agent most widely used and abused, and indeed, in Western cultures, alcoholism is still the most prevalent type of drug abuse. Ethyl alcohol is also the only potent pharmacologic agent whose use for nonmedical purposes is socially and culturally acceptable. However, daily use of these drugs is not necessarily abusive use or indicative of a state of dependence. For example, since drinking alcoholic beverages is socially acceptable, daily consumption is considered a normal part of the culture of many countries. Psychologic dependence on alcohol is discernible when the evening cocktail or the wine at dinner *is desired and missed when not available.* The development of dependence on alcohol is insidious, however, since the dependent state frequently goes unrecognized in its mild form; it becomes apparent only when daily consumption exceeds accepted norms and deviates from established cultural patterns. Medically prescribed barbiturates may also be taken daily for long periods without being considered abusive

Table 12-3. Minimal Doses of Commonly Used Central Nervous System
Depressants that May Lead to Physical Dependence and Tolerance

Drug	Minimal Dose
Pentobarbital	400 mg/day
Secobarbital	400 mg/day
Meprobamate	ca. 1.6−2.4 g/day
Glutethimide	ca. 2.5 g/day
Chlordiazepoxide	< 300 mg/day

Source: From *Drill's Pharmacology in Medicine,* 4th ed., edited by J. R. DiPalma. Copyright
© 1971, McGraw-Hill Book Company. Used with permission of McGraw-Hill Book Company.

drug use. Many individuals take barbiturates regularly in doses of 100 to 200 mg
for months or years without developing more than a mild psychic dependence on the
drug for the induction of sleep. Some people, however, find a need to increase the
dosage. And when the dosage of barbiturates is increased beyond the recommended
therapeutic level, the degree of psychic craving progressively and relentlessly increases
until, eventually, the drug becomes a major part of the user's existence. The development of tolerance and physical dependence is also gradual and, again, seems to be
induced only when the daily dose exceeds the therapeutically recommended dosage
(Table 12-3).

Thus, mild degrees of psychic dependence may develop to the central nervous
system depressant drugs when they are used in low or therapeutically recommended
dosage. Although this may lead to their continued use, drug administration may be
stopped without any serious subjective disturbances. When there is need for increased
drug consumption because of incomplete relief of anxiety and tension, then the development of tolerance enhances the need for more drug, and the development of
physical dependence reinforces compulsive use to avoid withdrawal symptoms.

The tolerance that develops to the central nervous system depressants is erratic
and incomplete and never reaches the degree observed with the opioids or amphetamines. The upper limit of the dose of barbiturate that may be tolerated varies
between 1.0 and 2.5 g per day orally. Drug-dependent individuals appear less intoxicated and less impaired in performance at a given blood level of drug than do nontolerant individuals. However, the lethal dose of any of these agents is not much
greater in the drug-dependent individual than in the nontolerant subject.

The most distinguishing feature of the alcohol-barbiturate type of drug dependence
is the abstinence syndrome that appears upon abrupt cessation of prolonged administration of high doses. The withdrawal symptoms are usually far more dangerous than
those resulting from withdrawal of the opiates or other agents of abuse to which physical dependence may be developed. However, the severity of symptoms depends on
the length of drug abuse and the degree of intoxication. In the typical course of withdrawal, symptoms begin within the first 24 hours after discontinuance of the drug,
reach their peak intensity within two to three days, but are self-limiting and usually
disappear within one to two weeks. During the first day of withdrawal there may be
headaches, anxiety, involuntary twitching of muscles, tremor of hands, weakness,

insomnia and nausea. During the next 48 hours the symptoms become progressively more intense: there may be a precipitous fall in blood pressure; fever; delirium characterized by disorientation, delusions and vivid visual hallucinations; and convulsions similar to those exhibited in grand mal epilepsy. The fever, delirium and convulsions are the most serious symptoms and have proved fatal in a number of instances.

NARCOTIC ANALGESICS

In legal parlance the term *narcotic* includes drugs with morphine-like activity, as well as marihuana and cocaine; the last two drugs are pharmacologically unrelated to morphine and induce entirely different states of dependence. In medicine, *narcotic* applies only to drugs having both analgesic and sedative action; the term essentially embraces only those drugs, either natural or synthetic, that have morphine-like pharmacologic activity. The term *narcotic analgesic,* used interchangeably with *opiate* or *opioid,* avoids the confusion inherent in the legal classification and is therefore better terminology to designate the morphine-like drugs.

The drugs classified as opioids, for which morphine is the standard of reference, include the natural opiates, their partially synthetic derivatives and wholly synthetic opiate-like drugs. Commonly used opioids include:

Natural opioids obtained from opium
  Morphine
  Codeine

Semisynthetic opioids
  Dihydromorphinone (Dilaudid)
  Heroin
  Methyldihydromorphinone (Metopon)

Synthetic opioids
  Phenazocine (Prinadol)
  Meperidine (Demerol)
  Anileridine (Leritine)
  Diphenoxylate (with atropine as Lomotil)
  Methadone (Dolophine)
  Levorphanol (Levo-Dromoran)

Synthetic opioids with low potency and low dependence liability
  Propoxyphene (Darvon)
  Ethoheptazine (Zactane)
  Pentazocine (Talwin)

Narcotic antagonists
  Nalorphine (Nalline)
  Levallorphan (Lorfan)

Although the opioids differ in chemical structure, in their analgesic potency and in their potential to become drugs of abuse, they have basically similar pharmacologic profiles (cf. pp. 461–463). Even the antagonists included in this group, when used alone, have pharmacologic actions like those of morphine. Only the important new antagonist naloxone differs in this respect from the other narcotic antagonists. The opioids are also alike in their ability to induce and maintain some degree of psychologic and physical dependence and to develop tolerance. With the exception of the narcotic antagonists, these agents may be substituted for one another to prevent the appearance of the withdrawal syndrome. And when this syndrome does occur, the signs and symptoms of abstinence are the same for all the opiates. These similarities permit describing the state of dependence developed to any opioid as "drug dependence of the morphine type."

Drug dependence of the morphine type is unique in that the *first* dose of an opioid may set in motion the mechanisms leading to psychologic and physical dependence and to the development of tolerance. Dependence can be initiated with small doses well within the therapeutic range; the intensity and rapidity with which dependence and tolerance develop varies with the agent but parallels the increase in dosage. This is very different from the dependence on the central nervous system depressants that develops gradually and then only when the daily dose is increased appreciably above therapeutic levels.

In contrast to the barbiturate-alcohol class of drugs, the opioids are *selective* depressants of the central nervous system. For example, doses of 5 to 10 mg of morphine may produce relief of pain without producing any change in the perception of other sensory stimuli (touch, light, sound and so forth); analgesia may occur before and often without sleep. Typically, however, analgesia is accompanied by drowsiness, mood alteration, mental clouding and some respiratory depression. An essential feature of the analgesic action of morphine is its ability to alter the *reaction* to pain, rather than merely to decrease the perception of the painful stimulus itself. The narcotic analgesics also relieve anxiety, tension and fear, the reactions evoked by the specific sensation of pain. Thus the patient, freed from suffering or distress, feels more comfortable and is able to tolerate the pain even when he knows it is still present.

The relief from worry, tension and fatigue, and the mental fogginess or "other-world" sensation produced by the opioids are interpreted by some subjects as pleasurable (euphoric). These effects account in large measure for the abuse potential of the narcotic analgesics. To the opiate abuser everything "looks rosy" and is "as it should be." However, the naive subject may find the effects of morphine quite unpleasant, with nausea, vomiting, itching and sweating as the predominant effects. In the compulsive drug user there is a state of drive satiation; the drug reduces hunger and diminishes the sexual drive. And, unlike alcohol, the opiates also suppress aggressive behavior. Violence is characteristic of the compulsive opioid user only when the drug is not available and he must resort to criminal activity to satisfy his craving. The rapid development of tolerance and physical dependence upon repeated administration reinforces the emotional need to continue taking the drug and to obtain it by any means.

The rate at which tolerance develops to the narcotic analgesics depends on the rate of administration, and it is significant only when administration continues on a more or less daily basis. However, the degree of tolerance may reach phenomenal proportions; some habitual users have been known to take as much as 5 g of morphine per day. Tolerance develops to all the effects which the chronic user considers desirable: analgesia, sedation and euphoria. Tolerance also develops to the respiratory depression produced by all the opioids. Since respiratory failure is the cause of death in opiate poisoning, this tolerance makes it possible for the compulsive user to satisfy his need with doses that would otherwise be lethal. Tolerance does not develop, however, to the effects on the pupil of the eye or on the gastrointestinal tract.

The severity of the abstinence syndrome upon discontinuance of opioid administration is determined by the degree of dependence developed. Although the symptoms of withdrawal are not nearly as serious as those seen upon withdrawal from alcohol or barbiturates, the morphine abstinence syndrome is nevertheless characterized by changes in all major organs and systems. Symptoms appear shortly before the time for the next scheduled dose, intensify over the next several days and then gradually subside and disappear within seven to ten days. The signs and symptoms include anxiety; restlessness; irritability; lacrimation; generalized body aches; insomnia; perspiration; dilated pupils (except upon withdrawal from meperidine); gooseflesh; hot flushes; nausea; vomiting; diarrhea; fever; increased heart rate and blood pressure; and abdominal and other muscle cramps. The vomiting and diarrhea, combined with the inability to retain water and food, lead to dehydration and loss of weight. All these symptoms, excepting dehydration and weight loss, can be suppressed by administering the drug of dependence or another narcotic analgesic. When the abstinence syndrome is precipitated by the administration of one of the narcotic antagonists, the symptoms are the same but the first signs appear within minutes and reach their peak within a half hour.

In drug dependence of the morphine type, the harm to the individual and society does not result from the direct pharmacologic effects of the drugs as it does in drug dependence of the barbiturate-alcohol type. Rather, ill health, personal neglect, social irresponsibility, economic loss and crime are the indirect consequences of the user's need to procure the drug at all costs. When the opiate-dependent individual is able to obtain his drug by legitimate means, or has adequate funds, and is also able to control his dosage, he can work productively, discharge social obligations and remain healthy. The capacity of the narcotic analgesics to induce *compulsive drug-seeking behavior* is their most malignant property; it is more pernicious than for the alcohol-barbiturate drugs with respect to the rapidity with which such behavior can be initiated in susceptible individuals by the repeated administration of small doses.

Some very exciting results of recent investigations hold the promise of rapid progress toward the disclosure of the mechanisms underlying the actions of opiates and opiate addiction. This new era in opiate research began with the development of efficient and practical methods for the detection of highly specific opiate binding sites in neuronal membranes. A partially purified, membrane-bound lipoprotein extracted from mouse brain has been found to exhibit a stereospecific binding of opiate agonists that is competitively inhibited by naloxone. Found only in vertebrates, these putative receptors are located primarily, but not exclusively, in the limbic system of the brain.

It is postulated that the receptor can exist in two conformations: the one with which an agonist interacts most readily initiates a pharmacologic response; the one to which an antagonist is preferentially bound, does not initiate such a response.

The isolation and identification of other putative receptors such as those for acetylcholine and insulin have also been accomplished recently using newly available, sophisticated, experimental techniques (cf. pp. 43–44). However, all of these promising results involved the characterization of membrane-bound receptors that interact with *endogenous* ligands recognized as functionally important. Why then should there be highly stereospecific receptors in mammalian brain that interact with chemicals of *exogenous* origin – with chemicals like the opiates that are entirely foreign to the body? The logical answer is that such receptors were not developed to bind opiates but are receptors for normal components of the body, for either endogenous molecules whose functional role is still undefined, or endogenous substances as yet undiscovered. Investigations using the latter conceptual approach proved highly successful. Less than five years after the disclosure of the existence of specific binding sites for opiate drugs, endogenous substances capable of binding and interacting as agonists at opioid binding sites have been discovered and characterized. These "endogenous opiates" are called *endorphins.* Endorphins have been extracted from the brain and pituitary gland of various animal species and from human pituitary gland and cerebrospinal fluid; all have been identified as **peptides** containing five to thirty amino acid residues.

Although the physiologic role of the endorphins has not been elucidated as yet, there are two sets of data that support the hypothesis that the endorphins may play a role in the control of emotional behavior. First of all, the greatest concentration in the brain of binding sites for opiates and endorphins is in the limbic system. Second, the narcotic analgesics relieve anxiety, tension and fear, the affective states evoked by pain and controlled by the limbic system.

"The most exciting outgrowth from this research could be the prospect that endorphin deficiency might play some role in narcotic addiction. Several laboratories are working to develop a radioimmunoassay that will permit the sensitive measurement of endorphins in body fluids. This capability might allow direct testing of a hypothesis that I advanced several years ago, that classical hormonal feedback mechanisms might act to suppress endogenous opioid synthesis when the receptors are occupied by an exogenous opiate like morphine. This hypothesis rests upon analogy to other endocrine and neuroendocrine systems, in which administration of an exogenous hormone (such as thyroid hormone) activates a homeostatic negative feedback that shuts down endogenous production (for example, of thyroid hormone by the thyroid gland). Sudden removal of the exogenous substance can expose the deficiency in endogenous synthesis; . . . thus, induced endorphin deficiency might play a part in the immediate or protracted abstinence syndrome. A more speculative hypothesis is that in some people a genetically determined endorphin deficiency could predispose to narcotic addiction. If this were true, it would be easier to understand the remarkably high rate of recidivism after abstinence, as well as the considerable success of maintenance (replacement?) treatment with surrogate opiates like methadone. In initiating the modern era of opiate maintenance for heroin addicts, Dole and Nyswander suggested that narcotic addiction is some sort of 'metabolic disease.'[5] It would be most interesting if this postulated disease proved to be an endorphin deficiency.

The opiates have been and remain among the most important and remarkably effective drugs known to man. Research of the past 5 years, building on the knowledge accumulated during prior decades, revealed the existence of specific opiate receptors and then of the endogenous peptide ligands that interact with them. The consequences of these advances for our understanding of pain mechanisms, affective disorders, and narcotic addiction are only beginning to unfold. Research in this field should remain lively for some time to come."[6]

STIMULANTS OF THE CENTRAL NERVOUS SYSTEM

Drugs may produce increased activity of the central nervous system either by blocking pathways which normally inhibit activity or by directly enhancing excitation. The drugs used for abusive purposes and classified as central nervous system stimulants act, in the main, by direct stimulation. In humans the cortical stimulation is seen as garrulousness, restlessness, increased motor activity and excitement. These stimulants also produce a lessened sense of fatigue, so that physical performance and work may be improved and prolonged when they have been impaired by fatigue or lack of sleep (cf. pp. 379–381). Prolonged use or use of large doses is nearly always followed by lethargy and mental depression.

The amphetamines and cocaine are the principal agents of abuse among the stimulants of the central nervous system (Table 12-4). They differ significantly in many of their pharmacologic actions but are remarkably similar in their subjective effects, toxic symptoms and present-day patterns of abuse. We shall therefore use amphetamine as the standard of reference for the group and indicate the ways in which dependence on cocaine differs from that for amphetamines.

The ability of the amphetamines to elevate mood, combat fatigue, reduce appetite and induce a general state of well-being accounts for their widespread use as stimulants and appetite suppressants. These effects are typical and occur even in those using the

Table 12-4. Commonly Abused Central Nervous System Stimulants

---

Amphetamines
  Dextroamphetamine (Dexedrine)
  Amphetamine (Benzedrine)
  Methamphetamine (Methedrine, Desoxyn)
Cocaine
Phenmetrazine (Preludin)
Diethylpropion (Tenuate, Tepanil)
Methylphenidate (Ritalin)
Mephentermine (Wyamine)

---

[5] Dole, V.P., and Nyswander, M. "Heroin addiction–a metabolic disease," *Arch. Intern. Med.* 120:19, 1967.

[6] Extract material from A. Goldstein. "Opioid peptides (endorphins) in pituitary and brain," *Science* 193:1081, 1976, by permission of author and publisher. Dr. Avram Goldstein, professor of pharmacology at Stanford University, and director of the Addiction Research Foundation, Palo Alto, California, is one of the pioneers and leaders in this area of research.

drugs for the first time. This is in contrast to the effects of the opioids, which many first-time users find unpleasant. These typical responses to the amphetamines also form the basis for their abuse potential. Many normal individuals take amphetamines in the course of treatment for obesity or depression and experience the drug-induced mood elevation, yet do not become compulsive drug users. Some patients introduced to the drugs in this way, however, develop varying degees of psychic dependence, since therapy commonly involves prolonged and continuous administration. Then, since tolerance develops, its sequel is the need to increase both the quantity and the frequency of administration in order to obtain the desired mood elevation. This phenomenon is similar to the development of dependence to medically prescribed barbiturates, except that the amphetamines induce only a mild type of physical dependence. The same pattern of abuse may be followed by long-distance drivers or students who use amphetamines to ward off sleep. However, the great majority of persons who abuse the amphetamines and other stimulants do so specifically for their euphoric effects. And this type of abusive use commonly involves the intravenous rather than the oral route of administration. In Western countries, cocaine, which is never used as a prescription drug, is almost always injected intravenously by the compulsive drug user. Among the Peruvian Indians of the high Andes, however, the centuries-old custom of chewing coca leaves is still prevalent. Although coca is freely available for the Indians, it is used most often for religious rituals and only occasionally for individual enjoyment.

Tolerance develops to many effects of the amphetamines, particularly to those which are most desired by the compulsive user. Although the tolerance develops slowly, it reaches such magnitudes that in order to obtain a state of elation, the habitual user may require doses several hundred-fold greater than the usual therapeutic dose. There have been reports of the use of more than 10 g of methamphetamine intravenously over a 24-hour period. (The therapeutic dose of methamphetamine is about 10 mg.) Such parenteral use of large doses can be particularly hazardous; intracranial hemorrhage associated with severe hypertension has occurred frequently.

Tolerance does not develop evenly to all the central nervous system effects, and the user may show increased nervousness and persistent insomnia as the dose of amphetamine is increased. After weeks or months of continued use, a toxic psychosis resembling schizophrenia may develop which is characterized by delusions and hallucinations, both auditory and visual. These psychologic disturbances may also appear within a day or two after ingestion of a single large dose, but usually disappear within a week after the drug is discontinued.

Cocaine is also employed in huge quantities by drug users — as much as 10 g per day. However, this excessive dosage is not indicative of the development of tolerance, since cocaine is so rapidly biotransformed that the effects of each administration may last only minutes. Nor is there cross-tolerance between cocaine and the amphetamine-like drugs. The use of large doses of cocaine is associated, however, with toxic psychoses similar to those seen with the amphetamines.

Abrupt discontinuance of the use of amphetamines does not lead to a physiologically disruptive state, and withdrawal of the drugs is never life-threatening. Upon abrupt withdrawal there is a period of prolonged sleep, lethargy and often a pre-cipitous depressive reaction. This state of depression, both psychic and physical, probably motivates continuation of drug use. There is a growing consensus that these symptoms, which appear regularly when the amphetamine-like drugs are discontinued, constitute a mild form of abstinence syndrome. Similar symptoms appear when the use of cocaine is abruptly terminated. But since tolerance does not develop to cocaine, these symptoms are not considered evidence for the development of physical de-pendence (cf. p. 350).

The harm to the individual and to society of the compulsive use of central nervous system stimulants arises during the toxic episodes induced by large doses. The com-pulsive user of the stimulant drugs has enhanced drives, in contrast to the decreased drives of the opiate user. The hyperactivity, the feeling of great muscular strength, the paranoid delusions and the auditory and visual hallucinations often combine to make the user a dangerous individual capable of committing serious antisocial acts. Chronic users of amphetamines are also prone to accidents, since they are unaware of their fatigue until it overcomes them at an inopportune time.

PSYCHEDELICS (HALLUCINOGENS)

The term *hallucinogen* designates a drug that acts on the central nervous system to produce a state of perception of objects with no reality or of sensations with no external cause. Among the commonly abused drugs included in this category are lysergic acid diethylamide (LSD); psilocybin and psilocin (from the Aztec mushroom); mescaline (from the peyote cactus plant); and marihuana.[7] However, drugs other than those classified as hallucinogens, such as the amphetamines and cocaine, can also in-duce illusions and delusions. The hallucinogens are also referred to as *psychotomi-metics* and *psychotogens*. The word *psychotomimetic* suggests that the effects pro-duced by the hallucinogens mimic the naturally occurring psychoses. These drugs do, indeed, produce effects similar to some of the symptoms of schizophrenia and manic-depressive psychoses, but there are also marked dissimilarities between the drug effects and the symptoms of disease. The term *psychotogen* indicates that a hallucinogen produces a psychotic state, but this may also be seen following the use of many other agents such as bromides, cardiac glycosides and heavy metals. Thus there are no clear distinctions between the hallucinogenic drugs of abuse and other classes of drugs act-ing on the central nervous system. The word *psychedelic,* meaning mind-manifesting, was coined to distinguish the hallucinogens from other classes of drugs which may, under certain conditions, produce similar effects. A psychedelic drug is defined as one that is self-administered for its capacity to *reliably* cause marked changes in mood, judgment and perception that are not, or cannot be, experienced except in dreams or religious trances. Thus the term *psychedelic* delineates the hallucinogens in terms of the purpose for which they are used. And, with the exception of atropine and scopol-amine, the psychedelics have little or no recognized therapeutic use.

---

[7]Diethyltryptamine (DET), dimethyltryptamine (DMT) and a number of other synthetic agents are also classified as psychedelics.

The characteristics of dependence on the various psychedelic agents are not sufficiently alike to permit them to be described as a single type. We shall discuss only the LSD and marihuana types.

Drug Dependence of the LSD Type

The state of dependence developed to LSD is also characteristic of the dependence developed to its related derivatives and to mescaline, psilocybin and psilocin. These agents differ in potency and duration of action but exhibit cross-tolerance to each other.

As little as 20 to 25μg of LSD may produce effects in susceptible individuals, and these may last from eight to twelve hours. The nature of the psychedelic state induced is not predictable in advance and is influenced by the setting of drug use as well as by the mood and expectations of the user. However, certain physical, psychologic and perceptual effects are included in most descriptions of the drug experience ("trip"), and these are summarized in Table 12-5. The perceptual changes are the most notable.

The patterns of abuse in the LSD group of drugs is different from that of most other drugs of abuse. The most common pattern is an occasional use at weekly or monthly intervals. Regular use of LSD following initial exposure is now the exception rather than the rule. Even among chronic users the drugs are rarely taken more than twice a week.

Although marked tolerance develops rapidly to the behavioral effects of LSD, it also disappears quickly. Since no physical dependence develops, the user has little compulsion to increase dose or to continue use to avoid the discomfort of its absence. The real and potential hazards of the psychedelic drugs lie in the unpredictability and unreliability of the effects which they may produce and in the frequency of unpleasant or disastrous experiences (bad trips). The syndromes produced by these psychedelics are psychologically harmful to the individual and may be manifested as either acute, recurrent or prolonged reactions.

The acute reactions, estimated to occur in about 10 per cent of those who experiment with LSD or related drugs, are of short duration and are usually treatable by reassurance or by sedative drugs or tranquilizers. The acute psychotoxic reactions may be characterized by uncontrollable excitement, confusion, or acute paranoia or all of these. The acute panic reactions appear as secondary responses to drug-induced

Table 12-5. The Major Effects Produced by the LSD Group of Drugs

Physical: Dizziness; increased heart rate; pupillary dilation; muscular weakness; numbness; tremors; dry mouth; nausea, vomiting; decreased appetite

Psychologic: Altered moods; inner tension relieved by laughing or crying; euphoria (sometimes dysphoria); sense of retardation of time; decreased ability to concentrate; difficulty in expressing thoughts and feelings; depersonalization; introspection; dream-like state; poor memory; rapid thoughts; impaired judgment; great anxiety and tension

Perceptual: Blurred vision; altered shapes and colors; great heightening of color intensity; increased acuity of hearing; colors are heard, sounds may be seen; perceptual distortion of space; organized visual illusions and hallucinations

effects. The sensory distortions and powerful emotions elicited by the drug produce in some individuals an overwhelming tension and anxiety, a fear of losing one's mind and an abject sense of helplessness. In the grip of such reactions the individual may expose himself to dangerous situations or engage in behavior that threatens his life. Deaths attributable to the direct actions of the drugs are unknown, but deaths by drowning, falling out of windows and walking into the path of automobiles have occurred. It is immaterial whether such deaths were accidental or suicidal.

Recurrent reactions may appear up to a year after the last use of drug and without further exposure to the psychedelic. They usually involve the spontaneous return of perceptual distortions and a reliving of the earlier traumatic experiences. These "flashbacks" may vary in length from a few seconds to a half hour, but occur unpredictably.

The prolonged reactions may be exhibited as chronic anxiety states or chronic psychoses. The former are a relatively common occurrence and are accompanied by time and space distortion, difficulty in functioning and depression stemming from the morbid or terrifying feelings or thoughts experienced during drug use. It is not certain whether the small number of individuals who develop prolonged psychotic reactions would have developed these same conditions in the absence of the use of psychedelic drugs.

Although the psychologic and social dangers associated with the use of LSD-like drugs are incontrovertible, the evidence for drug-induced chromosomal abnormalities and projected dangers to the unborn human remains equivocal. Since any drug used during gestation may entail a certain risk to the fetus, the better part of wisdom dictates the avoidance of psychedelics as well as other drugs during pregnancy.

The use of the LSD group of drugs has declined since 1967, perhaps as a consequence of the recognition of the real hazards attendant on their use. But current use of LSD and other psychedelic drugs among 12- to 17-year-olds is about 0.9 per cent, about twice that among older individuals.

Drug Dependence of the Marihuana Type

The hemp plant *Cannabis sativa* is the source of the ancient drug cannabis and its products, variously referred to as *hashish, charas, bhang, ganja, dagga,* and *marihuana.* Active ingredients are found in all parts of both male and female plants, with the highest concentration occurring in the flowers. The most potent natural supply of *cannabis* is the resinous exudate obtained from the flower clusters; in the Middle East and North Africa the resin is called *hashish.* In the United States, the term *marihuana* is used to refer to any part of the plant or its extracts. The drug is most commonly used in Western countries as a mixture of leaves and flowers incorporated into cigarettes.

The active ingredients in cannabis are tetrahydrocannabinols (THC); the particular isomer believed to be responsible for most of the psychologic effects characteristic of marihuana is delta-9-tetrahydrocannabinol (Δ^9-THC). This active ingredient has been synthesized, and data are now accumulating that implicate some of the metabolic products of Δ^9-THC as agents capable of producing central nervous system effects.

As with LSD, the subjective effects produced by marihuana are influenced by the state of mind, mood and expectations of the user and by the specific circumstances in which the drug is used. Alone and in a quiet setting, the user usually feels drowsy; in company, he is inclined to be talkative and hilarious. Experience also plays a role in the effects produced. Naive subjects appear to experience fewer of the subjective effects for which marihuana is used and more impairment of motor and intellectual ability than experienced smokers.

The content of active ingredients contained in materials available for smoking varies rather widely due to normal variation in the plant itself and to methods of preparing the cigarettes. However, the experienced smoker usually requires only one to two cigarettes to produce the effects desired. These are generally described as a sleepy, happy, dreamy state of altered consciousness, associated with uncontrollable and freely flowing ideas and changes in the perception of time, space, objects and sounds. When larger doses are taken, either as the crude preparation or as the purified Δ^9-THC, the subjective effects become remarkably like those elicited by LSD (Table 12-6). Whereas there appear to be few differences in the quality of the subjective effects induced by the two drugs, those induced by marihuana are usually milder and more predictable. Also, a much lower degree of tolerance is developed to the effects of marihuana than to those of LSD. But despite the similarity in their subjective effects, the two drugs show no cross-tolerance, a fact indicative of different mechanisms of action. Moreover, there are dissimilarities in the physiologic effects produced by the two drugs. Unlike LSD, marihuana has a sedative action, does not dilate pupils and does not significantly alter blood pressure.

Marihuana and alcohol are also frequently compared with each other, since the patterns of their social group use are similar. First, the recreational use of either drug in low or moderate doses does not necessarily lead to a state of drug dependence. Second, although low doses of both drugs tend to produce sedation in nonsocial use, in the group environment they induce a loquacious euphoria and increased sociability, often accompanied by hilarity. These effects are characteristic of a depression of inhibitory control mechanisms. As a consequence, judgment is impaired and motor skills affected, which make the user of low doses of either marihuana or alcohol a potential hazard behind the wheel of an automobile; these hazards are increased when there is concurrent use of both drugs, since marihuana and alcohol produce additive

Table 12-6: The Major Effects Produced by Tetrahydrocannabinol

Physical: Dizziness; increased heart rate; reddening of the conjunctivae ("red eyes"); dry mouth; nausea; vomiting; drowsiness; increased appetite

Psychologic: Altered mood; euphoria; elation; uncontrollable laughter; sense of retardation of time; decreased ability to concentrate; difficulty in expressing thoughts and feelings; depersonalization; introspection; dream-like state; poor memory (later good); rapid thoughts; impairment of judgment

Perceptual: Blurred vision; altered shapes and colors; heightening of color intensity; increased acuity of hearing; colors are heard, sounds may be seen; perceptual distortion of space; vivid hallucinations

impairment of performance of some motor tasks. In the use of marihuana, alterations in the perception of time and space may also contribute to decreased driving skills. However, the individual who is "high" on marihuana, unlike the user of alcohol, does not show ataxia, or motor incoordination, and thus does not alert those around him to his inability to function responsibly.

There are still other dissimilarities between the effects of low or moderate doses of marihuana and alcohol which may be of even more significance in their use. Marihuana, even when used in the group setting, tends to make the user introspective, whereas persons under the influence of alcohol behave like extroverts. Such differences in the behavioral response to the two drugs may account for the fact that the individual under the influence of marihuana is much less aggressive and violent and less likely to commit crime than is the person intoxicated with alcohol. Nor does the development of strong psychologic dependence drive the marihuana user to commit crime to appease his drug hunger. On the other hand, the smoking of only a few marihuana cigarettes can produce a temporary state of paranoia in some individuals, a side-effect rarely associated with the use of low doses of alcohol. Recent studies with synthetic tetrahydrocannabinol show that these psychotic reactions may also occur in some subjects who receive small doses of the pure chemical.

The continued use of high doses of either marihuana or alcohol may lead to a state of psychologic dependence. But the dependence on marihuana, unlike that on alcohol, is not characterized by the development of physical dependence or significant tolerance. There is, therefore, no characteristic abstinence syndrome when the use of marihuana is discontinued and no compulsion to continue its use to avoid discomfort. Individuals who have developed a strong psychologic dependence on marihuana display marked lethargy, inertia and self-neglect; they also may be subject to severe psychologic reactions. Whether such psychologic dependence is an emotional disorder introduced by the drug or a symptom of underlying emotional disturbance in the user cannot be stated with any factual certainty. More data of how marihuana produces its effects are needed before valid conclusions can be drawn.

Whereas the moderate social use of marihuana does not appear to be seriously deleterious, the effects of its long-term, chronic use are unknown. We do know that in some societies, the continued abuse of potent preparations, particularly hashish, has been associated with social degradation; it is not clear, however, which is the cause and which the effect. Again, more knowledge of the physical, personal and social consequences of the abusive use of marihuana is required before definitive judgments may be made. But it must be borne in mind that alcohol, the drug most widely used for social purposes, is also the drug most frequently abused in Western society. Although millions of people use alcohol for a temporary escape from reality and are able to control their drug use, other millions lose control over their intake and become drug-dependent. It is also interesting to note that alcoholism, known since biblical times, became a serious sociologic problem only after the invention of distillation and the introduction of alcoholic beverages more potent than the previously used wine or beer. The problems of opiate dependence and cocaine abuse were also magnified by technologic advances: the isolation of the pure drugs from their plant origin and the invention of the syringe. Now, not only have the active ingredients of *Cannabis sativa* been isolated in pure form, but Δ^9-THC has also been synthesized. Thus, until more factual knowledge is available, there is some justification for viewing the sequelae of the continued abuse of marihuana from the perspective of past experience with other drugs of dependence. It is also noteworthy that the use of marihuana is increasing, whereas the nonmedical use of other agents appears to have levelled off.

While efforts to gain a better understanding of the long-term consequences of the abusive use of marihuana are continuing, studies to determine its potential value as a therapeutic agent are also being carried out. There is presumptive evidence already available to indicate that marihuana may be effective in the treatment of some cases of glaucoma and in controlling the side-effects of cancer chemotherapy. There appears to be little hazard associated with the moderate, controlled use of marihuana and numerous studies have shown that both cannabis and Δ^9-THC have an extremely wide margin of safety. Therefore, if convincing data on therapeutic efficacy are obtained, marihuana may find acceptance as an agent safe for medical use.

SYNOPSIS

The drugs most likely to be used, if not compulsively abused, for nonmedical purposes are those which affect the central nervous system; they alter mood and behavior in ways that satisfy the emotional needs of certain individuals. The therapeutic agents most commonly used for the subjective effects they produce include alcohol, the sedative-hypnotics like the barbiturates, the narcotic analgesics, the amphetamines and cocaine. The agents without proven therapeutic usefulness that are most widely abused are LSD and marihuana. However, all these compounds represent only a fraction of the agents of both synthetic and plant origin that are involved in contemporary drug abuse.

All the agents used for subjective rather than medical purposes have one property in common: they are capable of eliciting in certain individuals a state of mind in which the user feels that the effects produced by the drug are necessary for his well-being. This psychologic dependence (formerly termed *habituation*) may range from a persistent desire for the drug to an undeniable compulsion to obtain and take the drug at any cost. This psychologic dependence develops in some, but not all, persons who use a drug repeatedly; these susceptible individuals are thought to have personality disturbances antecedent to drug use.

The development of psychic dependence on certain drugs, requiring their periodic or continuous administration, leads to an altered physiologic state. This condition of physical dependence (formerly termed *addiction*) is revealed only when the body is forced to do without the drug or, in the case of opioids, when a specific antagonist is administered. Tolerance, the need for increased dosage to produce the desired effect, is also induced by many of the drugs that create dependence, especially those that induce physical dependence. Physical dependence and tolerance are powerful factors in reinforcing the influence of psychologic dependence.

The particular type of dependence developed to a given drug may be characterized in terms of:

1. The degree of psychologic dependence induced
2. The presence or absence of physical dependence
3. The symptoms of the syndrome which develops when the drug inducing the physical dependence is discontinued
4. The degree of tolerance developed upon repeated administration

Strong psychologic and physical dependence accompanied by marked tolerance are characteristic of the states of dependence developed to the general depressants of the central nervous system and to the opioids. Alcohol and the barbiturates are the most commonly abused central nervous system depressants, but this group also includes nonbarbiturate sedative-hypnotics and the drugs classified as minor tranquilizers. The opioid category includes the natural and partially synthetic agents derived from opium as well as the wholly synthetic compounds. The barbiturate-alcohol type of dependence differs from dependence of the morphine type with respect to (1) the symptoms exhibited during drug use; (2) the course of development of dependence; (3) the withdrawal syndrome precipitated by discontinuance of drug administration; and (4) the limits of tolerance developed.

During chronic intoxication with barbiturates or alcohol, the user is accident-prone through incomplete development of tolerance to the sedative action and to the effects of the drugs on motor coordination. There is also impairment of mental acuity, confusion and increased emotional instability. Aggressiveness, violence and crime are associated with the use of the general depressants, not only in the user's efforts to procure his drug but also during the time he is under the influence of the drug. In contrast, the opioid user can function with reasonable efficiency both occupationally and socially as long as he is able to obtain an adequate supply of drug. With drug dependence of the morphine type, violence and crime are primarily related to the user's need to procure his drug.

Mild psychic dependence may occur with low or therapeutic doses of alcohol and barbiturates. However, strong psychologic dependence, physical dependence and tolerance develop only after continued use of doses above the socially acceptable or usual therapeutic levels of alcohol and barbiturates, respectively. On the other hand, dependence of the morphine type is created by doses within the therapeutic range and is set in motion by the very first dose. The symptoms of withdrawal from the alcohol-barbiturate class of drugs and from the opioids are extremely unpleasant and severe. But abrupt withdrawal from the general depressant drugs is much more dangerous than that from the opioids and may be life-threatening. The tolerance developed to the barbiturate-alcohol class of drugs is incomplete; there is considerable persistence of behavioral disturbances and little increase in the dose levels that produce toxic symptoms or death in nontolerant individuals. In contrast, marked tolerance develops to all the effects of the morphine-like drugs with the exception of their effects on the pupil and gastrointestinal tract.

The development of physical dependence is also characteristic of dependence of the amphetamine type. However, the degree of physical dependence developed to these central nervous system stimulant drugs is mild and is revealed upon withdrawal as a state of mental and physical depression. Dependence on other central nervous system stimulants, such as cocaine, or on the psychedelics, such as LSD and marihuana, does not involve physical dependence and, consequently, there is no characteristic abstinence syndrome. However, marked tolerance does develop with persistent use of the amphetamines and LSD. The continued use of high doses of marihuana also induces some tolerance, but there is no evidence of tolerance to cocaine even when it is used in huge quantities.

The high degree of psychic dependence developed to the amphetamines or cocaine can lead to a profound and dangerous type of drug abuse. Unlike the opiate user, the user of central nervous system stimulants is hyperactive and may respond by violence and criminal activity to the paranoid delusions associated with the toxicity induced by high doses. In contrast, the chief dangers associated with the use of the psychedelics, particularly LSD, are related to the individual rather than to society. There is no longer any controversy about the fact that the use of the LSD-type drugs entails significant psychologic hazards. The unpredictability of the outcome and the high risk of a bad drug experience, particularly in the unwary and unprepared, are now well recognized. Psychologic reactions also occur in some individuals who take small amounts of marihuana. Although the effects of marihuana are milder and more predictable than those of LSD, the long-term physical or psychologic effects of using marihuana are not yet known. It is currently believed that the chronic abuse of marihuana, as opposed to its periodic use, is primarily a symptom of emotional disturbance or mental instability. In light of our present knowledge, or lack of it, caution is indicated in the use of marihuana to avoid the risk of the development of psychologic dependence so characteristic of the social use of alcohol.

GUIDES FOR STUDY AND REVIEW

What is the basic cell unit of the nervous system? What is an afferent or sensory neuron? an efferent or motor neuron? What is a synapse? How is information transmitted from one unit of the nervous system to another? What are neurohumors and what is their function? What are the two most important chemicals identified as neurohumors outside the central nervous system?

The hypothalamus is concerned with the control and regulation of what important bodily functions? What is the functional role of the cerebral cortex in humans? the limbic system? What is the functional role of the reticular activating system (the RAS)? In general, how do various types of drugs influence the activity of the RAS and what is the result of such interaction? How can the effect of low doses of alcohol or barbiturates be explained in terms of their influence on the RAS?

What does the term *drug abuse* mean? What kinds of therapeutic agents and non-medicinal chemicals are commonly drugs of abuse? What do we mean by the term "drug misuse?"

What does the term *drug dependence* mean? Why is this a better term to use in connection with drugs of abuse than the older terms *drug addiction* and *drug habituation*? What are the two distinct and independent components of drug dependence?

What is psychologic dependence? What is physical dependence? Which of these two components of drug dependence is always present in the abusive use of drugs? Why? Can physical dependence develop to some drugs that are not drugs of abuse? Can physical dependence develop to some drugs of abuse under conditions which do not lead to drug dependence? What is the most characteristic feature of the state of physical dependence?

What is the relationship between the phenomena of drug tolerance and drug dependence? Can tolerance be produced to drugs that have little potential for abusive use? Does tolerance develop to all drugs that are drugs of abuse? With what types of drugs of abuse is the phenomen of tolerance almost invariably associated?

What drugs are included in the category of "general depressants of the central nervous system (CNS)"? What are the characteristics of the drug-dependent state that develops to this category of drugs? Does physical dependence develop to all these agents? What are the characteristic symptoms of withdrawal of these agents? How does the severity of the withdrawal syndrome associated with the alcohol-barbiturate type of drug dependence differ from that of the morphine type? How do the limits of tolerance developed to the general depressants of the CNS differ from those developed to the narcotic analgesics?

What drugs are included in the category of narcotic analgesics? What are the characteristics of the drug-dependent state that develops to this category of drugs? How does the course of development of dependence to the narcotic analgesics differ from that to the general depressants of the CNS? What is the outstanding difference between the morphine and alcohol-barbiturate types of drug dependence with respect to harm to the drug abuser and society when the drug may be obtained by legitimate means?

What are some of the commonly abused drugs classified as CNS stimulants? How does the drug-dependent state developed to amphetamine differ from that to cocaine, particularly with respect to physical dependence and tolerance? Why is the compulsive use of CNS stimulants a serious threat to the life of the drug abuser and to society?

How is the term *psychedelic* defined? How does the drug-dependent state developed to LSD differ from that to marihuana, particularly with respect to tolerance? How does the drug-dependent state developed to marihuana differ from that to alcohol?

SUGGESTED READING

Braude, M.C., and Szara, S. (eds.). *Pharmacology of Marijuana.* New York: Raven Press, 1976.

Brecher, E.M., and Eds. of Consumer Reports. *Licit and Illicit Drugs.* Mt. Vernon, N.Y.: Consumers Union, 1972.

Deneau, G.A., and Seever, M.H. Pharmacological aspects of drug dependence. *Adv. Pharmacol.* 4:143, 1964.

Eccles, J.C. *The Understanding of the Brain.* New York: McGraw-Hill, 1973.

Eddy, N.B., Halbach, H., Isbell, H., and Seevers, M.H. Drug dependence: Its significance and characteristics. *Bull. WHO* 32:721, 1965.

Efron, D.H. *Psychotomimetic Drugs.* New York: Raven, 1970.

Freedman, D.X. The psychopharmacology of hallucinogenic agents. *Annu. Rev. Med.* 20:409, 1969.

Freedman, D.X. The use and abuse of LSD. *Arch. Gen. Psychiatry* 18:300, 1968.

Guyton, A.C. *Textbook of Medical Physiology.* Philadelphia: Saunders, 1971. Chaps. 60 and 62.

Hicks, R.E., and Fink, D.J. (eds.). *Psychedelic Drugs.* New York: Grune & Stratton, 1969.

Ray, O.S. *Drugs, Society, and Human Behavior.* St. Louis: C.V. Mosby, 1972.

Schuster, C.R., and Thompson, T.T. Self-administration of and behavioral dependence on drugs. *Annu. Rev. Pharmacol.* 9:483, 1969.

Wallgren, H., and Barry, H., III (eds.). *Actions of Alcohol.* New York: American Elsevier, 1971.

Wittenborn, J.R., Brill, H., Smith, J.P., and Wittenborn, S.A. (eds.). *Drugs and Youth,* Proceedings of the Rutgers Symposium on Drug Abuse. Springfield, Ill.: Thomas, 1969.

13. HOW DRUGS ALTER PHYSIOLOGIC FUNCTION: A RECAPITULATION

When we first began our discussions of how drugs act on the living organism, we noted that most drugs have a chemical basis of action. The obvious exceptions are protective agents — such as the **demulcents** and **emollients** — which, when applied to the skin or mucous membranes, act by purely mechanical means to alleviate or prevent irritation; or osmotically active agents — for example, the cathartic magnesium sulfate and the diuretic urea — which act in a physical manner to retain water within the lumen of the gastrointestinal tract and renal tubules, respectively. But the mechanism of action of most drugs, either those acting locally or systemically, involves a chemical reaction between the drug and a functionally important constituent of the living system. The interaction may be as simple as the neutralization of gastric acidity by an orally ingested inorganic base, but for the great majority of drugs, the interaction is with a receptor. Yet, irrespective of whether a drug combines with a receptor or with an identifiable functional entity such as an enzyme, the end result of the interaction — the drug effect — is a *quantitative* alteration in a physiologic function or biochemical process. The *qualitative* nature of the drug effect is determined by the interacting component's functional role in the physiology of the organism. And it is the extent of our knowledge of the physiologic function subserved by the component with which the drug interacts and of the physicochemical basis of this interaction that delimits our understanding of the primary action of the drug.

Even though the primary actions of few drugs have been fully elucidated, it seems worthwhile to summarize succinctly what we know in general about the different types of mechanisms by which drugs may influence and alter biochemical processes and physiologic functions. We shall look first at the cell, and briefly review the ways in which drugs may affect the fundamental functions of protoplasm: metabolism, growth, adaptability and reproduction. We shall then turn our attention to the highly complex organization of cells called a human being. We shall exemplify how drugs influence the systems that regulate, coordinate and integrate the constituent parts so that they operate as a whole by considering the ways in which drugs affect the autonomic nervous system.

371

DRUG ACTIONS INFLUENCING THE FUNDAMENTAL PROPERTIES COMMON TO ALL CELLS

The characteristic unit of life is the cell; it is also the unit of structure and of development. This smallest unit of living matter has certain functions and displays certain properties which, taken together, are considered peculiar to viable organisms. In unicellular forms, in which the single cell is the entire organism, as well as in multicellular beings, these functions of the individual cell are the same, although they may be performed differently by different species. The cell assimilates and metabolizes; it takes in materials from its surroundings and chemically changes them into energy and new substances it needs and uses for repair, growth or reproduction. And for the maintenance of the dynamic equilibrium called "life," cells also possess adaptability, the property of reacting and adjusting, more or less successfully, to environmental changes. These manifold life activities of the cell are performed in an orderly, coordinated fashion, governed by the organization of its biochemical systems into specific cellular structures.

As we stated in earlier discussions of mechanisms of drug action, efforts to identify the various cellular substances and systems functioning to maintain the life of the individual cell have been particularly successful. Thus the mechanisms of action of many drugs that affect cell function by acting intracellularly to modify enzymic reactions essential for energy production, growth or reproduction have been elucidated. The sulfonamides, for example, compete with para-aminobenzoic acid (PABA) and interfere with its incorporation into folic acid, a metabolite essential for the normal growth of various species of bacteria (cf. p. 260). The antibiotic streptomycin inhibits the synthesis of normal proteins, an action that ultimately results in the death of the microorganism. Anticancer agents also act to damage vital cellular functions in a number of different ways and thereby inhibit the growth or replication of malignant cells (cf. p. 195).

These few examples illustrate an important point that bears repeating about the effects typical of drugs that are cytotoxic poisons (cf. p. 306). When the mechanism of drug action involves interference with the internal metabolic activities of a normally functioning cell, the effects produced are, almost without exception, harmful to the cell. Drugs with such actions are obviously useful, however, when they are employed by an economic species to eliminate an uneconomic species. Thus the value of the antimicrobial agents lies in the fact that they are *selectively toxic* to undesirable unicellular organisms; they act on a process essential either for reproduction or growth of the microorganism. The same process is either nonessential or nonexistent in the vital functions of most mammalian cells. Antitumor agents, however, have limited selectivity of action against undesirable, malignant cells and frequently attack rapidly proliferating normal mammalian cells (cf. pp. 306–307). And there are many other therapeutic agents, as well as nontherapeutic drugs, that produce serious, and sometimes fatal, complications in humans through their direct effects on vital functions of normal cells (cf. pp. 306–307). Some of the toxic symptoms of overdosage with aspirin, for instance, are attributable to the drug's effect on the normal cellular oxidation of glucose.

Drugs that act intracellularly may have salutary effects, however, when their actions are directed at enzyme systems functioning at other than normal levels. For example, dimercaprol (BAL, British antilewisite) may be effectively used as a specific antidote to restore the activity of cellular enzymes poisoned by mercury or arsenic (cf. pp. 333–335). Drugs that affect cellular metabolism may also be beneficially used in certain disease states characterized by aberrant enzyme activity. There is evidence to indicate, for instance, that most patients with gout produce too much uric acid. This normal waste material of humans (and certain other species) is the end product of the metabolism of purines derived, in turn, from the breakdown of the proteins of the cell nucleus. When the amount of uric acid in the blood is elevated, this relatively insoluble compound tends to deposit in the cartilage of various parts of the body. Allopurinol, a drug that inhibits an enzyme involved in the synthesis of uric acid, represents a rational approach to the therapy of gout aimed at decreasing the amount of uric acid produced.

Drugs may also act at the cell surface to disrupt structural integrity or to alter the rate of transport of substances essential for the metabolic activity of the cell. We have seen, for example, that in bacteria a rigid cell wall is a structure essential for maintaining the high osmotic pressure characteristic of these microorganisms (cf. p. 261). Interference with cell-wall formation, as by the action of penicillin or the cephalosporins, produces organisms that rupture when in their usual hypotonic environment. Agents such as nystatin and amphotericin B inhibit the growth of certain pathogenic fungi by disturbing the fundamental integrity of the cell membrane and allowing leakage of ions and various small water-soluble molecules from the cell interior. These agents display selective toxicity; they are effective against some but not all fungi and are without effect on bacteria, viruses or mammalian host cells. Their antifungal activity is known to depend on binding to sterols present in the membrane of only the drug-sensitive fungi, but how this drug binding disrupts the integrity of the membrane is not known (cf. p. 447).

DRUG ACTIONS INFLUENCING THE AUTONOMIC NERVOUS SYSTEM

Traditionally the nervous system is divided into central and peripheral parts, the *central nervous system* (CNS) consisting of the brain and spinal cord, and the *peripheral nervous system* comprising the cranial, spinal and peripheral nerves with their motor and sensory endings. The peripheral nervous system, in turn, is subdivided into the *somatic* and the *autonomic nervous systems.* The somatic nervous system innervates those parts of the body that are under voluntary control; it is concerned with consciously influenced functions such as movement of the muscles of locomotion and posture. In contrast, the autonomic nervous system (ANS) supplies all structures of the body except the skeletal muscles; it is concerned with the maintenance of homeostasis, does not require conscious activation and is largely automatic in its operation. Indeed, many of the organs innervated by the ANS can continue to carry out some of their functions when their nervous connections to the CNS are severed; intestinal segments can contract and the heart can beat and pump fluid even when completely removed from the body. However, only an intact ANS can provide the fine control of cardiac function, blood flow, digestion and other **visceral** or internal functions of the body essential for maintaining the internal environment within the limits compatible with life.

The classic division of the nervous system into central and peripheral and somatic and autonomic, although descriptively convenient, implies separations that really do not exist either anatomically or functionally. Skeletal muscles, for example, are supplied by motor nerve fibers that are axons of cells entirely within the CNS. And the normal functioning of the ANS is dependent on centers of integration within the brain such as those in the hypothalamus that regulate body temperature, water balance, fat and carbohydrate metabolism and other visceral functions (cf. p. 346). Whereas there are distinct differences between autonomic and somatic efferent neurons (Fig. 13-1, Table 13-1), the afferent components of these two systems are identical, and in the CNS there is extensive overlap between autonomic and somatic centers of integration. Somatic responses are always accompanied by visceral responses and visceral activity modifies somatic reactions. For instance, the sight and smell of a steak cooking over a charcoal fire stimulates the flow of saliva and gastric juices in preparation for ingestion and digestion; during digestion the increased blood flow through the gastrointestinal tract tends to decrease the capacity of skeletal muscle to do work. Thus the activities of the somatic and autonomic nervous systems are coordinated and interdependent.

Although the sensory components and the central control centers of the ANS are essential to its normal functioning, we shall confine our discussion to its efferent

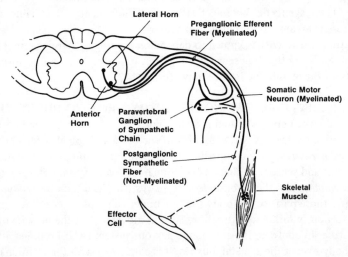

FIGURE 13-1. Cross-section of thoracic segment of spinal cord showing general arrangement of somatic and autonomic efferent neurons. Somatic neuron (solid line) has its cell body in the anterior horn and its axon terminal in skeletal muscle. Preganglionic fiber of sympathetic autonomic nervous system has its cell body in the lateral horn and synapses in ganglion outside spinal cord with postganglionic fiber (dashed line) to effector cell.

Table 13-1. Differences Between Autonomic and Somatic Motor Nerves

	Autonomic	Somatic
Structures innervated	All structures of the body except skeletal muscles	Skeletal muscles
Neuron in functional contact with effector		
Cell body	Completely outside CNS	Within CNS
Axon	Generally nonmyelinated	Myelinated
Effect of interruption of cerebrospinal nerve	Some automatic activity independent of innervation	Complete paralysis of skeletal muscle innervated

Table 13-2. Characteristic Differences Between the Sympathetic and Parasympathetic nervous systems

	Sympathetic	Parasympathetic
Origin of preganglionic fibers	Thoracic and upper lumbar segments of spinal cord	Brainstem and sacral segment of spinal cord
Ganglia	Near CNS	Near effector cell
Length of fibers		
Preganglionic	Short	Long
Postganglionic	Long	Short
Ratio of pre- to postganglionic fibers	High, may be 1:20 or more	Usually low — 1:1 or 1:2
Response to stimulation	Diffuse	Discrete
Preganglionic transmitter	Acetylcholine (ACh)	ACh
Postganglionic transmitter	Norepinephrine (most cases); ACh for sweat glands and blood vessels of skeletal muscles	ACh

pathways and **effector** organs. For it is only in the peripheral ANS that our knowledge of structure, physiologic function and biochemical processes is sufficient to explain the mechanisms by which drugs affect the system. To facilitate our understanding of these mechanisms, we shall briefly describe the most germane aspects of the anatomy and physiology of the efferent autonomic system and discuss the biochemical reactions underlying transmission of information within the system.

General Aspects of the Anatomy and Function of the Peripheral Autonomic Nervous System

On the motor side, the autonomic nervous system is separated into two main divisions, the *sympathetic* and the *parasympathetic.* The motor pathways of both systems consist of two neurons; the first, the *preganglionic* fiber has its origin within the brain or spinal cord but synapses with the second, the *postganglionic* fiber, outside the CNS. Most viscera are supplied with postganglionic fibers of both divisions. However, even though most viscera are functionally innervated by both the sympathetic and parasympathetic nerves, the actions of these two systems are almost always physiologically antagonistic (see Table 13-3). And albeit that the efferents of both divisions are

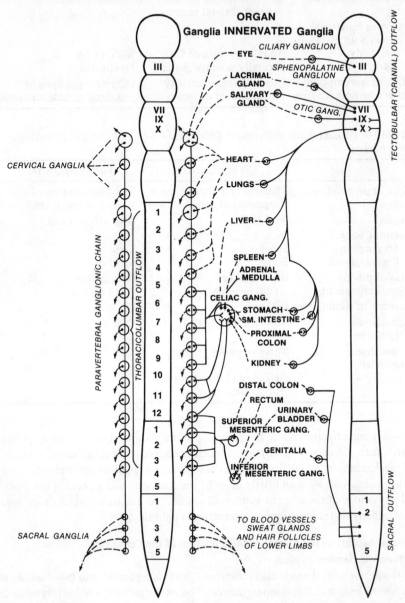

FIGURE 13-2. Schematic diagram of the two divisions of the autonomic nervous system. The diagram on the left shows the origin of the sympathetic nerves and the organs they innervate; that on the right shows the parasympathetic system and the organs it innervates.

similar in origin and number of neurons, their respective preganglionic fibers issue from entirely different segments of the CNS and synapse differently in relation to the viscera innervated. These and the other differences between the two divisions (noted below and summarized in Table 13-2) clearly establish that differentiation of the efferent ANS into two major divisions has both structural and functional significance.

Anatomical Considerations

SYMPATHETIC NERVOUS SYSTEM. The sympathetic division of the ANS is also called the *thoracicolumbar division* since the cells that give rise to its preganglionic fibers are located primarily in the thoracic and upper lumbar segments of the spinal cord (Fig. 13-2). The myelinated axons from these cells leave the spinal cord in the anterior nerve roots and synapse with postganglionic sympathetic nerves lying in ganglia outside the CNS. These synapses occur either in the ganglia of the paravertebral sympathetic chains that lie on each side of the spinal column throughout its length, or in special collateral ganglia such as the superior mesenteric ganglia. The paravertebral ganglia are connected to each other by nerve trunks; preganglionic fibers issuing from one level may pass up or down the chain before synapsing, or may synapse with more than one sympathetic ganglion en route. Thus a single preganglionic fiber may make contact with a large number of postganglionic fibers and one ganglion may be innervated by several preganglionic nerves. These ramifications of preganglionic and postganglionic fibers account in large part for the diffuse response that usually follows stimulation of the sympathetic division of the ANS.

PARASYMPATHETIC NERVOUS SYSTEM. The preganglionic fibers that issue from the midbrain, the medulla oblongata and the sacral part of the spinal cord comprise the parasympathetic or craniosacral division of the ANS (see Fig. 13-2). The ganglia in which these fibers synapse are in, on, or near the organs innervated and, consequently, the postganglionic fibers of the parasympathetic division are very short (Fig. 13-3). This anatomic arrangement of motor neurons largely accounts for the limited and discrete response that is characteristically evoked by stimulation of parasympathetic fibers.

Functional Considerations

As stated above, the autonomic nervous system is an important part of the complex machinery by which the body keeps its internal environment constant. It maintains body temperature, fluid balance and the ionic composition of the blood; it regulates, in whole or in part, respiration, circulation, digestion, metabolism, the secretion of various **exocrine** glands and, in general, all those bodily activities that are not under voluntary control and that ordinarily function below the level of consciousness. The fine and rapid adjustment to ever-changing internal and external environments, the coordinated response to emergencies or vigorous muscular activity, and the conservation and restoration of energy are made possible because the component parts of the ANS, the sympathetic and parasympathetic divisions, have distinct and contrasting functions (Table 13-3).

The sympathetic nervous system is normally active at all times. As a dynamic system, it is not only involved in the moment-to-moment control of homeostatic needs

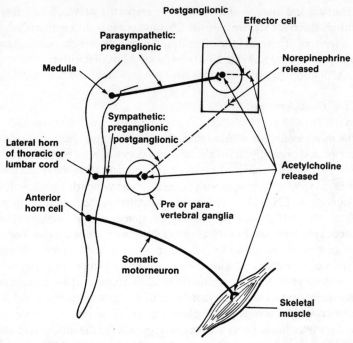

FIGURE 13-3. Schematic diagram of differences between sympathetic and parasympathetic neurons. Relatively short preganglionic fiber of sympathetic division originating in thoracic segment of cord is shown synapsing in ganglion outside central nervous system (CNS), a relatively long postganglionic fiber of sympathetic division terminates in an effector cell and releases norepinephrine on stimulation. Relatively long preganglionic neuron of parasympathetic division originating in medulla synapses in effector organ with relatively short postganglionic fiber. Somatic axon originating in lower segment of cord goes directly to skeletal muscle. Acetylcholine is released by preganglionic fibers of both sympathetic and parasympathetic nerves, by postganglionic parasympathetic fibers, and by somatic neurons.

during ordinary activity but is also capable of responding rapidly to emergencies and stressful situations. Anatomically the sympathetic division is geared to influence several organs simultaneously or to discharge as a unit and affect all the sympathetically innervated structures of the body. For example, in a situation that provokes fear or rage there is: an increase in heart rate, a rise in blood pressure, an increase in blood flow to skeletal muscles, a rise in the blood sugar concentration, a dilation of the bronchioles and increase in respiratory rate, a curtailment of gastrointestinal activity and dilation of the pupils of the eyes — all measures designed for "fight or flight." Many of these effects of massive discharge of the sympathetic system are reinforced by the epinephrine simultaneously released into the blood by the adrenal medulla.

   Although the sympathetic division is capable of so profoundly affecting the functional activity of the organism, this system and its associated adrenal medulla are not

Table 13-3. Basic Effects on Some Major Organ Systems Produced by Stimulation of Autonomic Nervous System

Effector	Sympathetic	Parasympathetic
Eye		
Pupil	Dilated	Constricted
Ciliary muscle		Contracted for near vision
Heart		
Rate (direct effect)	Increased	Decreased
Contractility	Increased	Slightly decreased or no effect
Bronchiolar smooth muscle	Relaxed	Contracted
Gastrointestinal tract		
Motility	Decreased	Increased
Sphincters	Constricted	Relaxed
Secretory activity	May be decreased	Increased
Salivary glands		
Secretory activity	Increased; thick mucous	Increased; watery, dilute saliva

essential to life. In the sheltered confines of the laboratory, the sympathectomized animal can continue a fairly normal existence. In the absence of sympathoadrenal functions, however, such an animal is much less resistant to environmental changes and is seriously deficient in protecting itself under stressful conditions.

The parasympathetic nervous system is concerned primarily with conserving and restoring energy. It slows the heart, lowers the blood pressure, constricts the pupil of the eye protecting the retina from excessive light, contracts the urinary bladder and the rectum for emptying of these organs, and aids in the digestion and absorption of nutrients by stimulating gastrointestinal movements and secretions. In general, the parasympathetic division controls functions essential for life. It is anatomically organized for discrete and localized actions on individual organs or regions; no useful purpose would be served were the parasympathetic system to participate in the massive discharge characteristic of the sympathetic division.

As we stated earlier, in most of the **smooth muscles** and visceral organs that are innervated by both divisions of the ANS the effects of the two systems are reciprocal. This is certainly the case, for example, in the heart, the bronchi, the gastrointestinal tract and the bladder (see Table 13-3). In other organs such as the salivary glands and pancreas, however, the influence of the two divisions is in the same direction — both stimulate secretion. And sometimes what appears functionally to be opposing actions may be the result of similar actions of the two divisions on opposing structures of the same organ. The involuntary adjustment of the eyes to changing light conditions is a case in point. The pupil of the eye dilates in response to sympathetic stimulation and constricts in response to increased parasympathetic activity. However, the nerve impulses of both divisions cause a muscle of the iris to contract; contraction of the radially oriented muscle innervated by sympathetic fibers produces dilation, and contraction of the circular muscle innervated by parasympathetic neurons produces constriction. Finally, it is important to point out that some organs are functionally innervated by only one division of the ANS: the adrenal medulla, spleen, sweat glands and probably the blood vessels of the viscera, skin and skeletal muscle are supplied only by the sympathetic division; focusing of the lens of the eye and lacrimation are controlled almost exclusively by the parasympathetic system.

Biochemical Aspects of Autonomic Nervous System Activity

The ability of the autonomic nervous system to elicit the appropriate, diffuse or discrete response to change in the internal or external environment depends upon the transmittal of information from sensors to effectors. The operation of this information system is partly electrical and partly chemical. Electrical phenomena account for the rapid transfer of information along the neuron; this passage of impulses along the nerve fiber to the nerve terminal is called *conduction. Transmission,* the process of passing information across a synapse from one neuron to another, or across a neuro-effector junction from nerve terminals to the cells innervated, is a chemical rather than an electrical process.

Transmission is mediated by specific chemical agents known as *neurohumoral transmitters* or *neurohumors*, which are synthesized in the neuron and stored in small vesicles at the axonal terminals (cf. p. 344). The sequence of events involved in neurohumoral transmission is as follows: (1) the arrival of the nerve impulse at the axonal terminals; (2) the release of the neurohumoral transmitter elicited by the nerve impulse; (3) diffusion of the transmitter across the synapse or neuro-effector junction; (4) combination of the transmitter with postjunctional receptors; (5) initiation of electrical or chemical activity in the postjunctional neuron or effector cell; and (6) destruction or removal of the neurotransmitter from the site of action.

The concept that nerves transmit their impulses across junctions by means of specific chemical agents is the foundation of the theory of neurohumoral transmission. This theory, which was first postulated at about the turn of the century[1] and which received direct experimental confirmation more than fifty years ago,[2] is now almost universally accepted. In the intervening years, however, only two agents have been identified and firmly established as neurotransmitters. These two are acetylcholine and norepinephrine.[3] The extensive data that have been collected concerning the details of

[1] T. R. Elliott, while a graduate student at Cambridge, England, postulated that sympathetic nerve impulses released an epinephrine-like substance and that this substance was the chemical step in junctional transmission. He published this hypothesis in *J. Physiol.* London, 32:401–467, 1905.

[2] Otto Loewi, who won the Nobel Prize in 1936 for work begun in 1921, established the first real proof of the chemical transmission of nerve impulses. The story of his brilliant research can be read in the words of Dr. Loewi, published a year before his death as "An Autobiographic Sketch" in *Perspectives Biol. & Med.* 4:3–25, 1960.

[3] See the footnote on page 344 which indicates that acetylcholine and norepinephrine have been established as neurotransmitters only in certain areas of the CNS.

chemical transmission in the peripheral nervous system have clearly shown that acetylcholine and norepinephrine each fulfill all the criteria of a putative neurotransmitter: (1) Acetylcholine and norepinephrine have been shown to be present at the axonal terminals of appropriate motor nerves. So too have the enzymes necessary for their synthesis and the structures required for their storage — two factors essential for ensuring that sufficient material will be available for release upon arrival of the propagated nerve impulse. (2) In experiments using isolated preparations, stimulation of appropriately innervated structures has led to the corresponding release of either acetylcholine or norepinephrine. The amounts of each compound recovered during periods of nerve stimulation were found to be in excess of those recoverable in the absence of stimulation. (3) The pharmacologic effects produced by the appropriate local administration of either acetylcholine or norepinephrine have been demonstrated to be identical with those elicited by stimulation of nerves containing the respective compound. (4) The responses elicited by stimulation of appropriate nerves or by the corresponding local administration of either acetylcholine or norepinephrine have also been shown to be affected by the same drugs and in like manner. (5) Finally, mechanisms have been identified for the rapid removal of acetylcholine and epinephrine from the immediate vicinity of their respective receptor sites. This termination of the action of the transmitters is essential if they are to be effective under dynamic conditions.

Thus acetylcholine and norepinephrine have gained acceptance as mediators in neurotransmission, since for each agent there is substantial evidence that: (1) it is present in the axon along with mechanisms for its synthesis, storage and destruction; (2) it is released from the nerve ending during stimulation; (3) the effects produced by its administration are the same as those in response to nerve stimulation; and (4) various drugs affect the responses to its administration and to nerve stimulation in the same way. Let us now examine in a little more detail the individual steps in transmission as they apply specifically to acetylcholine and to norepinephrine. We will then be ready to turn our attention to how the actions of **autonomic drugs** can be related to the individual events in neurohumoral transmission.

Acetylcholine

Acetylcholine has been identified and generally accepted as the chemical mediator at the axonal terminals of: (1) all preganglionic fibers of both divisions of the ANS and preganglionic nerves to the adrenal medulla; (2) all postganglionic fibers of the parasympathetic nervous system; and (3) some postganglionic fibers of the sympathetic nervous system such as those that innervate the sweat glands. Acetylcholine has also been clearly established as the chemical transmitter in all motor nerves of the somatic nervous system. Nerves that contain acetylcholine as the neurotransmitter are, by definition, *cholinergic nerves.*

The synthesis of acetylcholine is an example of the conjugation of a naturally occurring compound (cf. p. 146). Acetylcholine is the end product of the acetylation of choline, a normal dietary constituent as well as a compound that can be synthesized in the body from the amino acid serine. This conjugation reaction takes place in the axonal terminals of cholinergic nerves and is catalyzed by *choline acetyltransferase (choline acetylase)*, an enzyme that is also synthesized by the neuron.

The acetylcholine that is synthesized is stored in vesicles ("synaptic vesicles") in highly concentrated ionic form; it has been estimated that a single nerve terminal may contain 300,000 or more vesicles and that each vesicle may store from 1,000 to 50,000 molecules of acetylcholine.

When an impulse arrives at the nerve terminal, 100 or more of these vesicles synchronously discharge their content of acetylcholine, which then diffuses across the junctional cleft and combines with the specialized receptor of the postjunctional membrane. It is this binding of acetylcholine to its receptor that activates the next structure in the pathway (cf. pp. 42–43).

Destruction of the acetylcholine released in the process of cholinergic stimulation is accomplished by the enzyme acetylcholinesterase, which hydrolyzes the mediator to choline and acetic acid (cf. p. 141). So rapid is this hydrolysis at some sites that within milliseconds, the action of acetylcholine can be terminated and the postjunctional membrane again made responsive to nerve impulses. It is the strategic localization of acetylcholinesterase at the surface of postjunctional membranes that accounts for this rapid inactivation of the transmitter.

Norepinephrine

The role of norepinephrine as a neurohumoral agent is confined to postganglionic fibers of the sympathetic nervous system. Even within this system there are exceptions since, as noted above, the fibers to sweat glands and some vasodilator fibers

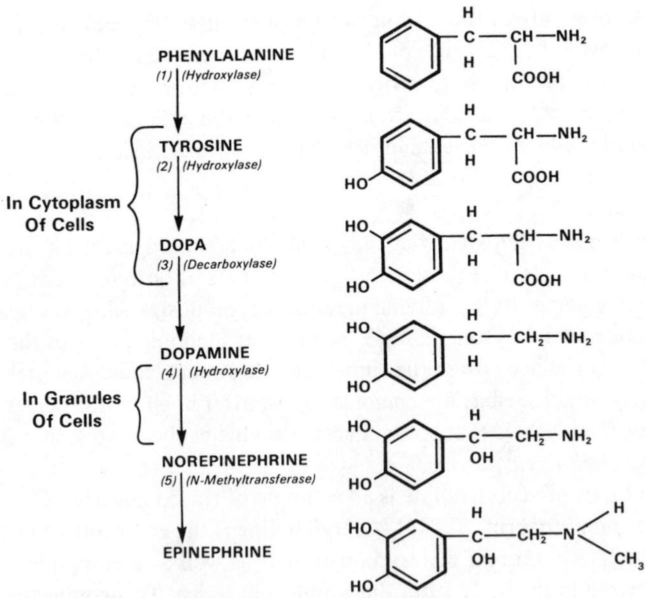

FIGURE 13-4. Synthesis of norepinephrine and epinephrine.

(found primarily in muscle) are cholinergic fibers. Nerves that release norepinephrine upon stimulation are called *adrenergic nerves.*

SYNTHESIS. The starting point for the synthesis of norepinephrine by the body is also an amino acid, but the total synthesis is more complicated than that for acetylcholine (Fig. 13-4). First of all, not all of the enzymes involved have the same locus of action: step 1 takes place outside the nerve terminals; steps 2 and 3 within the cytoplasm of the nerve ending; and step 4, the final step, within the storage granule (Fig. 13-5). Second, none of the enzymes in the sequence is specific for norepinephrine; the enzymes involved can catalyze similar reactions using other endogenous compounds and some drugs as substrates. For example, methyldopa, a drug used in the treatment of hypertension, not only inhibits the metabolism of dopa to dopamine (step 3) but can itself participate in steps 3 and 4 and be converted to methylnorepinephrine. We shall see later the pharmacologic significance of these interactions and how they can be used to explain mechanisms of drug action.

STORAGE AND RELEASE. The processes involved in the storage and release of the adrenergic transmitter are also more complicated than those for the cholinergic transmitter — some of the norepinephrine content of the nerve terminal exists as a dissociable complex within the storage granule. This form of the transmitter constitutes a *reserve pool* that is in equilibrium with an *intragranular mobile pool* of norepinephrine (pool MG in Fig. 13-5), which in turn is in equilibrium with the norepinephrine outside the storage granules, the *cytoplasmic mobile pool* (pool MC). The intragranular pools containing the more recently synthesized transmitter account for the norepinephrine that is released from adrenergic fibers in response to nerve stimulation.

DISPOSITION OF RELEASED NOREPINEPHRINE. Although there are two major enzymes, *catechol-O-methyl transferase* and *monoamine oxidase*, that can inactivate released norepinephrine (cf. pp. 148–149, 156), neither plays an important role in terminating the action of the adrenergic transmitter. Some small portion of the released norepinephrine diffuses away from the extracellular region and is metabolized, but the mechanism primarily responsible for the removal of norepinephrine from its receptor sites is the active reuptake by the axonal terminals. Obviously, this reentry into the nerve also conserves the transmitter and provides a source other than synthesis for maintaining adequate supplies in readiness for its functioning as a mediator of neurotransmission. Whereas diffusion along concentration gradients can account for the movement of released norepinephrine out of the axonal terminal, active transport processes are required for its reuptake: one transport system for reentry into the cytoplasmic pool and a second for active transport across the membrane of the granule to the intragranular mobile pool.

The various mechanisms for synthesis, storage, release and disposition of norepinephrine and their locations in the adrenergic nerve terminal are summarized in Figure 13-5.

Pharmacologic Considerations

Elucidation of basic cellular function and better understanding of drug action usually proceed in parallel. Thus, the validation of the role of acetylcholine and

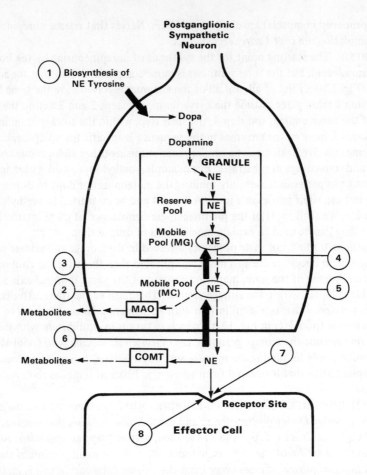

FIGURE 13-5. Schematic diagram of postganglionic sympathetic neuron showing sites of synthesis, storage release and metabolism of norepinephrine and the proposed sites of action of drugs that modify these processes. NE = norepinephrine; MAO = monoamine oxidase; COMT = catechol-O-methyltransferase. Heavy arrows symbolize active transport processes; light dashed arrows symbolize passive diffusion.

Sites of action that drugs can utilize to alter sympathetic activity and mechanisms by which the drugs act:

1. Interference with synthesis of transmitter: (a) inhibition of conversion of tyrosine to dopa, e.g., a-methyl-p-tyrosine; (b) enzymatic biotransformation of drug by same pathway utilized by NE, leading to synthesis of a "false transmitter," e.g., a-methyldopa competes with dopa; a-methyl-norepinephrine is formed and stored (see text).

2. Inhibition of monoamine oxidase leading to accumulation of norepinephrine at nerve ending, e.g., nialamide, tranylcypromine.

3. Blockade of active transport from cytoplasmic pool (MC) to intragranular stores, leading to depletion of latter and metabolism by monoamine oxidase of cytoplasmic norepinephrine, e.g., reserpine.

4. (a) Slow release of NE from storage granule, leading to depletion of transmitter, e.g., guanethidine; (b) Interference with release of granular stores of

norepinephrine in neurotransmission and the clarification of the sequence of events involved in the process at peripheral cholinergic and adrenergic terminals are of fundamental importance to pharmacology; the action of most drugs affecting the ANS can now be interpreted in terms of how they modify the synthesis, release, storage or disposition of a neurotransmitter, or stimulate or inhibit its interactions at receptor sites. The proposed sites of action of some drugs influencing transmission at an adrenergic junction are shown in Figure 13-5; Table 13-4 lists the individual steps in transmission at both cholinergic and adrenergic terminals and some representative agents that act at each point.

Drug Actions Influencing Transmitter Synthesis, Storage and Release
There are, of course, more ways in which drugs alter adrenergic transmission than cholinergic transmission, simply because the processes involved in the synthesis, storage and release of norepinephrine are more complex than those for acetylcholine. Let us, for example, consider the modes of action of hemicholinium, *a*-methyl-*p*-tyrosine (*a*-MT) and methyldopa, each of which interferes with neurotransmitter synthesis, thereby limiting the store of chemical mediator available for release. Hemicholinium blocks the synthesis of acetylcholine by inhibiting the active transport of choline from extracellular fluid into the cytoplasm of axonal terminals where the final step of synthesis occurs. *a*-Methyl-*p*-tyrosine blocks the synthesis of norepinephrine by inhibiting the enzyme responsible for the conversion of tyrosine to dopa (step 2 in Fig. 13-4). Methyldopa, on the other hand, is an inhibitor of norepinephrine synthesis because it effectively competes with dopa, the precursor of the normal transmitter, for the enzyme that catalyzes step 3 (Fig. 13-4). Since the enzymes involved in the synthesis of norepinephrine are relatively nonspecific, methyldopa can be decarboxylated and hydroxylated (steps 3 and 4, Fig. 13-4) to form *a*-methylnorepinephrine; the latter can be stored in granules and released by nerve stimulation, and, in general, act as a "false transmitter" at adrenergic receptor sites. It is a false transmitter only in the sense that it replaces the normal neurohumor. However, *a*-methylnorepinephrine has activity at neuroeffector junctions qualitatively identical to that of norepinephrine but quantitatively different at various sites of action.

There appear to be no drugs that interfere with the storage of acetylcholine in vesicles at the axonal terminal once it has been synthesized. And since little or none of the transmitter reenters the nerve terminal after its release, the available acetylcholine store is solely dependent on its synthesis. There are drugs that act, however, by pre-

---

norepinephrine in response to nerve stimulation, causing inhibition of adrenergic nerve activity, e.g., bretylium.

5. *Displacement of norepinephrine from cytoplasmic pool, leading to sympathomimetic effect, e.g., tyramine, ephedrine.*

6. *Blockade of active transport from extracellular fluid to cytoplasmic pool, causing augmentation of norepinephrine action at adrenergic receptor sites, e.g., cocaine, imipramine.*

7. *Activated by sympathomimetic agents, e.g., phenylephrine, isoproterenol, amphetamine.*

8. *Blocked by adrenergic blocking agents, e.g., propanolol, phenoxybenzamine.*

Table 13-4. Mechanisms of Drug Action in Relation to the Steps Involved in Neurohumoral Transmission at Cholinergic and Adrenergic Neuroeffector Junctions

Mechanism of Drug Action and Effect Produced	Neurotransmitter Involved	
	Acetylcholine	Norepinephrine
Inhibition of synthesis of transmitter leading to its depletion	Hemicholinium[a]	a-Methyl-l-p-tyrosine[a]
Biotransformation via same synthetic pathway as that of transmitter, leading to displacement of normal neurotransmitter by "false transmitter"	....	Methyldopa
Inhibition of active transport across membrane of storage granule, leading to depletion of transmitter	....	Reserpine
Inhibition of active transport across membrane of nerve terminal, leading to accumulation and potentiation of activity of transmitter at receptor sites	....	Cocaine, imipramine
Rapid release of transmitter from axonal terminal, leading to initiation of activity at effector sites	Carbachol[b]	Tyramine[a], ephedrine, amphetamine
Slow release of transmitter from storage granules, leading to depletion of transmitter	....	Guanethidine
Inhibition of release of transmitter, leading to inhibition of activity at effector sites	Botulinus toxin	Bretylium,[b] guanethidine
Inhibition of enzymatic destruction of neurotransmitter leading to accumulation and potentiation of activity of transmitter at receptor sites	Anticholinesterase agents (e.g., physostigmine, diisopropyl-phosphofluoridate (DFP)	Monoamine oxidase inhibitors (pargyline, tranylcypromine); (see text for discussion)
Combination with postjunctional receptor sites, leading to qualitatively same effects as produced by transmitter	Methacholine,[b] pilocarpine, nicotine,[a]	Epinephrine, phenylephrine, isoproterenol
Blockade of endogenous transmitter at postjunctional receptor sites, leading to inhibition of activity at effector sites	Atropine, trimethaphan	Propranolol, phenoxybenzamine

[a] Used only as an experimental tool.
[b] Largely supplanted in therapy by newer agents; still used as experimental tool.

venting the release of acetylcholine upon nerve stimulation. The extremely poor prognosis following poisoning by botulinus toxin, the most potent poison known, is attributable to its action in blocking the release of acetylcholine from cholinergic terminals throughout the nervous system; death, when it occurs, results from peripheral respiratory paralysis (cf. pp. 68, 84, 333).

In the case of adrenergic transmission, the rather complicated pattern of norepinephrine's storage and release provides a number of potential points for drug attack. For example, bretylium acts in a fashion analogous to that of botulinus toxin since the **adrenergic blocking agent** prevents the release of norepinephrine from intragranular pools in response to nerve stimulation. In contrast, some of the activity of the drug guanethidine mimics nerve stimulation and, by promoting the slow but prolonged release of the transmitter, depletes norepinephrine at adrenergic nerve endings. Reserpine also leads to depletion of the transmitter but it does this by blocking the active transport of norepinephrine from the cytoplasm into the intragranular pools; the adequate supply of transmitter within storage granules is dependent both on *de novo* synthesis and on recapture of norepinephrine previously released from the nerve terminal. The norepinephrine prevented by the action of reserpine from reentering the granule is largely destroyed by the monoamine oxidase present in the cytoplasm; the norepinephrine released from the granules by the action of guanethidine undergoes a similar fate. Thus, the long-lasting effects produced by both reserpine and guanethidine are very similar to those of an adrenergic blocking agent (e.g., bretylium) rather than those anticipated following the release of the adrenergic transmitter. On the other hand, agents such as tyramine, ephedrine and amphetamine that displace norepinephrine from its cytoplasmic mobile pool promote a rapid release of the transmitter and trigger action at the receptor site, that is, produce a **sympathomimetic** effect.

Drug Actions Influencing Transmitter Receptor Activity and Disposition of Transmitter

Drugs that act extracellularly can also produce their effects by a number of different mechanisms. In both the cholinergic and adrenergic systems there are a variety of agents that can combine with the receptors and mimic or antagonize the effects produced by the normal transmitter (see Table 13-4). At cholinergic nerve endings, the action of the acetylcholine released can be potentiated by anticholinesterase agents — drugs that inhibit its enzymatic destruction. In the adrenergic system, however, drugs that inhibit the extracellular enzyme catechol-O-methyl transferase or the intracellular monoamine oxidase, the two enzymes primarily responsible for the metabolism of norepinephrine, apparently produce little enhancement of the effects of norepinephrine. But, as noted before, drugs that inhibit monoamine oxidase can lead to accumulation of tyramine and this can have serious consequences when certain foods augment the normal body content of this sympathomimetic agent (cf. pp. 262, 286). Drugs such as cocaine and imipramine act extracellularly, however, to potentiate the action of norepinephrine at its postjunctional receptor sites; these agents inhibit the active reuptake of the transmitter from the extracellular fluid, the major process responsible for the termination of the effects of adrenergic stimulation.

General Significance of the Interaction of Drugs and Neurotransmitters

Many of the representative drugs listed in Table 13-4 are accepted therapeutic agents whose clinical usefulness is directly related to the manner in which they modify transmitter activity in the peripheral nervous system. For example, pilocarpine and physostigmine are useful in the treatment of glaucoma (cf. p. 89) because both agents increase the activity of the ocular muscles innervated by parasympathetic nerves; pilocarpine combines with the acetylcholine receptor and mimics the action of the transmitter, whereas physostigmine prevents the rapid destruction of and prolongs the activity of the acetylcholine released upon nerve stimulation. The therapeutic efficacy of reserpine and guanethidine also exemplifies the point under discussion. Although these two agents act by different mechanisms, their major therapeutic effects have been attributed to depletion of norepinephrine stores and to reduction of responses to sympathetic nerve activation.

In contrast to the examples just cited, the observed therapeutic effects of some other clinically useful drugs are not well correlated with their effects on the peripheral ANS. This is certainly the case for methyldopa, one of the principle drugs used to treat hypertension. There is, indeed, substantial evidence to show that methyldopa can deplete norepinephrine and act as a false transmitter at peripheral sympathetic nerves. Other available data, however, clearly indicate that the major blood pressure–lowering activity of methyldopa is not causally related to these actions or to any other effect on peripheral adrenergic transmitter activity. Currently it appears that the major hypotensive effect of methyldopa is due to its actions on the CNS. Corroborating data are being obtained to indicate that the therapeutic effects of methyldopa may be due to its interactions with putative neurotransmitters of the CNS similar to those demonstrated with the established, peripheral adrenergic neurotransmitter.

The anatomic and functional complexities of the CNS compared with those of the peripheral nervous system make it extremely difficult to obtain the evidence necessary to firmly establish a substance as a neurotransmitter in the CNS. Transmitter roles in the CNS have been proposed for acetylcholine, norepinephrine and dopamine (among other substances), and increasingly convincing evidence of central neurohumoral transmission is rapidly accumulating (cf. p. 344). When the transmitter roles of substances in the CNS receive direct validation, the precise mechanisms of drug action within the CNS will undoubtedly be elucidated, with the drugs serving as indispensable tools. For as Claude Bernard pointed out more than a century ago, the drug "becomes an instrument that dissects and analyzes the most delicate phenomena of the living machine."

GUIDES FOR STUDY AND REVIEW

What are cytotoxic poisons? What effects are typical of drugs that are cytotoxic poisons? When are drugs with cytotoxic actions useful? harmful? What property of antimicrobial agents makes them useful in treating economic species? What does the term "selective toxicity" mean?

What are the traditional subdivisions of the nervous system? of the peripheral nervous What are some examples of such therapeutic agents?

What are the traditional subdivisions of the nervous system? of the peripheral nervous system? Do these divisions have anatomic significance? functional significance?

How does the somatic nervous system differ from the autonomic nervous system? In what ways are these two systems similar?

What are the two major divisions of the autonomic nervous system? What are the major structural differences in these two systems? functional differences?

What factors account for the diffuse response of the sympathetic nervous system to stimulation? What factors account for the discrete and localized actions of the parasympathetic nervous system? What is the functional significance of this difference in the general type of response of the two systems?

How are the terms *conduction* and *transmission* distinguished from one another with respect to nervous activity? What are the mediators of transmission called?

What is the sequence of events involved in neurohumoral transmission? Which endogenous substances have been firmly established as neurotransmitters in the peripheral nervous system? What are the criteria that must be fulfilled for an endogenous material to be a neurotransmitter?

At which axonal terminals is acetylcholine the neurotransmitter? What is the name given to nerves that release acetylcholine?

How and where is acetylcholine synthesized? stored? released? metabolized? What factors are responsible for the termination of the action of acetylcholine?

At which axonal terminals is norepinephrine the neurotransmitter? What is the name given to neurons that release norepinephrine?

In general terms, how and where is norepinephrine synthesized? Does the entire synthetic process occur in one or more loci? Are the enzymes involved in the synthesis of norepinephrine specific or relatively nonspecific?

How and where is norepinephrine stored? released? metabolized? What factors are responsible for the termination of the action of norepinephrine?

In general, how may drugs that affect the autonomic nervous system produce their effects? How may drugs interfere with the synthesis of acetylcholine? norepinephrine? What are the consequences of such interference?

How may drugs interfere with the storage of norepinephrine? with its release? Are there drugs known to interfere with the storage or release of acetylcholine?

How may drugs influence transmitter receptor activity? disposition of transmitter? How does the disposition of acetylcholine differ from that of norepinephrine? What is the significance of this difference? How do drugs that inhibit the metabolism of acetylcholine affect activity at receptor sites? How do drugs that inhibit the enzymatic destruction of norepinephrine affect activity at receptor sites?

In general, what is the significance of the interaction of drugs and neurotransmitters?

SUGGESTED READING

Bennett, M.R. *Autonomic Neuromuscular Transmission.* London: Cambridge University Press, 1972.

Cotton, M. deV (ed.). Regulation of catecholamine metabolism in the sympathetic nervous system (N.Y. Heart Association Symposium) *Pharmacol. Rev.* 24:161, 1972.

Euler, U.S. von. Synthesis, Uptake and Storage of Catecholamines in Adrenergic Nerves. The Effect of Drugs. In H. Blaschko, and E. Muscholl (eds.) *Catecholamines. Handb. exp. Pharmak.*, Vol. 33, pp. 186–230. Berlin: Springer-Verlag, 1972.

Euler, U.S. von. Regulation of catecholamine metabolism in the sympathetic nervous system. *Pharmacol. Rev.* 24:365, 1972.

Hubbard, J.I. Mechanism of Transmitter Release. In J.A.V. Butler, and D. Noble (eds.), *Progress in Biophysics and Molecular Biology.* Oxford: Pergamon Press, 13:33, 1970.

Koelle, G.B. Current concepts of synaptic structure and function. *Ann. N.Y. Acad. Sci.* 183:5, 1971.

Kopin, I.S. Metabolic Degradation of Catecholamines. The Relative Importance of Different Pathways Under Physiological Conditions and After Administration of Drugs. In H. Blaschko, and E. Muscholl (eds.), *Catecholamines. Handb. exp. Pharmak.*, Vol. 33, pp. 271–282. Berlin: Springer-Verlag, 1972.

Michelson, M.J., and Ziemal, E.V. *Acetylcholine: An Approach to the Molecular Mechanism of Action.* Oxford: Pergamon Press, 1973.

Nachmansohn, D. The neuromuscular junction – the role of acetylcholine in excitable membranes. In G.H. Bourne (ed.), *The Structure and Function of Muscle* (2nd ed.), vol. 3, pp. 31–116. New York: Academic, 1973.

Potter, L.T. Synthesis, Storage and Release of Acetylcholine from Nerve Terminals. In G.H. Bourne (ed.), *The Structure and Function of Nervous Tissue*, vol. 4, pp. 105–128. New York: Academic, 1972.

Rang, H.P. (ed.). *Drug Receptors.* Baltimore: University Park Press, 1973.

Usdin, E. and Snyder, S. (eds.). *Frontiers in Catecholamine Research.* Oxford: Pergamon Press, 1973.

14. THE DEVELOPMENT AND EVALUATION OF NEW DRUGS

Until the early part of the nineteenth century, the only drugs available were crude preparations of plant, animal or mineral origin. The modern era of pharmacology was ushered in with advances in chemistry and the development of fundamental and essential methods of physiologic experimentation. The former permitted the isolation, purification and identification of active components of older preparations as well as the synthesis of new agents. And the development of experimental methods made it possible not only to distinguish worthless remedies from those that were useful, but also to determine how drugs produce their effects in the living organism.

Once given the necessary tools and techniques, pharamacology grew at an accelerating pace, paralleling the rapid advances in related disciplines and spurred on by the extensive research and development within the pharmaceutical industry itself. The proliferation of new drugs, the increased number of diseases that can be beneficially affected by drugs and the progress made in understanding the basic mechanisms of drug action are the tangible effects of this evolution. This growth reached its peak in the decade following World War II with the almost explosive expansion of basic research in the biomedical sciences. The rate of development, at least of new drugs, then declined and has now leveled off. But despite this recent decline, there are continuing advances being made and new agents are constantly being added to the therapeutic armamentarium. In this chapter we shall trace the development of a new drug from its genesis in the chemist's laboratory to its final acceptance as a safe and useful therapeutic agent (cf. Appendixes for drugs used in selected disorders).

DEVELOPMENT AND EVALUATION IN THE LABORATORY

The First Step — Discovering a Drug

Serendipity coupled with astute observations by alert investigators has played a role in the development of some very important drugs. The classic example is the discovery of penicillin by Fleming, which heralded the beginning of antibiotic therapy.[1] Such

---

[1] In 1928, Fleming noticed that a stray mold (genus *Penicillium*) on a plate culture of staphylococci had inhibited the growth of the bacteria.

chance observations occur rarely, so that almost all the new drugs available today are the original products of the research and development efforts of the large pharmaceutical firms. Leads for therapeutic discoveries have been and are being provided by both empiric and rational approaches: by the large-scale testing of natural or synthetic products and by the deliberate exploitation of side-effects of older agents, of unexpected clinical findings during the use of known drugs, or of newly discovered causes of disease.

Natural Products

During the first half of the twentieth century, natural products received only modest attention as potential sources of new drugs. However, interest in the study of plants was intensified in 1952 when reserpine was isolated from *Rauwolfia serpentina* and shown to be useful in the treatment of hypertension (cf. p. 477). Since preparations of *Rauwolfia* had been used in India for centuries for various therapeutic purposes, the discovery of its active principle stimulated the reexamination of folklore medicinals. While much of this folk medicine has provided only false clues to the pharmacologic value of plant remedies, some useful compounds have been discovered. For example, a study of the periwinkle plant (*Vinca rosea*), reputed to be beneficial in diabetes, did not disclose any compounds with antidiabetic activity, but did yield drugs effective against some types of cancer.

The investigation of natural products for potentially useful agents is ordinarily carried out by a relatively simplified procedure of extracting a sample of the material and testing the extract in a biologic system. Such a process is usually referred to as screening. This empiric approach is time-consuming since large numbers of compounds or random samples are tested to determine whether or not they possess exploitable pharmacologic activity. For example, thousands of samples of soil may be tested in the search for a new antibiotic. This seemingly inefficient approach is nonetheless valuable, since many chemical substances which soil microbes produce to suppress or destroy other microorganisms have been isolated and found to be therapeutically useful. The discovery of Mexican yams as an inexpensive source of starting materials for the synthesis of steroid hormones such as cortisone and progesterone is another example of how large-scale screening of natural products can lead to desirable end products.

Natural products remain the primary source of supply of many of our drugs of ancient heritage, for even though compounds like morphine have been synthesized in the laboratory, it is more economical to obtain them from their natural sources. Unlike the older preparations, however, these modern drugs of plant or animal origin are isolated and purified compounds. And drugs of natural origin like morphine and the digitalis derivatives, or the newer ones like antibiotics and hormones, continue to represent a large fraction of the total annual volume of drug sales.

Synthetic Chemicals

The products of the synthetic chemist's laboratory are the wellspring of the greatest number of new drugs; their potential pharmacologic activity is also discovered by screening processes. In the empiric approach, the screening process may involve a battery of experimental procedures to determine the total pharmacologic profile of a new chemical. Alternatively, groups of chemically related compounds may be put through a limited number of tests designed to reveal a specific type of activity, such as effect on blood pressure or kidney function. This so-called partially empiric approach, based on the concept of a relationship between structure and activity, has been utilized in several different ways, each of which has led to the synthesis of many valuable drugs.

One approach has been to systematically modify the molecular structure of an established drug in order to develop a congener that has more desirable properties than the original compound. The aim may be to improve the margin of safety, to eliminate a particular type of side-effect, to prolong or shorten the duration of action or to improve absorption from the gastrointestinal tract (Table 14-1). The success that may be achieved by such structural manipulation is dramatically illustrated by the development of the oral contraceptive agents. The synthetically modified estrogenic and progestational hormones have the same pharmacologic activity as the natural hormones. However, the partially synthetic derivatives, unlike the natural products, are effective when administered orally. The natural hormones are apparently metabolically degraded in the intestine or liver, or both, before they reach the systemic circulation. Thus the introduction of synthetically modified hormones which retain their activity when taken by mouth revolutionized gynecologic and contraceptive therapy.

It happens all too often that structural modifications of an existing drug yield congeners with pharmacologic profiles insignificantly different from that of the parent compound. Although these new agents offer little advantage over the drug already available, they are frequently marketed for competitive reasons and become "me-too" drugs. The practice is sometimes difficult to justify unless the "me-too" drug is less expensive to manufacture. On the other hand, a multiplicity of drugs with similar pharmacologic activity may represent therapeutic insurance for patients who are either unresponsive or allergic to other drugs within the group. Or, when resistance or tolerance develops to a particular drug, as for example in bacterial infections, the availability of "backstop" drugs — drugs of pharmacologic equivalence — may be exceedingly important.

At the same time, systematic modifications of the structure of an existing drug have frequently led to the synthesis of agents with therapeutic applicatio s or pharmacologic properties markedly different from those anticipated. Meprobamate, for example, was originally synthesized as a potential muscle relaxant. It was one of more than 1,200 derivatives investigated in a search for a long-acting successor to mephenesin, a muscle relaxant of short duration of action and unreliable absorption. Meprobamate was found to be effective orally, to have a satisfactory duration of action and to possess the looked-for muscle-relaxant activity. But it was also noted during the screening tests that meprobamate had the ability to allay anxiety without producing too much drowsiness. These latter pharmacologic properties account for its exploitation as a sedative to reduce tension and worry.

Table 14-1. Development of New Drugs by Modification of Older or Established Drugs

Established Drug	New Drug	Advantage of Newer Over Older Drug
Sulfanilamide	Sulfadiazine	Greater margin of safety
Procaine	Lidocaine	Effective when applied to body surfaces; little potential for allergic reactions; more stable to biotransformation at site of injection, hence longer acting
Procaine	Tetracaine	Much more potent, but relative therapeutic ratio with respect to lethal toxicity is only slightly increased
Phenylbutazone	Sulfinpyrazone	Greater selectivity of action as a uricosuric agent
Codeine	Dextromethorphan	Much greater selectivity of action as a cough suppressant; no analgesic properties and no abuse potential
Atropine	Atropine methyl nitrate (quaternary ammonium compound)	Fewer side-effects relative to the CNS because of decreased ability to penetrate into brain
Pentobarbital	Thiopental	Much faster penetration into brain due to increased lipid solubility, therefore useful as an intravenous anesthetic agent
Phenobarbital	Pentobarbital	Much more rapidly biotransformed, therefore shorter acting; faster onset of action due to increased lipid solubility; more useful as a sleep-inducing agent
Penicillin G	Phenoxymethyl penicillin	More completely absorbed from the gastrointestinal tract; more stable in acid medium
Penicillin G	Oxacillin	More completely absorbed from the gastrointestinal tract; not degraded by penicillinase, therefore useful against penicillin-resistant organisms
Morphine	Methadone	Less costly to produce; longer duration of action; effective by oral route

The ability of such an agent to produce sedation might well be regarded as a side-effect of the drug if one were looking merely for muscle-relaxant activity. Such a side-effect occurring by chance during a large-scale screening program might easily escape notice in the absence of a competent and alert investigator. But when careful observation is coupled with recognition of the potential usefulness of a side-effect, as it was in the case of meprobamate, new drugs may be discovered or new users found for older agents.

There are many significant advances in therapy that had their origin in the clues provided by the observed side-effects of existing drugs. For example, when sulfanil-amide was first introduced as an antibacterial agent, careful clinical observation indicated that it produces a slight increase in both the volume and pH of urine. Subsequently the drug was found to inhibit the enzyme carbonic anhydrase, which in turn was found to prevent the normal acidification of the urine (cf. pp. 126, 440). Structural manipulations led to the development of more potent carbonic anhydrase inhibitors, such as acetazolamide. Although the carbonic anhydrase inhibitors have limited usefulness as therapeutic agents, they played a significant role in the elucidation of normal kidney function. Moreover, further modification of the acetazolamide molecule produced the therapeutically important thiazide diuretics, of which chlorothiazide (Diuril) is the prototype (cf. pp. 440–441). A useful class of orally effective antidiabetic drugs also evolved from the antibacterial sulfonamides. The impetus for the development of these hypoglycemic agents was the clinical finding of a lowered blood sugar as a side-effect of the treatment of typhoid fever with a sulfonamide. It is noteworthy that these different structural modifications of sulfonamides eliminated their antibacterial activity and yielded diuretics with unimportant hypoglycemic activity or antidiabetic drugs without diuretic activity.

Probenecid is a good example of a drug developed for one purpose which later found a new and more important use. When penicillin was first introduced, its rapid elimination in the urine was of practical concern, since the antibiotic was both expensive and scarce. A systematic study was undertaken to find an organic acid that would compete with penicillin for the renal tubular secretory process and thereby inhibit penicillin's rapid loss from the body (cf. p. 219). Probenecid was the answer. It was also found that large doses of probenecid enhance the excretion of uric acid by inhibiting its reabsorption from the tubular urine. This uricosuric action of probenecid was usefully applied in the treatment of gout, a disease characterized by high levels of uric acid in the body (cf. p. 443).

The deliberate approach to achieve a specific pharmacologic objective has led to the development of a number of useful agents like probenecid which act by competitively antagonizing the actions of other drugs or of functionally important endogenous substances (cf. pp. 180–184). The search for new types of drugs may also be guided by rational concepts when the biochemical or physiologic abnormality underlying a disease state is revealed. The treatment of parkinsonism, for example, was dramatically changed in the last decade with the disclosure that the major defect in the disease is a decreased content of dopamine in certain areas of the brain. Dopamine itself cannot be used effectively to correct the biochemical defect, since it does not readily pass the so-called blood-brain barrier. But the drug levodopa does gain access to the brain where it is metabolically converted to dopamine.

The synthesis of effective drugs tailored to fit predetermined specifications occurs all too infrequently. However, the unquestioned success of levodopa as a new approach to the treatment of parkinsonism gives substance to the hope that more and more drugs will be developed from such sound theoretical considerations.

Studies in Animals

The Initial Evaluation of Potential Usefulness

The first tests a compound undergoes in animals are part of the initial screening to determine whether the agent has any biologic activity of potential pharmacologic interest. As already indicated, this may involve either a general, or profile, screen or a specific screen for a definite type of pharmacologic activity. In the general screen a small number of mice or rats are given several doses of the compound under consideration and are then observed for several hours or days. Careful observation at this stage may disclose unusual activity and provide leads to the kinds of pharmacologic action that might be worth pursuing. Frequently, these profile screens are standardized to yield reliable data at minimum cost and labor. An example of the kind of standardized procedure that might be used to categorize the central nervous system effects of a chemical compound is presented in Fig. 14-1.

Screening for specific types of pharmacologic activity may follow the clues provided by the profile screen or may be used at the outset when the compound to be tested has been fashioned for a particular purpose. The screen may be either organ-oriented or disease-oriented. In either case, the potential drug is used in experimental animal preparations designed to reveal changes in certain physiologic states or functions. For example, in the search for an agent useful in treating hypertension, anesthetized animals are prepared so that changes in blood pressure may be monitored in response to drug administration. Or if a potential antimalarial agent is being tested, the drug is administered to birds infected with the malarial parasite. In vitro screening procedures using isolated tissue or organ preparation (cf. pp. 172, 174) or specific enzyme systems may also serve to demonstrate an effect on some physiologic or biochemical function. The difficulty generally associated with any testing procedure, particularly with the disease-oriented test, is finding or producing in animals an exact counterpart of the physiologic state or disease seen in humans. Although there is little assurance that the drug's effect in the animal model will be duplicated in humans, these tests have predictive value and have been successfully employed to find new agents of benefit to humans. Normally, hundreds of compounds are screened before a potentially active drug is found.

Once a drug survives the initial qualitative assessment of its potential usefulness, it must be subjected to quantitative determinations of its potency and toxicity. The quantitative procedure used to determine the relationship between the dose administered and the magnitude of response is called a *bioassay*. A bioassay to determine the potency of a new agent compared with that of an established drug may have been part of the initial screening procedure. But now the purpose of the bioassay is mainly

Test CNS ACTIVITY AND ACUTE TOXICITY SCREEN **PERPHENAZINE** **Test No. P-3** **Chemist**

SPECIES: MOUSE	SEX: MALE
ROUTE: oral	WEIGHT (GM): 18–24
0.2%	2.0%
☒ SOL. ☐ INSOL.	☒ SOL. ☐ INSOL.
pH = 5	pH = 3
VEHICLE: H₂O	

1.18

mg/kg Dose (3 anim./dose)	Alertness	Visual Placing	Passivity	Stereotypy	Grooming	Vocalization	Restlessness	Irritability (Aggression)	Fearfulness	Reactivity (Envir.)	Spontaneous Activity	Touch Response	Pain Response	Startle Response	Straub Tail	Tremors	Twitches	Convulsions	Body Posture	Limb Position	Staggering Gait	Abnormal Gait	Righting Reflex	Limb Tone	Grip Strength	Body Sag	Body Tone	Abdominal Tone	Pinna	Corneal	IFR	Writhing	Pupil Size	Palpebral Opening	Exophthalmos	Urination	Salivation	Piloerection	Hypothermia	Skin Color	Heart Rate	Respir. Rate	Lacrimation	Misc.	No. Acute	No. Delayed
Normal Score	4	4	0	0	4	0	0	0	0	4	4	4	4	0	0	0	0	0	4	4	0	0	0	4	4	0	4	4	4	4	4	0	4	4	0	0	0	0	0	4	4	4	0		0	0
.01																																														
.03																																														
.10		3			•					3	3														3		3	3																		
.30		2								2	3	3								3			2	3	2		3	3	2	3	2			3												
1	1	2			5					2	2	1	1			1				3	1		3	3	1	2	2	2	2	2	1			2		1										
3	1	1				1				1	1	1	1			2				2	1		4	1	1	3	1	2	0	1	1			2		1										
10	0	1	5			1				1	1	0	1							1			7	1	1	8	0	1	1	0	1			1		1						3T	1			
30	0	0	8							0	0	0	1				1		P	0S			8	0	0	8	0	0	0	0	0			1		2						3T				
100	0	0	8							0	0	0	0						P	0S			8	0	0	8	0	0	0	0	0			1		2			1	3		2T	1			
300	0	0	8							0	0		0						P	0S			8	0	0	8	0	0	0	0	0					2						1T				
1000																																														

Figure 14-1. Scorecard for evaluating the central nervous system activity and acute toxicity of a potential therapeutic agent. The tests were conducted with groups of three mice, the dose for each group increasing by a factor of 3. The scale of scores for each sign or symptom ranged from 0 to 8, with 4 being assigned as the normal score. A higher score indicates an increase, a lower score a decrease in the particular behavior. The agent scored in this figure was evaluated as having sedative actions at doses that produced some changes in vital functions but were not lethal. (Courtesy of Dr. S. Irwin.)

to determine the relationship between the doses producing a desired effect and those eliciting an undesirable or toxic effect. At this stage of the evaluation, many drugs are found to be unsatisfactory for further trial, since their therapeutic indices indicate a small margin of safety between doses which yield desirable and undesirable effects.

The bioassay is also an essential feature of the standardization of impure drugs of natural origin, such as digitalis, heparin or hormones. The tests are carried out in strict conformity with the rigorous regulations set by appropriate public agencies. The Division of Biologic Standards of the Food and Drug Administration, for example, sets the standards for vaccines, serums and other so-called biologics; standards for hormones are set by the *United States Pharmacopeia.*

The Preclinical Evaluation of Safety and Efficacy

When a compound has been found in the profile or specific screening test and in confirmatory testing to produce an effect that suggests it is a potentially useful drug, it is selected for step-by-step, detailed and exhaustive in vivo (in animals) and in vitro studies. The aim of these preclinical studies is to obtain data on the drug's safety and efficacy sufficient to demonstrate that there will be no unreasonable hazard in initiating trials in human beings.

Regardless of the precise sequence, studies are carried out to determine the effectiveness of the drug in several species of animals (cf. pp. 257–260). While these studies are directed to the compound's major pharmacologic activity (e.g., analgesia), other experiments are conducted to determine its effect on various organ systems such as heart, lungs, kidneys, intestine, brain and muscle. A serious adverse effect on any of these organs can preclude further consideration of the compound as a therapeutic agent. The total process of gathering efficacy and safety data can take several years, and the drug may be discarded at any stage of the evaluation because of inadequate effectiveness or signs of toxicity.

Regulatory agencies have set stringent requirements for the kinds of data that must be submitted in order to obtain permission for trials in human subjects. In the United States, the regulatory authority is the Food and Drug Administration (FDA); similar agencies exist in most other countries. Guidelines issued by the FDA for studies of new drugs specify the number and types of animals to be used in tests of toxicity and efficacy. These guidelines are flexible and change from time to time as experience indicates the utility of newer or better approaches.

The preclinical studies are directed initially toward defining the safety of the drug. To this end, its acute, subacute and chronic toxicities are determined in several animal species (cf. pp. 303–305). The common measure of acute toxicity is the median lethal dose (LD50). It is usually determined, as previously described, by giving groups of animals single doses, some of which are lethal (cf. pp. 190–191). The toxic symptoms developed by the animals and the time at which they appear are also noted. Such observations may provide clues about the mechanisms of toxicity. For example, delayed death may be due to the toxicity of a metabolite rather than of the parent drug. At least three species of animals, one not a rodent, are used, and the acute toxicity is usually determined by more than one route of administration. These initial evaluations of toxicity give some indication of the species differences that may be anticipated, the harmful effects that may be expected and the dosage at which they may be evoked. They have little predictive value, however, unless accompanied by longer-term studies using measures of toxicity other than death.

The subacute toxicity studies must be conducted in at least two animal species, one of which must be a nonrodent. The duration of treatment usually lasts from four to thirteen weeks. In each species at least three dose levels are employed, varying from near-therapeutic doses to a level sufficiently high to produce clear-cut toxicity. The drug is administered one or more times daily by the route(s) to be used in the human trials. Routine laboratory examinations, such as hematologic studies and tests of liver and kidney function, are carried out during the period of observation. At the termination of the study, the animals are sacrificed and thorough pathologic examinations are made of organs and tissues.

Chronic toxicity studies must be carried out in at least three species, only one of which is usually a rodent. These studies last from a minimum of six months to two years or longer, depending on the intended duration of drug use in humans. Three dose levels are commonly employed, varying from a nontoxic but greater-than-therapeutic dose to a level high enough to produce a toxic response upon repeated administration. These chronic studies permit many correlated observations to be made which are not practical during the short-term studies. For example, the effect of the drug on food consumption, body weight and growth may be assessed. Again, routine laboratory tests are made at intervals during the long period of drug administration in order to evaluate the possibility of deleterious effects on various bodily functions. Some animals are sacrificed periodically for gross and histologic postmortem examinations. Potential carcinogenic activity is also assessed in specially designed experiments. Extensive reproduction experiments are carried out in rats and rabbits to detect any alterations in the reproductive cycle or any harmful effects on the unborn. Tests for potential teratogenic effects became a routine part of drug toxicity studies only after the thalidomide catastrophe of 1961 focused attention on the need for evaluation of the special effects of drugs upon the fetus. These special animal tests and the longer chronic toxicity studies may be conducted concurrently with the initial studies in human subjects. This is particularly true when the drug is intended only for short-term use in humans.

Emphasis in the preclinical phase of investigation is placed on toxicity studies, since adequate scientific evidence must be secured to demonstrate that the drug is safe for human trial under the conditions proposed for its use. The efficacy of the drug does not have to be proved before permission is granted to initiate human studies. But, even though it is recognized that a drug's effect on animals is only predictive of benefit in human disease, the rationale for its proposed use in humans must be documented by animal experimentation. Thus, preclinical tests are also carried out to define more explicitly the drug's full spectrum of pharmacologic properties, and its absorption, distribution, biotransformation and excretion.

The rate and extent of absorption and excretion are usually determined during the course of the subacute toxicity studies by following the changes in plasma concentration of the drug after oral and parenteral administration. Measurements of plasma concentration following intravenous administration provide some information of the extent of tissue distribution as well. And the temporal relationship between plasma concentrations of the drug and its pharmacologic actions may suggest the way in which the drug produces its effect. For example, a lack of relationship may indicate that the drug acts through a metabolite. Measurements of the change in plasma concentration of drug (or metabolites) during the chronic toxicity studies may help to determine whether drug accumulation or enzyme induction occurs upon repeated administration. Additionally, organs and tissues may have to be analyzed directly for their content of drug or metabolites. In order for any of these biochemical studies to be conducted, it is obvious that a sensitive and specific method must be available or developed for the determination of the drug and its metabolite(s) in animal tissues.

At this stage of drug development, the studies of absorption and elimination performed in animals are only preparatory to carrying out similar studies in humans when human trials are authorized. Detailed investigation of how the body affects the drug is not warranted at this point, since it has limited value in incipient clinical studies. Additional animal studies are usually conducted concurrently with clinical studies. However, preliminary data on the fate of a drug in animals may provide an opportunity to determine which species more closely resembles man and, thus, which species may provide toxicity data more directly related to man.

The Formulation of the Drug Product

Before proceeding to a discussion of clinical studies, mention must be made of the formulation of the drug product to be used in treating patients. Drugs are not administered as such but are formulated as liquids, capsules, tablets or injectable solutions. The formulation contains an excipient such as lactose if it is a capsule or tablet, a solvent of some sort for liquids or injectables, a preservative, coloring agent and so forth. The formulated product provides greater ease in administering the correct dosage, and proper formulation can enhance absorption, whereas improper formulation can retard absorption even to the point of decreasing drug efficacy. The appropriate drug formulation can give the drug product stability so that it does not deteriorate with age as rapidly as it otherwise might.

Formulation studies usually begin early in the investigation of a promising compound, and data are obtained by administration of the drug product to animals and by in vitro studies. The final formulation may have to be adjusted after clinical trials are started.

CLINICAL STUDIES

When a compound passes pharmacologic, toxicologic and biochemical tests in animals, the crucial question arises, "What does it do in humans?" Many adverse effects produced by drugs simply cannot be discerned in animals. For example, symptoms such as nausea, dizziness, headache, ringing in the ears, heartburn and depression would not be recognized in animal studies. In fact it has been estimated that at least half the undesirable effects seen most frequently in the widespread use of drugs can be ascertained *only* during human trial. Moreover, for many human diseases and illnesses there are no reliable animal models. This is particularly true for noninfectious diseases such as parkinsonism and arthritis. Thus, no matter how extensive the studies in animals may be, they can only complement, not take the place of, trials in human subjects. Species variation, which may be manifested as qualitative or quantitative differences in the pharmacodynamics or pharmacokinetics of drug action, or both, necessitates the use of human subjects to obtain evidence of the clinical safety and efficacy of a drug.

The initial trials in humans of a potentially useful agent must, obviously, be carried out with extreme caution by qualified investigators in carefully planned studies. Yet only in the last forty years has federal legislation been enacted to regulate the manner in which drugs are introduced for human use. The first law, enacted in 1906 as the Federal Food, Drug and Cosmetic Act, was concerned only with standards of purity for drugs already on the market. It designated *The Pharmacopeia of the United States* and *The National Formulary* as the compendia of official standards and empowered the federal government to enforce these standards and require that a drug possess the purity and strength claimed for it. However, it was not until 1939 that new drugs had to be judged safe for their intended use before they could be sold. The Federal Food, Drug and Cosmetic Act of 1938 required, for the first time, that manufacturers submit a new drug application to the FDA for review and approval of studies undertaken to demonstrate the safety of the newly proposed therapeutic agent. It took the death of more than one hundred people in the "elixir of sulfanilamide" disaster of 1937 to gain passage of the law. The so-called elixir of sulfanilamide contained diethylene glycol as a liquid vehicle in the absence of any investigation of the toxicity of this solvent. Diethylene glycol produces severe kidney and liver damage; death results from kidney failure or respiratory failue due to pulmonary edema. Today, an accepted remedy, even one used for years, is considered to be a "new drug" if manufactured in a new form, and it requires evaluation by the FDA.

The Kefauver-Harris Drug Amendment of 1962 changed the 1938 act to include a requirement that the manufacturer provide "substantial evidence" that a new drug is not only safe but also effective. The law defines substantial evidence as "adequate and well-controlled investigations, including clinical investigations, by experts qualified by scientific training and experience to evaluate the effectiveness of the drug involved." The efficacy provisions were also made retroactive to include products marketed between 1938 and 1962. Agents marketed under the 1938 act constitute a large percentage of the drugs prescribed today — about 4,000 preparations sold by 237 companies.[2] But the 1962 law and subsequent amendments to the 1938 act did more than require a demonstration of the substantial efficacy of a drug before it could be marketed. These laws also increased governmental regulatory authority (1) to ensure that adequate preclinical studies are completed before human studies

---

[2] The review of these drugs has been carried out under the auspices of the National Academy of Sciences — National Research Council. Thirty panels of experts, each responsible for particular categories of disease, have carried out surveys of the effectiveness of the 1938–1962 drugs based on information submitted by the drug manufacturers.

are initiated, and (2) to provide greater control and surveillance over the distribution and clinical testing of investigational drugs.

Before starting tests of a new drug in humans, the sponsor (usually a pharmaceutical firm, sometimes an individual physician or a research institute) must supply the Investigational New Drug (IND) Branch of the Division of New Drugs within the Bureau of Medicine with the information specified by the Federal Food, Drug and Cosmetics Act. This application form is known as the "IND." A new drug is defined as (1) any chemical or substance not previously used in humans for the treatment of disease; (2) combinations of approved drugs or of old drugs, even though the individual components are not new drugs; (3) the employment of an approved drug for uses other than those approved; (4) a new dosage form of an approved drug; and (5) even the use of a drug in vitro as a diagnostic agent when its use will influence the diagnosis or treatment of disease in a human patient.

The IND submitted to the FDA contains the results of all the preclinical investigations carried out in animals, including complete toxicity data, the full pharmacologic spectrum of the drug and any studies of absorption, distribution, biotransformation and excretion. In addition, the IND must provide the following information:

1. Complete composition of the drug, its source and manufacturing data with details of all quality control measures employed to assure exact reproducibility of manufacture and identification of all ingredients.
2. Specifications of the dosage forms to be given to humans.
3. A description of the investigations to be undertaken, including the doses to be administered, the route and duration of drug administration and the specific clinical observations and laboratory examinations to be performed.
4. The names and qualifications of, and the facilities available to, each investigator who will participate in the initial studies (phase 1).
5. Copies of all informational material supplied to each investigator (the data sheets supplied to the investigator incorporate the data submitted in the IND itself).
6. An agreement from the sponsor to notify the FDA and all investigators if any adverse effects arise during either the continuing animal studies or human tests.
7. Agreement to submit annual progress reports.
8. Certification that "informed consent" will be obtained from the subjects or patients to whom the drug will be given.

Investigations in humans may begin as soon as the FDA has indicated its approval, or thirty days from submission of the IND if no formal notice has been received. The clinical studies are divided into three phases, the first two of which are described as clinical pharmacology.

Conditions Essential to the Proper Execution of Clinical Studies

Before any investigational drug is used in human beings, the law requires that the physician "obtain the consent of such human beings or their representatives except when it is not possible or when in his professional judgment it is contrary to the best interest of such human beings." The basic elements of informed consent include (1) a fair explanation of the procedures to be followed, including an identification of those which are experimental; (2) a description of the attendant discomforts and risks; (3) a description of the benefits anticipated; (4) a disclosure of appropriate alternative procedures that would be advantageous for the subject; (5) an offer to answer any inquiries concerning the procedures; and (6) an instruction that the subject is free to withdraw consent and to discontinue participation in the project at any time. In the early phases of trials in human subjects there can be no exceptions to the rule of obtaining consent, since the drug is being administered primarily for the accumulation of scientific data. Only in later stages of testing, where patients are given a new drug for *treatment,* may exceptional circumstances warrant drug administration without informed consent. The law defines these exceptions as situations "where as a matter of professional judgment exercised in the best interest of a particular patient under the investigator's care it would be contrary to the patient's welfare to obtain his consent." Thus, although large numbers of subjects participate in clinical studies, almost every patient involved is fully informed of the actions of the drug, the purpose of the study and the benefits to be derived from it.

Additional procedures for safeguarding the rights and welfare of human subjects participating in clinical trials of drugs have been established by many institutions where such studies are being performed. These procedures are a direct outgrowth of the policies of the Department of Health, Education, and Welfare (HEW). The HEW stipulates that "no grant or contract for an activity involving human subjects shall be made unless the application for such support has been reviewed and approved by an appropriate institutional committee." Subsequent to the formation of such committees, many institutions decided that it was their responsibility to safeguard the welfare of all human subjects, not just those involved in activities supported by HEW funds. As a result most clinical studies in the United States are initiated only after an institutional review committee has carefully examined applications, protocols or descriptions of the proposed studies and arrived at an independent determination of possible risks. Favorable recommendation is given when this review determines that (1) the rights and welfare of the subjects involved are adequately protected; (2) the risks to an individual are outweighed by the potential benefits to him or by the importance of the knowledge to be gained; and (3) that informed consent has been obtained by methods that are appropriate and adequate.

Women with child-bearing potential are never subjects for clinical trials unless the appropriate teratologic studies in animals have been completed. Such studies must show that administration of ten to twenty times the therapeutic dose produces no teratogenic or toxic effects on the embryo or fetus and no adverse effects on the mother. Also, with the obvious exception of trials of new contraceptive drugs, no women are used as subjects when pregnant or if they are likely to become pregnant either during or immediately after the clinical study.

In any experiment, the aim is to establish the reliability of and confidence in the outcome of the study by ruling out error and providing a standard of comparison. Thus clinical studies are usually conducted as *controlled* experiments. Whereas what constitutes an adequately controlled study of a new drug in humans varies, by necessity, with the nature of the drug and drug effect being evaluated, there are certain indispensable requirements for all clinical studies. An adequate number of subjects must be used, and the drug effect(s) must be evaluated by appropriate and sensitive methods. The new drug must be concurrently compared with a reference drug over a range of doses. The data must be collected without bias and subjected to valid statistical analysis.

The efficacy of a new drug can be evaluated, with rare exception, only by comparison with one or more accepted agents as standards of reference. The rare exception occurs, for example, when a new drug produces cure of a previously fatal disease, as when the mortality rate of miliary-meningeal tuberculosis was reduced from 100 to 5 per cent by streptomycin. In most instances, however, the patients are randomly assigned to two or more experimental groups; each group is then treated with a different drug, either the new drug or the older agent(s) available for the specific illness.

To minimize the bias of the patient or investigator, or both, many of the clinical trials are conducted as *single-blind* or *double-blind* studies. A single-blind study is one in which the patient is unaware of the nature of the medication. This does not mean, however, that the new drug is administered without informed consent. The patient is informed that the drug can be properly tested only in a controlled fashion and that, on a randomly selected basis, some patients will receive the new drug while others receive different treatments. In a double-blind study, both the patients and the investigators who supervise the patients and evaluate the data are unaware of which medication has been assigned to a particular individual. The medication each patient received is revealed only after all evaluations of drug effects have been completed. Then the comparisons between the new drug and the standard preparation(s) can be made on the basis of unbiased observations. Properly designed studies using sufficiently large numbers of patients and appropriate statistical analysis of the differences between treatment groups can reveal whether the new agent is inferior, superior or equal to the established treatment. Studies under blind conditions are particularly important in evaluating the efficacy of drugs which produce subjective effects, such as relief of pain.

A new drug is also frequently compared with a placebo (cf. p. 264) as an aid in distinguishing pharmacologic effects from those which are temporally correlated with the mere administration of the drug. However, the use of placebo controls is necessary and appropriate only under certain circumstances. Placebos have a rightful place in studies carried out on normal, healthy volunteers in which the active drug is of no direct therapeutic benefit to the subject. This is also a particularly helpful design when the subjective effects of a drug are under study. Placebos are equally appropriate, if not essential, in studies of wholly new drugs for which there are no existing counterparts. For example, the efficacy of an entirely new vaccine in preventing an infectious disease could hardly be assessed in the absence of a placebo group to determine the normal concurrent incidence of the infection. Placebo controls are not permissible, however, when it means withholding a drug from a group of patients who would benefit from its use. Therefore placebos have no place in studies of a new drug in patients suffering from conditions for which an effective drug is already available. The new drug should properly be compared with the existing drug.

Studies in Normal Individuals: Phase 1 of the FDA Regulations

In phase 1 the studies are conducted under carefully controlled conditions in a comparatively small number of subjects, mainly healthy volunteers. The investigator, usually a trained clinical pharmacologist, must be able to evaluate human toxicologic and pharmacologic data. The primary objective of this necessarily cautious phase of the investigation is to determine a safe and tolerated dosage in humans. However, observations of pharmacologic activity, toxicity (if it occurs), absorption, metabolism and excretion may also be made during phase 1. Measurements of blood and urinary levels of the new drug are particularly important at this stage if the drug appears to be ineffective in humans. Only with such data can the investigator decide whether the deficiency is in drug action rather than in a lack of absorption or too rapid elimination.

Limited Studies in Patients: Phase 2 of the FDA Regulations

When encouraging results are obtained in phase 1, the studies designated as phase 2 may be started. Additional pharmacologic studies in animals may also be necessary to indicate the safety of entering this second phase of clinical investigation. Phase 2 consists of initial trials of the value of the drug in the treatment or prevention of the disease for which it is intended. The drug is administered to a limited number of patients under careful supervision to determine its safety and effectiveness. Here the clinician needs to be familiar with the conditions to be treated, the drugs used in these conditions and the methods of their evaluation.

These are, perhaps, the most crucial tests in the development and evaluation of a new drug. The decision to proceed with extensive trials in large populations must be made on the basis of the data obtained in a relatively small number of patients. It is at this point that additional studies of the rates of absorption, metabolism and excretion in individual patients may facilitate further investigations. Evidence of the drug's safety or efficacy may depend on the ability to demonstrate that some patients metabolize or excrete the drug so slowly that high plasma levels lead to toxicity or, conversely, that some patients eliminate the drug so rapidly that effective plasma levels cannot be attained. However, the need or utility of carrying out more or less extensive metabolic studies is guided by the characteristics of the drug under study. For example, when the pharmacologic effect can be measured by following changes in prothrombin time, blood sugar, blood uric acid and so forth, the need for determining plasma concentrations of the drug may be less critical. Thus, flexibility in the design of additional studies is most desirable at this stage of investigation. Trained and capable investigators can then carry out the kinds of studies that will do the most to ensure safe and effective drug use. However, any changes in the original protocol require the submission of amendments to the IND, and may require review by institutional review committees.

Large-Scale Controlled Studies: Phase 3 of the FDA Regulations

Studies on a limited number of normal subjects and patients are primarily aimed at ascertaining whether a new drug merits further investigation. The figures in Table 14-2 indicate that a large percentage of the INDs originally submitted to the FDA are discontinued by the sponsor of the new drug or preparation. It is likely that many of these projects are terminated during initial studies and before extension of the clinical testing to phase 3. But when the data obtained in phases 1 and 2 provide reasonable assurance of the safety of the drug and a promise of clinical efficacy, proposals are made for the extensive trials of phase 3. The studies in the final phase must yield data on which the sponsor and the FDA can base a decision that the drug is marketable as safe and effective for its intended use. Thus, in phase 3, controlled clinical trials are conducted by a sufficient number of qualified investigators on a large enough population of patients to obtain the necessary data to substantiate claims of safety and efficacy. As many as 150 clinicians may participate in these studies, and the patients under their supervision usually number over 1,500 and may even exceed 3,000.

At the beginning of phase 3, the IND must be revised to reflect any modifications in the investigations to be undertaken. The FDA must also be informed of the qualifications of the new investigators who have agreed to study the drug under the con-

Table 14-2. Tabulation of the Number of Original INDs[a] Submitted, INDs Discontinued, Original NDAs[b] Submitted,[c] NDAs Approved[d] and New Molecular Entities Approved[e] by FDA for Calendar Years 1963–1976

Year	Original INDs Submitted	INDs Discontinued by Sponsor	Original NDAs Submitted	NDAs Approved	New Molecular Entities
1963	1066	6	192	71	12
1964	875	215	160	70	16
1965	761	306	221	50	17
1966	715	580	216	50	16
1967	671	627	128	74	18
1968	859	564	108	56	7
1969	956	482	60	39	10
1970	1122	....	87	53	17
1971	923	116/	256	68	13
1972	902	452	272	42	9
1973	822	311	149	77	16
1974	802	399	129	80	18
1975	876	472	137	61	13
1976	885	524	127	98	24

[a]Applications submitted to FDA for permission to begin investigations in humans.
[b]NDA = New Drug Application.
[c]Applications submitted to FDA for permission to market a new drug.
[d]New drugs marketed as totally new entities or as revisions of older drugs.
[e]Newly discovered drugs.
Source: Food and Drug Administration, Public Health Service, Department of Health, Education and Welfare; courtesy of Stanley A. Stringer, Chief, Product Coordination Staff, New Drug Evaluation, Bureau of Drugs.

ditions specified in the IND. In addition to experienced clinical pharmacologists, physicians who are not specialists may serve as investigators so that a broad background of experience may be secured in a large number of patients.

The value of carrying out extensive studies on the biotransformation of a new drug during phase 3 is largely dictated by the usefulness of such information in the evaluation of safety and efficacy. However, more detailed studies are usually carried out at this time to determine the drug's capacity to bind to plasma proteins, to induce or inhibit enzymes and to interact in various ways with other drugs.

THE NEW DRUG APPLICATION (NDA)

The clinical studies of phase 3 are completed when, in the opinion of the sponsor, sufficient data have been collected to permit the judgment that the drug is safe and effective. There are no hard and fast rules on what constitutes "safety" or "efficacy"; these qualities must be judged in relation to the specific clinical conditions for which the drug is to be used. For example, a lesser degree of efficacy and a smaller margin of safety are acceptable for an agent to be used to treat cancer than for a drug to treat a self-limiting, nondebilitating and nonfatal disease. In the latter case, or when an effective drug of the same type is already available, efficacy in a high proportion of patients and a low incidence of adverse effects would have to be demonstrated. When the sponsor is convinced that the data obtained in phase 3 studies justify approval of the drug as safe and effective for the use(s) intended, a New Drug Application (NDA) is submitted. Usually at least four years or more will have elapsed between the time the drug was picked out of the original pharmacologic screen and the date of completion and filing of its NDA.

The NDA contains all the chemical, pharmacologic, clinical and manufacturing data that have been collected since research on the drug was initiated. In some cases, the NDA may also contain data of bioequivalence and bioavailability as defined[3] and

---

[3] (a) Pharmaceutical equivalents: drug products that contain identical amounts of the identical active drug ingredient, i.e., the same salt or ester of the same therapeutic moiety, in identical dosage forms, but not necessarily containing the same inactive ingredients, and that meet the identical compendial or other applicable standard of identity, strength, quality, and purity, including potency and, where applicable, content uniformity, disintegration times and/or dissolution rates. (b) Pharmaceutical alternatives: drug products that contain the identical therapeutic moiety, or its precursor, but not necessarily in the same amount or dosage form or as the same salt or ester. Each such drug product individually meets either the identical or its own respective compendial or other applicable standard of identity, strength, quality, and purity, including potency and, where applicable, content uniformity, disintegration times and/or dissolution rates. (c) Bioequivalent drug products: pharmaceutical equivalents or pharmaceutical alternatives whose rate and extent of absorption do not show a significant difference when administered at the same molar dose of the therapeutic moiety under similar experimental conditions, either single dose or multiple dose. Some pharmaceutical equivalents or pharmaceutical alternatives may be equivalent in the extent of their absorption but not in their rate of absorption and yet may be considered bioequivalent because such differences in the rate of absorption are intentional and are reflected in the labeling, are not essential to the attainment of effective body drug concentrations on chronic use, or are considered medically insignificant for the particular drug product studied. (d) Bioavailability: the rate and extent to which the active drug ingredient or therapeutic moiety is absorbed from a drug product and becomes available at the site of drug action. (From *Fed. Reg.* 42:1624, 1977.)

determined by the procedures included in the 1977 amendment to the Federal Food, Drug and Cosmetic Act. Traditionally, physical and chemical tests were used to demonstrate that a drug product met the appropriate standards of strength, quality and purity and had its purported identity. With the development of biopharmaceutics and pharmacokinetics, however, it became possible to characterize a drug product more fully by determining its biologic availability. Therefore, standards for certain drug products were amended to include bioequivalence and bioavailability requirements. Bioequivalence data are required whenever there is evidence that drug products containing the same active drug ingredient or therapeutic moiety and intended to be used interchangeably for the same therapeutic effect are not or might not be bioequivalent drug products (cf. p. 87). In vivo bioavailability data must be included in the NDA unless other information is sufficient to permit the FDA to waive this requirement. However, in vivo bioavailability data are always required for certain classes of drugs such as anticoagulants, anticonvulsants, antibacterials, cardiac glycosides, and tranquilizers.

The Medical Evaluation Branch of the Division of New Drugs within the Bureau of Medicine is responsible for receiving and evaluating the NDA and is required to act on the application within 180 days. Theoretically, if the NDA is "complete," it will be promptly approved and then the new agent may be marketed. What is more frequently the case, however, is that the application is considered "incomplete." The sponsor is informed of the specific data that are lacking, and he has the opportunity to resubmit the NDA with the additional required information or studies. He may also request a hearing when there is disagreement with the conclusions reached by the professional staff of the Bureau of Medicine. A negative ruling following a hearing may be appealed to the courts. It is obvious from the figures in Table 14-2, however, that a sizable number of NDAs fail to gain FDA approval.

The data in Table 14-2 also clearly indicate that new molecular entities, i.e., active moieties not yet marketed in the United States by any drug manufacturer either as a single entity or as part of a combination product, represent less than 25 per cent of all the new drugs approved for marketing between 1963 and 1976. The majority of the NDAs approved are for either a new salt, new formulation, new indication for use, or new combination of drugs previously marketed by the same or different sponsor, or for a drug that duplicates an already marketed drug product. Of the 206 new molecular entities approved in this thirteen-year period, only 53 have been evaluated as offering "important therapeutic gain" and 73 as offering "modest therapeutic gain" by the FDA. In making this type of evaluation, the FDA considered only the degree of therapeutic gain deemed to have been offered by the drug at the time of its introduction in the light of available therapeutic alternatives, without reference to subsequent experience. The criteria used were (1) *important therapeutic gain*; the drug may provide effective therapy or diagnosis (by virtue of greatly increased efficacy or safety) for a disease not adequately treated or diagnosed by any marketed drug, or provide markedly improved treatment of a disease through improved efficacy or safety (including decreased abuse potential); (2) *modest therapeutic gain*; the drug has a modest, but real advantage over other available marketed drugs, e.g., somewhat greater effectiveness, decreased adverse reactions, less frequent dosing in situations in which frequent dosage is a problem.

The manufacturer's responsibilities do not end when a drug has finally been approved for marketing, but continue well into the period of its general clinical use. Although there is no accepted definition of this phase of FDA regulations, the term *phase 4* is commonly applied to all aspects of investigation that follow the granting of an NDA and the general availability of a new drug in widespread clinical use. The sponsor's claims of drug efficacy and safety that are to appear in brochures or advertising are reviewed and approved by the FDA. Reports concerning current clinical studies must be sent to the FDA every three months during the first year, every six months in the second year and annually thereafter. These reports must also include information about the quantity of drug distributed and copies of mailing pieces, labeling and, for a prescription drug, advertising. Any unexpected side-effects, injury, toxic or allergic reactions, or failure of the drug to exert its expected pharmacologic action that is made known to the manufacturer must, in turn, be transmitted to the FDA. Thus the FDA has responsibility not only for assuring that drugs are safe and effective before being marketed, but also for continued surveillance of those drugs long after their introduction into general clinical use.

CONCLUDING REMARKS

There is little doubt that the steps taken to improve the standards of drug development and evaluation have provided increased protection to both the test subject and the consumer. But with all these safeguards, no new drug — or, for that matter, no established drug — is completely free of hazard. Nor can more and more regulatory control hope to achieve this end; indeed, the effects of greater restrictions in drug development and evaluation might serve to deny the public the benefits of improved drug therapy. Given the unique genetic makeup of each person and the pharmacologic individuality this confers, there will always be some people who respond to a drug in an unexpected manner. And the more widespread the use of a drug, the greater will be the number of incidents of drug ineffectiveness or drug toxicity. But the risks inherent in the use of any drug can be minimized if drug use, whether by physician or patient, is always based on current knowledge of the general principles and concepts of pharmacology.

> Knowledge is the root and practice is the bough and there is no bough without a root behind it, although roots may be found which can as yet boast no boughs.
>
> *Moses Maimonides*

GUIDES FOR STUDY AND REVIEW

How are new therapeutic agents discovered? What are the sources of therapeutic agents?

How are chemicals evaluated initially for their potential usefulness as therapeutic agents? What is a bioassay and how is it used to evaluate potential drug effectiveness and safety?

What kinds of information, in general, must be available about a potential therapeutic agent before clinical trials in humans can be initiated? What agency in the United States decides whether trials in humans can begin? When was this made law? What is an IND?

What do we mean by "informed consent" with respect to the use of investigational drugs in humans? Are there any conditions under which informed consent for administration of an investigational drug is not needed? What regulations protect women with child-bearing potential?

How is the efficacy of a new drug evaluated? What kinds of drugs serve as a standard of reference? What is a single-blind study? a double-blind study?

When is the use of a placebo appropriate in the clinical trial of a new drug? When is its use inappropriate?

What subjects are generally used and how extensive are the clinical trials in phase 1 of the FDA regulations? in phase 2? in phase 3? What is the NDA and when is it submitted? Must efficacy as well as safety of a new drug be demonstrated? by law? When can a new agent be placed on the market? What responsibilities does the sponsor of the new drug have after it is placed on the market? How do the regulations for marketing new therapeutic agents resemble those for registering new economic poisons?

SUGGESTED READING

Bohonos, N., and Piersma, H.D. Natural products in the pharmaceutical industry. *BioScience* 16:706, 1966.

Brodie, B.B., and Reid, W.D. The Value of Determining the Plasma Concentration of Drugs in Animals and Man. In B.N. La Du, H.G. Mandel, and E.L. Way (eds.), *Fundamentals of Drug Metabolism and Drug Disposition.* Baltimore: Williams & Wilkins, 1971. P. 328.

Burger, A. Approaches to drug discovery. *N. Engl. J. Med.* 270:1098, 1964.

Burns, J.J. Application of Metabolic and Disposition Studies in Development and Evaluation of Drugs. In B.N. La Du, H.G. Mandel, and E.L. Way (eds.), *Fundamentals of Drug Metabolism and Drug Disposition.* Baltimore: Williams & Wilkins, 1971. P. 340.

Gaddum, J.H. Biological Assay. In *Pharmacology* (6th ed.). Revised by A.S.V. Burgen and J.F. Mitchell. London: Oxford University Press, 1968. P. 195.

Gaddum, J.H. Bioassays and metabolism. *Pharmacol. Rev.* 5:87, 1953.

Goldenthal, E.J. Current views on safety evaluation of drugs. *F.D.A. Papers* 2:13, 1968.

Gosselin, R.A. The status of natural products in the American pharmaceutical market. *Lloydia* 25:241, 1962.

Ladimer, I., and Neuman, R.W. (eds.). *Clinical Investigations in Medicine: Legal, Ethical and Moral Aspects.* Boston: Boston University Law-Medicine Research Institute, 1962.

Lasagna, L. The Drug Industry and Medicine Avenue. In *The Doctor's Dilemmas.* New York: Harper & Row, 1962. P. 131.

May, C.D. Selling drugs by "educating" physicians. *J. Med. Educ.* 36:1, 1961.

Report of Drug Research Board, Committee on Problems of Drug Safety, National Academy of Sciences—National Research Council. Application of metabolic data to the evaluation of drugs. *Clin. Pharmacol. Ther.* 10:607, 1969.

Roll, G.F. On politics and drug regulation. Center for the Study of Drug Development, University of Rochester Medical Center, Rochester, New York: Publication Series: PS—7701, Jan. 1977.

Talalay, P. *Drugs in Our Society.* Baltimore: Johns Hopkins University Press, 1964.

Turner, R.A. *Screening Methods in Pharmacology.* New York: Academic, 1965. P. 22.

Vane, J.R. A Plan for Evaluating Potential Drugs. In D.R. Laurence and A.L. Bacharach (eds.), *Evaluation of Drug Activities: Pharmacometrics.* New York: Academic, 1964. Vol. 1, p. 23.

Wardell, W.M. Introduction of new therapeutic drugs in the United States and Great Britain: An international comparison. *Clin. Pharmacol. Ther.* 14:773, 1973.

Wolstenholme, G., and Porter, R. (eds.). *Drug Responses in Man* (A Ciba Foundation Symposium). Boston: Little, Brown, 1967.

World Health Organization Scientific Group. *Principles for Pre-Clinical Testing of Drug Safety* (WHO Technical Report Series No. 341). Geneva: World Health Organization, 1966.

Zaimes, E., and Ellis, J. (eds.). *Evaluation of New Drugs in Man.* New York: Macmillan, 1965.

GLOSSARY

acid A molecule, ion or other entity that acts as a proton or hydrogen ion donor; a substance that ionizes in solution to form hydrogen ions; any substance that contains hydrogen capable of being replaced by basic radicals (cf. base).

additive effect A term ordinarily used to describe the combined effects of two drugs, acting simultaneously, which elicit the same overt response by the same mechanism of action. As in summation (q.v.), the total effect is equal to that expected by simple addition. The magnitude of the combined effect must be within the capacity of the system to respond. Ex.: the combined effect of aspirin and phenacetin to relieve pain.

adrenergic blocking agent An agent that selectively inhibits certain responses to adrenergic nerve stimulation and to epinephrine, norepinephrine and other sympathomimetic drugs.

adrenergic nerve A nerve that releases norepinephrine when it is stimulated, i.e., most postganglionic fibers of the sympathetic nervous system (cf. cholinergic nerve).

affinity A measure of the effectiveness of the interaction of a drug and its receptor. The greater the affinity of a drug, the greater its propensity to bind with a given receptor; the greater the affinity of a drug, the smaller the concentration of drug needed to produce the same intensity of response as that of a drug with a lesser affinity for the same receptor.

allergic response An adverse response to a foreign chemical resulting from a previous exposure to that substance. It is manifested only after a second or subsequent exposure and then as a reaction different from the usual pharmacologic effect of the chemical. Since a minute amount of an otherwise safe drug may elicit the allergic response, the term *hypersensitivity* is frequently used to describe the sensitization reaction. However, *hypersensitivity* should not be used to designate the allergic response, since it may be confused with the extreme *sensitivity* displayed by certain individuals in whom very small doses of a drug elicit the intensity of pharmacologic effect primarily seen only at higher doses (cf. antibodies, antigen).

analgesic drug An agent that relieves pain without producing a loss of consciousness. In the latter respect, an analgesic differs from an anesthetic drug (q.v.).

413

anesthetic drug (Gr. *an*, "not," + *aisthesis*, "feeling")   An agent that causes reversible loss of feeling or sensation. General anesthesia affects the entire body, causing not only loss of sensation but also loss of consciousness. Local anesthetics cause loss of sensation only in the particular area where they are applied, by blocking the transmission of nerve impulses from the affected area.

angina pectoris   A syndrome characterized by a transient interference with the flow of blood, oxygen and nutrients to heart muscle and associated with severe pain.

anthelmintics   Drugs used to rid the body of worms (helminths).

antibiotic   A chemical substance or metabolic product that is produced by micro-organisms and that destroys or prevents the growth of other microorganisms.

antibodies   Substances in the tissues or fluids of an organism that act to antagonize specific foreign bodies. The first exposure of the body to a foreign antigen triggers certain cells to elaborate specific antibodies — large proteins identified as specific immunoglobulins. Subsequent exposure to the same (or a related) antigen leads to an immune response characteritzed by an increase in the amount of the induced antibody. The type of response to the antigen-antibody inter-action differs radically for different antigens and in different hosts; it is inde-pendent of the pharmacologic effects produced by the eliciting drug but is determined by the mediators released by the antigen-antibody complex (cf. allergic response).

antidote   Any chemical agent used to overcome the action or the effects of a poison.

antigen   A substance which, when introduced into the body, is capable of inducing the formation of antibodies and subsequently of reacting in a recognizable fashion with the specific induced antibodies. All proteins foreign to the organ-ism may be antigens; many purified polysaccharides and simpler chemical groups (such as drugs) also can become antigenic when coupled to proteins. The relatively simple compounds — haptens — that do not by themselves stimu-late antibody formation may react specifically with the antibody after the latter is formed.

antirheumatic agent   A drug effective in the treatment of acute rheumatic fever.

antiseptic   A chemical agent with bacteriostatic action that inhibits the growth of microorganisms but does not necessarily kill them.

ataxia   Lack of normal coordination of muscular movement, especially inability to coordinate voluntary muscular movements.

autonomic drug   Any agent that has its primary action on any part of the autonomic nervous system or on autonomic effector cells.

bactericide (disinfectant, germicide)   An agent that is capable of producing rapid death of microorganisms. *Disinfectant* and *germicide* are used more frequently for agents killing microorganisms on inanimate objects, but all three terms are synonymous (cf. antiseptic).

base   A molecule, ion or other entity that acts as an acceptor of protons or hydrogen ions; a substance that ionizes in solution to form hydroxyl ions; any substance that has the property of neutralizing acids to form salts; any substance that can replace the hydrogen of an acid (cf. *acid*).

bioassay A procedure for determining the quantitative relationship between the dose of a drug and the intensity of the biologic response it evokes. Bioassays are used (1) to determine the potency of a drug relative to another drug or a standard of reference, or (2) to standardize preparations of impure drugs.

bioavailability The rate and extent to which the active drug ingredient or therapeutic moiety is absorbed from a drug product and becomes available at the site of drug action (as defined by FDA regulations).

biochemical antagonism *See* drug antagonism.

bioequivalent drug products Pharmaceutical equivalents or pharmaceutical alternatives whose rate and extent of absorption do not show a significant difference when administered at the same molar dose of the therapeutic moiety under similar experimental conditions, either single dose or multiple dose (as defined by FDA regulations).

biotransport The translocation of a solute from one side of a biologic barrier to the other side, the transferred solute appearing in the same form on both sides of the biologic barrier.

ceiling effect The maximum intensity of a specific effect that can be produced by a given drug, regardless of how large a dose is administered. The maximum effect produced by a given drug may be less than the maximum response of which the reacting tissue is capable or less than the maximum effect that can be produced by another drug.

certain safety factor (CSF) A number which is an assessment of the relative safety of a drug or of its selectivity of action. The CSF is derived from the extremes of the quantal dose-effect curves of the effects to be compared, e.g., LD1/ED99, the ratio of the lowest lethal and highest therapeutic levels of response (cf. standard safety margin, therapeutic index, selectivity).

chemical antagonism *See* drug antagonism.

chemical teratogens Chemicals that produce abnormalities of fetal development when administered to a pregnant animal.

cholinergic nerve A nerve that releases acetylcholine when it is stimulated, i.e., all motor nerves of the somatic nervous system, all preganglionic fibers of the autonomic nervous system, all postganglionic fibers of the parasympathetic division and a few postganglionic fibers of the sympathetic division (cf. adrenergic nerve).

competitive antagonism *See* drug antagonism.

conduction The passage of an impulse along an axon or muscle fiber (cf. transmission).

congener A drug that belongs to a group of chemical compounds having the same parent compound.

Controlled Substances Act An act passed by the United States Congress under the title *Comprehensive Drug Abuse Prevention and Control Act of 1970* to replace the *Harrison Narcotic Act of 1914.* This act codifies the regulations covering drugs subject to abuse and divides narcotic and other drugs into five schedules according to legitimacy of medical use and potential for abuse. Schedule I contains those that have a high abuse and *no* currently accepted therapeutic use in the U.S., e.g., heroin, marihuana, LSD, peyote and mescaline. Drugs listed in Schedule I may be obtained only for research or chemical analysis. Schedule II lists drugs that have a high abuse potential with severe psychic or physical dependence liability, e.g., opium, morphine, codeine, meperidine and other narcotic analgesics; cocaine; straight amphetamines and metamphetamines; phenmetrazine (Preludin); methylphenidate (Ritalin); methaqualone; amobarbital: pentobarbital; and secobarbital. Schedule III contains drugs that have an abuse potential less than those in schedules I and II but may lead to moderate or low physical or high psychologic dependence, e.g., glutethimide (Doriden); methyprylon (Noludar); nalorphine; chlorphentermine; barbiturates (except those listed in another schedule); paregoric or any other compound mixture containing limited quantities of morphine, codeine or other narcotic analgesics. Schedule IV contains drugs that have a low abuse potential and lead to only limited physical or psychologic dependence compared to drugs in schedule III, e.g., barbital and phenobarbital, chloral hydrate, meprobamate, paraldehyde, chlordiazepoxide (Librium) and diazepam (Valium). Schedule V lists drugs with an abuse potential less than those in schedule IV, e.g., preparations (except paregoric) of narcotics mixed with nonnarcotic active medicinal ingredients. All persons who manufacture, sell, prescribe or dispense the substances covered by the law must be licensed and registered by the Bureau of Narcotics and pay an annual registration fee. Until the act of 1970, the law was enforced by the Treasury Department, Bureau of Internal Revenue. The 1970 act transferred the control of law enforcement to the Department of Justice, Bureau of Narcotics and Dangerous Drugs.

convulsion An involuntary, generalized contraction of muscle, usually having its origin in disturbed function of the central nervous system. In clonic convulsions the gross, rhythmic, coordinated movements of different parts of the body are characterized by alternating contraction and relaxation of opposing (reciprocally innervated) muscle groups. In tonic convulsions, an intense contraction is maintained in all muscle groups.

coordinate covalent bond *See* covalent bond.

covalent bond The chemical bond formed between two atoms when the atoms share a pair of electrons. A covalent bond can result from the sharing of electrons supplied by one atom only, the resulting bond being called a coordinate covalent bond. The covalent bond is about twenty times stronger than the ionic bond (q.v.).

cross-dependence The ability of one drug to suppress the manifestations of physical dependence induced by another drug and to substitute for the other in maintaining the physically dependent state.

cross-sensitization The phenomenon whereby the initial exposure to a drug may elicit an allergic response in an individual previously sensitized to a different but related drug or environmental chemical.

demulcents Substances of high molecular weight that form aqueous solutions capable of alleviating irritation, particularly of mucous membranes and abraded surfaces, e.g., acacia (gum arabic), glycerin.

disintegration time The time required for a tablet to break up into particles of smaller or specified size under carefully controlled experimental conditions. The degree of compression of the tablet and the type of binders used influence disintegration time. Rapid disintegration does not ensure rapid absorption, but the absorption of drugs that are rapidly transferred across a barrier may be rate-limited by a long disintegration time (cf. dissolution time).

dissolution time The time required for a given quantity or fraction of drug to go into solution from a solid dosage form. Since solution of the drug is preliminary to absorption, slow dissolution may be rate-limiting for drugs that are rapidly absorbed.

diuretic A drug that increases the volume of urine excreted.

dosage The total quantity of drug to be administered over a period of time in order to produce a desired effect. Thus the usual oral dosage of penicillin is 500 mg to 2 g, given in individual doses of 125 to 500 mg four to six times a day.

dosage form The physical state in which a drug is dispensed.

dose The amount of drug needed at a given time to produce a particular biologic effect.

dose-effect curve (dose-response curve) Graphic representation of the mathematical expression of the relationship between dose (the independent variable) and effect (the dependent variable). One of the most basic principles of pharmacology states that the intensity of response elicited by a drug is a function of the dose administered, i.e., a larger dose produces a greater effect than a smaller dose, up to the limit of the capacity of the biologic system to respond. The term *graded* is applied to the type of relationship in which the responding system is capable of showing a progressively increasing effect with increasing concentration of drug. The term *quantal* is applied to the type of relationship in which the number or proportion of individuals responding by a particular, stated response (all-or-none) increases as the dose increases.

drug abuse The excessive and persistent use, usually by self-administration, of any drug without due regard for accepted medical practice. The vast majority of drugs of abuse are agents that act on the central nervous system to produce profound effects on mood, feeling and behavior.

drug antagonism Any interaction between two drugs in which the conjoint effect of the two agents is less than the sum of the effects of the drugs acting separately.

Pharmacologic antagonism is observed when a drug — the antagonist — reduces the effect of another drug — the agonist — by preventing the latter from combining with its receptor. Pharmacologic antagonism is competitive when the antagonist combines reversibly with the same binding sites as the agonist and can be displaced from these sites by an excess of the agonist. Pharmacologic antagonism is noncompetitive when the effects of the antagonist cannot be overcome by increasing concentration of the agonist.

Physiologic or functional antagonism is observed when two agonists, acting at different sites, counterbalance each other by producing opposite effects on the same physiologic function.

Biochemical antagonism is observed whenever one drug indirectly decreases the amount of a second drug that would otherwise be available to its site of action in the absence of the first drug (the antagonist). Biochemical antagonism is the converse of synergism (q.v.).

Chemical antagonism is simply the reaction between an agonist and an antagonist to form an inactive product. The agonist is inactivated in direct proportion to the extent of chemical interaction with the antagonist.

drug dependence A condition in which the user has a compelling desire to continue taking a drug either to experience its effects or to avoid the discomfort of its absence. *Drug dependence* is a general term that is applicable to all types of drug abuse (q.v.). It has been substituted for the terms *drug addiction* and *drug habituation.*

Psychologic dependence (psychic dependence, psychic craving, compulsive abuse) is a condition characterized by an emotional or mental drive to continue taking a drug, the effects of which the user believes are necessary to maintain his sense of optimal well-being. When the desire to continue taking the drug becomes a psychic craving or compulsion, the user may become preoccupied with drug taking and drug procurement; such behavior is termed *drug-seeking behavior or compulsive drug use.*

Physical dependence is an altered or adaptive physiologic state produced in an individual by the repeated administration of a drug. That physical dependence has been induced during the prolonged use of a drug is revealed only when the drug is abruptly discontinued or when its actions are diminished by the administration of a specific antagonist.

drug misuse The occasional nonmedical use (as opposed to the persistent nonmedical use in drug abuse) or the inappropriate medical use of drugs for purposes or conditions for which they are unsuited, or their appropriate use in improper dosage.

drug resistance A state of decreased response, or complete lack of response, to drugs that ordinarily inhibit cell growth or cause cell death. Drug resistance is therefore a phenomenon which, by definition, may be associated only with drugs used to eliminate (1) an uneconomic species, such as insects, bacteria or other parasites, or (2) rapidly growing cells, such as cancer cells in higher organisms.

drug tolerance A condition of decreased responsiveness which is acquired after prior or repeated exposure to a given drug or one closely allied in pharmacologic activity. Tolerance is characterized by the necessity of increasing the size of successive doses in order to produce effects equal in magnitude or duration to those achieved initially. Alternatively, it is an inability of the subsequent administration of the same dose of a drug to be as effective as was the preceding dose.

The term *tachyphylaxis* is used to describe the acute development of tolerance to the rapid, repeated administration of a drug.

effector Organ or cell that responds in a characteristic manner to a stimulus.

emetic A substance that induces vomiting.

emollients Fats or oils used for their local, protective or softening action of the skin, e.g., olive oil, white petrolatum, lanolin.

endocrine Denoting an organ or structure whose function is to secrete into the blood or lymph a substance (hormone) that has a specific effect on another organ or part.

enteral Pertains to administration of drugs into any part of the gastrointestinal tract, i.e., oral administration (swallowing of the drug), sublingual administration (under the tongue) and rectal administration (cf. parenteral).

enzyme A protein catalyst, a product of living cells, which accelerates biochemical reactions but remains apparently unchanged by the process.

equivalent A term used in chemistry to connote equal combining power. The equivalent weight of an element is its atomic weight divided by its valence (q.v.) in the particular reaction under consideration. A gram-equivalent weight is the equivalent weight of an element (or formula weight of a radical) divided by its valence. A solution containing one gram-equivalent of a particular constituent of the solute in a liter of solution is called a normal solution.

excipient An inert substance used to give a pharmaceutical preparation a suitable form or consistency.

exocrine Denoting a gland that discharges its secretion through a duct opening on an internal or external surface of the body, e.g., lacrimal gland, salivary gland.

first-order kinetics The kinetics characteristic of a reaction whose velocity is proportional to the concentration of a single substance. In an enzyme reaction there are two reactants: the substrate and the enzyme. However, in the intact organism the enzyme concentration usually remains constant so that only the changing substrate concentration influences the rate of metabolism or biotransformation. Enzyme systems display first-order kinetics at concentrations of substrate which do not saturate the binding sites of the enzyme. Similarly, drug-receptor interactions display first-order kinetics at drug concentrations which do not lead to 100 per cent receptor occupancy. The rates of migration of substances across biologic barriers also display first-order kinetics when the mechanism of translocation is passive diffusion or when the mechanism is facilitated diffusion or active transport and the quantity of solute to be transferred does not saturate the carrier (cf. zero-order kinetics).

galenical A *medicinal* prepared by extracting one or more active constituents of a plant.

germicidal *See* bactericide.

hapten A simple chemical capable of binding rather firmly with a protein conjugate to form a product that has antigenic properties (cf. antigen, antibodies, allergic response).

homeostasis The maintenance of the constancy of the body's optimal internal environment with respect to the composition, pH and osmotic pressure of the body fluids.

hormone (Gr. *hormonaein,* "to stimulate") A specific chemical substance secreted by cells in one part of a living organism which in various ways influences the growth, development or behavior of other cells remote from the source of the hormone.

hydrogen bond The chemical bond formed between a strongly electronegative atom and a hydrogen atom which is already bound by an ionic or covalent bond to another strongly electronegative atom such as oxygen, fluorine or nitrogen. The strength of the hydrogen bond is less than that of a true ionic bond.

hydrolysis A chemical reaction in which a compound is cleaved by the addition of a molecule of water.

hydrostatic pressure The pressure (force per unit area) exerted by water or an aqueous system normal to the surface on which it acts. In a moving fluid, the static pressure is measured at a right angle to the direction of flow.

hyperosmotic *See* osmotic effect.

hypertonic *See* isotonic.

hypnotic A drug that produces a state clinically identical with sleep by means of an action on the central nervous system (cf. sedative, anesthetic drug).

hyposmotic *See* osmotic effect.

hypotonic *See* isotinic.

idiosyncratic response A genetically determined abnormal response to a drug. The response may take the form of extreme sensitivity to low doses or extreme insensitivity to high doses of a drug which administration ordinarily produces qualitatively similar effects only at much higher or much lower doses, respectively. Or the drug reactions may be qualitatively different from the usual effects observed in the majority of subjects. The discontinuity of a frequency-response curve is characteristic of the idiosyncratic response and distinguishes this type of reactivity from the normal resistance to high doses of a drug or sensitivity to low doses (cf. sensitivity).

interstitium Structures such as cells and fibers lying between other structures and forming a supporting framework of tissue that binds together the organs that form the animal.

ionic bond The chemical bond formed between two atoms by the outright transfer of one or more electrons from one atom to the other. The strength of this bond depends on the distance between the two ions and diminishes as the square of the distance between them.

isotonic Pertaining to solutions which have the same osmotic pressure (are isosmotic) as the reference standards and which do not cause any volume change in cells. Solutions which induce a net loss of water from cells are *hypertonic*; conversely, solutions which cause cells to take up water are *hypotonic* with respect to the cell contents.

law of mass action When a chemical reaction reaches equilibrium at a constant temperature, the product of the active masses on one side of the chemical equation divided by the product of the active masses on the other side of the equation is a constant, regardless of the amount of each substance present at the beginning of the action. Thus for the ionization of an acid:

$$HA \rightleftharpoons [H^+] + [A^-]$$

$$\frac{[H^+] \times [A^-]}{[HA]} = A \text{ constant}$$

ligand An organic molecule that donates the necessary electrons to form coordinate covalent bonds with metallic ions. The term is also used to indicate any ion or molecule that reacts to form a complex with another molecule, frequently a macromolecule.

lipid A broad term used to include all the ether-soluble, water-insoluble substances obtained from plant and animal sources. According to W.R. Bloor's definition: (1) Simple lipids are esters of fatty acids and various alcohols, classified as (a) fats and oils when they are esters of glycerol, a three-carbon, straight-chain alcohol with three hydroxyl groups, and (b) waxes when they are esters of alcohols other than glycerol. (2) Compound lipids are esters of fatty acids and alcohols containing additional groups: (a) phospholipids, containing a phosphoric acid group; (b) glycolipids, containing a carbohydrate and a nitrogen-containing compound but no phosphoric acid group; and (c) others, such as sulfolipids. (3) Derived lipids are compounds derived from the preceding groups and having the general properties of the lipids; the derived compounds include fatty acids, glycerol, sterols and long-chain alcohols.

materia medica The material or substances used in the composition of remedies for the treatment of disease. Also, the branch of medical science that deals with the sources, nature, properties and preparations of drugs.

median effective dose The smallest dose required to produce a stated effect in 50 per cent of the population, usually designated by the abbreviation *ED50*. When death is the response, the ED50 is termed the *median lethal dose*, or LD50. Depending on the stated response, the median effective dose can also be designated AD50, the median analgesic dose; CD50, the median convulsive dose; etc.

mEq The abbreviation for milliequivalent, one thousandth of a gram-equivalent weight (cf. equivalent).

mM The abbreviation for millimole, one thousandth of a mole (q.v.).

molarity Pertaining to molecules, or to moles per unit volume; thus a molar solution is one containing one gram-molecular weight of solute per liter of solution.

mole One gram-molecule of any substance, i.e., the expression in grams of the molecular weight of a substance; a gram-molecular weight (cf. molarity).

narcotic In medicine, the term *narcotic* applies only to drugs having both an analgesic and a sedative action. In legal parlance, the term includes drugs with morphine-like activity as well as marihuana and cocaine. The term *narcotic analgesic,* used interchangeably with *opiate* or *opioid* (q.v.), avoids the confusion inherent in the legal classification.

narcotic analgesic *See* opioid.

neuroeffector junction A junction between a neuron and an effector organ or cell such as a smooth muscle of the pupil of the eye, or a gland cell (cf. synapse).

neuromuscular junction A junction between a somatic motor neuron and a skeletal muscle fiber.

noncompetitive antagonism *See* drug antagonism.

nonpolar A nonpolar compound is one in which the centers of positive and negative charge almost coincide, so that no permanent dipole moments are produced. Nonpolar compounds do not ionize or conduct electricity.

normal equivalent deviation (NED) A multiple (1, 2, 3, etc.) of the standard deviation. The quantal log dose-response curve may be transformed to a straight line when the data are replotted on coordinates in which the ordinate is expressed as normal equivalent deviation. Each per cent responding is converted to an NED, i.e., to the corresponding multiple of the standard deviation:

NED	Per Cent Response	Prob
−3	0.1	2
−2	2.3	3
−1	16	4
0	50	5
+1	84	6
+2	97.7	7
+3	99.9	8

A further refinement of the use of the NED as an expression of the percentage response in quantal dose-effect curves involves the elimination of the positive and negative signs by the expedient of adding 5 to each NED value. This new unit is called a *probit* (from contraction of the term *probability unit*).

nucleic acids A group of complex compounds of high molecular weight that occur in all plant and animal cells and in viruses. Nucleic acids are made up of long chains of nucleotides which are composed of four characteristic groups: (1) heterocyclic bases of the purine type; (2) heterocyclic bases of the pyrimidine type; (3) a carbohydrate, being either a ribose (five-carbon sugar) or a desoxyribose (ribose with one oxygen atom removed); and (4) phosphoric acid. Nucleic acids containing ribose are known as ribonucleic acids (RNA); the principal bases in RNA are the purines adenine and guanine and the pyrimidines cytosine and uracil. Nucleic acids containing desoxyribose are called desoxyribonucleic acids (DNA); the principal bases are adenine and guanine and the pyrimidines cytosine and thymine. The nucleic acids are intimately involved in the mechanisms of self-duplication which are basic to life and by which hereditary characteristics are transmitted from cell to cell.

opioid A drug having both an analgesic and a sedative action; the term essentially embraces only those drugs, either natural or synthetic, that have morphine-like pharmacologic activity. Synonymous with *narcotic analgesic* and *opiate*.

osmotic effect The effect produced on the net movement of water when two solutions of unequal concentrations are separated by a semipermeable membrane which permits freer passage of water than of the dissolved substances. The direction of movement of water will be from the solution in which the water molecules are *more concentrated* (the more *dilute* solution, i.e., the solution containing fewer molecules of solute) to the solution in which the water molecules are *less concentrated* (the more *concentrated* solution, i.e., the solution containing more molecules of solute). The measure of the tendency of solvent to pass from the more dilute solution to the more concentrated solution is the *osmotic pressure*; osmotic pressure is the force or pressure required to prevent osmotic flow of water into a given solution.

Any two solutions that have the same osmotic pressure are *isosmotic*. Solutions which have a greater osmotic pressure than a given reference solution are *hyperosmotic*; solutions which have a smaller osmotic pressure than a given reference solution are *hyposmotic* (cf. isotonic).

oxidation A chemical reaction in which oxygen is added to a compound or, by extension, the proportion of oxygen in a compound is increased by the removal of other groups (cf. reduction).

parenteral Pertains to administration of drugs into any part of the body other than the gastrointestinal tract (cf. enteral), e.g., subcutaneous, intramuscular or intravenous injection; topical application to the skin or mucous membranes; inhalation through the lungs.

partition coefficient The measure of the tendency of a solute to distribute itself between two phases, expressed as the ratio of the solute's concentration in one phase to its concentration in the second phase. An example is the lipid/water partition coefficient, the ratio of a solute's concentration in a lipid phase (fat-solvent) to its concentration in water after the system has come to equilibrium.

peptide Any member of a class of compounds of low molecular weight that yield two or more amino acids on hydrolysis. Formed by the loss of water from the NH_2 and COOH groups of adjacent amino acids. Peptides form the constituent parts of proteins.

pH (Fr. *puissance d'hydrogen,* "power of hydrogen") A chemical symbol used to express acidity and alkalinity in terms of the concentration of hydrogen ion. The pH equals the negative logarithm of the H^+ concentration in gram-atoms per litter, i.e., the logarithm of the reciprocal of the H^+ concentration. The concentration of H^+ in pure water at 25°C is taken as the point of neutrality. Water ionizes to only a slight degree, and the concentration of H^+ is 10^{-7} M; the concentration of hydroxyl ion (OH^-) is also 10^{-7} M. Since the H^+ and OH^- ions are in equilibrium with nonionized water molecules, the law of mass action is applicable; i.e., the product of the concentrations of the two ions must be a constant. This constant, the *ion product of water,* has a value of 1×10^{-14} at 25°C. As the ion product must be valid in any solution in which water is present, this constant may be employed to calculate the concentrations of H^+ and

OH⁻ ions present in such solutions. Thus pH values may range from 0 to 14, number less than 7 indicating acidity and numbers greater than 7, alkalinity.

pharmaceutical alternatives   Drug products that contain the identical therapeutic moiety, or its precursor, but not necessarily in the same amount or dosage form or as the same salt or ester (as defined by FDA regulations).

pharmaceutical equivalents   Drug products that contain identical amounts of the identical active drug ingredient, i.e., the same salt or ester of the same therapeutic moiety in identical dosage forms, but not necessarily containing the same inactive ingredients.

pharmacogenetics   The scientifc study of genetic factors which account for individual differences in the response to drugs.

pharmacokinetics   The branch of pharmacology that deals with the study of the factors which influence the magnitude of drug effect by determining the amount of drug at its various sites of action as a function of time after drug administration.

pharmacologic antagonism   *See* drug antagonism.

phospholipids   Compound lipids that are esters of fatty acids and alcohols containing a phosphoric acid group (cf. lipid).

physiologic antagonism   *See* drug antagonism.

placebo   An inert substance, such as the sugar lactose, which is used as a sham drug. The placebo has no inherent pharmacologic activity but may produce a biologic response by virtue of the factor of suggestion attendant upon its administration.

plasma clearance (renal)   The volume of plasma needed to supply the amount of a specific substance excreted in the urine in one minute. The clearance of a substance which is completely filterable and which is neither reabsorbed nor secreted by the renal tubular cells measures the glomerular filtration rate. A substance which is so rapidly secreted by the renal tubular cells that it is almost completely cleared in one passage through the kidney can be used to measure the total amount of plasma flowing through the kidney.

polar   A polar compound is, in general, a compound that exhibits polarity, or local differences in electrical properties, and has a dipole moment associated with one or more of its interatomic valence bonds. Polar compounds associate readily in most cases. In the most general use of the term, polar compounds include all electrolytes, most inorganic substances and many organic ones.

polymer   A compound formed by two or more molecules of a simpler compound, the relative amount of each element remaining the same. The meaning of this term has also been extended to denote any one of a number of compounds composed of the same elements or radicals and related in such a way that the molecular formulas are in the relation of whole-number multiples of each other.

population   A collection of items defined by a common characteristic. Examples would be all individuals responding to the administration of atropine by an increase in the diameter of the pupil of the eye; all doctors living in New York City; all parts produced by a machine in one day.

potency A comparative expression of drug activity measured in terms of the dose required to produce a particular effect of given intensity relative to a given or implied standard of reference. Potency, like affinity, varies inversely with the magnitude of the dose required to produce this effect. If two drugs are not both capable of producing an effect of equal magnitude, they cannot be compared with respect to potency; for example, the analgesic potency of aspirin cannot be compared with that of codeine, since no dose of aspirin can relieve pain of certain intensities which are effectively relieved by codeine (cf. ceiling effect).

proteins Highly complex molecules that are universally present in all living matter. All proteins are built from the same subunits, the amino acids, which are joined together by primary bonds to form long chains. The bond, called a peptide bond, $-CONH-$ is formed between the carboxylic acid group, $-COOH$, of one amino acid and the amino group, $-NH_2$, of another amino acid, with the splitting out of water. A single protein molecule may consist of a chain of a hundred or more subunits made up of twenty different kinds of amino acids recurring many times along the length of the chain. The sequence in which the amino acids occur along the chain is characteristic for each protein. Some proteins, called conjugated proteins, contain other chemical groups in addition to amino acids. Nucleoproteins consist of proteins combined with nucleic acids; lipoproteins consist of proteins combined with lipids.

reduction A chemical reaction in which oxygen is removed from a compound or in which the alteration leads to a decrease in the proportion of oxygen in a compound (cf. oxidation).

sedative An agent that can induce a state of drowsiness at a dose that does not produce sleep.

selectivity The capacity of a drug to produce one particular effect in preference to other effects – to act in lower doses at one site than those required to produce effects at other sites. Selectivity can be measured by the same ratios used to assess drug safety. Selectivity should not be confused with potency. Potency is a comparative measure of the capacity of *several* drugs to produce an effect of equal intensity, whereas selectivity is a comparative measure of the propensity of a single drug to produce several effects (cf. specificity, certain safety factor, standard safety margin, therapeutic index).

sensitivity The ability of a member of a population, relative to the abilities of other members of the same population, to respond in a qualitatively normal fashion to a particular dose of a drug. Sensitivity may be measured or described in terms of the normal distribution curve or the dose-effect curve in which a wide range of doses may separate the most sensitive from the least sensitive individuals. The individuals lying to the left of the median are the most sensitive, those to the right, the least sensitive. Any individual responding with a given preselected response to a dose of a drug is said to be sensitive to the drug. Individuals responding at the extremes of a normal distribution curve should not be confused with individuals showing an idiosyncratic response. The characteristic feature in the idiosyncratic response to low or high doses is a discontinuity from the normal distribution of dose sensitivities.

side-effect Any effect other than that for which a given drug is administered. The intensity of the side-effect is a function of the dose administered. A particular effect of a drug may be a side-effect under certain circumstances or the desired therapeutic effect under others; e.g., dryness of the mouth is a side-effect of atropine when the drug is being used to decrease gastric secretion in the treatment of peptic ulcer. When atropine is used to decrease salivation, dryness of the mouth is the therapeutic effect and decreased gastric secretion the side-effect (cf. idiosyncratic response, toxic effect, allergic response).

smooth muscle The effector organ of much of the autonomic nervous system. *Multi-unit* smooth muscle such as that of the iris of the eye, the piloerector muscle of the cat, and probably vascular smooth muscle has innervation similar to skeletal muscle; the nerve supply is excitatory and the organ displays little or no spontaneous or rhythmic activity. *Visceral* smooth muscle contracts spontaneously and rhythmically but this activity can be modified by autonomic nerves that either inhibit or enhance the intrinsic activity.

specificity The capacity of a drug to manifest its effects by a single mechanism of action. A drug is said to have specificity, even though it may produce a multiplicity of effects, if all the effects produced are due to a single mechanism of action. Atropine, for example, has great specificity of action since it antagonizes only the actions of acetylcholine (or other drugs closely resembling acetylcholine) at the acetylcholine receptor. The widespread distribution of the acetylcholine receptor accounts for the multiplicity of effects (or nonselectivity) of the action of atropine (cf. selectivity).

standard deviation A measure of dispersion of variability about the mean value of a distribution. The standard deviation has no verbal definition and is defined only by its formula:

$$\text{SD, or } s = \sqrt{\frac{\Sigma(x-\bar{x})^2}{n}}$$

where x = the arithmetic average
$(x-\bar{x})$ = the deviation, the difference between an individual number and the average
$\Sigma(x-\bar{x})^2$ = the sum of all the deviations squared
n = number of observations

standard safety margin A number which is an assessment of the relative safety of a drug or of its selectivity of action. The standard safety margin has the dimension of per cent; it is the percentage by which the dose effective in virtually all of a population (the ED99) has to be increased to produce a lethal effect in a minimum number of the population (The LD1). Thus the standard safety margin is equal to $\dfrac{(LD1 - ED99)}{ED99} \times 100$

(Cf. certain safety factor, therapeutic index, selectivity.)

stereoisomers Two substances of the same composition and constitution that differ only in the relative spatial position of their constituent atoms and/or groups. The isomerism may be due to the relative spatial position of groups attached to atoms joined by a double bond (geometric isomerism), or it may be due to the presence of one or more asymmetric atoms, i.e., a quadrivalent atom of carbon, silicon, etc., to which four different atoms or radicals are attached and which therefore possess spatial geometric forms that cannot be superimposed, but are in fact mirror images.

summation The algebraic sum of the individual effects of two drugs acting simultaneously which elicit the same overt response, regardless of the mechanism of action of each of the drugs, e.g., the combined effect of aspirin and codeine in relieving pain, in which the two drugs act by different mechanisms; or the combined effect of aspirin and phenacetin in relieving pain, in which case the two drugs apparently act on the same receptors (cf. additive effect, synergism).

sympathomimetic An adjective describing (1) an effect that resembles the response to stimulation of adrenergic nerves, or (2) an agent whose effects, in general, are similar to those elicited by adrenergic stimulation.

synapse The junction between two neurons as occurs in ganglia (cf. neuroeffector junction, neuromuscular junction).

syndrome The complete picture of a disease, including all the signs and symptoms.

synergism The situation in which the combined effects of two drugs acting simultaneously is greater than the algebraic sum of the individual effects of these drugs. The term is usually reserved for those cases in which two drugs act at different sites and one drug, the synergist, increases the effect of the second drug by altering its biotransformation, distribution or excretion. An example would be the exaggerated response to tyramine in individuals being treated with monoamine oxidase inhibitors (cf. summation, additive effect).

tachycardia Excessive rapidity in the action of the heart; the term is usually applied to a heart rate above 100 beats per minute.

tachyphylaxis *See* drug tolerance.

therapeutic index A number which is an assessment of the relative safety of a drug or of its selectivity of action. A therapeutic index is ordinarily computed from the quantal dose-effect curves describing data obtained in experiments with animals. The term usually refers to the ratio LD50/ED50, the ratio of the dose required to produce a lethal effect in 50 per cent of the population to the dose required to produce the desired therapeutic effect in 50 per cent of the population. The larger the ratio, the greater the relative safety of the drug. However, the LD50/ED50 ratio is not sufficient for a true assessment of drug safety, since median doses tell nothing about the slopes of the dose-response curves being compared or the degree of overlap of the curves (cf. certain safety factor, standard safety margin, selectivity).

threshold dose The dose of a drug just sufficient to produce any preselected intensity of effect. If the preselected effect is the first detectable effect, the threshold dose is the smallest dose required to produce a detectable effect. The dose required to produce a 50 per cent decrease in heart rate may be considered a threshold dose if the preselected effect is a 50 per cent decrease in heart rate.

tinctures Alcoholic or hydroalcoholic solutions of the active principles of drugs, e.g., paregoric.

toxic effect An effect of a drug on an organism that is deleterious to the well-being or life of the organism. A toxic effect may be a side-effect or undesired effect under some circumstances but under other circumstances may be the desired effect. A toxic effect is a side-effect when a drug is being used as a therapeutic agent in the prevention, treatment or diagnosis of disease. A toxic effect is the desired effect, and not a side-effect, when the drug is being used to eradicate microorganisms, pests or malignant cells and does so without harm to the user.

Toxic effects may be classified on the basis of rate of onset, duration of symptoms, and rate of intake of the chemical. Acute toxicity is the type that occurs when absorption is rapid and when exposure is sudden and severe. Subacute toxicity results from frequent, repeated exposure over a period of several hours or days to a dose of drug that is insufficient to produce toxic effects when given as a single dose. Chronic toxicity is the type that usually occurs from repeated exposure over a long period to a substance which has a tendency to accumulate in the body.

transmission The passage of an impulse across a junction; the process by which a nerve ending activates the next structure in the pathway (cf. conduction).

uricosuric agent A drug that increases the excretion of uric acid in the urine.

valence The property of an atom or radical to combine with other atoms or radicals in definite proportions. The valence of an atom or radical is designated by a number representing the proportion in which a given atom or radical combines. The standard of reference is hydrogen, which is assigned a valence of 1; and the valence of any given atom or radical is then the number of hydrogen atoms, or their equivalent, with which the given atom or radical combines. Many elements have more than one valence, and their compounds are classified and designated accordingly. The number of electrons in the outer shell of an atom determines the valence or valences of the atom. By gaining, losing or sharing these outer-shell electrons, atoms combine to form molecules.

Van der Waals forces Weak attractive forces between any two neutral atoms or atomic groupings. The force of attraction is inversely proportional to the seventh power of the distance between the atoms.

viscera (plural of viscus) The large interior organs in the three great cavities of the body (abdomen, pelvis, thorax), especially in the abdomen.

volume of distribution or **apparent volume of distribution** The volume of body fluid in which a drug appears to be dissolved. In a normal lean, 70-kg male, the whole body water comprises about 40 liters. The extracellular water is about one-third of the total, or about 12 liters, 3 liters of which is the volume of circulating plasma-water.

zero-order kinetics The kinetics characteristic of a reaction that proceeds at a constant rate independent of the concentrations of reactants. Enzyme reactions display zero-order kinetics at levels of substrate which saturate the binding sites of the enzyme. In analogous fashion, drug-receptor interactions become zero order when the concentration of drug at the receptor produces complete receptor occupancy, and facilitated diffusion or active transport becomes zero order when the concentration of solute saturates the carrier mechanism (cf. first-order kinetics).

APPENDIXES

APPENDIX 1
Locally Acting Drugs Affecting
the Gastrointestinal Tract

I. **Gastric Antacids**
A. **Definition.** Chemical substances that on ingestion react locally with the hydrochloric acid of the gastric contents to lower acidity (raise pH)
B. **General Considerations**
  1. **Effects**
    a. Increase in gastric pH. The activity of an antacid is dependent upon the total acid-combining capacity of the compound and the length of time it remains in the stomach. The commonly used antacids do not make the gastric contents alkaline enough to damage gastrointestinal tissue.
    b. Reduction of the protein-digestive action of pepsin at about pH 4. The reduction in pepsin activity is sufficient to decrease the corrosive action of gastric juice on an ulcerative lesion, but not to suppress completely the digestion of food proteins. At pH 7 to 8, pepsin becomes completely inactive.
    c. Increase in rate of stomach emptying. The higher the pH is raised, the more rapidly the stomach empties. Antacids are expelled into the intestine with the rest of the stomach contents.
  2. **Classification**
    a. **Systemic.** Antacids that form compounds which are soluble in gastric and intestinal secretions. The products formed are readily absorbed.
    b. **Nonsystemic.** Agents that interact with HC1 to form relatively insoluble compounds. The reaction products are not absorbed to any degree and therefore have little, if any, systemic effect.
      (1) **Buffer antacids.** Agents that limit the rise in pH of the gastric contents to less than neutrality, usually only to about pH 4
      (2) **Nonbuffer antacids.** Agents that have the potential for elevating the pH of gastric contents to 7 or above
  3. **Uses**
    a. **Therapeutic.** For the treatment of peptic ulcer and hiatal hernia

433

The therapeutic objective is to raise gastric pH to about 4 from its normal range of 1 to 2 in order to relieve pain (the pain of peptic ulcer is reasonably well established to be the result of the action of the acid on the lesion). At pH 4, the decrease in the activity of pepsin also contributes to the decreased corrosive action of gastric juice on the lesion.

   b. **Popular.**   For the treatment of indigestion (upset stomach; sour stomach; heartburn; acid indigestion). Antacids are one of the groups of widely advertised nostrums used most extensively, and usually inappropriately, by the general public.

C. **Systemic Antacids**
   1. **Agents**
      a. Sodium bicarbonate (Bellans; Soda Mint; Resolve)
      b. Sodium citrate. Common constituent of many proprietary preparations that "fizz." The preparations that contain sodium bicarbonate and citric acid react in solution to form sodium citrate and release carbon dioxide.
   2. **Effects**
      a. May increase gastric pH to 7 or greater and provoke rapid gastric emptying
      b. Readily absorbed; increases the concentration of sodium bicarbonate in blood, producing systemic alkalosis and electrolyte disturbances which burden the kidney with electrolyte readjustments. Systemic alkalosis may be characterized by loss of appetite, weakness, mental confusion and, rarely, tetany.

D. **Nonsystemic Antacids**
   1. **Buffer Antacids**
      a. **Agents**
         (1) Aluminum hydroxide gel (Amphojel; Creamalin)
         (2) Aluminum phosphate gel (Phosphaljel)
         (3) Other aluminum-containing compounds (Alglyn; Rolaids)
         (4) Magnesium trisilicate (U.S.P.)
         (5) Magnesium trisilicate with aluminum hydroxide gel (Gelusil; Tums)
      b. **Effects**
         (1) In the stomach, the relatively insoluble buffer antacids react slowly with hydrochloric acid to form chloride salts and reduce gastric acidity. The chloride salts react with alkaline intestinal secretions to form insoluble salts (e.g., aluminum carbonate) which are excreted in the feces.
         (2) Aluminum-containing antacids have a constipating effect.
         (3) Magnesium-containing antacids have a laxative effect (many proprietary preparations combine aluminum and magnesium antacids to counteract each other's effect on intestinal motility).

2. **Nonbuffer Antacids**
   a. **Agents**
      (1) Calcium carbonate (U.S.P.)
      (2) Magnesium oxide (U.S.P.)
      (3) Magnesium hydroxide (Milk of Magnesia)
      (4)*Calcium carbonate with magnesium trisilicate (Chooz; BiSoDol)
      (5)*Magnesium oxide with aluminum hydroxide (Aludrox; Maalox; Di-Gel)
   b. **Effects**
      (1) Chloride salts are formed in the stomach upon reaction with acid; in the intestine, chloride is converted to insoluble carbonate or other insoluble compounds which are excreted in the feces.
      (2) Calcium antacids, like aluminum antacids, have a constipating effect.
      (3) Calcium carbonate may cause "acid rebound," i.e., enhanced rate of gastric acid secretion secondary to antacid administration. Calcium-ion stimulates the release of the hormone gastrin, which, in turn, stimulates gastric acid production.

II. **Digestants**
   A. **Definition.** Drugs that promote the process of digestion in the gastrointestinal tract
   B. **Therapeutic Use.** In the treatment of conditions characterized by a lack of one or more of the substances that normally digest foodstuffs; for replacement therapy in deficiency states
   C. **Agents.** Hydrochloric acid; pepsin; bile salts and acids

III. **Laxatives and Cathartics**
   A. **Definition.** Laxatives and cathartics are orally administered agents that promote intestinal evacuation. Although the two terms are frequently used interchangeably, they are more properly used to imply different intensities of effect. Laxative effect suggests the excretion of a soft, formed stool and may result from increased motor activity of the intestine or simply from changes in the water-content of the stool. Cathartic effect implies a more fluid evacuation and is invariably the result of increased intestinal motor activity; cathartics may be administered in doses that produce only a laxative effect.
   B. **Uses and Contraindications**
      1. **Therapeutic Uses of Cathartics**
         a. In cases of drug and food poisoning, to flush the offending substance from the intestinal tract (saline cathartics, such as sodium sulfate, are often used for this purpose)
         b. To empty the gastrointestinal tract prior to radiologic examination of abdominal organs and prior to *elective* bowel surgery (castor oil is the traditional agent)

---

*Contain buffer antacids.

      c. To expel intestinal parasites and the drugs (anthelmintics) used to treat these parasitic infestations

  2. **Therapeutic Uses of Laxatives**

      a. To keep the stool soft and to prevent irritation and straining in patients with hernia (before and after surgery), cardiovascular disease or rectal disorders (emollient laxatives generally used)

      b. In the temporary treatment of chronic functional constipation when other measures are inadequate

  3. **Contraindications**

      a. In all cases of constipation associated with organic disease

      b. In all cases of gastrointestinal cramps, colic, nausea, vomiting or other symptoms of appendicitis or any undiagnosed abdominal pain

C. **Classification.**   Cathartics and laxatives are generally classified on the basis of their general mechanism of action as stimulant and saline cathartics and as bulk-forming and emollient laxatives.

D. **Stimulant Cathartics (Irritant Cathartics)**

  1. **Agents**

      a. Castor oil (Neoloid)

      b. Cascara sagrada (Nature's Remedy); senna (Gentlax; Senokot; Swiss Kress)

      c. Phenolphthalein (Evac-U-Gen; Ex-Lax; Feen-a-mint; Phenolax); bisacodyl (Dulcolax)

  2. **Site of Action.**   With the exception of castor oil, the effects of these agents are limited primarily to the large intestine and are produced only after a delay of 6 hours or more. Castor oil acts in the small intestine and, as a consequence, usually produces its cathartic effect within 3 hours.

  3. **Mechanism of Action.** The increase in motor activity of the intestine is thought to result from local irritation of the intestinal mucosa or from a selective action upon the intestinal smooth muscle or nerve networks within the intestinal wall.

    Castor oil itself is nonirritant but, when acted upon by intestinal digestive enzymes (lipases), it is converted to glycerol and ricinoleic acid, and the latter agent produces the cathartic effect.

  4. **Undesirable Effects**

      a. May cause griping, intestinal cramps, increased mucus secretion and excessive fluid evacuation

      b. Phenolphthalein may produce allergic reactions in sensitive individuals.

E. **Saline Cathartics**

  1. **Agents**

      a. Magnesium salts: magnesium sulfate (epsom salt); milk of magnesia

      b. Sodium salts: sodium sulfate (Glauber's salt); sodium phosphate (Sal Hepatica)

      c. Potassium sodium tartrate (Rochelle salt)

  2. **Site of Action.**   Throughout small and large intestine

3. **Mechanism of Action.** The saline cathartics are soluble salts that are only slightly and slowly absorbed from the digestive tract. Their presence in the intestinal lumen leads to a retention of water by osmotic forces. The resulting increase in bulk of the intestinal contents serves as a mechanical stimulus to increase intestinal motor activity.

4. **Effects**
   a. Full doses of saline cathartics produce a semifluid or watery evacuation in 3 to 6 hours.
   b. Some absorption of the saline cathartics does occur, but this causes little untoward effect if kidney function is adequate. If urinary excretion is reduced or absorption increased, the accumulation of magnesium ion in the body may lead to central nervous system depression.

F. **Bulk-forming Laxatives**
   1. **Agents**
      a. Methylcellulose (Cellothyl; Hydrolose; Mucilose Compound)
      b. Plantago or psyllium seed (Konsyl; Metamucil; Plova; Serutan)
      c. Sodium carboxymethylcellulose (SCMC)
   2. **Site of Action.** Throughout small and large intestine
   3. **Mechanism of Action.** The various natural and semisynthetic polysaccharides and cellulose derivatives dissolve or swell in water and the resulting increase in bulk of the intestinal contents acts as a mechanical stimulus. These agents also form an emollient gel or viscous solution that serves to keep the fecal material soft and hydrated.
   4. **Effects**
      a. The laxative effect is usually apparent in 12 to 24 hours but full effect is not manifest until 2 to 3 days of medication.
      b. Essentially devoid of systemic effects since these laxatives are excreted almost quantitatively in the feces
      c. If adequate fluids are not taken with the bulk-forming laxatives, they can cause fecal impaction and intestinal obstruction.

G. **Emollient Laxatives**
   1. **Agents**
      a. Mineral oil (liquid petrolatum; Petrogalar)
      b. Dioctyl sodium succinate (Colace; Doxinate)
   2. **Site of Action.** Throughout small and large intestine
   3. **Mechanism of Action.** Promote defecation merely by softening the feces, without either direct or mechanical stimulation of intestinal motor activity
   4. **Adverse Effects**
      a. Mineral oil is a lipid solvent and when administered with or directly after meals may interfere with the absorption of essential fat-soluble substances and lipid-soluble drugs.
      b. If drops of swallowed mineral oil coating the pharynx gain access to the lungs, a lipid pneumonia may result.

APPENDIX 2
Drugs Influencing Renal Function

I. Diuretics
  A. **Definition.** An agent that increases the volume flow of urine
  B. **Osmotic Diuretics**
    1. **Agents**
       Urea
       Mannitol
    2. **Site of Diuretic Action**
       Primarily in the proximal tubule where tubular urine remains isosmotic
    3. **Mechanism of Action**
       Increase in volume of tubular urine due to osmotic pressure exerted by
       the large amount of excess solute that is not absorbed. Increased volume
       leads to increased rate of urine flow which allows less time for reabsorp-
       tion. Increased volume causes decrease in Na^+ concentration in tubular
       urine which makes active transport of Na^+ more difficult and less ef-
       ficient $-$ Na^+ has to be transported against a higher than usual concentra-
       tion gradient. End result: increased rate of elimination of water and
       proportionally increased rate of elimination of Na^+ and Cl^-
    4. **Route of Administration**
       Urea $-$ oral route
       Mannitol $-$ intravenous route
    5. **Untoward Reactions**
       Little if any when properly administered. Urea may produce nausea and
       vomiting.
  C. **Xanthines as Diuretics**
    1. **Agents**
       Theophylline (in tea)
       Caffeine (in coffee, cola soft drinks, kola nuts)
       Theobromine (in cocoa)
    2. **Site of Diuretic Action**
       No single locus of action, but appears to be primarily in proximal tubule

438

3. Mechanism of Diuretic Action

Increase in glomerular filtration rate partly responsible, but diuresis can occur in the absence of any increase in glomerular filtration rate. Tolerance to diuretic effect of the xanthines is easily developed.

D. Mercurial Diuretics

Mercurial diuretics have been largely replaced by newer agents but are important from the historical point of view. All mercurial diuretics are organic compounds containing mercury.

1. Agents

Many, but the most commonly used are:

Meralluride (Mercuhydrin)

Mercaptomerin (Thiomerin)

The pharmacologic actions and therapeutic uses of all the agents are so similar that they can be discussed as a group.

2. Site of Diuretic Action

Various segments of the nephron — *not* a single site of action. Evidence for actions in ascending limb of loop of Henle

3. Mechanism of Action

Inhibition of Na^+ reabsorption; inhibiton of active Cl^- reabsorption in ascending limb of loop of Henle

4. Route of Administration

Intramuscular. Subcutaneous and oral administration produce local irritation.

5. Fate in the Body

  a. **Absorption.** Incompletely absorbed from gastrointestinal tract
  Theophylline or other xanthines added to parenteral preparations improve absorption by decreasing ability of mercurials to combine with tissue proteins at site of injection.

  b. **Metabolism and excretion.** Up to 95% of an administered dose of organic mercurial recovered in urine in 24 hours

  c. **Distribution.** Organic mercurials can be detected, even after prolonged administration, only in the liver, spleen and kidney.

  The inorganic compound, mercuric chloride, is a poor diuretic. This can be explained on the basis of distribution. $HgCl_2$ is concentrated in organs other than the kidney and is excreted slowly. However, when $HgCl_2$ is combined with a suitable carrier such as cysteine, $HgCl_2$ becomes a relatively potent diuretic and its excretion and distribution become like that of the organic mercurials.

6. Untoward Effects

The classic symptoms of systemic mercury poisoning are not likely to be a problem in the use of mercurial diuretics. These symptoms are only likely to appear when an organic mercurial diuretic is used injudiciously in individuals with primarily inadequate renal function.

Cysteine and other monothiols can reverse some of the toxic effects of mercurials without preventing the diuretic effects. The dithiol dimercaprol (BAL) readily reverses both the acute and chronic toxic effects of mercurials, organic and inorganic, and also antagonizes the diuretic action of the mercurials.

E. The Sulfonamide Derivatives — Carbonic Anhydrase Inhibitors

1. Agents

Acetozolamide (Diamox). Limited usefulness as a diuretic but important because of its role in the development of fundamental renal physiology and pharmacology

2. Site of Action

In the proximal and distal tubules where H^+ from tubular cell is exchanged for Na^+

3. Mechanism of Action

Inhibition of carbonic anhydrase.

Carbonic anhydrase accelerates the equilibrium reaction:

$$H_2O + CO_2 \rightleftharpoons H_2CO_3 \rightleftharpoons H^+ + HCO_3^-$$

Dissociation of H_2CO_3 in the tubular cell yields free H^+ which is necessary for reabsorption of HCO_3^- from tubular urine. When carbonic anhydrase is inhibited, H^+ is supplied in insufficient amounts and too slowly for the exchange reaction to occur at a normal rate. When the rate of exchange of Na^+ for H^+ is decreased, the reabsorption of HCO_3^- is inhibited. Net result: diuresis with increased HCO_3^- and Na^+ excretion. As HCO_3^- is eliminated, amount of HCO_3^- delivered to kidney decreases and the amount of H^+ available, even in the absence of carbonic anhydrase activity, is sufficient to exchange with Na^+, combine with the HCO_3^- and account for reabsorption of all HCO_3^- filtered. Thus action of acetozolamide is limited; duration of action is only about 24 hours.

4. Fate in the Body

Well absorbed when administered orally. Excreted by the kidney within 24 hours

5. Untoward Reactions

Few of serious nature

F. Sulfonamide Derivatives — Benzothiadiazine Derivatives

1. Agents

Many, but the most commonly used are:

Chlorothiazide (Diuril)

Hydrochlorothiazide (Esidrix)

All benzothiadiazines have qualitatively the same properties, but differ among themselves quantitatively; therefore, can be discussed as a group. Synthesized as an outgrowth of studies on carbonic anhydrase inhibitors, but agents vary widely in their ability to inhibit carbonic anhydrase.

2. **Site of Diuretic Action**

Not fully determined as yet, but principal effect is close to the origin of the distal convoluted tubule

3. **Mechanism of Diuretic Action**

All agents act predominantly to inhibit Na^+ reabsorption by the kidney tubule. Those agents which are relatively potent inhibitors of carbonic anhydrase also act via this mechanism. However, the diuretic potency of the thiazides is *unrelated* to their carbonic anhydrase inhibitory activity.

The *pattern* of electrolyte excretion is dependent on the presence or absence of carbonic anhydrase inhibitory activity. The compounds with more potent carbonic anhydrase inhibitory activity, such as chlorothiazide, will produce, in addition to the increased NaCl excretion, an increase in HCO_3^- and K^+ excretion. Those derivatives with weak carbonic anhydrase inhibitory activity will not produce as large an increase in HCO_3^- excretion. However, *all potent* diuretics which inhibit Na^+ reabsorption deliver more Na^+ to the site of exchange of Na^+ for K^+ and H^+ in the more distal portions of the nephron. As a consequence, more exchange of Na^+ for K^+ and H^+ takes place. The greater the carbonic anhydrase inhibitory activity of the thiazides, the less H^+ available to exchange for Na^+, and the more K^+ will be exchanged for Na^+.

The various derivatives of benzothiadiazine differ not only in potency (size of dose needed to produce a maximum effect) but also in the amount of NaCl excreted at the maximally effective dose.

4. **Pharmacologic Effects Other Than Diuresis**

a. **Therapeutically useful effects**

(1) **Hypotensive effect.** Used as hypotensive agents either alone or in association with other agents

b. **Untoward reactions**

(1) **Excessive loss of K^+.** The loss of K^+ is of special importance in digitalized patients, in patients with liver disease, in patients receiving adrenocortical steroids.

(2) **Hyperglycemia.** May aggravate established diabetes mellitus or bring to light latent diabetes. Symptoms provoked by thiazides are reversible on stopping the drugs.

(3) **Uric acid retention.** Thiazides in therapeutic doses block uric acid secretion by the renal tubule. Use of thiazides may precipitate gout. Effect is quickly reversed on stopping the drugs.

(4) **Other effects.** Skin rashes

5. **Route of Administration.** Oral

6. **Fate in the Body.** Chlorothiazide is incompletely absorbed from the gut, but other agents are well absorbed.

All agents are excreted fairly rapidly by the kidney so that duration of action is about 12 to 24 hours.

G. Aldosterone Antagonists — Spirolactones

1. Agents
Spironolactone (Aldactone)

2. Site of Action
In the kidney at sites where the hormone aldosterone has its activity — primarily in the distal tubule

3. Mechanism of Action
Spirolactones are structurally related to aldosterone and competitively block the stimulating effects of aldosterone on the exchange of Na^+ for K^+ and H^+.

4. Route of Administration
Spironolactone in the form first introduced was incompletely absorbed from the gut, but in the more recent, finely dispersed small particle form, spironolactone is much better absorbed and is effective in about a quarter of the dose of the original material. This is an excellent example of how *pharmaceutical formulation* may greatly alter the activity of a drug.

5. Untoward Reaction
Appear to be relatively nontoxic

6. Therapeutic Uses
Although spirolactones alone may produce a diuresis in some cases, delivery of a relatively large amount of Na^+ to the distal part of the nephron is essential for full effect, and this is achieved by the concomitant administration of another diuretic which increases Na^+ delivery to the distal tubule. The spirolactone ensures that Na^+ is not reabsorbed or exchanged for K^+ or H^+ under the influence of aldosterone. Therefore, the chief use of the spirolactones is in combination with other diuretics to counteract the loss of K^+ and enhance the excretion of Na^+.

H. High-ceiling Diuretics — Potent, Widely Used Agents

1. Agents
Ethacrynic acid
Furosemide

2. Site of Action
Proximal and distal tubules, and in medullary portion of loop of Henle

3. Mechanism of Diuretic Action
Inhibit Na^+ reabsorption by the kidney tubule at all sites of active Na^+ reabsorption. Inhibit active Cl^- reabsorption in ascending limb of loop of Henle

4. Routes of Administration
Oral and intravenous

5. Fate in the Body
a. **Absorption.** Appear to be satisfactorily absorbed from GI tract
b. **Excretion.** Excreted in urine and in feces via bile. Excretion by kidney is blocked by probenecid.

6. **Side-effects**

Effects related to diuretic activity. Such potent diuretics that their use can lead to:

Excessive loss of K^+ and/or Cl^-

Dehydration

Elevated blood uric acid, precipitation of gout

General fatigue and muscle cramps (reversed by K^+)

II. Uricosuric Agents

A. **Definition.** Agents that increase the renal excretion of uric acid

B. **Agents.** Probenecid; sulfinpyrazone (Anturane)

C. **Site of Action.** Renal tubular cell, primarily in proximal tubule

D. **Mechanism of Action.** Inhibit the active reabsorption of uric action by the renal tubular cells

E. **Route of Administration.** Oral

F. **Fate in the Body.** Well absorbed. Highly bound to plasma protein, but actively secreted into urine by tubular cells. Unless urine is markedly alkaline, probenecid is almost completely reabsorbed from tubular urine. Therefore, long duration of action

G. **Effects**

1. Cause uric acid to be excreted at a rate sufficient to keep up with the rate of its formation in the body

2. Inhibit active tubular secretion of other organic acids such as para-aminohippuric acid (PAH), penicillin and ethacrynic acid by competing for same transport process

H. **Therapeutic Uses**

1. In the treatment of chronic gout

2. As an adjunct in penicillin therapy in diseases which require very high doses of penicillin

APPENDIX 3
Chemotherapy

I. General Considerations

Chemotherapy deals with the treatment of disease by chemical agents that can produce a toxic effect upon the disease-causing organism without producing undue harm to the host. Drugs used in the treatment of parasitic (microbial, viral, fungal, helmintic, etc.) and neoplastic diseases are termed *chemotherapeutic agents*. An *antibiotic* is a chemical substance produced by a microorganism that suppresses the growth of or directly kills another microorganism.

The goal of chemotherapy is to kill or to assist the body in the elimination of rapidly dividing, invading cells. This can be accomplished with minimal or no injury to the normal cells of the host by exploiting qualitative or quantitative differences between the biochemistry of invading cells and that of normal host cells. The more fundamental and the greater the difference between invading and host cells, the greater is the *selective toxicity* and the smaller is the likelihood of injury to the host.

There are many different types of neoplastic diseases and bacterial or other infections. These different types have differing sensitivities toward chemotherapeutic agents, so that each agent has its own spectrum of diseases against which it is effective.

Disease-causing cells have the capacity to become resistant to drugs which initially inhibited their growth (see pp. 267–271).

II. Antimicrobial Agents

A. Drug-Parasite Interactions

1. Spectrum of Activity.   Refers to the range of specific microbes capable of being inhibited by a particular agent. The spectrum of activity of a drug is dependent to some degree on the dose administered. A *narrow*-spectrum antimicrobial agent is one that primarily affects a limited number of different microorganisms. Examples of narrow-spectrum antibiotics: penicillin; erythromycin. A *broad*-spectrum drug is one capable of inhibiting a wide variety of microorganisms. Examples of broad-spectrum antibiotics: tetracyclines; streptomycin.

444

2. **Type of Activity.** Classification is based on the dosage used in therapeutics, not on the *in vitro* potential activity of an agent.
   a. **Bacteriostatic.** The ability of an agent to inhibit multiplication and growth of microorganisms. Examples of bacteriostatic agents: sulfonamides; tetracyclines; chloramphenicol; para-aminosalicylic acid (PAS).

   Prevention of bacterial growth suppresses the infection or total bacterial cell population, thus enabling the normal defense mechanisms of the host (white blood cells, tissue phagocytes, and antibodies) to eradicate the disease.
   b. **Bactericidal.** The ability of a drug not only to inhibit growth but also to kill the parasite. Examples of bactericidal agents: penicillin; streptomycin; cephalosporins; bacitracin. Eradication of disease still depends to some degree on the activity of host defense mechanisms.

   In general, bactericidal activity is associated with those agents that act by disrupting the synthesis or function of the microbial cell wall or cell membrane.
3. **Activity Resulting from Combining Antimicrobial Agents**
   a. **Additive effect.** Usually obtained by combining two bacteriostatic agents or two bactericidal agents
   b. **Antagonist effect.** May result from combination of a bacteriostatic agent with a bactericidal agent, since most bactericidal drugs act maximally on multiplying bacteria and bacteriostatic agents depress bacterial multiplication. However, results of combining bactericidal and bacteriostatic agents are unpredictable.
   c. **Delay in emergence of resistant organisms.** Combinations may delay the emergence of organisms resistant to either agent in the combination. Delay of emergence of resistant organisms is particularly important when long-term therapy is needed or in diseases caused by organisms that develop resistance rapidly. Example: the use of para-aminosalicylic (PAS) acid to delay resistance of tuberculous organisms to isoniazid, streptomycin, or rifampicin when therapy may continue for as long as 2 years.
4. **Mechanism of Antimicrobial Action**
   a. Inhibition of bacterial cell wall synthesis (penicillins; cephalosporins; bacitracin)
   b. Inhibition of bacterial protein synthesis (erythromycin; tetracyclines; chloramphenicol; streptomycin; lincomycin)
   c. Inhibition of bacterial synthesis of essential nonprotein metabolites (sulfonamides; PAS; isoniazid)
   d. Alteration of permeability of cell membrane (polymyxin B)
B. **Untoward Effects of Antimicrobial Therapy**
   1. Development of resistant organisms
   2. Development of *superinfection* as a result of changes in the normal

microbial population of the intestinal, upper respiratory and genitourinary tracts. Superinfection is the appearance of a new infection by pathogenic microorganisms or fungi during antimicrobial therapy of a primary disease.

3. Interference with normal nutrition, e.g., reduction of intestinal microflora may decrease availability of vitamin K since considerable quantities of this essential nutrient are synthesized by intestinal bacteria.

4. Development of drug allergy from known or unknown exposure (see pp. 271–274)

5. **Specific Drug Toxicities**
   a. **Sulfonamides.** Decreased solubility of conjugated drug may lead to precipitation in urinary tract (see p. 148); blood disorders can occur in individuals with certain genetic enzyme deficiences (see pp. 253–255).
   b. **Penicillin.** One of the least toxic agents known, but can produce convulsion in very high doses
   c. **Tetracyclines.** Since the tetracyclines can form complexes with calcium, they can be incorporated into tissues that are actively laying down calcium (teeth and bones), and can cause mottling and discoloration of teeth.
   d. **Streptomycin** (also neomycin, paramomycin, kanamycin, gentamicin). Can cause nerve damage leading to hearing loss and disturbances in the nonacoustic part of the inner ear (vestibular apparatus), which functions to orient the body during movement
   e. **Chloramphenicol.** Can depress the blood-cell-forming tissues in bone marrow

C. **Host Factors Determining Response to Antimicrobial Agents**
   1. **Age.** Impaired ability of the very young or elderly patient to biotransform or excrete drugs (see pp. 243–247)
   2. **Genetic Enzyme Deficiencies.** E.g., in biotransformation of isoniazid (see pp. 251, 254); in enzymes of red blood cells producing idiosyncratic responses to sulfonamides (see pp. 253–255)
   3. **Pregnancy.** Increased risk to both mother and fetus
   4. **Impaired Liver or Kidney Function.** Drug toxicity due to altered rate of drug elimination
   5. **Impaired Defense Mechanisms of Body**
      a. Due to disease: e.g., cancers of various types
      b. Due to drugs: e.g., anticancer agents; corticosteroids

D. **Misuses and Causes of Failure of Antimicrobial Drug Therapy**
   1. Treatment of untreatable infections: e.g., 90% of viral infections of upper respiratory tract; measles; mumps
   2. Treatment of fever of undetermined origin or an undiagnosed condition
   3. Improper dosage: excessive amounts leading to drug toxicity; suboptimal doses; adequate doses but given for too short a period of time
   4. Self-medication with a drug that "just happened to be around the house."

All antimicrobial agents, like any other therapeutic agents, may produce serious and even fatal reactions. *These drugs must never be taken without medical direction and supervision.*

III. Antifungal Agents

A. Treatment of superficial infections: e.g., tinea (ringworm) infections confined to the epidermis, hair and nails
 1. **Topically Administered Agents**
   a. Undecylenic acid (Desenex; Mycodecyl; Pedzyl): primarily fungistatic and has undoubted benefit in retarding growth of (but not eradicating) *tinea pedis* (athlete's foot)
   b. Tolnaftate (Dermoxin; Tinactin): highly effective in a variety of fungal infections of the skin
 2. **Systemically Administered Agent.** Griseofulvin, an antibiotic, is the only systemic agent available for treatment of superficial infections.
B. Treatment of deep infections: e.g., candidiasis (thrush); infection involving the mucus membranes, gastrointestinal tract and other visceral organs
 1. Nystatin, an antibiotic; fungistatic and fungicidal, depending on concentration. Useful treatment for candidiasis (thrush) infections that can be reached by topical application to mucus membranes of various body orifices. Not absorbed to any useful extent, but has local effect in bowel lumen. Not given parenterally.
 2. Amphotericin B, an antibiotic, given parenterally (not absorbed orally) for systemic fungal infections. Adverse reactions occur in all patients and there is a high incidence of serious and toxic side-effects. However, before the availability of amphotericin B, certain fungal infections were 100% fatal. Therefore, a certain degree of toxicity in its use is acceptable.

IV. Antiviral Agents

A few drugs that can prevent or cure viral illnesses are now available.
A. Amantadine: Used to prevent influenza A_2 infection
B. Idoxuridine: Used topically in the eye or on the skin for relief and cure of herpes simplex virus and other DNA-viruses
C. Methisazone: Used to prevent smallpox in persons who have been in contact with the disease (not approved for general use in USA but used in England)

V. Antiseptics and Disinfectants

A. **Definitions**
 1. *Antiseptics* are substances that are applied to living tissue to kill or prevent the growth of microorganisms.
 2. *Disinfectants* are bactericidal drugs that are applied to inanimate objects.
 3. *Germicides* are agents that are toxic to microorganisms in general when applied to living tissue or inanimate objects; term is frequently used to cover both antiseptics and disinfectants.
B. **Mechanisms of Action**
 1. Coagulation of protein
 2. Destruction of normal permeability characteristics of cell membrane

3. Poisoning of enzyme systems of cell (cf. p. 439)

In many cases, germicides destroy microorganisms in such a non-selective manner that normal host cells may also be injured (see p. 306).

C. Agents
1. Phenols
    a. Hexachlorophene: Incorporated into soaps but evidence is lacking for the effectiveness and safety of use as an "aid to personal hygiene"; 3% solutions used for reducing bacterial counts on surgeons' hands and forearms
    b. Cresol: Soapy emulsion (Lysol) used as disinfectant and antiseptic
2. Acids
    a. Boric acid: Mildly antiseptic; does not irritate skin or delicate tissues
    b. Benzoic acid: Weak, tasteless nontoxic bacteriostatic agent used extensively as a preservative in food and drink in a concentration of 0.1%
3. Surface-active Agents
    a. Anionic agents.   Include common soaps; owe their action primarily to dislodging bacteria in the skin
    b. Cationic agents.   Benzalkonium (Zephiran); cetylpyridinium (Ceepryn; Cepacol). Commonly used for antisepsis of skin and disinfection of instruments; included in various proprietary preparations such as mouthwashes, etc.
4. Oxidizing Agents
    Hydrogen peroxide, extensively used for cleaning wounds
5. Heavy Metals
    Thimerosal (Merthiolate), primarily bacteriostatic, used as cutaneous antiseptic; silver nitrate, used as prophylactic in eyes of newborn infants to prevent disturbances caused by gonococci
6. Alcohols
    Ethyl and isopropyl alcohol are bactericidal and extensively used as skin antiseptics
7. Halogens
    a. Iodine: Possesses high bactericidal and vericidal activity
    b. Chlorine: Chlorine-releasing compounds used principally to sterilize water for sanitization

VI. Antiprotozoal Agents
The infectious diseases of humans that are commonly caused by protozoa include: malaria; amebiasis; trypanosomiasis (sleeping sickness); trichomoniasis (a venereal disease). Malaria and amebiasis are the most common protozoal diseases; they are worldwide diseases and afflict hundreds of millions of persons.

A. Antimalarial Drugs
The malarial parasite is a protozoan of the genus *Plasmodium*, four species of which are known to infect humans. The insect vector is the female *Anopheles* mosquito (the disease may also be transmitted from one human

to another through a transfusion of blood containing malarial parasites or by syringes and needles contaminated with parasite-containing blood). Each parasite of the four species has a sexual cycle in the mosquito and an asexual cycle in the tissues and blood of humans. The efficacy of drugs in the prevention and treatment of malaria is related to the species of infecting parasite and to its stage of development.

The principal agents employed in therapy:

1. Chloroquine
2. Primaquine
3. Chloroguanide
4. Pyrimethamine

The mechanism of action of chloroquine and primaquine, as well as the older agents, quinine and quinacrine (Atabrine), is in large part completely nonspecific. They interact with, and alter the properties of, both microbial and mammalian DNA. Whatever selective toxicity they possess depends upon selective accumulation at the intracellular milieu of the parasite. These agents act rapidly, however, and sensitive strains develop resistance to them with relative difficulty.

The mechanism of action of chloroguanide and pyrimethamine is much more selective than that of the above group but resistance to their action can be obtained more readily. Chloroguanide and pyrimethamine inhibit the utilization of folic acid within the cell; they are effective against the plasmodial enzymes at doses lower than those that affect mammalian cells.

B. Amebicides

Amebiasis is caused by *Entamoeba histolytica.* There are two principal phases in its life cycle, the *cystic* and the *trophozoite.* Ingested cysts liberate the trophozoite in the intestine. The trophozoite is motile and can penetrate the intestine, eventually reaching the liver; it is the trophozoite that causes the intestinal and extraintestinal forms of amebiasis. While the parasite remains in its cystic form within the lumen of the bowel there may be little or no disturbance to the well-being of the host. However, it is the cyst excreted in the feces that is the potential source of infection to the host or to others.

The goal of therapy in amebiasis is to kill the trophozoite forms wherever they may exist: 1) In the bowel, cysts cease to be produced when all trophozoites are killed, thereby inhibiting the spread of the infection to other tissues or organs of the host as well as to other persons; 2) Killing trophozoites at sites other than the intestine eradicates the extraintestinal forms of the disease.

Drugs poorly absorbed from the GI tract are used to treat mild or asymptomatic intestinal infections, e.g., diiodohydroxyquin (Enterosept). Chloroquine, which has no effect on the intestinal form of the disease, is used for hepatic amebiasis, since the drug localizes in the liver in a concentration several hundred times greater than that in plasma. The newer agent metronidazole is useful in the treatment of mild-to-severe intestinal disease as well as in the extraintestinal forms of the disease.

VII. Anthelmintic Drugs

A. General Considerations

Anthelmintics are drugs used to rid the body of parasitic worms (helminths); anthelmintics may act locally to expel the helminths from the gastrointestinal tract or to combat systemic infestations. Worm infections represent the most common parasitic disease in the world — they affect half of the world's population.

Worms parasitic for humans include: tapeworms (cestodes), roundworms (nematodes), and flukes (trematodes). The different species vary with respect to bodily structure, physiology, habitat in the human host and sensitivity to drugs.

Parasitic worms are harmful to the host for a number of reasons:

1. Worms may cause injury to the tissues and organs by blockade due to their size and number: e.g., roundworms may cause gut obstruction; filariae may block lymphatic channels and cause massive edema.
2. Heavy infestations may interfere with nutrition by robbing the host of food.
3. Toxic substances made by the parasite may be absorbed by the host.
4. They may make the host more susceptible to secondary infections by bacteria.

Intestinal worm infections in general are more easily treated than those in other locations in the body: The worms need not be killed by the drug, and the drug need not be absorbed when given orally. The treatment of worms in tissues or organs other than the intestine is more difficult because they must be killed or critically injured so that they may be destroyed and eliminated from the tissues and ultimately from the body. Since drugs used to treat extraintestinal infestations must reach the site of infestation, the drugs must either be given parenterally or be absorbed when given orally with consequent greater danger to the host if the drugs are toxic. In general, localization of worms in tissues makes them highly resistant to chemotherapeutic attack.

None of the anthelmintics used currently are effective against all worms. Each agent has its own spectrum of activity and identification of the type of parasitic infection is essential before chemotherapy begins. Selective toxicity for the parasite is achieved either by exploiting quantitative biochemical differences between parasite and host or by limiting access of the drug to the host.

B. Mechanisms of Anthelmintic Activity

1. Paralysis of musculature of worms resulting in relaxation of the worms' hold on the intestinal mucosa and their subsequent expulsion by normal

bowel evacuation or following use of cathartics. Agents having this mechanism of action: piperazine; hexylresorcinol
2. Inhibition of oxidative metabolism: e.g., pyrvinium (cyanine dye); niclosamide
3. Interference with carbohydrate metabolism: e.g., niridazole; compounds containing antimony (tartar emetic)
4. Inhibition of ova production (probably by inhibiting DNA replication): e.g., chloroquine; niridazole

VIII. Anticancer Agents

There are two outstanding differences between microbial infections and neoplasms that account for the failure of cancer chemotherapy to achieve the same dramatic success as microbial chemotherapy.

A. Use of drugs in the treatment of an infection allows the normal host defense mechanisms to eliminate the infecting agent. In contrast, the body appears to possess no effective defenses against most neoplastic cells, so that sucessful treatment of the disease presumably depends upon the destruction of every neoplastic cell. However, in several human neoplasms, the detection of "foreign" antigens suggests that immunologic defenses of the host may play an important role in long-term remissions.

B. The many *qualitative* differences between microbial cells and those of the host favor the development of selectively toxic drugs that inhibit growth or kill infecting organisms with minimal or no injury to host cells. In contrast, with one exception, only *quantitative* differences are known between neoplastic cells and host cells; this allows for only a moderate degree of drug selectivity and does not permit the inhibition of cancer cells without producing harm to those host cells which also normally undergo rapid division.

The use of the enzyme asparaginase in the treatment of human leukemia takes advantage of the only qualitative difference discovered to date between the metabolism of normal and malignant tissue. Certain human leukemic cells require the amino acid asparagine as an essential growth factor, whereas most normal tissues synthesize their own asparagine. The enzyme asparaginase catalyzes the hydrolysis of asparagine and deprives the malignant cells of an essential amino acid, thus causing cell death without similarly damaging normal cells. The use of asparaginase as an effective anticancer agent is limited to those few leukemias involving cells heavily dependent on asparagine for growth.

Differences in rate of metabolism and reproduction are the most important exploitable differences between neoplastic cells and host cells. But those host cells that normally undergo rapid division are also vulnerable to anticancer drugs; e.g., epithelial cells in the gastrointestinal tract and skin, and the tissues involved in blood cell formation. Toxic effects of anticancer drugs usually include, therefore, ulceration of the GI tract, skin rashes, loss of hair and decrease in the number of circulating blood cells. Susceptibility to microbial infections usually increases, since many antineoplastic agents also suppress the immune response. Other consequences of the growth-inhibiting properties of antineoplastic agents are fetal abnormalities, with resulting defects in development, or fetal resorption. These adverse effects can be produced by virtually all the drugs that have been specifically developed for the treatment of cancer. Many drugs also produce specific untoward effects.

C. **Mechanism of Action.** The final pathway of all cancer growth is through an aberrant nucleic acid sequence leading to more rapid cell growth. Anticancer drugs produce their effects by interfering in one way or another with DNA replication or nucleic acid synthesis. Thus the ability to inhibit protein synthesis is the pharmacologic effect common to all anticancer drugs. The various drugs used to treat cancer may be classified according to the mechanism by which they produce this inhibition of protein synthesis.

1. **Alkylating Agents.** Highly reactive chemicals that inhibit cell division by binding to DNA and causing abnormal cross-linking of the DNA strands. This cross-linking makes DNA excessively stable and incapable of its usual reactivity and of carrying out its normal function.

    Nitrogen mustard (mechlorethamine), the first and most widely used alkylating agent, must be injected i.v. because it is so highly reactive. The newer agents, derivatives of nitrogen mustard (e.g., chlorambucil; melphalan, etc.), have the advantage of being somewhat less reactive and therefore able to be given orally; they are also well absorbed from the GI tract.

2. **Antimetabolites.** Chemical substances that are specific antagonists of normal substrates in the metabolic reactions of living organisms. An antimetabolite exerts its effect by interacting with a particular enzyme in such a manner as to prevent the enzyme from promoting a specific biochemical reaction. All of the antimetabolites that are anticancer drugs selectively inhibit one or more enzymatic steps which are critical for the synthesis of DNA.

    a. **Folic acid antagonists.** Interfere with nucleic acid synthesis by inhibiting the enzyme that converts folic acid to the form in which the folic acid participates as a coenzyme in the biosynthesis of nucleic acids.

        Methotrexate is the most commonly used agent.

    b. **Purine antagonists.** Structural analogs of the natural purines; do not act directly but are metabolically incorporated into ribonucleotides which then become the active inhibitors of a number of critical reactions involving nucleotide synthesis. This process is referred to as "lethal synthesis."

        6-Mercaptopurine is the most important of the antipurine drugs.

    c. **Pyrimidine antagonists.** Agents that interfere with normal pathways of pyrimidine biosynthesis. They act in a manner analogous to that of antipurines. The antipyrimidines are not active by themselves but

are incorporated into ribonucleotides and the fraudulent ribonucleotides inhibit an enzyme critical to the formation of DNA.

d. **Antibiotics.** Actinomycin D forms a complex with DNA and blocks
DNA-dependent synthesis of mRNA.

APPENDIX 4
Drugs Used to Alter the
Perception of and Response to Pain

THE NATURE OF PAIN

> Remember that pain has this most excellent
> quality: if prolonged it cannot be severe, and if
> severe it cannot be prolonged.
> > Seneca (4? B.C.E. – C.E. 65),
> > from *Moral Epistles to Lucilius,* XCIV

Pain, the symptom that most commonly brings a patient to consult a physician or
dentist, is certainly the most intrusive of all symptoms. Although pain is one of our
most useful sensations, indicating the presence and frequently the location of disease,
and alerting us to threats of bodily injury, it often exceeds its protective function and
becomes destructive. Relief of pain is, therefore, one of the great objectives in medicine.

Webster's dictionary[1] defines pain as "a basic bodily sensation induced by a noxious
stimulus, received by naked nerve endings, characterized by physical discomfort (as
pricking, throbbing, or aching) and typically leading to evasive action." This definition recognizes several of the important phenomena that are associated with pain. It
recognizes that the simple "stimulus-response" concept – of stimuli activating receptors and giving rise to sensory impulses that are translated into a sensation or
perception – is an integral part of the totality termed *pain*. The word "basic" incorporates the fact that, except for the very rare cases of individuals afflicted with
congenital generalized analgesia, all humans are born with the gift of pain perception.

The dictionary definition also reflects the consensus of neurophysiologists that
there are specific receptors for pain which are simple, unencapsulated, free nerve
endings without specialized structure. Pain receptors are present in skin, mucus membranes, skeletal muscles, blood vessels, visceral organs and in most other areas of the
body with the exception of the parenchyma of the lung and cerebral cortex. But
these receptors are unlike the more specialized sensory receptors such as those for
heat or cold, since pain receptors respond to a variety of stimuli, including mechanical

---

[1] *Webster's New Collegiate Dictionary.* Springfield, Mass.: G.&C. Merriam Co., 1973.

(pressure or stretching), thermal, electric and chemical. As the word "noxious" implies, however, painful sensations are elicited in healthy tissue by these various means only when the stimuli are relatively strong and potentially damaging. Pain receptors in different areas, moreover, are frequently more sensitive to one type of stimulus than another; the viscera, for example, are fairly insensitive to cutting, whereas cutting the skin is usually painful.

The inclusion of the phrase "leading to evasive action" in the Webster definition acknowledges that the total phenomenon of pain involves more than the physiology of the perception of pain — the awareness of a painful stimulus. It also involves the reaction to the stimulus. The physiology of pain perception is complex, since it involves discriminative capacity to identify the location, the onset, the intensity and the duration as well as the physical characteristics of the eliciting stimulus. Yet the physiology of the perception of pain may be almost the same in all mammals. But the reaction to pain is highly individualized in humans. It is determined by social mores, by the psychic state of the individual and by emotions and the individual's interpretation of the painful stimulus in terms of past and present events. The complete pattern of response to painful stimuli is, to some extent, also learned behavior, unlike pain perception, which is innate. Children, for example, react to pain much as their parents do. Animals kept isolated during the period of weaning to adulthood and deprived of normal sensory and social experiences learn very slowly, or not at all, to avoid painful stimuli after their release into a normal environment. Litter mates reared normally learn quickly to avoid the same painful stimuli. The reaction to pain is also influenced by the significance of the pain to the individuals. Athletes, for instance, who suffer injuries during a competition have shown a remarkable ability to postpone reaction to the painful stimulus until the excitement of the competition is over.

Since pain is such a complex phenomenon, it should be obvious that there are many ways to relieve pain and that the means to be used depend upon its cause — if it can be identified:

1. Removal of the cause: e.g., restoration or extraction of an aching tooth; neutralization of gastric acid in peptic ulcer
2. Using physical measures: e.g., the application of heat, cold or pressure to a painful area. This type of procedure takes advantage of the fact that pain impulses can be modified and decreased through the generation of other concomitant stimuli, for example, the application of a liniment as a counterirritant.
3. By distraction of attention to the painful stimulus: e.g., the use of auditory stimuli — stereophonic music, sounds resembling a waterfall — in dental surgery. The converse is also true, i.e., the absence of distracting environmental stimuli enhances the perception of pain. This is apparent to anyone who has gone to bed unaware of an aching muscle or tooth and then gradually begins to perceive the painful condition.
4. By hypnotic suggestion
5. By the use of drugs, including pharmacologically inactive substances, i.e., placebos

(cf. pp. 262–264). Any drug that can alter the physiology or the subjective appreciation of pain can give relief from pain. Thus analgesia or the relief of pain can be effected anywhere along the pain pathways – in the pathways involved either in the perception of, or in the reaction to, pain.

Perception – the awareness of a painful stimulus – is not dependent on consciousness but is dependent on intact afferent pathways: on receptors; sensory nerves conducting the impulses to the brain and the thalamus, where perception occurs. If a drug acts at any point along this pathway to interrupt the transfer of information to the brain, then pain cannot be perceived.

The reaction to pain – the "pain experience" – is a much more complex phenomenon requiring consciousness and occurring at the highest level of the brain – the cortex. Here, too, drugs can offer relief by altering the response to pain. Thus the use of agents that relieve anxiety – the so-called minor tranquilizers – can lower the subject's reaction to pain.

The following sections discuss the principal classes of drugs used to treat pain. We start with those agents that alter the perception of pain: (1) the local anesthetics that block nerve conduction and prevent afferent impulses from reaching the CNS; (2) the nonnarcotic, antipyretic-analgesics that inhibit perception by peripheral actions at receptors as well as by actions within the CNS. We then consider the narcotic analgesics that interfere relatively selectively with the reaction to painful stimuli. Finally we discuss ethanol and general anesthetic agents that nonselectively alter perception and reaction to painful stimuli by their general CNS depressant action.

Suggested Reading
Stravino, V. D. The nature of pain. *Arch. Phys. Med. Rehab.* 51:37, 1970.
Winter, C. A. The Physiology and Pharmacology of Pain and Its Relief. In G. deStevens (ed.), *Analgetics*, Vol. 5, *Medicinal Chemistry*. New York: Academic, 1965. P. 10.

LOCAL ANESTHETICS
I.   **Definition.** Local anesthetics are drugs that produce a reversible loss of sensitivity to pain in the restricted area to which they are applied.
II. **Chemistry.** The clinically useful *injectable* local anesthetics are, almost without exception, *amines*. The structural configuration most consistently associated with effective agents is that of an *aliphatic* chain of two or more carbons, one end of which bears a hydrocarbon nucleus and the other an amino group:

$$R_1 - (CH_2)_n - N \Big\langle {R_2 \text{ (alkyl group)} \atop R_3 \text{ (hydrogen or alkyl group)}}$$

hydrocarbon   amine
nucleus

III. **Pharmacodynamics**
A. **Site and Mechanism of Action.**   Site of action is the nerve fiber. Local

anesthetics act by blocking nerve conduction — by inhibiting impulse transmission along the nerve(s) from the point of drug application to the organs, tissues or other nerves that are usually stimulated by the blocked nerve(s). Local anesthetics produce this inhibition of impulse transmission by interfering with the normal permeability of the nerve fiber.

B. **Local Actions**
   1. Local anesthetic activity
   2. Effect on local blood vessels
      a. Arteriolar vasoconstriction with cocaine
      b. Arteriolar vasodilatation with all other agents

C. **Systemic Actions**
   1. **On Cardiovascular System**
      a. Can produce a fall in blood pressure
      b. Can depress the muscle of the heart and slow impulse conduction. This property is of practical importance since some local anesthetics are used to suppress cardiac arrhythmias.
   2. **On CNS**
      Involves both stimulation and depression. Stimulation may be manifested by restlessness, apprehension, tremors which may progress to convulsions. Central stimulation is followed by depression and death is usually due to respiratory failure.

IV. **Fate in the Body**
   A. **Absorption.** Dependent on mode of administration, on physicochemical properties of individual agent and on presence of vasoconstricting agents
   B. **Distribution.** No selective deposition in tissues. Cross placenta
   C. **Biotransformation.** See pp. 156—157.
   D. **Excretion.** Metabolites and unchanged portion of drug are excreted in urine

V. **Modes of Administration**
   A. **Topical or Surface.** Application of solutions, ointments or sprays to skin or mucus membranes. Blocks nerve fiber terminals
   B. **Infiltration.** Injection into the intradermal layer or subcutaneous tissues. Blocks small nerve fibers or their terminals
   C. **Nerve Block.** Injection into immediate vicinity of the nerve supplying the area to be anesthetized
   D. **Spinal.** Injection into the spinal fluid

VI. **Toxicity.** Except for allergic or idiosyncratic reactions, is predictable and a result of overdosage. Thus, cardiovascular collapse and CNS stimulation and depression with respiratory failure may be expected as the toxic effects of overdosage.

VII. **Commonly Used Agents**
   A. **Amides**
      Lidocaine
      Dibucaine
   B. **Esters**
      Procaine

Tetracaine

Butacaine

Benzocaine — lacks terminal amino group and used only topically

ANALGESICS

I. Antipyretic Analgesics (Nonnarcotic Analgesics)

A. General Considerations

An analgesic drug is a substance that, through its action upon the nervous system, serves to reduce or abolish suffering from pain without producing unconsciousness. An antipyretic drug is a substance which reduces an elevated body temperature.

Certain agents possess both analgesic and antipyretic properties. They are, therefore, grouped together in one classification and divided into subgroups on the basis of their chemical structure.

1. The Derivatives of Salicylic Acid

Sodium salicylate

Acetylsalicylic acid (aspirin)

2. The Derivatives of Aniline

Phenacetin (acetophenetidin)

Acetaminophen (paracetamol, Tylenol, Tempra, APAP)

3. The Derivatives of Pyrazolon

Antipyrine

Aminopyrine (Pyramidon)

Phenylbutazone (Butazoladine)

B. Mechanism of Analgestic Action

The way in which pain is alleviated by these agents is not definitely known. The salicylates alleviate pain by acting both in the CNS and at the periphery to modify the cause of pain at the site where the pain originates. The sensation of pain is believed to be associated with the liberation or generation of endogenous substances, such as the prostaglandins (see p. 459), in response to other endogenous compounds like bradykinin. The salicylates inhibit the synthesis of prostaglandins and, as a result, prevent the sensitization of pain receptors. There is some evidence to indicate that the mechanism of action of other antipyretic-analgesics may be the same as that of the salicylates.

The agents fulfill at least *one criterion* of the *ideal analgesic*: they have *selectivity* of action. In analgesic doses they cause no mental disturbance, anesthesia or changes in modalities of sensation other than pain. But, they are *not ideal* analgesics because they relieve pain of only low intensity, whether localized or widespread in origin, particularly pain of: headache, muscles or joints, or other pains arising from external structures rather than from viscera.

C. Mechanism of Antipyretic Effect

Normal body heat is maintained within limits by a balance between the *heat-producing* and *heat-dissipating* mechanisms of the body. The peripheral mechanisms of production and loss of body heat are regulated by certain nuclei in the hypothalamus. The action of the antipyretics is mainly on the hypothalamus and not peripherally on blood vessels or sweat glands. Evidence for this is that high sectioning of the spinal cord prevents the anti-pyretic drugs from lowering the temperature of fevered animals. There is also evidence to indicate that certain fevers are caused by endogenous sub-stances (pyrogens) released from white blood cells; these pyrogens act on the temperature-regulating center in the hypothalamus. The temperature-elevating effect of pyrogen is inhibited by aspirin and acetaminophen, prob-ably by inhibition of the synthesis of prostaglandins whose synthesis is stimu-lated by pyrogens.

The antipyretic action is usually rapid and effective in *febrile* patients, but can *rarely* be demonstrated when the body temperature is *normal*. The antipyretics act to increase heat loss in febrile individuals by:
1. Increasing peripheral blood flow through peripheral vasodilatation.
2. Producing a shift in water to the bloodstream with a corresponding dilution of the blood
3. Increasing perspiration

D. **The Salicylates**
The salicylates have some important pharmacologic actions in addition to their analgesic and antipyretic actions. Some of these provide the basis for additional therapeutic uses of the salicylates and others are largely responsi-ble for the untoward effects seen in some patients.
1. **Anti-inflammatory Action**
The salicylates reduce the
pain,
immobility,
swelling and
inflammation of the joints in acute rheumatic fever and rheumatoid arthritis.

So rapid and dramatic is the benefit obtained in the polyarthritis of acute rheumatic fever that salicylates can be employed in the differen-tial diagnosis of the condition. The mechanism of this action is poorly understood but recent studies have suggested that the action of aspirin and other nonsteroidal anti-inflammatory drugs may also involve the inhibition of the synthesis of prostaglandins. The prostaglandins represent a series of naturally occurring acidic lipids with powerful pharmacologic activity including activity in inflammation and immune phenomena. Aspirin blocks the synthesis of prostaglandins in a variety of human and animal tissues.
2. **Uricosuric Action**
Salicylates increase uric acid excretion by specific inhibition of tubular reabsorption of urate; this action forms the basis for their use in the treatment of gout. Although the salicylates can still be used for this

purpose, newer agents, such as probenecid, are preferred for the chronic therapy of gout, since doses of more than 5 grams a day of salicylate must be employed to produce uric acid excretion.

3. **Side-Effects**

The nontherapeutic effects are important considerations when salicylates are being used in treatment of acute rheumatic fever or gout for which very large doses are used.

a. Gastrointestinal effects: Include gastric irritation, nausea and vomiting. These effects are due to both an action on the CNS and a local gastric effect.

b. Prolong bleeding time at ordinary analgesic doses; in large doses, over 6g/day, reduce prothrombin levels.

c. Effects on respiration: Disturbances in acid-base balance. Salicylates stimulate respiration directly and indirectly. These effects are of paramount importance because they contribute to the serious acid-base balance disturbances that characterize poisoning by this class of compounds. The direct effect is produced by stimulation of the respiratory center in the medulla and the indirect effect is a result of alterations in the metabolism of carbohydrates, proteins and fat.

d. In addition to these effects of salicylate overdosage, there may be other effects which can jeopardize the patient. These take the form of a series of reactions called salicylism — resembling the side-effects seen with large doses of quinine. The symptoms consist of: headache, dizziness, ringing in the ears (tinnitus), dimness of vision and mental confusion.

   As the dosage is increased, the symptoms become more severe — there is increased CNS stimulation, which may be followed by depression, stupor and coma.

   These symptoms occur along with the disturbances in acid-base balance and gastrointestinal symptoms.

e. Allergic reaction:
   Skin rash — most frequent
   Edema
   Asthma — less frequent but more than 16% of asthmatics show increased symptoms after aspirin

4. **Fate of Salicylates**

a. **Absorption** (see pp. 79, 87, 88)
   Rapidly and chiefly absorbed from the upper intestinal tract. Absorption of both Na-salicylate and aspirin occurs from the stomach itself, particularly if the pH is low. This is, again, an example of the fact that the unionized form is more quickly absorbed. However, absorption is faster for both these agents in the upper part of the small intestine.

b. **Biotransformation** (see pp. 147, 157, 217–219)

E. **Derivatives of Aniline**

Phenacetin

Acetaminophen

Only used as *analgesic* or *antipyretic* agents; they do not have anti-inflammatory activity. These agents do not differ in their analgesic and anti-pyretic actions from the salicylates but they do have different important side-effects.

1. **Side-Effects**

In the process of their biotransformation, the derivatives of aniline give rise to a compound which can oxidize hemoglobin to methemoglobin. Methemoglobin does not have the O_2-combining properties of hemo-globin. The degree of methemoglobinemia is directly related to the dose of the aniline derivatives administered.

Chronic therapy with aniline derivatives, such as phenacetin (which is contained in many proprietary preparations), has been implicated in the production of kidney damage. Occasional use of phenacetin or related compounds does not lead to renal damage.

2. **Biotransformation**

The major portion of these compounds is excreted as a conjugate of the parent compound. Phenacetin is converted to acetaminophen in body and acetaminophen appears to be the active agent of greater potency although phenacetin also has some analgesic activity.

F. **Pyrazolon Derivatives**

Antipyrine

Aminopyrine

Phenylbutazone

Aminopyrine and phenylbutazone have antirheumatic activity. Phenyl-butazone also has uricosuric activity. These agents are not often used because of potentially serious side effects: high incidence of depression of formation of certain blood cells, especially with aminopyrine.

II. **Narcotic Analgesics – Opioids**

A. **Definition** (see p. 355)

B. **Agents** (see p. 355)

C. **Pharmacodynamics:** All of the opioids share the same pharmacologic proper-ties and differ from each other only quantitatively with respect to analgesic potency, duration of action, etc. The opioids exert a number of extremely diverse effects on most of the systems and tissues in the body. Their major effects are on the CNS and GI tract.

Morphine is the prototype of the opioids.

1. **Analgesic Effect.** Highly selective; little, if any, alteration of any other sensory phenomena

a. Elevation in threshold for pain perception demonstrated experimentally in both humans and animals.

b. Alteration in the reaction to pain; relief of anxiety, tension and fear associated with pain (see p. 356).

c. Mechanism and site of analgesic action. Mechanism unknown (cf. pp. 357–358). Site of action: large number of centers in brain are affected; alterations in the reticular activating system are important since this system integrates all the responses to pain through its projections to the cortex (see p. 348).

d. The analgesic effect cannot be separated from the sedative effect due to the overall CNS depression produced by the opioids. Sedative effects are most profound in patients in bed at time of medication. The decrease in anxiety and relief of distress may produce euphoria in some patients.

2. **Respiratory Effects.** The respiratory center is very sensitive to morphine and its surrogates; severe respiratory depression rarely seen with clinical doses; death from morphine overdosage is due to respiratory depression.

3. **Cardiovascular Effects.** Little effect on blood pressure or heart rate in supine patient given low therapeutic doses. Most narcotic analgesics decrease capacity of cardiovascular system to respond to stress of gravitational shifts. Thus, when supine patient assumes head-up position, there may be a fall in blood pressure (orthostatic or postural hypotension) and fainting may occur. The release of histamine by morphine and other opioids may play a role in hypotension.

4. **Antitussive Effects.** All opioids can suppress the cough reflex by suppressing the cough center in medulla. Codeine: drug of choice in the U.S. Dextromethorphan (Romilar): a newer synthetic that is a good antitussive and exhibits no analgesic activity and fewer other effects of the narcotic analgesics

5. **Stimulatory Effects**

a. Nausea and vomiting: Caused by stimulation of emetic center secondary to direct stimulation of the chemoreceptor trigger zone (CTZ) in medulla. After initial stimulation, morphine will depress CTZ. A major side-effect of opioid therapy

b. Miosis (pin-point pupils): Caused by stimulation of the pupilloconstrictor centers of the motor nerve controlling pupillary diameter. Miosis characteristic of, and diagnostic for, intake of all narcotic analgesics except meperidine (pethidine, Demerol). Tolerance does not develop to this effect.

c. Gastrointestinal tract: Marked constipation due to contraction of sphincters, increased muscular tone and decreased propulsive movements; delays stomach emptying. Tolerance does not develop to these effects.

d. Effects on biliary tract: Contraction of bile duct and increased pressure in biliary system; narcotic analgesics, therefore, contraindicated in gallbladder disease

6. Miscellaneous Effects
    a. Causes constriction of bronchi; contraindicated in severe asthma.
    b. Renal effects: In therapeutic doses, no significant effect; with larger doses there is an antidiuretic effect mediated in part by the stimulation of pituitary secretion of the antidiuretic hormone (ADH) and in part by an increased tone of the bladder musculature which results in the retention of urine.

D. Fate in the Body
    1. Absorption. Morphine well absorbed but rapidly conjugated in liver. Codeine well absorbed and less rapidly biotransformed in liver; therefore a large proportion of oral dose of codeine reaches systemic circulation.
    2. Distribution. Morphine is rapidly distributed; however, little of total reaches brain but little is needed for CNS effects; heroin and codeine more completely distributed to brain.
    3. Biotransformation. (See p. 146.) Conjugation with glucuronic acid main pathway for morphine.
    4. Excretion. 7-10% of total morphine excreted in feces, remainder in urine.

E. Toxicity
    1. Acute. Characterized by coma, pin-point pupils, severe respiratory depression. Treatment is usually with narcotic antagonists, compounds that are specific competitive pharmacologic antagonists.
    2. Chronic. (See pp. 355–359.)

ALCHOHOL AND GENERAL ANESTHETIC AGENTS
I. General Considerations
Changes in the excitability of the central nervous system (CNS) occur in a gradual continuous fashion; [decreases from normal progress from sedation to coma and increases in excitability range from mild hyperexcitability to severe convulsions.] Drugs that have the ability to produce graded CNS depression with the administration of progressively larger doses are classified as *general depressants of the CNS*. (Analogously, drugs that increase excitability on this continuum as a function of dose are called *general CNS stimulants* [see Appendix 6: Drugs Used in the Treatment of Mental Disorders].) The action of the general CNS depressants is relatively *nonselective*, affecting total brain function, in contrast to *selective* depressants such as the antipyretic-analgesics which act at a restricted locus to lower elevated body temperature.

    The ability to depress excitability at all levels of the CNS is a property shared by many compounds of diverse chemical structure including: methanol and ethanol and other aliphatic alcohols; cyclopropane and ether and other gaseous and volatile anesthetics; and barbiturate and nonbarbiturate sedative-hypnotic drugs. It is most probable that all of the CNS effects produced by these agents are the result of a depressant action on excitable cells. However, the mechanism by which the neuronal depression is brought about is unknown.

Various physical or metabolic effects, particularly inhibition of either energy consumption or production or both, have been implicated but not proved to be the basis of the neuronal depression (cf. pp. 45–46.) When an excitatory effect on some function is observed following low doses of a CNS depressant, in general it too is the result of neuronal depression — but of an inhibitory system. Depression of a system inhibitory to a particular function increases the level of excitability of other neurons involved in that function. The so-called stimulant effect of ethanol is an example of this release from inhibition (cf. pp. 352–353).

The effects of the general CNS depressant drugs are additive not only with each other but also with the physiologic state at the time of drug administration. A given amount of ethanol, for example, will produce less sedation and drowsiness when consumed at a party than when imbibed in a quiet, nonsocial environment. The effects of the general CNS depressants can also be antagonized by other drugs, but this antagonism is physiologic rather than pharmacologic (cf. pp. 286–287). For example, general CNS stimulants such as caffeine or nikethimide can counteract the respiratory depression produced by large doses of the general CNS depressants. Antagonism between the stimulants and depressants is brought about by opposite effects on the same physiologic function but not by opposition at the same site(s) of action. As a result, normal function cannot be entirely restored. The practice of using CNS stimulants to counteract the severe respiratory depression of intoxication by general depressants has been largely discontinued; measures that stress intensive supportive care have met with much greater success in such poisonings (cf. pp. 326–329).

Individual general CNS depressant drugs differ from one another primarily with respect to potency. For instance, the concentration of anesthetic in the blood that is needed to produce surgical anesthesia is much less for halothane than for ether. However, it is important to note that although the potency of a drug is a relatively unimportant characteristic (cf. pp. 178–180), the lack of potency may limit the maximum effect that can be achieved therapeutically. The low potency of nitrous oxide, for example, limits its usefulness as a safe, general anesthetic gas; the concentration that must be inhaled in order to produce anesthesia does not provide for adequate oxygenation. Consequently, nitrous oxide can be used for only very short procedures or in conjunction with other more potent agents.

The pattern of events that occur as an individual is exposed to progressively increasing concentrations of a general CNS depressant is fairly predictable. The signs and symptoms that appear with increasing depth of depression permit the anesthesiologist to determine when conditions are favorable for surgical procedure and when a reaction constitutes a danger signal. The pattern of deepening CNS depression differs in specific ways for specific agents. But the "stages" and "signs" of anesthesia represent a framework upon which to build the exceptions for individual agents. The pattern of depression based on the signs produced by the action of anesthetics on different excitable tissues is arbitrarily divided into the following stages of anesthesia:

Stage I — Analgesia. The first stage is characterized by analgesia and amnesia and lasts until consciousness is lost. It is associated with depression of the ascending reticular activating system and of the relay systems in the thalamus. The areas of the brain concerned with message storage and retrieval are also susceptible to depression at this stage.

Stage II — Delirium. This stage, characterized by loss of consciousness and control, begins with unconsciousness and ends with the loss of the eyelid reflex. The excitement of this stage involves the depression of additional areas in the brainstem and cerebellum. Purposeless movements and vomiting may occur; pupils are usually widely dilated, there is hyperreaction to stimuli, and breathing is irregular. This stage is neither useful nor desirable clinically.

Stage III — Surgical Anesthesia. This stage, which involves progressive loss of reflexes and muscle tone, ends with cessation of spontaneous respiration. It is usually divided into four phases which are differentiated on the basis of the character of respiration, the presence or absence of certain reflexes, the eyeball movements and pupillary diameter.

Stage IV — Respiratory Paralysis. Complete respiratory paralysis occurs, which leads to and ends with complete circulatory failure.

II. Aliphatic Alcohols

A. Definition

The generic term *alcohol* designates an important class of organic compounds that are hydroxyl (-OH) derivatives of aliphatic (straight-chain) hydrocarbons. The compounds may have one or more hydroxyl groups. The important compounds in this class include methanol, ethanol, ethylene glycol (dihydroxy) and glycerol (the trihydroxy compound derived from the digestion of fats). When the simple term *alcohol* is used, it ordinarily refers to ethanol (ethyl alcohol).

B. Physicochemical Properties

The physicochemical properties of the aliphatic alcohols are extremely well correlated with their pharmacologic activity and their fate in the body (cf. pp. 56–57).

Ethanol is a universal solvent; it is able to dissolve substances that are soluble in water and in organic solvents. As a result, ethanol is widely used as a pharmaceutical agent in preparations of pure drugs from crude extracts and in compounding of solutions for medicinal use.

C. Pharmacology

1. Actions on the CNS

Although ethanol is not used as a general anesthetic agent, the events that occur as an individual is exposed to progressively increasing concentrations can be described by the same pattern used for general anesthetics. The stages and planes of general anesthesia exemplified by ethanol intoxication are presented in Table A-4 along with the blood alcohol content associated with each level of depression. The degree of CNS depression is directly related to the blood alcohol content because equilibrium between blood and brain tissue occurs very rapidly.

Table A-4. Stages and Planes of General Anesthesia Exemplified by Alcohol Intoxication

Stage and Plane	Whiskey Dose (oz/hr)	Blood Alcohol (mg/100 ml)	Function Impaired	Physical State	Neurologic Status[1]			
					Conditioned Reflexes	Superficial[2] Reflexes	Deep[3] Reflexes	Spontaneous Function
I	1-4	0-100	Judgment; fine coordination	Happy; boastful; "sociable"	+++ → ++	+++	+++	+++
	4-12	100-300	Motor coordination; static reflexes; pain perception	Staggers; slurred speech; analgesia; amnesia	++ → +	+++	+++	+++
II	12-16	300-400	Voluntary response to sensation	Emotional; restless; helpless	+ → 0	++++	++++	++++
III, i	16-24	400-600	Sensation; voluntary movement; progressive loss of protective reflexes	Comatose	0	+ - ++	+++	+++
ii					0	0 - +	+ - ++	+++
iii					0	0 - +	0 - +	++
iv					0	0	0	+
IV	24-30	600-900	Spontaneous respiration; cardiovascular regulation	Dead	0	0	0	0

[1] +++ essentially normal function
++++ hyperexcitability; increased response
++ or + progressively decreasing functional response
0 total absence of function
[2] e.g., eyelid reflex
[3] e.g., pupillary response to light

The pharmacologic significance of ethanol lies not only in its direct action upon the individual who consumes it, but also in its indirect action in decreasing the ability of that individual to carry on societal responsibilities. Such considerations are of particular importance from the standpoint of operation of an automobile (cf. pp. 216–217). Impairment of visual acuity and reaction time occur in early stage I, at blood levels of ethanol much below 100 mg/100 ml, the level above which an individual is considered legally intoxicated in most states in the U.S. Many investigations, using laboratory testing methods that give quantitative rather than subjective clinical evaluations, have shown that:

Dose of whiskey, oz.	Blood ethanol, mg/100 ml	Function impaired
0.5	15	Vision
1 – 1.5	30 – 40	Fine muscle coordination
2 – 3	80	Reaction time (slowed)
4	100	Judgment

2. Actions on Other Systems

a. **The gastrointestinal tract.** Hypertonic solutions stimulate acid production in stomach, delay gastric emptying and promote injury to surface epithelium. Chronic alcoholics have malabsorption of many substances including fat, folic acid, thiamine and Vitamin B_{12}.

b. **The liver.** The chronic use of alcohol is associated with the accumulation of fat in the liver. There is considerable evidence to indicate that this deposition of fat is an indirect result of the biotransformation of ethanol itself. The oxidation of ethanol takes place by a series of steps (cf. pp. 214–215) and in each of these steps some energy is made available to the body – the oxidation of 1 gram of ethanol yielding a total of 7 calories. The energy liberated by the metabolism of ethanol can be utilized by the body in the same way as energy from the oxidation of food substances. In the sense that ethanol is a source of energy it, too, is a food, but ethanol supplies only one compound that can enter into normal anabolic reactions – acetate. Some of the acetate required by the body is furnished by the oxidation of fatty acids. The oxidation of ethanol decreases the need for oxidation of fatty acids and promotes the preferential synthesis of the fatty acids to fats. Thus in addition to the nutritional deficiencies commonly associated with excessive or chronic use of alcohol, alcohol itself may be a factor in the etiology of alcoholic liver disease.

The nonmicrosomal enzyme alcohol dehydrogenase is predominantly responsible for the oxidation of ethanol (cf. pp. 154, 156) and for the time course of ethanol elimination (cf. pp. 213–217). However, up to 20%

of the ethanol in the body may be oxidized through an alternate pathway, the microsomal ethanol oxidizing system (MEOS) associated with the smooth endoplasmic reticulum (cf. pp. 152–154). Although the MEOS plays only a minor role in the elimination of ethanol, it takes on considerable importance during chronic ethanol consumption or multiple drug use. The MEOS, like many other microsomal enzyme systems, is inducible and its activity can be increased by the chronic administration of ethanol itself or by other drugs. As a consequence, during chronic ethanol consumption there is an increase in the rate of metabolism of that fraction of ethanol oxidized by MEOS. This can explain a part of the tolerance to ethanol that develops in alcoholics. Chronic consumption of ethanol can also induce other microsomal enzymes and thereby accelerate the rate of biotransformation of other drugs such as meprobamate and pentobarbital. This can explain the well-known fact that alcoholics often have an increased tolerance to a variety of drugs. This increased tolerance, however, is only seen in the *sober* alcoholic. In the presence of ethanol the activity of a variety of microsomal enzymes is *inhibited* rather than accelerated. Thus the drinking alcoholic as well as the inebriated individual is *more* susceptible to the effects of other CNS depressants. The effects produced by the coadministration of ethanol and meprobamate, for example, are synergistic (cf. p. 286), i.e., the degree of CNS depression observed is greater than the algebraic sum of the individual effects of ethanol and meprobamate. This can be attributed to the inhibition by ethanol of the biotransformation of meprobamate.

   c. **The kidney.** Ethanol produces diuresis by inhibiting the secretion of antidiuretic hormone (cf. pp. 132–133).

3. **Fate in the Body**

   a. **Absorption.** (See pp. 52, 79, 82–83.)

   b. **Distribution.** Ethanol distributes very rapidly to the total body water, and equilibrates very rapidly with its target organs. Therefore, ethanol blood concentration may be used to estimate the level of ethanol in the brain. The equilibrium between the concentration of ethanol in the expired air and in blood is also attained rapidly and, thus, ethanol blood levels can be estimated by measuring its concentration in expired air.

   c. **Elimination.** (See pp. 214–217.)

D. **Pharmacologic Actions of Other Aliphatic Alcohols**

The ability of the aliphatic alcohols to produce CNS depression increases with increasing molecular weight and is directly proportional to their lipid solubility. Methanol, the first member of the homologous series, is a less potent depressant than ethanol, but is potentially more toxic because methanol ingestion can lead to blindness (cf. p. 234).

APPENDIX 5
Sedatives and Hypnotics

I. **Definitions**
   A. A *sedative* is a drug that produces a mild degree of nonselective depression
      of the central nervous system (CNS) by decreasing the response of an in-
      dividual to all sensory modalities.
   B. A *hypnotic* is a drug that produces more nonselective depression of the CNS
      than the sedative and that induces a state resembling natural sleep.
II. **General Considerations**
   The difference between sedatives and hypnotics is only quantitative. These
   agents have in common the ability to produce all degrees of depression of the
   CNS, starting with mild sedation and progressing through hypnosis, anesthesia,
   coma and death from respiratory failure. The different effects are a function
   of the dose of the drug administered. The designation of a particular agent
   for use as a sedative, hypnotic or anesthetic is determined by its physicochemical properties.
   The general depressants of the CNS that are classified as sedatives-hypnotics
   include the barbiturates and many other compounds of diverse chemical structures. The major pharmacologic effects of the barbiturates and the nonbarbiturates are confined to the CNS and there appears to be little fundamental difference in the mode of action of these two subclasses of sedative-hypnotic drugs.
III. **The Barbiturates**
   A. **Physicochemical Properties**
      The barbiturates have the following general structural formula:

Of the more than 2500 barbiturates that have been synthesized, only about 15 are currently available in the U.S. and of these only the following are official drugs (listed in the *United States Pharmacopeia* or *The National Formulary*):

1. **Long Acting**
   Phenobarbital (Luminal), U.S.P.
   Mephobarbital (Mebaral), N.F.
   Metharbital (Gemonil), N.F.
2. **Short-to-Intermediate Acting**
   Pentobarbital (Nembutal), U.S.P.
   Secobarbital (Seconal), U.S.P.
   Butabarbital (Butisol), N.F.
   Amobarbital (Amytal), N.F.
   Talbutal (Lotusate), N.F.
3. **Ultra-short Acting**
   Thiopental (Pentothal), U.S.P.
   Methohexital (Brevital), U.S.P.
   Thiamylal (Surital), N.F.
   Hexabarbital (Sombulex), N.F.

Only those compounds in which oxygen is the substituent at "X" are properly termed *barbiturates*. However, compounds such as thiopental and thiamylal in which sulfur replaces the oxygen at X are also referred to as barbiturates, specifically as *thiobarbiturates*.

Changes in structure that produce changes in lipid solubility usually influence the time course of drug action in a highly predictable manner. In general, structural changes that increase lipid solubility yield compounds with a relatively faster onset and shorter duration of action, a greater tendency to bind to proteins, a more rapid rate of biotransformation, and a slower rate of excretion (Table A-5). Thus lipid solubility (which is influenced by extent of ionization) is the most important factor affecting the distribution and fate of barbiturates. And since onset and duration of action are dependent on the rates of drug entry into and out of the CNS, lipid solubility also usually determines the choice of barbiturate for a particular therapeutic application. Highly lipid-soluble compounds such as thiopental are used primarily as anesthetic agents, because a state of anesthesia is induced within seconds after administration of a single intravenous dose and recovery of consciousness occurs within 5 to 15 minutes. The short-to-intermediate–acting barbiturates distribute to the CNS much more slowly than the ultra-short-acting drugs, but rapidly enough to induce sleep within 15–30 minutes after oral administration. Thus these agents find their principal utility as hypnotics but are also used for sedation in doses $\frac{1}{3}$–$\frac{1}{4}$ the hypnotic dose. Drugs such as phenobarbital diffuse across biologic barriers at slow rates; effective concentrations in the brain are obtained within 1–2 hours after oral administration and persist for 8–12 hours. The long-acting

Table A-5. Relation between Physicochemical Factors and Pharmacokinetic Behavior of Representative Barbiturates

Characteristics	Phenobarbital	Pentobarbital	Secobarbital	Thiopental
Partition coefficient of nonionized form, methylene chloride/water	3	39	52	580
Per cent bound to plasma protein at pH 7.4	2	35	44	65
Onset of activity	Slow (60–120 min. after P.O.)	Rapid (15–30 min. after P.O.)	Rapid (15–30 min. after P.O.)	Very rapid (1–2 sec. after I.V.)
Duration of action, hr. (approximate)	8–12	3–5	3–4	0.25–0.5
Per cent of dose excreted unchanged in urine	27–50	Negligible	Negligible	Negligible
Plasma half-life, hr	24–96	21–42	20–28	3–8

barbiturates are used principally in the treatment of epilepsy, although phenobarbital is still frequently employed as a daytime sedative or as a hypnotic in hospitalized patients.

B. Pharmacologic Properties

1. Mechanisms and Sites of Action

The barbiturates reversibly depress the activity of all excitable cells and tissues by an action on or in a membrane. The exact mechanism of action is unknown, although many diverse mechanisms have been proposed. The brain is particularly sensitive, so that when barbiturates are employed in therapeutic doses, there is very little effect on other excitable tissues such as those in the heart or skeletal muscle. The barbiturates act at all levels of CNS but selectively affect the reticular activating system (RAS) (cf. pp. 348, 353). It is this selective depression of the ascending RAS that has been shown to be responsible for the sleep induced by the barbiturates and other sedative-hypnotic drugs.

2. Actions

a. On the CNS

All of the barbiturates are capable of depressing CNS excitability on a continuum graded through sedation, hypnosis, general anesthesia and coma.

In general, barbiturate-induced sleep resembles natural sleep, but the time spent in REM (rapid eye movement) sleep is reduced. The REM phase occupies about 20–25% of sleep time and is associated with dreaming. Individuals deprived of REM sleep usually exhibit a rebound increase in REM sleep when the drug is withdrawn and this rebound may manifest itself in nightmares and feelings of having slept poorly.

All barbiturates, because of their ability to depress the CNS on a continuum, can inhibit convulsions that arise in disease states such as tetanus or that are produced by drugs such as strychnine. However, phenobarbital, mephobarbital and metharbital, unlike other barbiturates, have selective anticonvulsant activity at low doses and are useful agents in the symptomatic treatment of epilepsy.

The barbiturates, even those used as anesthetic agents, are unlike the gaseous or volatile anesthetics since in subanesthetic doses the barbiturates have no analgesic effect. Indeed, the barbiturates cannot be relied upon to induce sleep in patients experiencing severe pain and may even produce an overexcited reaction to painful stimuli.

b. On other systems

In oral sedative and hypnotic doses, the barbiturates do not produce significant effects on cardiovascular or other peripheral functions; the effects on respiration resemble those of natural sleep.

3. Untoward Effects

a. The barbiturates are relatively safe and effective drugs when administered in therapeutic doses. Undesirable side-effects and severe toxicity are manifested as a continuation of the therapeutic effect (cf. pp. 193–194) and are usually the result of improper use or incorrect choice of agent.

   b. Development of tolerance (cf. pp. 279–283, 351, 354).

   c. Development of dependence (cf. pp. 352–355).

C. Fate in the Body

1. Absorption (cf. pp. 79–80, 82–83).

The barbiturates are efficiently absorbed from the various segments of the gut and from muscle. (The barbiturates are too irritating to be given by the subcutaneous route.) Rates of absorption are directly correlated with lipid solubility.

2. Distribution

The barbiturates readily diffuse across all biologic barriers at rates determined by their physicochemical characteristics and regional blood flow (cf. pp. 104, 208, 234–236).

3. Elimination

Biotransformation, urinary excretion and tissue redistribution are the processes responsible for the termination of action of the barbiturates by removing them from their sites of action. Lipid solubility is the most important factor determining which of these processes plays the major role in the termination of drug action and elimination from the body.

The action of the ultra-short-acting drugs is terminated primarily as a result of redistribution from brain to lean tissues and then to fat (cf. pp. 231–236); biotransformation (cf. pp. 161–163) accounts for their elimination from the body since these highly lipid-soluble drugs are readily reabsorbed from the tubular urine.

The action of the short-to-intermediate–acting barbiturates is terminated primarily by biotransformation to inactive metabolites which are excreted in the urine. The long-acting phenobarbital is eliminated by both biotransformation and urinary excretion. Only barbital is dependent primarily on renal excretion for its removal from the body.

IV. Nonbarbiturate Sedatives and Hypnotics

A. Agents

Chloral hydrate

Paraldehyde

Ethinamate (Valmid)

Glutethimide (Doriden)

Methaqualone (Quaalude)

As indicated earlier all of the above agents resemble the barbiturates with respect to their differential effects on various functions. Therefore we will note below only the aspects of each agent that are different from those of the barbiturates.

B. Chloral Hydrate

Unpleasant tasting and smelling and, therefore, administered orally in a preparation that masks its taste.

Chloral hydrate is biotransformed to trichloroethanol (cf. p. 156) and the parent drug and its metabolite are equally potent CNS-depressant agents.

C. Paraldehyde

Unpleasant odor and taste. Between 11 and 28% is excreted unchanged by the lungs, and because of its odor, its use has been largely restricted to hospitalized patients.

D. Methaqualone

Methaqualone possesses antispasmodic, local anesthetic and weak antihistaminic activity in addition to its sedative-hypnotic actions. It also has antitussive activity equivalent to codeine but resembles the barbiturates in its lack of analgesic activity.

APPENDIX 6
Drugs Used in the Treatment
of Mental Disorders

I. **Antipsychotic Drugs.** Agents used to improve mood and behavior of psychotic patients without excessive sedation and without causing addiction.
Phenothiazine derivatives:
  Chlorpromazine
  Thioridazine
Haloperidol
Lithium salts
Reserpine

A. **Phenothiazine Derivatives.** The phenothiazines not only act on the CNS but, in therapeutic doses, also exert significant effects upon other organ systems. The phenothiazines have important effects on the autonomic nervous system, including blockade of the actions of epinephrine and nor-epinephrine at sympathetic receptors and of acetylcholine at postganglionic parasympathetic receptors. This group also possesses antihistaminic and antiserotonin activity. Chlorpromazine (CPZ) is the prototype drug; it is the agent most widely used and differs from other phenothiazines only quantitatively with regard to primary action on the CNS and side-effects.

1. **CNS Effects**

   a. CPZ depresses the sensory input to the reticular formation and raises the threshold for stimuli impinging on the reticular formation. This sensory impairment produces a considerable degree of *sedation*. The sedative effect differs from that of the barbiturates since there is no ataxia or incoordination with CPZ and the subject can be easily aroused.

   b. Gross behavioral effects: Apparent indifference or slowing of responses to external stimuli, diminution of initiative and of anxiety without a change in state of waking or consciousness or of intellectual abilities. After single doses to normal subjects, there is impairment of performance of tasks that require attention but little effect on tests requiring intellectual function. Barbiturates and meprobamate affect preferentially those tasks that are dependent on intellectual functioning. On chronic administration of CPZ to patients, there is improvement in performance on tests, especially those tests requiring a great deal of attentive behavior.

    c. CPZ depresses the chemoreceptor trigger zone (CTZ) and is particularly effective against the nausea and vomiting induced by certain drugs and disease states. It is *not* effective in motion sickness.

    d. CPZ disrupts temperature-regulatory mechanisms in the hypothalamus; there is a resulting tendency for body temperature to fall, if subject is in a cool environment. CPZ also depresses centers involved in the control of blood pressure.

    e. CPZ can cause a variety of motor disorders ranging from involuntary muscle movements (tremors) to muscle weakness and fatigue. Some of these effects resemble the symptoms of Parkinson's disease.

2. **Effects on Autonomic Nervous System**

CPZ produces vasodilatation and a fall in blood pressure due to blockade of sympathetic receptors and to inhibition of hypothalamic regulatory centers. Blockade of postganglionic parasympathetic receptors results in dry mouth (inhibition of salivary secretion).

3. **Other Effects**

    a. Mild antihistaminic activity

    b. Endocrine system: CPZ reduces urinary levels of gonadotropins, estrogens and progestins. CPZ may block ovulation and induce lactation.

4. **Side-effects and Toxic Reactions**

    a. Many of the side-effects, such as dry mouth and muscular disorders, are due to actions described above. The most troublesome side-effect is postural hypotension; tolerance usually develops to this effect and generally disappears after the first days of treatment.

    b. The most dangerous effects of CPZ treatment are those resulting from allergic reactions. These include skin eruptions, disorders in blood-cell formation and jaundice due to obstruction of the normal flow of bile.

5. **Therapeutic Uses**

    a. For treatment of psychotic disorders such as schizophrenia

    b. As an antiemetic to treat nausea and vomiting in radiation sickness and other diseases or emesis produced by drugs such as nitrogen mustards and tetracyclines

    c. In the control of intractable hiccoughs (mechanism of action is unknown)

B. **Haloperidol**

Similar to CPZ; no clinical advantages over phenothiazines but useful in those patients who tolerate phenothiazines poorly

C. **Lithium Salts**

Used in the treatment of manic disorders (manic stage of manic-depressive psychosis). Can also prevent relapses in the depressed or hypomanic patient. Mechanism of action unknown.

In therapeutic doses, patients may complain of fatigue and muscular weakness. Slurred speech, ataxia and tremor of hands are commonly noticed. Serious toxic effects are associated with high plasma levels; the CNS is primarily affected.

D. Reserpine

First antipsychotic drug introduced into therapy; replaced by newer agents; used today mainly to treat hypertension.

1. CNS Effects

Low doses: Sedation and a marked calming effect

High doses: May increase severity and frequency of seizures in epileptic patients and may cause seizure in patients with no history of convulsive disorders

2. Effects on Autonomic Nervous System

Decreases blood pressure and heart rate; increases gastrointestinal motility and hydrochloric acid secretion; produces miosis. These effects are due to a decrease in sympathetic activity and the concomitant enhancement of parasympathetic activity. The decrease in activity of sympathetic nervous system is the result of depletion of stores of epinephrine and norepinephrine in many organs, including brain, heart, blood vessels and adrenal medulla. Reserpine depletes norepinephrine stores by preventing active transport of the neurohormone into granules from cytoplasm of nerve-endings (see pp. 383–387). Reserpine also depletes the body's stores of serotonin. It has been claimed that each of the biologic amines affected is involved in reserpine's effects on the CNS, but the available evidence is still equivocal.

II. Antianxiety Drugs

Meprobamate (Equanil; Miltown)

Chlordiazepoxide (Librium)

Diazepam (Valium)

In patients suffering from worry and tension, the use of antianxiety drugs for daytime sedation has sometimes proved helpful and desirable. The drowsiness and relief of tension, similar to that produced by alcohol and barbiturates, are generally felt to be pleasant.

The pharmacology of all of these agents is much the same and closely resembles that of the barbiturates. They are somewhat safer than the barbiturates in that dose-effect curves for the antianxiety drugs are less steep. Although the continuous use of the antianxiety drugs leads to physical dependence, the probability of developing such dependence is much less than that seen with the barbiturates.

The antianxiety drugs produce muscular relaxation by an action in the CNS (not on the muscle). These agents also increase appetite.

Side-effects include: nausea, skin rash; impairment of libido; blood disorders.

Chlordiazepoxide and valium are also used extensively in the treatment of the alcoholic. Success here is probably because they substitute for alcohol and thus attenuate the alcohol withdrawal syndrome.

These agents are not effective in the treatment of psychoses.

III. Antidepressant Drugs

Monoamine oxidase (MAO) inhibitors

Nialamide

Tranylcypromine

Imipramine

CNS stimulants (see pp. 359–361)

Amphetamines

Methylphenidate (Retalin)

Depressive disorders range from mild despondency to severely retarded states and suicidal risks. Treatment usually includes psychological support and an attempt to alter the stressful social situations. Electroshock therapy is possibly the most effective treatment for depression, but has fallen into disrepute in the United States, where the treatment for severe depression is with antidepressant drugs such as imipramine or the MAO inhibitors. The clinical effectiveness of these agents has been difficult to assess, but there is some indication that they are useful in depressions characterized by marked retardation. These agents have a delayed onset of action, up to several weeks, which makes them of little value in suicidal patients.

A. Monoamine Oxidase Inhibitors (cf. p. 262)

The MAO inhibitors block the *intracellular* metabolism of naturally occurring amines such as epinephrine, norepinephrine, serotonin and tyramine. The chronic administration of MAO inhibitors results in the accumulation of these amines in various tissues including the brain, liver and sympathetic nerves. However, the MAO inhibitors inhibit not only the enzyme for which they are named but many other enzymes as well.

1. Pharmacologic Effects

a. Behavioral effects are seen as an elevation of mood in certain depressed mental states; it takes several days or weeks for this effect to be discernible in depressed patients. *The relationship between MAO inhibition* (resulting in accumulation of amines, e.g., norepinephrine, 5HT in brain) *and the therapeutic actions of these drugs is not firmly established.*

b. Cardiovascular effects

Either hypotension or hypertension may be produced depending on the dose, duration of use, co-medication or ingestion of tyramine-containing foods. The postural hypotension that occurs with the use of all MAO inhibitors cannot, at present, be attributed to enzyme inhibition.

MAO inhibition is responsible, however, for the acute toxicity that develops when certain exogenous amines are ingested either as drugs (ephedrine) or as components in foods (tyramine in cheese). (See pp. 262, 290–291.)

     c. Other effects: Dry mouth, constipation, insomnia, nervousness

         Because of their general enzyme-inhibiting properties, the MAO inhibitors also prolong and intensify the effects of CNS depressants such as barbiturates and alcohol, and narcotic analgesics such as meperidine.

  2. Therapeutic Uses. Reserved for those patients not helped by non-MAO inhibitor antidepressant drugs and used only in hospitalized patients.

B. Imipramine

Prototype drug for group of antidepressant drugs with *no* MAO inhibitor activity. These compounds are closely related to the phenothiazines in structure and in pharmacologic activity.

  1. Effects on CNS

    The effects resembling those of the weaker phenothiazines include mild sedation, potentiation of CNS depressants. Unlike the phenothiazines, imipramine augments the CNS effects of amphetamine and atropine.

    In contrast to the sedation produced in normal subjects, depressed patients respond with an elevation of mood, increased mental alertness and physical activity, improved sleep patterns and appetite and a reduction in morbid preoccupation with self-destruction.

  2. Other Effects. Imipramine possesses distinct parasympathetic postganglionic blocking activity which is manifested as dryness of the mouth, constipation and urinary retention, blurred vision. Postural hypotension and mild jaundice may also occur.

  3. Imipramine and related compounds are the drugs of choice in the treatment of depression; used in outpatient treatment.

C. CNS Stimulants

  1. Amphetamines and Derivatives

    The amphetamines (amphetamine, dextroamphetamine and methamphetamine) produce their effects in part by a direct action on sympathetic receptors and in part by mediating the release of norepinephrine from stores in sympathetic nerve terminals. Phenmetrazine (Preludin) and diethylpropion (Tenuate; Tepanil) are also sympathomimetic amines which share the pharmacologic and toxic effects of the amphetamines.

    a. Peripheral effects: Vasoconstriction and increase in blood pressure. Except for a marked contraction of the urinary bladder sphincter making urination difficult, other smooth muscle effects are not notable, e.g., bronchial muscle is relaxed but not sufficiently to be of therapeutic value.

    b. CNS effects

      (1) The effects of a single dose of amphetamine may be manifested as a general alerting action: increased alertness, attentiveness and wakefulness and a decreased sense of fatigue. Generally there is an elevation of mood, often elation and euphoria, although mentally retarded patients do not display euphoria and some patients

may even feel dysphoric or be sedated. Amphetamine will improve performance of simple tasks when there is boredom, fatigue or lack of motivation; performance of complicated tasks is worsened by amphetamine.

The general alerting action is associated with stimulation of the reticular formation and lowering of the threshold to sensory stimuli. This effect on the CNS is a direct effect and not one mediated by the release of norepinephrine.

After chronic use, over 2–4 days, a model paranoid psychosis characteristic of amphetamine abuse is seen. There is some sleep deprivation but not enough to explain the psychosis. The paranoid psychosis is comparable to a true natural psychotic state (this is unlike the psychoses induced by LSD and mescaline). The amphetamine psychosis is normally self-limiting, reversing within 24–48 hours. Intervention, if necessary, is with chlorpromazine. One cannot "talk the patient down" as is possible with bad trips on LSD or mescaline. After chronic use, a state of depression occurs.

(2) The appetite depressant (anorexiant) effect of amphetamine which may result in weight loss is primarily due to appetite suppression rather than an increased rate of tissue metabolism or motor activity. Tolerance develops to this effect; if doses are raised to overcome tolerance, undesirable side-effects can occur.

(3) In normal subjects, usual doses of amphetamine do not appreciably increase respiration. When respiration is depressed by centrally acting drugs, amphetamine may stimulate respiration.

c. Fate of amphetamine

Well absorbed from GI tract. Distributed to brain.

Amphetamines are not biotransformed by MAO but are oxidized by microsomal enzyme systems.

Urinary excretion is dependent on urine pH; increased rate of excretion with acid pH.

d. Therapeutic uses

To be used with caution if not contraindicated in presence of hypertension, cardiac and cerebrovascular disease, hyperthyroidism, and in emotionally unstable individuals predisposed to drug abuse. Contraindicated in pregnancy since there is a risk of congenital anomalies in the fetus.

(1) In the treatment of obesity; use should be limited to short-term therapy to help patient in establishing a dietary regimen.

(2) In the treatment of narcolepsy (a condition characterized by brief attacks of deep sleep). Tolerance does not appear to develop to these agents in the treatment of narcolepsy.

(3) In the treatment of mild mental disorders such as mood

disturbances, chronic nervous exhaustion. This use is controversial.

(4) In the treatment of the hyperkinetic child. The basis for improvement is not understood and the beneficial effects of the amphetamines are paradoxical.

2. Other Agents

Methylphenidate (Ritalin) and pipradol (Meratran) have much the same pharmacologic activity and toxicity as the amphetamines but produce fewer peripheral sympathomimetic effects. Methylphenidate is often used instead of amphetamine for treatment of hyperkinetic children since it has better social acceptance.

APPENDIX 7
Weights and Measures

METRIC SYSTEM

The metric system, the system of weights and measures used in science, is also the official measuring system of the *United States Pharmacopeia,* the Council on Pharmacy of the American Medical Association and other governing bodies. It is also the measuring system prescribed by law in most European countries.

The metric system is a decimal system, and its basic units of measurement can be subdivided or multiplied to form secondary units that differ from each other by some power of 10. The prefixes used to designate subdivisions of the units are from Latin, and those used to designate multiples are from Greek (Table A-7-1).

The basic metric units of measurement are: the *meter,* the unit for linear measurement; the *liter,* the unit for capacity or volume; and the *gram,* the unit for mass or weight. The meter (m) is defined as the distance between two lines at $0°C$ on a platinum-iridium bar known as the International Prototype Meter deposited at the International Bureau of Weights and Measures. The liter (L) is defined as the volume of 1 kilogram of pure water at $4°C$ and 760 mm Hg pressure. Originally the liter was designated as the contents of a cube whose sides measure 1 decimeter, or 10 centimeters. It was intended that the liter be identical with the volume contained in 1,000 cubic centimeters (cc). However, the liter was found to be 1,000.028 cc. The difference is so small that, for all practical purposes, the liter may be considered equal to 1,000 cc, and the thousandth part of a liter, the milliliter, equal to 1 cubic centimeter. The gram (g) is defined as the weight of 1 milliliter of water at $4°C$ and 760 mm Hg pressure.

APOTHECARY SYSTEM

The apothecary system of weights and measures is largely being replaced by the metric system. These two systems are used interchangeably, however, for some older drugs. Table A-7-2 gives some of the units of weight and volume in the apothecary system. Table A-7-3 lists some of the more commonly employed approximate metric and apothecary equivalents. When liquids are prescribed to be used by patients who do not have chemical measuring equipment, the directions on the prescription are

482

usually given in terms of common household measuring utensils. Table A-7-4 lists the volume of some convenient kitchen utensils in terms of approximate metric and apothecary equivalents.

Table A-7-1.   Metric System of Weights and Measures

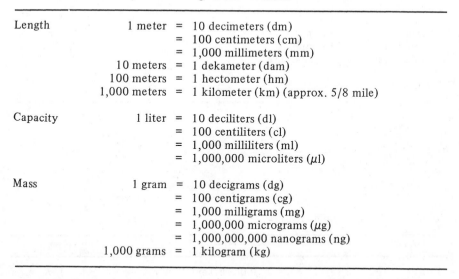

Length	1 meter	=	10 decimeters (dm)
		=	100 centimeters (cm)
		=	1,000 millimeters (mm)
	10 meters	=	1 dekameter (dam)
	100 meters	=	1 hectometer (hm)
	1,000 meters	=	1 kilometer (km) (approx. 5/8 mile)
Capacity	1 liter	=	10 deciliters (dl)
		=	100 centiliters (cl)
		=	1,000 milliliters (ml)
		=	1,000,000 microliters (μl)
Mass	1 gram	=	10 decigrams (dg)
		=	100 centigrams (cg)
		=	1,000 milligrams (mg)
		=	1,000,000 micrograms (μg)
		=	1,000,000,000 nanograms (ng)
	1,000 grams	=	1 kilogram (kg)

Table A-7-2.   Apothecary System of Weights and Measures

Weight	60 grains	=	1 dram
	480 grains or 8 drams	=	1 ounce
	12 ounces	=	1 pound
Volume	60 minims	=	1 fluidram
	8 fluidrams	=	1 fluid ounce
	16 fluid ounces	=	1 pint
	2 pints	=	1 quart
	4 quarts	=	1 gallon

Table A-7-3.   Commonly Used Approximate Metric and Apothecary Equivalents

Metric		Apothecary
1 milligram	=	1/60 grain
1 gram	=	15 grains
1 kilogram	=	2.2 pounds (avoirdupois)
1 milliliter	=	15 minims
60 milligrams	=	1 grain
30 grams	=	1 ounce
0.06 milliliter	=	1 minim
30 milliliters	=	1 fluid ounce
500 milliliters	=	1 pint
1,000 milliliters	=	1 quart

Table A-7-4.   Household Measures

Utensil	Metric	Apothecary
1 drop	0.06–0.1 ml	1 – 1 $\frac{1}{2}$ minims
1 teaspoonful[a]	5 ml	1 $\frac{1}{3}$ fl. dram
1 tablespoonful	15 ml	1 fl. ounce
1 wineglass	60 ml	2 fl. ounces
1 waterglass	250 ml	8 fl. ounces

[a]The capacity of the household teaspoon varies considerably. The American Standards Association has established an American Standard Teaspoon for household purposes, containing 4.93 ± 0.24 ml; the *U.S.P.* specifies that this teaspoon may be regarded as containing 5 ml.

INDEX

Abel, John Jacob, 12, 13, 15
Absorption, 73–99. *See also specific drug*
  duration of action and, 207, 226–228, 237,
    244
  epithelial barrier to, 77
  formulation of drugs and, 87–89, 210, 400
  gastrointestinal, 74–89
    antidotes in prevention of poison ab-
      sorption, 328, 332–333
    drug interactions and, 287, 289, 290, 293
    from large intestine, 84
    lymphatics and, 74–75
    from oral cavity, 77–78
    pH and, 62–63, 77, 79–80
    pinocytosis and, 68, 84
    from rectum, 78, 84
    from small intestine, 80–84
    of solid drugs, 84–89
    from stomach, 62–63, 78–80, 83
    stomach emptying rate and, 78, 83, 98,
      290, 293
  genetic abnormalities in, 253, 255–256
  from intramuscular sites, 97–98, 226–227
  rate of, 209–211
    administration route and, 117, 205, 210–
      211, 236–237
    blood flow and, 76, 95–96, 97, 99
    dosage forms and, 210–211
    elimination and, 227, 245
    first-order kinetics, 209–210, 237
    time course of action and, 226, 236–237
    toxic effects and, 327–328
    zero-order kinetics, 210–211, 237
  from respiratory tract, 91–94
  from skin, 89–91
  from subcutaneous sites, 95–97
Abstinence syndrome, 349. *See also* With-
    drawal syndrome
Abuse of drugs. *See* Drug abuse and depend-
    ence

Acetaminophen (paracetamol), 461. *See
    also* Antipyretic analgesics
Acetanilid, effect of age on biotransforma-
    tion of, 243
Acetazolamide, 395, 440
  mechanism of action, 440
Acetic acid, ionization of, 60
Acetophenetidin. *See* Phenacetin (Aceto-
    phenetidin)
Acetylation, 145, 146, 148
  genetic abnormalities in enzymes for, 251,
    252, 254
  interspecies variation in, 258
  toxicity of sulfonamides produced by, 148
Acetylcholine, 42–43, 381–382
  atropine and effects of, 180–182, 195–196,
    197, 335, 386
  cholinesterases and, 141, 142, 159, 335, 387
  dose-response curves for, 172–177
  drugs mimicking activity of, 486, 487
  mechanism of action, 33, 42–43, 381–382
  in nerve impulse transmission, 344, 380–
    382, 385, 386, 387, 388
  receptor isolation, 43, 358
  release of, 378, 382
  storage of, 382
  structure and receptor interaction, 43
Acetylcholinesterase, synthesis of, 381–382
  competition for sites on, 141, 142, 159
  inhibitors of, 386, 387
Acetylsalicylic acid. *See* Aspirin. *See also*
    Salicylates
Acid(s), as local toxic agents, 305. *See also*
    Electrolyte(s) *and specific acid, e.g.,*
    Acetic acid
Actinomycin D, 453
Action, law of mass. *See* Mass action, law of
Active transport, 66–67
  age and, 244
  into bile, 139

Active transport—*Continued*
  in choroid plexus, 108–110
  drug absorption and, 84
  rate of absorption and, 209
  urine formation and, 124–133. *See also* Excretion, renal, of drug
Acute toxicity, 303–304, 309. *See also* Toxicity, evaluation of
Addiction, drug, defined, 342. *See also* Drug abuse and dependence
ADH. *See* Antidiuretic hormone (ADH)
Adipose tissue
  DDT storage in, 106, 236
  drug storage in, 233, 234–236
  effect on drug dosage, 242, 293–294
Administration of drug doses. *See* Dose; Dose-effect (dose-response) curve; Dose-response relations
  routes, 74–76, 98–99, 226–228. *See also specific route, e.g.,* Oral administration
Adrenergic blocking agents, 384–385, 386
Adrenergic nerves, 383
Aerosols, use of, 93
Afferent arteriole, renal, 122
Afferent (sensory) neurons, 343, 374
Affinity of drug for receptor, 176, 177–178, 199
Age. *See also* Children and infants
  absorption and, 243, 245
  biotransformation and, 243, 245, 246–247
  body composition and, 242
  poisoning incidence and, 322–326, 332
  renal excretion and, 244, 245–246, 295
  response to drugs and, 243–247, 293
  toxicity of organic nitrites and nitrates and, 246–247
Air, excretion in inspired, 93, 94, 118
Air quality standards, 320–321
Albumin, drug binding to, 105. *See also* Protein binding
Alcohol. *See* Alcohol abuse and dependence; Ethyl alcohol; Methyl alcohol
Alcohol abuse and dependence, 352–355. *See also* Ethyl alcohol
  acceptability of, 353
  cross-tolerance to drugs in, 283, 291
  incidence of, 353
  marihuana dependence vs., 364–365
  opioid dependence vs., 356, 357, 367
  physical dependence, 351, 354–355
  psychologic dependence, 351, 353–354
  tolerance and, 280, 283, 351, 354
  withdrawal syndrome, 351, 354–355, 367
Alcoholism. *See* Alcohol abuse and dependence
Alcohols, aliphatic
  definition, 465
  pharmacologic action of, 468

physicochemical properties of, 56, 57, 465
Aldosterone, inhibition of, 442
Allergy, 271–279, 296–297, 311
  cross-sensitization and, 277
  dose and, 277–278
  hypersensitivity vs., 272
  idiosyncracy vs., 277–279
  immune mechanism and, 272–274, 297
  incidence of, 276–277, 278, 297, 307
  manifestations of allergic reaction, 274–276, 308
  mediators and, 273, 274, 297
  toxicity vs., 277–279
Alpha-methyldopa, 384, 385, 386
Alpha-methyl-*p*-tyrosine, 384, 385, 386
Aluminum-containing antacids, 434
Alveoli, pulmonary, 68, 91–92, 93
Amebicides, 449–450. *See also specific drug, e.g.,* Chloroquine; Diiodohydroxyquine; Emetine; Metronidazole
American Conference of Government Industrial Hygienists toxicity guides, 314
American Drug Index, 25
Amines
  ionization of, 60, 61
  oxidation of, 153–154, 155
Amino acids
  active transport of, 67, 125
  as conjugating agents, 145, 146, 147
Aminopyrine (Pyramidon), 458, 461
  effect of age on biotransformation of, 243
Ammonia
  industrial environmental limits of, 314
  ionization of, 39, 60
  toxicity of concentrated gas, 305
Amphetamine(s), 479–481
  abuse of, 359–361
    intravenous use in, 360
    physical dependence, 351, 360–361, 367
    psychologic dependence, 351, 360
    tolerance in, 351, 360, 368
    withdrawal syndrome in, 351, 360, 367
  biotransformation of, 153, 155, 258, 480
  effects on
    autonomic nervous system, 386, 479
    central nervous system, 359, 479–480
  elimination of, 221, 332, 480
  inhibitor of tyramine metabolism, 159
  reflex action and, 345
  site of action
    in central nervous system, 347, 480
    at periphery, 386, 479
  therapeutic uses, 360, 480–481
  toxic effects of, 344, 360
Amphotericin B, 447
Analgesic drugs, 458–463. *See also specific drug*
  cumulative toxicity of mixtures of, 305

incidence of poisoning by, 322, 325
narcotic, 355, 461–463. *See also* Opioid(s)
nonnarcotic, 458–461. *See also* Antipyretic analgesics
Anaphylaxis, 275
Anesthetic drugs. *See* General anesthetics; Local anesthetics
Animal studies of drugs, 396–400. *See also* Evaluation of drugs; Toxicity, evaluation of
Antacids, 433–435
adverse interactions of, 287, 290
classification of, 433
nonsystemic, buffer and nonbuffer, 433–435
systemic, 433, 434
effect on absorption of drugs, 290
in gastric acid neutralization, 34, 45, 433
therapeutic uses, 433–434
Antagonism, drug, 180–184, 287, 289, 290, 332–336. *See also* Enzymes, induction of *and* inhibition of
of acetylcholine-atropine, 180–181, 195–196, 197, 335, 386
biochemical, 285, 286–287, 288–289, 291, 385–387
chemical, 287, 289, 290
classified, 180, 196, 285, 286–287
competitive, 180–182
of diphenhydramine-histamine, 180–182, 196
drug-receptor interactions and, 180–184, 199, 285
of epinephrine-dibenamine, 183
log dose-effect curves, 180–184, 199, 335
noncompetitive, 182–184, 199
of parathion-cholinesterase, 183–184
pharmacologic, 180–184, 199, 285, 286, 333, 335–336
physiologic (functional), 285, 286, 328
of sodium transport
by mercurials, 439
by benzothiadiazine derivatives, 440–441
by high-ceiling diuretics, 442–443
of spironolactone-aldosterone, 442
in therapy of poisoning, 332–336
Anthelmintics, 450–451
mechanism of action of, 256, 450–451
Antianxiety drugs, 477–478. *See also specific drug, e.g.,* Chlordiazepoxide (Librium); Diazepam (Valium); Meprobamate (Equanil, Miltown)
Antibacterials, 444–447. *See also* Antibiotic(s) *and specific drug, e.g.,* Sulfonamides
Antibiotic(s), 444–447. *See also specific agent, e.g.,* Penicillin
in cancer chemotherapy, 453

combinations of, 445
host factors and, 446, 447
isolation from soil microbes, 392
mechanism of action of, 445
misuse of, 446–447
resistance to, 267–271, 295, 296
selective toxicity and, 444
spectrum of activity of, 444–445
untoward effects of therapy with, 445–446
Antibodies, 266. *See also* Allergy
allergy and, 272–274, 276, 279, 297
Anticancer drugs, 451–453
alkylating agents, 452
antagonists of
folic acid, 452
purine, 452
pyrimidines, 452–453
mechanisms of action of, 452–453
resistance to, 267, 270, 271, 294, 296
selective toxicity of, vs. antibacterials, 451
toxicity and, 195, 407
Anticoagulants. *See also specific drug, e.g.,* Heparin
adverse interactions of, 163, 288–289, 290
binding by cholestyramine, 290
hemorrhage and overdoses, 307
phenobarbital and therapy with, 162–163
Antidepressants, 478–479. *See also* Monoamine oxidase inhibitors *and specific drug, e.g.,* Amphetamine; Imipramine; Tranylcypromine
interactions of, 262, 286, 288, 290-291
Antidiabetic drugs, 288–289, 290, 395. *See also* Insulin
Antidiuretic hormone (ADH), 126, 132–133
Antidote(s), 326, 332–336. *See also specific agent, e.g.,* Atropine; Charcoal
complexing agents, 332, 333, 335–336
in elevation of threshold of toxicity, 333, 335–336
first-aid measures, 328, 330–331
hazards of, 336, 337
nonspecific, 328–332
in prevention of poison absorption and distribution, 329, 332, 333, 334
in removal of poison from site of action, 333, 335
specific, 332–336
universal, 329
Antifungal agents, 447. *See also specific drug, e.g.,* Griseofulvin
Antigen(s), 266. *See also* Allergy
allergy and, 272–274, 276–277, 279
drugs as, 273–274
Antihistaminics. *See also specific drug, e.g.,* Diphenhydramine (Benadryl)
toxic effects in children, 307

Antihistaminics—*Continued*
uses in allergy, 279, 297
Antimalarials, 448–449. *See also specific drug,
e.g.,* Chloroguanide; Chloroquine; Primaquine; Pyrimethamine; Quinacrine (Atabrine); Quinine
resistance to, 270, 271
Antimony compounds, 451
species difference in response to, 261
Antipyretic analgesics, 458–461. *See also
specific drug, e.g.,* Salicylates
aniline derivatives, 461
definitions, 458
mechanism of action
of analgesics, 458
of antipyretics, 458–459
pyrazalon derivatives, 461
salicylates, 459–461
Antipyrine, 461
Antiseptics, 447–448. *See also specific drug,
e.g.,* Phenol
mechanism of action, 447–448
toxic effects, 306
Antiviral agents, 447
Apomorphine, vomiting induction and, 329, 345
Apothecary system of weights and measures,
482–484
Apparent volume of distribution. *See* Volume of
distribution
Application site. *See* Route of administration
Arabs, medicine of early, 5–7
Arginine monohydrochloride in urine acidification, 332
Aromatic amines as carcinogens, 309
Asbestos, cumulative toxicity of, 304, 316, 317
Ascorbic acid in urine acidification, 332
Aspirin. *See also* Salicylates
absorption of, 79, 87, 88, 460
biotransformation of, 146, 147, 157, 217–
219
elimination of
dose and, 217–219
urinary, metabolites of, 218
incidence of allergy to, 276
incidence of poisoning with, 324–326
ionization of, 59
potency as analgesic, 179, 180
toxicity of, 372, 460
Association areas of cerebral cortex, 347
Atabrine. *See* Quinacrine (Atabrine)
Atropine
acetylcholine and effects of, 180–181, 195–
197, 335, 386
as antidote for organic phosphate poisoning,
333, 335
effects of gastric emptying, 290
genetic determinants of biotransformation,
248, 249

as psychedelic, 361
pupil and, 31, 32
site of action, 32, 195
specificity of action, 195–197
topical administration and effects of, 197
Atropine esterase, atropine biotransformation
and, 248–250
Autonomic nervous system, 373–388. *See also*
Acetylcholine; Norepinephrine; Parasympathetic nervous system; Sympathetic
nervous system
divisions of, 375–377
drugs affecting neurotransmitters in, 383–
388
functional organization of, 375–380
inactivation of, 384–385, 386, 387–388
neurotransmitters of, 380–383
release of, 384–385, 386
significance of, 388
somatic nervous system vs., 373–375
storage of, 384–385, 386
synthesis of, 384–385, 386

Bacterial resistance to drugs. *See also* Resistance,
drug *and specific drug*
mechanisms of, 269–271, 295
origin of, 267–269
BAL. *See* Dimercaprol (BAL)
Barbiturates. *See also* Sedatives and hypnotics
and specific drug, e.g., Phenobarbital
absorption of, 79–80, 83, 473
abuse and dependence, 352, 355
degrees of, 353–354
opioid dependence vs., 356, 357
tolerance and, 279, 280, 281, 282, 283, 354
withdrawal syndrome, 349, 351, 354–355,
367
albumin-binding of, 105
central nervous system and, 348, 352–354,
472
medullary respiratory center, 345
reticular activating system, 348, 472
classification of, 470
distribution of, 473
elimination of, 473
hypnotic vs. sedative, 469
interactions with ethyl alcohol, 291, 468
maternal administration and neonate, 112
pharmacokinetics and physicochemical properties of, 470–471
poisoning
dialysis in, 332
incidence of, 322
mortality from, 303, 322
toxicity of, 472–473
Benadryl. *See* Diphenhydramine (Benadryl)
Benzene, 145, 305
industrial environmental limits, 314, 315

Benzocaine, 458
Benzpyrene biotransformation, 162, 280
Bernard, Claude, 9, 10, 11, 14, 36–37, 46
Bicarbonate ion, 126–127
  kidney and, 124, 126–127, 132
    acetazolamide and reabsorption of, 440
    chlorothiazide and, 441
  in normal plasma, 119
  pH of urine and, 133
Bile, secretion and circulation of, 137–138
Bioassay, 396, 398
Biochemical antagonism, 285, 286
  multiple-drug therapy and, 288–289
  in specific antidotal therapy, 334
Bioequivalence, requirements for, 87, 407–408
Biologic half-life, 212, 238
  cumulative toxicity and, 233–236, 304
  distribution to body fluids and, 222–223
  duration of drug action and, 223
  elimination rate and, 212, 222–224, 238
  multiple-dose schedules and, 228–233, 238
Biopharmaceutics, defined, 9
Biotransformation, 117, 139, 165. See also
    Biochemical antagonism; Synergism
  age and, 243, 244, 245, 246
  allergy and, 276–277
  of aspirin, 217–219
  of atropine, 243–244, 246
  as catalyzed reaction, 140
  chemical pathways of, 144, 158, 165
    major, 157–158
    nonsynthetic reactions in, 149–154, 165.
      See also Hydrolysis; Oxidation; Reduction
    species differences in, 257–260
    synthetic reactions in, 144–149, 165. See
      also Conjugation and specific reaction,
      e.g., Acetylation; Methylation
    synthetic vs. nonsynthetic, 150, 151, 152
  drug resistance and, 270–271
  enzymes, mediators of, 140–142. See also
    Enzyme(s)
  enzyme induction and, 160–165, 270
  enzyme inhibition and, 158–160, 334
  of ethanol, 156, 214–216
  genetic factors in. See Enzyme(s), genetic
    abnormalities of
  pathologic conditions and, 295
  pharmacologic activity and, 150, 151
  rate, 142–144, 212, 214–219, 290–291
    alterations of, in treatment of poisoning,
      334
    drug concentration at site of action and,
      144, 205, 206
    first-order kinetics, 212
    potential for constant rate of, 144, 212
    substrate and enzyme concentration and,
      142–144, 158
    zero-order kinetics, 214–219

response to drugs and, 150, 151, 214, 216,
    288–289, 294–295
sites of, 144
synergism and, 286
of thiopental, 235
tolerance and, 280, 282, 295
Biotransport, 49–51, 69. See also Transport;
    Transport mechanisms
Bishydroxycoumarin. See Dicumerol (Bishy-
    droxycoumarin)
Blake, James, 11–12, 14
Blood. See also Hemoglobin; Plasma
  circulation. See Blood flow
  coagulation, 33, 34, 162–163, 197
  drug levels in. See Blood drug levels
  drugs and pathologic changes in, 306, 310
  effects of allergens on, 275
  oxygen, carbon monoxide inhalation and,
    303–304
  renal regulation of constituents, 119
  volume of. See Blood volume
Blood-brain barrier, 108
Blood drug levels. See also Distribution of drugs
  age and, 244–245
  capillary permeability and, 100, 102
  concentration at site of action and, 207–208
  "decay" curve of, 212
  distribution volume and, 222–223
  duration of action and, 207–208, 224
  in elimination rate determination, 211–212
  excretion rate and, 135–137, 219–223, 236
  intensity of drug effect and, 207–208
Blood flow, 74. See also Circulation, of blood
  cerebral, 107–110
  portobiliary, 138
  pulmonary, 92–93
  rate of
    absorption rate and, 76, 84, 95–96, 97, 99
    distribution rate and, 73, 76, 102, 104
    urinary excretion rate and, 135–137, 244,
      295
  renal, 121, 122–123
  vasomotor factors in, 33
Blood pressure
  capillary, on venous vs. arterial side, 101
  effects of rapid intravenous injections on, 98
  histamine and, 286
  hypothalamic regulation of, 346
  medulla and, 345
Blood volume
  distribution and, 102–105
  plasma volume as per cent of, 102
  renal regulation of, 119
Body fluids
  distribution to, 74, 102–105, 223
  drug concentration, distribution and, 242
  drug dosage and, 242, 293–294
  drug response and, 262, 293–294

Body fluids—*Continued*
  pH, 62, 63
    bicarbonate ion and, 126
    response to drugs and, 262
  regulation of, 118–119, 346
  total body water, 242
Body size, dosage and, 242–243, 247
Body temperature, 29, 30, 31
  hypothalamic regulation, 346
  response to drugs and, 262
Body type, body composition and, 242
Body weight, dosage and, 242, 247
Bond(s)
  covalent, 38–39
  in drug-receptor interactions, 37–44,
    105
  enzyme-substrate interactions and, 140–
    141
  hydrogen, 39–40, 54–55
  ionic, 38
  in nonreceptor drug binding, 105–107
Bone
  drug storage in, 106, 233
Botulinus toxin, poisoning by, 67, 82, 333
  interaction with acetylcholine, 386, 387
Bowman's capsule
  anatomy of, 119, 120, 121, 122
  urine formation and, 123, 124
Brain
  blood-brain barrier, 108
  blood supply, 107–110
  cerebrospinal fluid, 108–110
  choroid plexus, 109–110
  diffusion across capillaries, 107–108
  drug distribution to, 98, 107–110, 208,
    234–236
  structural and functional relations in, 342–348
Brainstem, functional anatomy of, 345
Brexylium, 384, 385, 386, 387
British Pharmaceutical Codex (B.P.C.), 24
British Pharmacopoeia (B.P.), 24
Bromide
  cumulative toxicity of, 233–234, 334
  distribution of, 104
  sodium chloride as poisoning antidote, 334
Buchheim, Rudolf, 11, 12, 14
Butacaine, 458
Butazolidin. *See* Phenylbutazone (Buta-
    zolidin)

Caffeine
  central nervous system and, 347
  as diuretic, 438–439
  incidence of allergy to, 276
Calcium carbonate, 435. *See also* Antacids
Calcium disodium edetate (EDTA)
  extracellular reactions of, 34
  for heavy metal poisoning, 34, 333, 335

Cannabis, 363–366. *See also* Marihuana
    (marijuana)
Capillaries, 95–96, 100, 102
  absorption rate and, 92–93, 95–96, 97
  distribution and, 100–102, 107–110
  endothelium, permeability of
    in brain, 107–110
    drug binding and, 106, 135
    hepatic, 101
    intramuscular, 97
    molecular size and, 100–101, 122
    pores in, 101
    to proteins, 68, 101, 122–123
    pulmonary, 92, 93, 94
    renal, 101, 122–123
    subcutaneous, 95–96
Carbohydrates as conjugating agents, 144
Carbon dioxide
  air pollution by, 319
  formation and hydration in kidney, 126–127
  industrial environmental limits, 315
Carbon monoxide
  air pollution by, 319
  industrial environmental limits, 315
  poisoning, 303–304, 335
    oxygen as antidote, 333, 335
Carbon tetrachloride
  industrial environmental limits, 315
  poisoning, 309
Carbonic anhydrase
  carbon dioxide hydration and, 126
  inhibitors, 395, 440–441
    in urine formation, 440
Carcinogens, 112, 162, 305, 309. *See also*
    Anticancer drugs
  assessment of potential, 308–309, 399
  organs affected by, 317
  in workplace, 316, 317
  standards for, 316
Cardiovascular system. *See also specific topic,*
    e.g., Blood flow
  allergic manifestations in, 275
  angina pectoris, 78
  hypothalamus and, 346
  medulla and, 345
  rapid intravenous injections and, 98
  toxic effects of drugs and, 307
Carrier mechanisms
  active transport and, 66, 292
  facilitated diffusion and, 64–66, 69
Cathartics, 435–437. *See also* Laxatives
  adverse effects of interaction of, 289
    contraindications, 436
    defined, 435
  in antidotal therapy, 329
  mechanism of action of, 45, 49, 436, 437
  saline, 436
  stimulant, 436

therapeutic use, 435–436
untoward effects, 436, 437
Caustics (corrosives), local toxicity of, 305–306
Cell membrane, 53–59, 68–69
active transport across, 65, 66, 69
composition of, 53–55
Davson-Danielli model of, 54, 55–57
diffusion through, 55–66, 100–102. *See also* Diffusion
facilitated diffusion, 64–66, 69
filtration through, 68, 69
lipid/water partition coefficient, 56–57, 58
molecular size and, 58–59
mosaic model of, 55, 69
passive diffusion, 56–64
pinocytosis through, 67–68
pore theory of, 59, 69, 101
structure and function and, 53–55, 68, 69
of weak electrolytes, 59–63, 69
Cell(s). *See also* Cell membrane
cytotoxic (protoplasmic) poisons of, 306, 372–373
filtration through spaces between, 68
sites of drug action in, 33, 34, 35–44, 46, 271, 372–373
receptors in, 35–42, 46
solubility of compounds and penetration into, 56–57
without receptors, 45, 46
Central nervous system. *See also* Brain; Central nervous system, drugs affecting
afferent (sensory) and efferent (motor) neurons, 343
autonomic nervous system vs., 373–375
evaluation of effects of new drugs on, 396, 397
feedback mechanisms, 345, 348
functional organization of, 342–348, 374
impulse transmission in, 343–344
Central nervous system, drugs affecting. *See also* Drug abuse and dependence
actions on medullary reflex center, 345
depressants, 352–355, 463–474. *See also* General anesthetics; Sedatives and hypnotics *and specific drug, e.g.,* Alcohol; Barbiturates; Opioids
cortical activity and, 347
frequency of adverse effects from, 307
psychedelics (hallucinogens), 351, 361–366, 368. *See also* Lysergic acid diethylamide (LSD); Marihuana (marijuana)
stimulants, 348, 351, 359–361, 367, 368, 479–481. *See also specific drug, e.g.,* Amphetamine(s)

tolerance and, 279, 280, 281–283. *See also* Tolerance
Cephaloridine, interaction with probenecid, 292, 445
Cerebellum, functional anatomy of, 345, 346
Cerebrospinal fluid (CSF), 108–110
circulation of, 108, 109, 110
distribution by, 108–110
formation of, 109, 110
Cerebrum, functional anatomy of, 346–348
Certain safety factor, defined, 192, 201
Ceruloplasmin, effects of deficiency of, 253, 256
Charcoal, as antidote, 329
Chemical antagonism, 285, 287
in therapy of poisoning, 332, 333, 334
Chemotherapy, agents used in
amebicides (q.q.v.), 449–450
anthelmintics (q.q.v.), 450–451
antibacterial (q.q.v.), 444–447
anticancer (q.q.v.), 451–453
antifungal (q.q.v.), 447
antimalarial (q.q.v.), 448–449
antiseptics and disinfectants (q.q.v.), 447–448
antiviral (q.q.v.), 447
Children and infants. *See also* Age
drug passage over placental barrier, 110–112, 247
enzyme systems in, 243, 245–247
hemoglobin conversion to methemoglobin, 246
incidence of poisoning in, 323–325, 332
passive diffusion in, 245
response to drugs in
blood concentration and duration of action, 244–245
cumulative toxicity and time-response relation, 244–245
therapeutic implications, 244–246
transport mechanisms in, 244
Chloral hydrate
abuse of, 352
as sedative-hypnotic, 469
biotransformation of, 156, 473–474
dependence on, 351
physical properties of, 473
Chlorambucil, 452
Chloramphenicol (Chloromycetin)
bacteriostatic activity of, 445–446
biotransformation and toxicity in infants, 245–246
blood disorders and, 310, 446
Chlordiazepoxide (Librium), 20, 477
abuse and dependence, 351, 352
tolerance to, 332
Chloride ion, 119
active transport (reabsorption), 129, 130, 442
renal excretion and reabsorption, 126

Chloroform, 40, 45
Chloroguanide
  as antimalarial drug, 448–449
  mechanism of action, 449
Chloromycetin. See Chloramphenicol
    (Chloromycetin)
Chlorophenothane (DDT), 236
  accumulation in adipose tissue, 104, 236
  toxicity of, 236
Chloroquine, 449
  in amebiasis of, 449
  as anthelmintic, 451
  as antimalarial drug, 448–449
  binding to nucleic acids, 106, 449
  gastric emptying and absorption and, 290
  mechanism of action, 449
  resistance to, 270, 271
  storage in liver, 106
Chlorothiazide (Diuril)
  binding by cholestyramine, 290
  blood levels of uric acid and, 292
  development of, 395
  as diuretic, 440–441
  mechanism of action, 441
  pharmacology of, 440–441
Chlorpromazine, 475–476
  as antipsychotic drug, 475–476
  hepatotoxicity of, 307, 476
  hypothalamus and, 328
  pharmacology of, 475–476
Cholesterol, effect of cholestyramine on, 287
Cholestyramine, 287
  binding of bile acids, 287
  binding of drugs, 290
Cholinergic nerves, 381
Cholinesterase
  atypical, 251, 252
  methacholine-acetylcholine competition
    for sites on, 141, 142, 159
  organic phosphate insecticides and, 223, 335
  parathion and effect of, 183–184
Choroid plexus, 109–110
Chromosomes, 248
Chronic toxicity, 304–305. See also Cumu-
    lative toxicity; Toxicity, evaluation
    of
Cigarette smoking
  psychologic dependence on, 349
  smoke in
    biotransformation of benzpyrene and,
      161, 162
    respiratory effects of, 94, 305
Ciliary movement in respiratory tract, 94
Cinchona, quinine from, 1, 29
Circulation
  of blood. See also Blood flow
    capillary wall as barrier to entry into,
      92, 93, 95

discovery of, 9
intravenous drug administration in poor,
    98
maintenance of, in poisoning, 328
time for complete cycle, 98
tourniquet for slowing entry into, 96–
    97
of cerebrospinal fluid, 109, 110
of lymph, 74
Clark, A. J., 11, 171
Clinical studies of new drugs, 400–409
  blind studies, 404
  conditions essential for, 402–404
  drug formulation and, 400
  large-scale controlled, 406–407
  in normal individuals, 405
  placebo controls in, 264, 404–405
  quantal response in, 185
  reference standards in, 404
  regulations concerning, 401–403, 406–
    408, 409
Coagulation of blood
  heparin and, 34, 197
  phenobarbital and anticoagulant therapy,
    162–163
Cocaine
  abuse and dependence, 351, 359–361
    dosage in, 360
    intravenous use in, 360
    psychologic dependence, 349, 351
  dose-response curves of, 176, 177
  interactions with norepinephrine, 384–
    385, 386, 387
  ionization of, 59, 60
  as vasoconstrictor, 33
Codeine. See also Opioids
  antitussive effects, 462
  biotransformation of, 146, 151, 463
  gastric emptying and absorption of, 290
  medullary center depression by, 345
  potency as analgesic, 178, 179
  summation of effects of aspirin plus, 284
Colchicine, 27, 28
Collecting ducts and tubules of kidney
  anatomy of, 121, 122
  in urine formation, 132–133
Compendia of drug standards, 20, 22, 23–
    25, 401
Competitive drug antagonists, 180, 199
Competitive inhibition, 159
Compulsive drug use, 349. See also Psycho-
    logic drug dependence
Concentration gradient. See also Diffusion
  diffusion and, 51–53, 62, 63, 64, 65, 66,
    68, 209
  transcapillary movement and, 101
Congener(s), in drug development, 393
Conjugation, 144–149

with acetic acid, 148
  interspecies variation in, 258
with amino acids, 146, 147
  glutamine, 147
  glycine, 145, 146, 147
    aspirin biotransformation and, 211, 213
  sulfate (cysteine), 145, 146, 148
center for, 144, 145–147, 158
with glucuronic acid, 144
  aspirin biotransformation and, 217, 218
  interspecies variation in, 258
Constant-rate absorption, 210–211
Contraceptive agents, sustained release
    preparations of, 89
Controlled experiments in drug evaluation,
    404–405
Controlled Substances Act, 329
Coordinate covalent bond, 39, 60, 61
Copper, ceruloplasmin and absorption and
    distribution, 253, 256
Corpus callosum, 346
Corrosives, local toxicity of, 305–306
Cortex, cerebral
  barbiturate-alcohol type of drug
      dependence and, 353
  excitation and inhibition of, 347–348
  functional anatomy of, 346–348
Cortex, renal, anatomy of, 120, 122
Covalent bond, 38–39
  drug-receptor interactions and, 41, 42
Cross-dependence, 352
Cross-sensitization, 277
Cross-tolerance, 283. See also Tolerance
Cumulative toxicity, 233–236, 309–310
  biologic half-life and, 233, 304
  of bromide ion, 233–234, 333, 334
  carcinogenicity and, 305
  in children and infants, 244–245
  determination in animals, 399
  in disease states, 262
  elimination rate and, 233–234
  of lead, 233, 304
  lipid solubility and, 233, 234–236
  of thiopental, 234–236
  tissue redistribution and, 234–236
Curare
  absorption of, 83
  action of nicotine and, 37
  site of action of, 10–11, 37
Cyanide poisoning, 304
  antidotal treatment, 332, 334
  oxygen utilization by cells and, 306
Cytotoxic agents, 306, 372–373

Daries, Peter John Andrew, 9
Davson-Danielli cell membrane model, 54, 55, 57

DDT. See Chlorophenothane (DDT)
"Decay" curve of drug concentration in
    blood, 212
Deferoxamine for iron poisoning, 332, 333
Dependence, drug. See Drug abuse and de-
    pendence
Depot preparations of drugs, 96, 97
  absorption rate of, 211
Depressants, 352–355, 463–468, 469–474.
    See Central nervous system, drugs af-
    fecting
Detoxification, significance of term, 139.
    See also Biotransformation
Development of new drugs, 391–396. See
    also Evaluation of drugs
  formulation of drug products, 400
  by modification of existing drugs, 393–
      395
  from natural products, 392
  from synthetic products, 392–396
Dialysis in poisoning, 332
Diazepam (Valium), 477
Dibenamine, epinephrine effect and, 183
Dibucaine, 457
Dicumarol (Bishydroxycoumarin)
  adverse interactions of, 289
  phenobarbital biotransformation and, 162–
      163
Diethylstilbesterol, maternal use and effect
    on offspring, 112
Diffusion. See also Cell membrane, diffusion
    through
  concentration gradient and, 51–53, 68
  facilitated, 64–66, 69, 84. See also Facilitated
      diffusion
  ionization degree and, 62–63, 69
  lipid solubility and, 55–57
  from maternal to fetal blood, 110–112, 247
  molecular size and, 58–59
  passive, 61–64, 73. See also Passive dif-
      fusion
  transcapillary, 100–102, 102–105
    in brain, 107–108
    drug binding and, 106, 135
Digestants, 435
Digestion
  bile acids and, 137–138
  drugs affected by reactions of, 84, 98
Digitoxin
  dose-response relations, 191, 192, 194
  half-life of, 223, 231–232
Dihydromorphinone (Dilaudid). See Hydro-
    morphone (Dilaudid)
Diiodohydroxyquin, 449
Dilantin. See Phenytoin (Dilantin)
Dilaudid. See Hydromorphone (Dilaudid)
Dimercaprol (BAL), for heavy metal
    poisoning, 333, 335

Dioctyl sodium succinate, 437
Dioscorides, Father of Materia Medica, 4,
    5, 6
Diphenhydramine (Benadryl)
  histamine effects and, 181-182, 196
  selectivity of action, 196
Discontinuity of frequency-response curves,
    249-250
Disintegration of solid drugs and absorption,
    85-87
Dissolution of solid drugs
  absorption and, 84-85, 86, 87
  particle size and, 85, 86, 87
Distal segment (distal convoluted tubule)
    of kidney
  anatomy of, 121, 122
  site of action of diuretics, 441, 442
  urine formation and, 132-133
Distribution of drugs, 73, 74, 99-113. See
    also Blood drug levels; Tissue redis-
    tribution
  absorption compared with, 100
  antidotes and poison distribution, 332,
    333, 334
  biologic half-life and, 222, 223
  from blood to brain, 107-110
  blood flow and vascularity and, 104
  blood level and, 207-208, 222
  body fluid concentration and, 242
  to body fluids, 102-105, 222
  capillaries and, 100-102
  cerebrospinal fluid in, 108-110
  drug binding and, 105-107
  drug interactions and, 286, 288-289, 290,
    293-294
  genetic abnormalities in, 253, 256
  from mother to fetus, 110-112, 247
  physiologic variables and, 262
  selectivity and, 197
  volume of, 102-105, 222-223
Diuretic(s), 438-443. See also specific drug,
    e.g., Acetozolamide; Chlorothiazide;
    Ethacrynic acid; Furosemide; Hydro-
    chlorothiazide; Mannitol; Mercury;
    Spironolactone; Urea; Xanthines
  adverse interactions of, 281
  types of
    aldosterone antagonists, 442
    benzothiadiazines, 440-441
    carbonic anhydrase inhibitors, 440
    high-ceiling, 442-443
    mercurials, 439-440
    osmotic, 438
    xanthines, 438-439
  urine pH and, 285
Dopamine
  inhibition of synthesis of, 383
  norepinephrine synthesis and, 382, 384

parkinsonism and, 395-396
Doriden. See Glutethimide (Doriden)
Dosage form. See also Formulation of drugs
  in formulation of new drugs, 400
Dose. See also Dose-effect (dose-response)
    curve; Dose-response relations
  alcohol effects and, 214, 216, 217, 353,
    465-467
  allergy and, 277, 279
  in amphetamine and cocaine abuse, 360
  of aspirin, elimination and, 217-219
  in barbiturate abuse, 352-354
  blood levels of drugs and, 208, 218, 220,
    224
  body weight and size and, 242-243, 247
  calculation of average, 242
  clinical studies in determining, 405
  duration of action and, 224, 228, 236
  elimination time and, 218-219, 238
  form of dosage and, 84-89
  frequency schedules, 228-232
  idiosyncrasy and size of, 279
  in LSD abuse, 362
  marihuana effects and, 347, 364, 365
  sex and, 247
  time-response and multiple doses, 228-239
  time-response and single, 224-228
  tolerance and, 279, 354, 360
  toxicity and. See Dose-response relations
Dose-effect (dose-response) curve. See also
    Dose-response relations
  graded, 172-184, 198-200
    affinity and, 176-178
    drug antagonism and, 180-184, 199
    graphic representation, 172, 173, 175-
      178, 179, 181, 182, 183, 199
    log dose-effect curve, 175-178, 179, 181,
      182, 183, 199
    potency of drugs and, 178-180, 199
  quantal, 184-197, 200, 201
    assumptions in, 184, 200
    certain safety factor and, 192, 194
    graded response and, 191, 192
    median of, 187
    normal distribution curve, 185-187, 200
    in safety evaluation, 191-195, 200, 201
    selectivity of drug action and, 195-197
    S-shaped (sigmoid) curve, 189, 190, 191
    standard deviation of, 188-189, 200
    standard safety margin and, 193
    therapeutic ratio and, 191, 192
    threshold dose, 185
Dose-response relations, 9, 169-201. See also
    Dose; Dose-effect (dose-response) curve
  average vs. representative, 188, 200
  derivation of, 171-172, 198
  genetic factors in, 247-257. See also Genetic
    factors

individual variations in, 187–191, 200
mass action law and, 170–175, 178, 198–199
side-effects, 191, 194–195. *See also* Side-effects
toxic, 191. *See also* Toxicity
Double-blind study, 404
Drug abuse and dependence, 341–368
abuse and dependence related, 342
agents involved in, 351
amphetamines, 359–361. *See also* Amphetamine(s)
barbiturate-alcohol type, 352–355. *See also* Alcohol abuse and dependence; Barbiturates
central nervous system depressants, 352–359
central nervous system stimulants, 359–361
cocaine, 359–361. *See also* Cocaine
cross-dependence of drugs in, 352
general characteristics of, 348–351
LSD, 361–363, 364, 366. *See also* Lysergic acid diethylamide (LSD)
marihuana, 363–366, 368. *See also* Marihuana (marijuana)
maternal, neonate and, 112
opioids, 355–359, 367. *See also* Opioid(s)
physical dependence, 349–350, 351, 367–368. *See also* Physical drug dependence
psychedelics (hallucinogens), 361–366
psychologic dependence, 348–349, 350, 351, 366, 367. *See also* Psychologic drug dependence
tolerance and, 279, 350, 351, 366. *See also* Tolerance *and specific drug*
withdrawal syndrome and, 349, 351. *See also* Withdrawal syndrome *and specific drug*
Drug addiction, 342. *See also* Drug abuse and dependence *and under specific drug*
Drug allergy. *See* Allergy
Drug antagonism. *See* Antagonism, drug
Drug habituation, defined, 342. *See also* Drug abuse and dependence
Drug misuse, 341. *See also* Drug abuse and dependence
Drug-receptor interactions. *See also* Dose-effect (dose-response) curve
of acetylcholine, 33, 42–43, 380–382
affinity of drug for receptor, 176–178, 199
antagonism, 180–184, 199, 280. *See also* Antagonism, drug
atomic structure and, 37–38
autonomic nervous system and, 384–388. *See also* Autonomic nervous system, drugs affecting neurotransmitter in
bonds in, 37–44, 105
covalent bonds, 38–39, 41–42

hydrogen bonds, 39–40, 41, 42, 43, 46
ionic bonds, 38, 46
Van der Waal's forces and, 40, 41, 42, 43, 46
character of, 37–38, 40–44
drug resistance development and, 270, 271, 296
enzyme-substrate binding compared with, 140–141
of epinephrine and norepinephrine, 43–44, 380–381, 382–385
genetic factors and, 253, 256, 296
mass action law and, 170–175, 178, 198–199
potency of drugs and, 178–180, 199
selectivity of, 195–196. *See also* Selectivity of drugs
significance of, in autonomic nervous system, 388
specificity of, 49, 140, 195–196. *See also* Specificity of drugs
stability of, 40–41, 46
three-dimensional aspects of, 43–44, 46
tolerance and, 279, 280, 281–283
Drug toxicity. *See* Toxicity
Duration of action, 207. *See also* Time-response relations
absorption rate and, 226, 237
age and, 244–245
biologic half-life and, 223
blood drug level and, 207–208, 223
dosage form and, 228
dose and, 223–224, 228, 238–239
doubling dose and, 223–224
elimination rate and, 211–224, 292
enzyme inhibition and, 160
genetic abnormalities and, 251, 252, 253, 254
protein binding and, 106
species variation in, 259
of thiopental, 235
tolerance and, 280
Durham-Humphrey Act of 1952, 19
Dyes
diffusion through membranes, 51–52
in liver function tests, 139

Economic toxicology, 18
applications of, 260–261, 311–313
Edema, pharmacologic response in, 294, 295
EDTA. *See* Calcium disodium edetate (EDTA)
Effective dose, median (ED50), 188, 200
determination in animals, 189–191
in evaluation of drug safety, 191–194
selectivity of drug action and, 196
Efferent (motor) neurons, 343
autonomic vs. somatic, 374–375

Efferent (motor) neurons—*Continued*
  sympathetic vs. parasympathetic, 375–377, 378
Egypt, medicine in ancient, 1–2
Ehrlich, Paul, 11, 13, 14, 36, 41, 137
Electrolyte(s). *See also specific ion, e.g.,* Sodium ion
  biliary transport of, 139
  ionization
    of amines, 61
    of weak, 59–63, 69
  of normal blood plasma, 119
Elimination. *See also* Biologic half-life; Biotransformation; Excretion
  absorption and, 227–228, 237, 244–245
  of amphetamines, 221
  of aspirin, 217–219
  blood level and rate determination, 211–212
  of ethanol, 212, 213, 214–216
  first-order kinetics in, 212, 219, 237, 238
  multiple-dose schedule and rate of, 228–233
  of penicillin, 220–221, 222
  of salicylates, 216–219
  time-response relations and, 211–224, 237–238
  toxicity and, 327–328, 334–335
    cumulative toxicity, 233–234, 236, 304–305
  of waste products, 118
  zero-order kinetics in excretion or biotransformation and, 212, 219, 238
Embolism, danger of, in intravenous route, 98
Emetine, 450
Endocrine system. *See also* Hormones
  function of, 342
  hypothalamic regulation of, 346
Endorphins, 358–359
Endothelium. *See* Capillaries, endothelium
Enteral administration, 76
Enteric coatings for drugs, 87–88
Enterohepatic circulation, 138–139
Environmental factors, drug response and, 18, 263, 304, 309–310
Environmental Protection Agency (EPA), 318–319
  air quality standards of, 318–319, 320–321
  in pesticide registration, 312
Environmental toxicology, 18, 318–319, 320–321
Enzyme(s), 140–144. *See also* Biotransformation
  age and enzyme systems, 243, 246
  cofactors and, 140

constitutive, 270
  deficiencies in infants, 243, 246
  drug resistance and, 270–271
  genetic abnormalities of
    in erythrocyte, 250, 252, 253, 254–255
    of functional systems, 250, 252–253, 254–255
  induction of
    drug therapy and, 160–165
    species variation in, 291
    tolerance and, 280, 282
  inhibition of, 158–160
    heavy metals in, 306
  ions and activity of, 140
  kinetics, 142–144
  microsomal, 152–154. *See also* Microsomal enzymes
  mode of action of, 140–142
  species variations in, 258–260, 291
  specificity of, 141–142
Ephedrine
  interaction with norepinephrine, 384, 385, 386, 387
  interspecies variation in biotransformation of, 258
  tolerance to, 280, 282
Epidermis, 89, 90. *See also* Skin
Epinephrine
  allergy and, 297
  combination with receptors, 43, 44, 386
  conversion of norepinephrine to, 149, 382
  dibenamine and, 182–183
  inactivation of, 146, 149, 156
  ionization of, 61
  thyroid hormone and response to, 262
Epithelium
  absorption and, 74, 77
  alveolar, 92, 93
  of large intestine, 84
  of oral cavity, 77
  of skin, 89, 90
  of small intestine, 80, 81, 82
  spaces between cells of, 100
  of stomach, 78
Epsom salts (magnesium sulfate), 45, 49, 436–437
Equanil. *See* Meprobamate (Equanil; Miltown)
Erythromycin, 444
Erythrocytes
  diffusion of glucose into, 64
  genetic abnormalities in enzyme systems, 252, 254–255
Estradiol, 149
Ethacrynic acid, 442–443
Ethanol. *See* Alcohol abuse and dependence; Ethyl alcohol
Ether, 13, 45, 352

Ethereal sulfate synthesis, 148. *See also* Sulfate conjugation
Ethinamate (Valmid), 473
Ethyl alcohol, 463–468. *See also* Alcohol abuse and dependence
  absorption of, 52, 53, 82, 83
  adverse interactions of, 288, 291
  as antidote for methanol poisoning, 333, 334
  as antiseptic, 448
  biotransformation of, 156, 214–217
  blood level of
    absorption and, 52, 53
  central nervous system depression by, 352–355, 463–468
    ascending reticular activating system, 348, 353
    cortical depression, 348
    medullary respiratory center, 345
    stages and planes of general anesthesia, 466
  distribution of, 468
  dose-response relations, 185, 189, 216, 353, 466, 467
  effect on microsomal enzymes, 291, 467–468
  elimination
    in expired air, 118
    rate of, zero-order kinetics, 214–217
  incidence of poisoning by, 322
  industrial environmental limits, 315
  interactions with barbiturates, 219, 468
  pharmacology of, 463–468
    effects on central nervous system, 465–467
    effects on gastrointestinal tract, 467
    effects on kidney, 468
    effects on liver, 467–468
Ethyl biscoumacetate (Tromexan), species variation in biotransformation, 259
Evaluation of drugs. *See also* Development of new drugs; Food and Drug Administration (FDA)
  animal studies in
    data use and interpretation of, 259, 260, 310–311, 316, 399, 400
    initial, 396–398
    preclinical, 398–400
    side-effects in, 400–401
  clinical studies, 400–409. *See also* Clinical studies of new drugs
  continuing, 409
  history of, 9–10, 11
  interspecies variation and, 257–260
  investigational new drug application (IND), 360–361
  new drug applications (NDA), 402, 405–407
  toxicity, 301–303, 310–311. *See also* Safety of drugs; Toxicity, evaluation of

Excretion, 117, 118–139, 165
  in enterohepatic cycle, 118, 137–139, 165
  of lipid-soluble drugs, 133, 165
  physiologic variables and, 262
  pulmonary, 94, 118
  renal, of drug, 118, 133–137. *See also* Urine formation
    absorption rate and, 292
    age and, 243–245
    biologic half-life of drugs and, 222–224, 237–238
    blood flow and, 133–134, 136–137, 295
    blood level of drugs and, 219–224
    clearance studies, 135–137
    drug response and, 291, 292, 295–296
    first-order kinetics in, 219, 220
    glomerular filtration in, 133–134, 165, 219, 244, 295–296
    increase in poisoning, 333, 334
    protein binding and, 106, 133, 222
    rate, 135–137, 219–224, 237–238, 295–296
    tubular reabsorption in, 133–134, 165, 228, 295–296
    tubular secretion in, 134–135, 165, 219, 223, 244, 395
    uric acid agents affecting, 443
    zero-order kinetics in, 219
Excretion ratio, 137
Extracellular extravascular fluid
  compartments in brain, 108, 109
  drug distribution and concentration in, 102, 103–104
Extracellular sites of drug action, 33–35, 45–46
  without receptors, 45–46
Eye
  drugs and pupil size, 31–32, 462
  effects of autonomic stimulation on, 379

Facilitated diffusion, 64–66, 69
  carrier concept of, 65–66, 69
  drug absorption and, 84, 209
Fats, digestion and absorption of, 137
FDA. *See* Food and Drug Administration (FDA)
Feces, drug excretion in, 88, 118, 139
Federal Food, Drug and Cosmetic Act, 401
Federal Insecticide, Fungicide, and Rodenticide Act, 311
Federal regulations for
  air quality, 318
  drugs. *See* Food and Drug Administration
  economic poisons, 311–313
    label requirements, 312, 313
    toxicity criteria, 313
  industrial environmental contaminants, hazards of, 313–317

Federal regulations for—*Continued*
  pesticides, 311–313
  toxic substances, 318
  water, 318
Fetus
  distribution between mother and, 110–112
  teratogens and, 112, 308, 399, 403
Fever(s), quinine for malarial vs. nonmalarial, 29, 30, 31
Filtration, 68, 69, 101
  glomerular. *See* Excretion, renal, of drug
First aid for poisoning, 330–331
First-order kinetics
  of absorption, 209–210, 237
  of elimination, 212, 219, 237–238
    of biotransformation, 212
    of drug excretion, 219, 237
  of enzyme reactions, 143–144
Folds of Kerckring, small intestine, 80, 81
Folic acid (pteroylglutamic acid)
  antagonists of, in cancer therapy, 452
  PABA and, 260
Food and Drug Administration (FDA), 19, 20, 310
  guidelines for animal tests, 398–400
  IND on drugs and, 402, 406, 407
  National Clearinghouse for Poison Control, 325–326
  new drug application (NDA), 406, 407–408
  regulations for clinical studies, 400–408
  standards for biologicals, 398
Foodstuffs
  allergy to, 273
  drug interactions with, 290
  drug response and, 262
Forensic toxicology, 19
Formulation of drugs
  drug particle size and dissolution, 84–85
  enteric coatings, 87–88
  inert ingredients, 85–86
  new products, 400
  silicon rubber preparations, 89
  sustained-release medications, 88–89, 96, 97, 99, 211
Frequency schedules of drug administration, 228–233
Functional antagonism. *See* Physiologic (functional) antagonism
Furosemide, 442–443

Galen (Greek physician), 5, 8
Ganglia, 343, 376, 377, 378
Gases
  excretion in expired air, 118
  incidence of poisoning by, 319, 320
  threshold limits of poisonous gases, industrial, 314–316
  toxic effects of, 303–304, 305
Gastrointestinal tract. *See also specific structure, e.g.,* Stomach
  absorption from, 77–89. *See also* Absorption, gastrointestinal
  cathartic actions on, 45, 49
  drug administration into. *See* Oral administration
  drug excretion by, 88, 118, 137–139, 165
  effects of autonomic stimulation on, 379
  gastric acid neutralization, 34, 45
  hypothalamic regulation of, 346
  locally acting drug affecting
    antacids, 433–435
    cathartics, 435–437
    digestants, 435
    laxatives, 437
  poison removal from, 329, 330–331
  toxic effects of drugs on, 306
General anesthetics
  abuse of, 433
  administration of, 93, 210–211
  chemical diversity of, 45
  distribution from maternal blood to fetus, 111–112
  mechanism of action, 45, 46
  pharmacology of, 463–465
  stages and signs in, 464–465
Generic drug names, 19–21
Genes, 248
Genetic factors, 247–261
  in atropine biotransformation, 248–249
  biotransformation processes and. *See* Enzyme(s), genetic abnormalities of
  continuous vs. discontinuous variations, 249–250
  drug absorption and distribution and, 255–256
  idiosyncratic drug responses and, 247–248
  interspecies variation and, 257–261
  receptors and, 256
  resistance and. *See* Resistance, drug
Germicides. *See also* Antiseptics
  nonreceptor action of, 45
  toxicity of, 306
Glaucoma
  drug use in, 89
  marihuana and, 366
Glomerulus, renal
  anatomy of, 120–122
  capillary endothelium of, 122
  filtration in, 68, 122–123, 124, 133–134, 165
    determination of rate, 135–136
    drug excretion rate and, 137, 219
    in infants, 244
  function assessment of, 135–136

Glucose
    active transport in kidney of, 125
    antimony and biotransformation of, 261
    facilitated diffusion into erythrocytes of, 64
    genetic abnormality in metabolism of, 255
Glucuronic acid conjugation, 145, 146, 147
    in aspirin biotransformation, 218
    interspecies variation in, 258
    microsomal enzymes and, 154
        phenobarbital and, 164
    in newborn, 245
    physicochemical properties of conjugates, 147
Glutamine conjugation, 145, 147
Glutethimide (Doriden), 473
    abuse of, 352
    adverse interactions of, 289
    enterohepatic cycle and, 139, 147
    tolerance to, 280
Glycine conjugation, 145, 146, 147
    in aspirin biotransformation, 218
Gonococcus, sulfonamides and resistance to, 268
Gout
    side-effects of diuretic therapy
        chlorothiazide, 440
        high-ceiling diuretics, 443
    treatment with
        probenecid, 395, 443
        salicylates, 459–460
        sulfinpyrazone, 443
Graded dose-response relation, 172–184, 198–200. See also Dose-effect (dose-response) curve, graded
Greece, medicine in ancient, 2–5
Griseofulvin, 447
Guanethidine, 386, 387

Habituation, drug, 342. See also Drug abuse and dependence
Half-life. See Biologic half-life
Hallucinogens (psychedelics), 361–366
    cross-tolerance of, 362
    dependence and abuse, 351, 361–366, 368. See also Lysergic acid diethylamide (LSD); Marihuana (marijuana)
Halogens, as antiseptics, 448
Hapten, 274
Harvey, William, 9, 14
Hashish, 341, 363
Heavy metals, 8. See also specific metal, e.g., Lead
    as antiseptics, 448
    as carcinogens, 317
    enzyme inhibition by, 159, 306
    percutaneous absorption of, 91
    poisoning, 35, 306, 333, 335

Hemoglobin
    conversion to methemoglobin, 246–247, 250, 252, 254–255
    genetic variations in, 254–255
    oxygen binding with, 44
    oxygen-carbon monoxide competition for binding with, 304, 335
    susceptibility of fetal hemoglobin to oxidation, 246–247
    three-dimensional structure of, 44
Heparin
    chemical antagonists of, 287
    extracellular action of, 33–34
    selectivity and toxicity of, 197
Heroin dependence, 355–359
    maternal, effect on fetus, 112
Hexobarbital biotransformation
    effect of age, 243
    interspecies variation, 259
Hexylresorcinol, 451
High-ceiling diuretics, 442–443
Hippocrates, 2, 3–4
Histamine
    as allergy mediator, 273, 274
    biotransformation of, 149
    blood pressure and, 182, 286
    capillary permeability and, 101
    diphenhydramine and effects of, 181–182, 196, 286
    morphine and release of, 281, 462
    as vasodilator, 33
History of pharmacology, 1–15, 391
Homeostasis, 118–119
Hormones. See also specific hormone, e.g., Thyroxine
    enzyme induction by, and effect on drugs, 164
    oral contraceptives, 393
    standardization of, 398
    sustained-release preparations, 94, 211
Hyaluronidase, 96
Hydrochlorothiazide, 440–441
Hydrocortisone, allergy and, 297
Hydrogen bond, 39–40
    drug-receptor interactions and, 41, 42, 43
    enzyme-substrate interactions and, 140
    groups able to form, 54–55
Hydrogen ion concentration (pH)
    of body fluids, 62
        bicarbonate ion and, 126–127
        response to drugs and, 262
    ionization or weak electrolytes and, 61–62
    in mouth, 77
    in small intestine, 80
    in stomach, 79
        absorption of strychnine and, 63
        enteric coatings and, 87–88

Hydrogen ion concentration (pH)—*Continued*
  of urine, 133-134, 291, 332. *See also* Urine,
    pH of
Hydrolysis, 146, 149, 156-157
Hydromorphone (Dilaudid)
  drug abuse and dependence, 355-359
  potency as analgesic, 178-179
Hydrophilic groups of cell membrane, 54-
    55, 69
Hydrophobic groups of cell membrane, 54-
    55, 69
  solubility and, 57
Hypersensitivity
  allergy compared with, 272
  confusion in term use, 277
Hypnotics. *See* Sedatives and hypnotics
Hypothalamus, functional anatomy of, 346

Idiosyncracies, drug, 247-257. *See also* Genetic
    factors
  allergies vs., 272-279, 297
  biotransformation abnormalities and, 248-
    249, 251, 254
  drug absorption and distribution abnormal-
    ities and, 255-256
  incidence of, 277
Imipramine,
  as antidepressant, 478-479
  effects of, on central nervous system,
    479
  interactions of, 284, 289
    with norepinephrine, 384, 385
Immune mechanism in allergy, 272-274
  immunoglobulins, 272
IND (Investigational New Drug), 402, 406,
    407
India, medicine of ancient, 1, 2, 3
Inducible enzyme. *See* Enzyme(s), induction
    of
Inert constituents of drugs, 85
Infants. *See* Children and infants
Infectious drug resistance, 268-269
Information sources on drugs, 21-25
Informed patient consent for clinical studies,
    402-403
Inhalation therapy, 76, 93-94, 99
Injections of drugs, 76. *See also* Intramuscular
    (I.M.) administration; Intravenous (I.V.)
    administration; Subcutaneous (S.C.)
    administration
Insecticides. *See also* Malathion; Parathion;
    Pesticides
  percutaneous absorption of, 91
  resistance to, 270, 271, 295
Insulin
  digestive enzymes and, 98
  discovery of, 13
  sustained-release, 96, 211

Interactions, drug, 283-293. *See also*
    specific topic, e.g., Antagonism, drug
  biotransformation and, 288, 289, 290-
    291
  classification of, 284-287
  gastrointestinal absorption and, 287, 289,
    290, 293
  protein-binding, effect on distribution and,
    288-289, 290
Interstitial fluids. *See* Body fluids
Intestine, 137. *See also* Large intestine; Small
    intestine
Intracellular fluid
  in brain compartments, 109, 110
  drug distribution and concentration in,
    103, 104
Intracellular sites of drug action, 33, 35-44,
    46, 270, 271
  resistance and availability of, 270, 271
Intramuscular (I.M.) administration, 97, 99
  absorption and, 97, 226-227
  advantages and disadvantages, 97, 99
  of depot preparations, 97
  onset of action and, 226-227
Intravenous (I.V.) administration, 9, 97-
    98, 99
  advantages of, 97, 99
  of central nervous system stimulants, 360
  distribution to brain and, 98
  elimination rate and, 211-212
  embolism and, 98
  hazards of, 98, 99
  in poor circulation, 98
  time course of action and, 227
Intrinsic factor, absorption of vitamin B_{12}
    and, 253, 255-256
Inulin
  age and half-time of elimination of, 244
  in plasma clearance studies, 135-136
Iodide ion, distribution of, 104
Ion(s). *See* Ionization *and specific ion, e.g.,*
    Sodium ion
Ionic bond, 38
  drug-receptor interactions and, 41-42
  enzyme-substrate interactions and, 140
Ionization
  of amines, 61
  of ammonia, 39, 61
  distribution to brain and, 107, 109-110
  equilibrium constant in, 60-61
  pH and, 61-62
    physiologic variables and, 262
  rate of diffusion and, 62-63, 70
  transcapillary diffusion and,
    101
  of weak electrolytes, 59-63, 70
Ipecac, 329
Iron, poisoning by, 332, 333

Isoniazid
  biotransformation, abnormalities of, 251, 254
  mechanism of action, 445

Journals of pharmacology, 22–23

Kefauver-Harris Drug Amendment of 1962, 401–402
Kidney. See also specific portion, e.g., Glomerulus, renal
  action of diuretics on, 438–443
  anatomy of, 119–123
  artificial, 13
  blood vessels of, 99, 121, 122–123, 131
  cumulative toxicity of analgesic mixtures, 305
  drug biotransformation, 144
  drug response in disease, 262, 304, 307
  excretion by. See Excretion, renal, of drug; Urine formation
  function tests, 135–137, 244
  functions of, 101, 119
  tonicity of interstitial fluid of, 130–131
Kinetics
  of enzyme-substrate interactions, 142–144
  of facilitated diffusion, 64–65
  first-order, 143–144. See also First-order kinetics
  zero-order, 144. See also Zero-order kinetics

Langley, J. N., 11, 36, 37
Large intestine
  absorption from, 84
  rectal administration of drugs, 84, 99
Latency period of drugs, 205–206
Laxatives, 435-436, 437
  contraindications, 436
  defined, 435
  therapeutic use, 436
  types of
    bulk-forming, 437
    emollient, 437
Lead, poisoning by,
  air quality standards vs., 233, 319
  antidotal therapy, 34, 333, 335
  cumulative toxicity of, 233, 304
  incidence in children, 324
Lethal dose, median (LD50), 188, 200
  evaluation of, in animals, 185–191, 398–399
    for chemicals not intended for use in humans, 311–313
    for therapeutic agents, 185–191
  therapeutic and lethal effect related, 191–195, 200–201
Levodopa for parkinsonism, 395–396
Librium. See Chlordiazepoxide (Librium)

Lidocaine (Xylocaine)
  dose-response curves of, 176, 177
  local anesthetic activity of, 456–457
Limbic system, 346, 358
Lipid(s), of cell membrane, 53–55, 56–59, 69, 70. See also Lipid solubility
Lipid solubility, 57
  cumulative toxicity and, 233, 234–236
  diffusion and, 56–59, 60, 62, 63, 102
  distribution to brain and, 107
  excretion and, 135, 165, 222–223
  gastric absorption and, 79–80
  microsomal enzymes and, 150
  onset of drug action and, 225
  transcapillary movement and, 100, 104
Lipid/water partition coefficient, 57
  diffusion across cell membrane and, 56, 57
Liver
  bile secretion by, 118, 137–139
  biotransformation and, 78, 84, 144
  blood flow through, 78, 84, 101–102, 138
  chloroquine storage in, 106
  drug response in disease of, 262, 307
  excretion by, 118, 137–139
  function, tests of, 139
  microsomal enzymes of, 153–154
  permeability of capillaries (sinusoids), 101–102
Loading (priming) dose, 229, 231, 232, 238
Local anesthetics, 96, 456–458. See also Cocaine; Lidocaine (Xylocaine); Procaine (Novocaine)
  chemistry, 456
  definition, 456
  modes of administration, 457
  pharmacodynamics, 456–457
    actions on cardiovascular system, 457
    actions on central nervous system, 457
  toxicity, 457
Local toxicity, 305–306
Loop of Henle
  anatomy of, 121, 122, 129
  importance in formation of hypertonic urine, 129–132
  urine formation and, 129–132
LSD. See Lysergic acid diethylamide (LSD)
Lung(s)
  absorption in, 91–94, 99
  alveoli of, 92–93, 94
  blood flow through, 92–93
  cigarette smoke and, 94, 305
  drug administration through, 76, 93–94, 99
  excretion by, 93, 94, 114
  removal of particulate matter by, 94
  water loss through, 93
Lymphatic system, 74–75

Lysergic acid diethylamide (LSD), dependence, 361–363
  dangers associated with use, 362–363, 368
  major effects of, 362
  psychologic dependence on, 350, 351, 362–363
  tolerance to, 350, 351, 368

Magendie, François, 9, 10, 14
Magnesium-containing antacids, 434, 435
Magnesium sulfate (Epsom salts), 45, 49, 436–437. See also Laxatives and Cathartics
Maintenance dose, 229. See also Multiple dose schedules
Malaria. See Chloroquine; Quinacrine (Atabrine); Quinine
Malathion
  biotransformation of, 163–164
  insect resistance to, 271
  percutaneous absorption of, 91
  toxicity of, 164, 301, 304
Mannitol, osmotic diuretic action of, 438
Marihuana (marijuana), 363–366, 367–368
  dosage and effect of, 364, 365
    vs. alcohol, 364–365
    vs. LSD, 364
  patterns of use, 364
  potential value in therapy, 366
  psychologic dependence on, 351, 364–365
  sources of, 363
  tetrahydrocannabinols and effects of, 363–364
  tolerance to, 351, 364
Mass action, law of, 60–61
  dose-response relation and, 170–175, 178, 198–199
  enzyme reactions and, 142–143, 171, 180
  protein binding and, 105
  weak electrolytes, ionization and, 60–61
Materia medica, history of, 1–8
Mechanism of drug action, 34–44, 46. See also Drug-receptor interactions; Selectivity of drugs; Site of drug action; Specificity of drugs
  chemical structure of drug and, 11, 36, 46
  interaction with function molecules and, 35
  receptors and, 35–44, 46. See also Drug-receptor interactions
  without receptors, 45–46
Mechlorethamine, 452
Median, 188, 200
Median effective dose (ED50), 188. See also Effective dose, median (ED50)
Median lethal dose (LD50), 188. See also Lethal dose, median (LD50)

Mediators
  allergy and, 273, 274, 297
  of biotransformation, 140–144. See also Enzyme(s)
Medical ethics, 2, 3–4, 402–405
Medical Letter on Drugs and Therapeutics, The, 25
Medieval medicine and pharmacy, 5–8
Medulla, renal, anatomy of, 120, 121
Medulla oblongata, functional anatomy of, 345
Melphalan, 452
Membrane(s), 53
  cell. See Cell membrane
Meprobamate (Equanil, Miltown), 477
  abuse and dependence, 351, 352
  adverse interactions of, 289
  development of, 393
  in treatment of anxiety, 477
  tolerance to, 280, 351
6-Mercaptor urine, 452
Merck Index: An Encyclopedia of Chemicals and Drugs, The, 25
Mercury, percutaneous absorption of, 91
Mescaline, 362
Metabolism. See Biotransformation
Metacholine, cholinesterase and, 141–142, 159
Methanol. See Methyl alcohol
Methaqualone, 474
Methemoglobin formation
  agents causing, 252
  as antidote in cyanide poisoning, 334
  hemoglobin conversion to, 246, 250, 252, 254–255
Methotrexate, 452
Methyl alcohol
  biotransformation of, 156, 334
  poisoning
    dialysis in, 332
    ethanol as antidote for, 334
    immediate vs. delayed effects of, 309
Methylation, 145, 146, 148–149
Methylcellulose, 437
Methylphenidate (Ritalin), 481
Metric system of weights and measures, 482–484
Meyer, Hans H., 56, 57
Microsomal enzymes, 152–154
  activity and drug effect, 295
  age and, 243
  biochemical antagonism and, 291
  biotransformation and, 146, 152–154
  dual effect of ethyl alcohol on, 291, 467–468
  induction of, 160–165

inhibition of, 291
lipid-soluble substrates and, 153-154, 160, 165
liver disease and, 294
tolerance and induction of, 279-280
Microvilli of small intestine, 80, 81, 82
Midbrain, functional anatomy of, 345
Milk, drug excretion in, 118
Miltown. *See* Meprobamate (Equanil; Miltown)
Mineral oil, 437
Mode of action. *See* Drug-receptor interactions; Mechanism of drug action
Modern Drug Encyclopedia, 25
Molecular size
passive diffusion and, 58-59, 63, 69
transcapillary movement and, 101-102
Monoamine oxidase inhibitors, 478-479.
See also specific drug, e.g.,
Tranylcypromine
interaction with antidepressants, 284, 288-289
norepinephrine and, 384, 386, 387
tyramine in foods and, 262, 286
Monomolecular reaction, 143. *See also* First-order kinetics
Mood-altering drugs. *See* Antidepressants; Depressants; Stimulants; *and specific drug*
Morphine, 461-463
absorption, 463
biotransformation of, 146
distribution to brain, 463
effects on
cardiovascular system, 462
cough reflex, 462
eye, 31, 32, 462
respiration, 462
endorphins and, 357-359
gastric emptying and absorption and, 290, 462
histamine release by, 281
isolation from opium, 10, 392
maternal dependence, infant in, 112
pharmacodynamics of, as prototype, 461-463
physical dependence on, 356-359
potency as analgesic, 178-179, 461-462
reaction to pain and, 354, 461-462
site of action, 31-33, 357-359
thyroid hormone and response to, 262
tolerance to, 279, 281, 283, 356-357
toxicity, narcotic antagonists and, 279, 313, 349, 357, 463
Mosaic cell membrane model, 55, 69
Motor (efferent) neurons, 343. *See also* Autonomic nervous system
autonomic vs. somatic, 374, 375
parasympathetic vs. sympathetic, 375-378

Mouth
absorption from, 74, 78
epithelium of, 77
pH in, 77
Multiple dose schedules
cumulative toxicity and, 233-236
elimination kinetics and selection of, 228-233
maintenance dose, 229-232, 238-239
priming dose, 229-232, 238-239
Multiple drug dosage. *See* Interactions, drug
Muscarine, mushroom poisoning and, 83, 84
Muscles (skeletal)
innervation of, 373, 374, 375, 378
nicotine and contraction of, 36-37
paralysis by curare, 10-11, 37
Mushroom poisoning, 83, 84
Mutations, 250
development of drug resistance by, 267-271

Nalorphine
morphine toxicity and, 279, 357
Narcotic(s), 355. *See also* Opioid(s) *and specific drug, e.g.,* Morphine
Naloxone, 356
physical dependence on, 349
National Clearinghouse for Poison Control (FDA), 325-326
National Formulary, The, 20, 22, 24, 401, 470
Natural products, new drug development from, 392
Neomycin
allergy to, 301
toxicity of, 446
Nephron. *See also specific structure, e.g.,* Loop of Henle
absorptive surface area of, 122
anatomy of, 119-122
Neuromuscular junction, action of curare at, 11, 36-37, 374, 378. *See also* Autonomic nervous system
Neuron (nerve cell), 343
New drug application (NDA), 407-409
New Drugs (Council on Drugs of the A.M.A.), 24-25
Nialamide, 384, 478
Niclosamide, 451
Nicotinamide biotransformation, 149
Nicotine
absorption of, 79, 91
curare and action of, 36-37
Niridazole, 451
Nirvanol. *See* Phenylethylhydantoin (Nirvanol)
Nitrates, age and toxicity of, 246-247

Nitrites
  age and toxicity of, 246–247
  for cyanide poisoning, 334
  sensitivity to in genetic abnormalities, 252–253, 254
  tolerance to, 280, 283
  as vasodilators, 33
Nitrogen mustard, 97–98, 452
Nitroglycerin
  sublingual, in angina pectoris, 78
  tolerance to, 281
  as vasodilator, 33
Nitrous oxide, 45
Nomenclature of drugs, 19–21
Noncompetitive drug antagonism, 159, 180, 182–184, 199
Nonelectrolytes, passive diffusion of, 59, 69
Nonprescription ("over-the-counter") drugs, 19
Nonproprietary drug names, 20–21
Nonselective toxicity, 306
Norepinephrine, 382–388
  antagonists of receptors for, 384–385, 386, 387
  conversion to epinephrine, 148–149, 382–383
  histamine effects and, 286
  inactivation of, 149, 383, 384–385
  ionization of, 60–61
  as neurohumor, 344, 380, 381–385
    drugs influencing, 384–385, 386, 387–388
    drugs mimicking, 384, 385
  release of, 383, 384–385
    drugs influencing, 384–385, 386
  storage of, 383, 384–385
    drugs influencing, 384–385, 386
  synthesis of, 382, 383, 384
    drugs influencing, 384, 385, 386
Normal frequency distribution, 185–187
Novocain. See Procaine (Novocain)
Nucleic acids, chloroquine interactions with, 106
Nystatin, 447

Occipital lobe, cerebral, 347
Occupational Safety and Health Act, 314
Occupational Safety and Health Administration (OSHA), toxicity standards, and carcinogens, 315, 316
Occupational toxicity, 313–318
  cancer in, 314, 316, 317
  incidence of, 313
  standards, 314–315
Official drug names, 20
Onset of drug action. See Time-response relations

Opioid(s), 461–463. See also specific drug, e.g., Morphine
  analgesic action of, 461–463
  dependence and abuse, 351, 355–359, 367–368
  barbiturate-alcohol type of dependence vs., 356, 357
  behavior in chronic, 356
  dosage in, 357
  effects of, 357
  tolerance to, 351, 356–357
  withdrawal syndrome, 351, 357, 358, 367
  medullary respiratory center and, 345
  pain and, 356, 461–462
  pharmacology of, 461–463. See also Morphine
  similarities and differences between, 356, 461–463
Opium, 28
  history of use, 1, 2, 5, 8, 27, 341
  morphine isolation from, 10, 392
Oral administration
  absorption
    after dissolution and disintegration of solids and, 84–88
    from gastric mucosa, 78
    interactions involving, 287, 290
    intestinal, 80, 82–84
    rate of, 209–211
    stomach emptying rate and, 79, 83, 98, 290, 293
    water ingested with tablets and, 87, 88
  contraindications for, 84, 98
  duration of action and, 237
  economy of, 98
  hepatic passage of drugs into circulation after, 84, 98
  onset of drug action and, 226
  of sustained-release medications, 88–89
Oral cavity. See Mouth
Oral contraceptives, development of, 393
Organic acids, tubular secretion of, 126, 128, 134–135, 296, 395
Organic phosphate insecticides, poisoning therapy. See also Malathion; Parathion
  atropine in, 333, 335–336
  pralidoxime in, 320, 333, 335
Osmotic effect, 45, 119
"Over-the-counter" (nonprescription) drugs, 19
Overton, Ernest, 56–57
Oxidants, as air pollutants, 319, 320
Oxidation
  enzymes in, 146, 151, 154–156
    microsomal enzyme systems, 146, 152, 154, 155
  in newborn, 243

oxidative reactions of ethanol, 215, 291, 468
Oxygen
    as antidote for carbon monoxide poisoning,
        333, 335
    carbon monoxide displacement of, 304
    hemoglobin combination with, 246, 335
    as respiratory stimulant, 99
    utilization by cells in cyanide poisoning,
        306

Pain. See also Antipyretic analgesics; General
        anesthetics; Local anesthetics; Opioids
    drugs used to treat, 454-468
    nature of, 454-456
Para-aminobenzoic acid (PABA)
    antigenicity of, 276-277
    folic acid synthesis in bacteria and, 260
    sulfa drug competition with, 260, 271
Para-aminohippuric acid (PAH)
    age and elimination of, 244
    clearance studies with, 137
Para-aminosalicylic acid (PAS), 445
Paracelsus (Theophrastus Bombastus von
        Hohenheim), 5, 7-8, 14, 18, 302
Paracetamol. See Acetaminophen (para-
        cetamol)
Paraldehyde, excretion from lungs, 118, 474
Parasites, drug resistance of, 267-271
Parasympathetic nervous system, 375, 377.
        See also Acetylcholine
    anatomy of, 375, 376, 377
    drugs affecting, 385-388
    pharmacologic significance of, 388
    functions of, 377, 379-380
    neurotransmitter in, 380-382
    sympathetic nervous system vs., 375, 377-
        380
Parathion
    cholinesterase and effects of, 183-184
    percutaneous absorption of, 91
    treatment of poisoning from, 333, 335-
        336
Parenteral administration, 74. See also In-
        halation therapy; Intramuscular (I.M.)
        administration; Intravenous (I.V.)
        administration; Subcutaneous (S.C.)
        administration; Topical application
Parietal lobe, cerebral, 347
Parkinsonism, levodopa in, 395-396
Particulate matter, pulmonary removal of,
        94
Passive diffusion, 51-64, 69, 73
    in children and infants, 245
    concentration gradient and, 52-53, 69, 209
    drug absorption and, 77, 79-80, 82-84,
        91, 93, 94
    energy in, 52, 68
    ionization and, 62-63, 69, 133-134

lipid solubility and, 56-59. See also Lipid
        solubility, diffusion and
    lipid/water partition coefficient and, 57-59
    membrane structure and, 53-55, 69
    molecular size and, 58-59, 63, 69
    of nonelectrolytes, 56, 57, 69
    rate, factors in, 52-53, 69
    reabsorption of drugs from tubular urine,
        133-134, 219, 223
    of weak electrolytes, 59-63, 69
Pathologic conditions, biotransformation in,
        296
Peak effect of drugs, 207
    rate of absorption and, 227, 244-245
    tolerance and, 280
Penicillin
    agencies of sensitization to, 277
    albumin binding of, 105
    allergic reactions to, 275, 301
    bacterial resistance to, 270-271
    bactericidal action of, 444-446
    depot preparations of, 97, 226-227
    discovery of, 391
    duration of action, 226-227
    elimination of, 220, 222
        probenecid and, 292, 395
        renal tubular secretion in, 134
    inappropriate use of, 341
    onset of action and administration route,
        226
    relative safety of, 301
    selective toxicity for bacteria, 260-261,
        445
    spectrum of activity, 444
    toxicity of, 446
    transport and entry into brain, 110
Pentazocine, dose-response curve of, 209.
        See also Narcotic(s)
Pentobarbital. See also Sedatives and
        hypnotics
    absorption, 82-83
    abuse and dependence, 352-355
    as hypnotic, 470
    pharmacokinetics and physicochemical
        properties of, 471
Per os administration, 76. See also Oral ad-
        ministration
Permeability. See Diffusion
Pernicious anemia, 255-256
Pesticides, evaluation of toxicity of, 311-
        312. See also Insecticides
pH, 62. See also Hydrogen ion concentration
        (pH)
Phagocytosis, 68, 94
Pharmaceutical chemistry, 19
Pharmacodynamic tolerance, 279, 280, 281,
        283
Pharmacodynamics, 17-18

Pharmacogenics, 248-257. *See also* Genetic factors
Pharmacognosy, 19
Pharmacokinetics, 205. *See also* Time-response relations
Pharmacologic antagonism, 180-184, 286. *See also* Antagonism, drug
Pharmacology, divisions of, 17-19
Pharmacology for Physicians, 25
Pharmacopeia, first official, 7
Pharmacopeia of the United States of America, The (U.S.P.), 20, 22, 23, 398, 401
Pharmacopoeia Internationalis, The (Ph.I.), 24
Pharmacotherapeutics, 19
Pharmacy, 19
Pharynx, 91
Phenacetin (Acetophenetidin), 146, 151, 155, 279, 458, 461
Phenobarbital. *See also* Sedatives and hypnotics
    absorption, 82, 83, 210
    abuse and dependence, 352-355
    anticoagulant therapy and, 159-160
    binding by cholestyramine, 290
    biotransformation of, 146, 147, 155
    central nervous system and, 348, 469, 472
    dose-response relations of, 190-191, 193-194
    elimination of, 473
    glucuronide synthesis stimulation in the newborn and, 164
    interactions of, 283, 287, 289
    mechanism and site of action, 472
    pharmacokinetics and physicochemical properties of, 470-471
    poisoning, 134
    relative safety of, 191-194, 301
    time course of action, 208, 210, 225
    tolerance to, 280
    toxicity of, 472-473
Phenolphthalein, enterohepatic cycle and, 147
Phenol, 448
    as antiseptic, 447-448
    conjugation of phenol, 145, 148
Phenothiazines, 475
    as antipsychotic drugs, 475-476
    pharmacology of, 475-476
    toxicity of, 307, 476
Phenylbutazone (Butazolidin), 461
    absorption of, 86, 87
    blood disorders and, 308, 461
    drug displacement from plasma proteins and, 289, 290
    effects of, 461
    renal tubular secretion of, 134

variations in dissolution and disintegration in brands of, 86, 87
Phenylethylhydantoin (Nirvanol), incidence of allergy to, 276
Phenylthiourea, taste thresholds for, 256, 257
Phenytoin (Dilantin), 146, 161, 347
Phospholipids of cell membrane, 53
Physical drug dependence, 349-351. *See also* Drug abuse and dependence; Withdrawal syndrome
    on alcohol, 351, 352, 354-355
    on amphetamines, 351, 360-361
    on barbiturates, 349, 351, 354-355
    development of, 366
    dosage of barbiturates and, 354
    on narcotic analgesics, 351, 357
    psychologic dependence and, 349-350, 351
    tolerance and, 366
    withdrawal syndrome and, 349
Physicians' Desk Reference to Pharmaceutical Specialties and Biologicals (P.D.R.), 25
Physiologic factors, response to drugs and, 261-262
Physiologic (functional) antagonism, 286
Pilocarpine, sustained release in glaucoma, 89
Pinocytosis, 51, 67-68, 69
    capillary permeability and, 101
    drug absorption and, 84
Piperazine, 451
Pipradol (Meratran), 481
Placebo(s), in drug evaluation, 264, 404-405
Placebo effect, 262-264, 404-405
Placenta in distribution between mother and fetus, 110-112
Plantago (psyllium seed), 437
Plasma. *See also* Blood
    drug distribution and concentration in, 102, 103, 104-105. *See also* Blood drug levels
    drug transformation in, 144, 157
    electrolytes of normal, 115
    pH variations in, 63
    proteins, drug binding to, 105-106, 288-289, 290, 294
    renal regulation of constituents, 119
    volume as percent of total blood volume, 102
Plasma clearance, measurement of renal, 135-137
P. O. administration. *See* Oral administration
Poison Control, National Clearinghouse for, 325-326
Poison Prevention Packaging Act of 1970, 325
Poisoning. *See also* Toxicity
    by absorption through skin, 91

acute vs. chronic, 303–305
antidotal therapy, 326–336. *See also* Antidote(s)
botulinus toxin, 68, 84
by chemicals not for use in humans, 311–317
cyanide, 304, 332, 334
environmental aspects of, 18, 318–319
  standards for air quality, 320–321
FDA poison control centers, 325–326
by heavy metals, 35, 306, 333, 334
immediate vs. delayed effects of poisons, 304–305
incidence of, 319–326
  age distribution of, 323–325
  therapeutic agents in, 323–326
iron, 332
lead, 34, 45, 233, 304, 324
by mushrooms, 84
prevention, 331
Poison(s), 302, 304. *See also* Poisoning; Toxicity
cytotoxic (protoplasmic), 306, 372–373
economic aspects of use, 18, 260–261, 311–313
selective toxicity of, 309–310
standards for in workplace, 313–314, 315
Pollutants Standard Index, 319, 320
Polycyclic hydrocarbons as carcinogens, 309
Pons, functional anatomy of, 345
Pores
in endothelium of renal capillaries, 101
pore theory of cell membrane, 59
Potassium ion, 119
excretion, 124, 128, 132
  exchange with sodium ion in kidney, 128, 132
  reabsorption and, 124, 128
Potency of drugs, 178–180. *See also* Doseeffect (dose-response) curve
Pralidoxime as antidote for organic phosphate poisoning, 335
Pregnancy
as contraindication to clinical drug studies, 403
distribution between mother and fetus in, 110–112, 247
drug use in, 112, 247, 308
teratogenic agents in 112, 308, 399, 403
Pressure gradient, 68
in kidney, 123
transcapillary movement and, 101
Primaquine
erythrocyte enzymes and response to, 253, 255
mechanism of action, 449
use in malaria, 448–449
Primary amines, 60–61

Priming (loading) dose, 229. *See also* Multiple dose schedules
Primitive medicine, 1–2, 341
Probenecid, 395, 443
cephaloridine excretion and, 292
penicillin excretion and, 292, 395
uricosuric action of, 395, 443
Procaine (Novocain)
allergy to, 276–277
biotransformation of, 146, 157
dose-response curves, 176, 177
list of proprietary names for, 21
local anesthetic activity of, 456–458. *See also* Local anesthetics
Procaine penicillin, duration of action of, 226, 228
Propionylcholine, dose-response relations of, 172, 173, 176
Proprietary (trade) drug names, 20, 21
Prosthetic groups of enzymes, 140. *See also* Enzyme(s)
Protein(s). *See also specific type of protein, e.g.,* Enzyme(s)
absorption of, 68, 84
in allergic reactions, 68, 273–274
binding. *See* Protein binding
of cell membrane, 54–55, 69, 70
charged groups in, 34
drug resistance development and, 271
enzyme stimulation and synthesis of, 161–162
genetic abnormalities in, 251–256
  of functional systems, 252–253, 254, 255
liver and, 101
plasma, 119
structure and drug interactions with, 34, 36, 43–44
transcapillary movement, 68, 101
Protein binding, 105–106
biliary active transport and, 139
drug interactions by competition for sites of, 290, 294
excretion of drugs and, 133, 135, 222
to hapten in antigen formation, 274
Protoplasmic poisons, 306, 372–373
Proximal segment (proximal convoluted tubule) of kidney
anatomy of, 121, 122
tubular secretion and, 128
urine formation and, 125–129
Psilocin, 361, 362
Psilocybin, 361, 362
Psychedelics (hallucinogens), 361–366. *See also* Lysergic acid diethylamide (LSD); Marihuana (marijuana)
Psychic drug dependence, 348. *See also* Psychologic drug dependence

Psychologic drug dependence, 348–351. *See
    also* Drug abuse and dependence *and
    specific drug, e.g.,* Barbiturates
  on alcohol, 349, 351, 353–354, 367
  on amphetamines, 351, 360, 368
  on barbiturates, 351, 354
  on cigarette smoking, 349
  on cocaine, 360, 368
  on LSD, 351, 362
  on marihuana, 349, 351, 365, 368
  on narcotic analgesics, 351, 356
  personality maladjustments and, 350
  physical dependence and, 349–350, 351
  tolerance and, 366
Psychologic factors. *See also* Psychologic drug
    dependence
  clinical new drug studies and, 263, 404–405
  placebo effect and, 262–264, 404–405
Psychotomimetic, 361. *See also* Hallucino-
    gens (psychedelics)
Psychotogen, 361. *See also* Hallucinogens
    (psychedelics)
Pteroylglutamic acid (folic acid), PABA
    and, 260–261
Pyramidon. *See* Aminopyrine (Pyramidon)
Pyrimethamine
  as antimalarial drug, 448–449
  mechanism of action, 449
Pyrvinium, 451

Quantal dose-response relation, 184–197,
    198, 200–201. *See also* Dose-effect
    (dose-response) curve, quantal
Quantatative drug reactions. *See* Dose-effect
    (dose-response) curve; Time-response
    relations
Quaternary ammonium compounds, 42
  absorption, 84
  biliary transport and elimination, 139
  renal tubular secretion, 134–135
  selectivity of, 197
Quinacrine (Atabrine), biologic half-life of, 223
Quinine
  antacids and absorption of, 284
  cinchona bark as source of, 29
  distribution of taste thresholds for, 256, 257
  fever and, of malarial vs. nonmalarial origin,
    29, 30
  renal tubular secretion, 134
  site of action, 29, 30

Radioactive isotopes, fetus and maternal ex-
    posure to, 112
RAS (ascending reticular activating system),
    345, 348
Reabsorption, renal tubular. *See also* Sodium
    ion; Water
  active, 124–125, 130–132

  half-life and, 217
  passive, of drugs, 133–134, 213, 217–218,
    232
  passive, of solutes, 124–125
  pH of urine and, 133–134, 285, 289
  rate of, 134, 289
Receptor(s), 35–44, 46
  drug interactions with. *See* Drug-receptor
    interactions
  history of concept of, 36–37
  isolation of, 43–44
  putative for morphine, 358–359
Rectum
  absorption in, 84
  as drug administration route, 82, 84,
    99
Red blood cells. *See* Erythrocytes
Reduction, enzymes in, 146, 152, 156
Reference standards in evaluation of drugs,
    361–362
Reflexes
  amphetamines and, 326
  medullary control of, 326–327
Religion and magic in medicine, 2–3, 4, 6, 8
REM (rapid eye movement) sleep, effect of
    drugs on, 472
Remington's Pharmaceutical Sciences, 24
Reserpine, 477
  effects on autonomic nervous system, 384,
    386, 387, 477
  effects on central nervous system, 477
  Rauwolfia, source of, 392
Resistance, drug, 267–271
  acquired, 267
  of bacteria to drugs, 267, 271
  clinical consequences of, 267–268, 393
  genetic factors in, 268–269
  to insecticides, 265, 270, 271
  mechanisms of, 269–271
    decreased affinity of drug for target site,
      270, 271
    decreased intracellular availability, 270,
      271
    elaboration of inactivating enzymes, 270
  mutants and, 268
  to penicillin, 270
  prevention of, 269
  to sulfa drugs, 270, 271
  transfer of, 268–269
Respiration. *See also* Respiratory tract
  hypothalamic regulation of, 346
  inhibition in poisoning, 303–304, 328
  medulla and, 345
  oxygen in stimulation of, 99
Respiratory tract. *See also* Lung(s); Respira-
    tion
  absorption through, 76, 91–94, 99
  air passage through, 93

allergic reactions in, 275
asthma, 94, 99
cilia of, 94
deposition of particles in, 93–94
drug administration through, 76, 93–94, 99
excretion through, 94, 118
structure of, 91–93
Reticular activating system (RAS), 345, 348, 472, 475, 480
Reviews on drugs, list of, 22–23
Rome, medicine of ancient, 4, 5
Route of administration, 74, 76–77, 98–99. *See also specific route, e.g.,* Oral administration
Rubella, fetus and maternal, 112

Safety of drugs, 191–195, 200–201. *See also* Clinical studies of new drugs; Dose-effect (dose-response) curve; Toxicity
Safety packaging of drugs, 325
Salicylates, 458–460. *See also* Aspirin
adverse interactions of, 288–289, 290
biotransformation of, 146, 147, 157–158
dose and elimination of, 217–218
excretion of, 134
formation from aspirin, 216
mechanism of action
as analgesic, 458
as anti-inflammatory drug, 459
as antipyretic, 458–459
poisoning, 324–325, 332
toxicity of, 460
uricosuric activity, 459–460
Salicyluric acid formation, 218
Saliva, 77, 118
Schistosomiasis, antimonials in, 261
Schmiedeberg, Oswald, 11–12, 14, 84
Scopolamine, 341
Screening for new drugs, 396–397
Secobarbital. *See also* Sedatives and hypnotics
absorption, 79–80
abuse, 352
as hypnotic, 470
pharmacokinetics and physiochemical properties, 471
Secondary amines, 60, 61
Secondary receptors, 105
Secretion, renal tubular, 128, 134–135, 219, 223, 244
age and, 244
rate of, 137
Sedative(s), abuse and dependence, 351, 352–355
Sedatives and hypnotics, 469–474. *See also* Barbiturates *and specific drug, e.g.,* Phenobarbital

barbiturates, 469–473
classification, 470
effects of, 472
fate in body, 473
mechanism and site of action, 472
pharmacokinetics and physiochemical properties of, 470–471
toxicity of, 472–473
hypnotic vs. sedative, 469
nonbarbiturates, 473–474
Selective toxicity, 302
of poisons, 309–310
of therapeutic agents, 260–261, 307–309, 444, 451
Selectivity of drugs, 41, 195–197
of atropine, 197
of diphenhydramine, 196
distribution and, 197
of drug-receptor interactions, 195–197
of heparin, 197
importance of, 197
quantal dose-response relation and, 196, 201
route of administration and, 197
side-effects and, 197
for site of action, 35, 40, 41, 46, 195–196
therapeutic usefulness and, 307, 444
toxicity and, 302, 307–309, 310
Semipermeable membrane, 49, 50, 51
Sensory (afferent) neurons, 343, 374
Serotonin (5-hydroxytryptamine), nerve impulse transmission and, 344
Sertürner, Frederick W. A., 10, 14
Sex
body composition and, 242
drug dosage and, 247
Sex-linked traits, 248
Side-effects, 191, 195–197. *See also* Allergy; Toxicity
evaluation in animals, 400–401
incidence of, 307, 310–311
potential usefulness of, 395
in safety assessment, 195
selectivity and specificity and, 195–197
as toxicity criterion, 195
Silent receptor, 105
Silica, cumulative toxicity of, 304
Silicon rubber, use in sustained release preparations, 89
Single-blind study, 404
Single doses of drugs, time-response relations and, 224–228
Sinusoid(s), blood flow through hepatic, 101
Site of drug action, 31–35. *See also* Cell(s), sites of drug action in; Extracellular sites of drug action; Intracellular sites of drug action

Site of drug action–(*Continued*)
  antidotes in removal of poisons from, 333, 334–335
  of atropine, 31, 32
  concentration at, 205, 206
    absorption and, 74–77, 205, 206
    biotransformation and, 205, 206
    blood level and, 207–208
    distribution and, 73, 74
    excretion rate and, 205, 206
    toxicity and, 327–328
  of curare, 11, 36–37
  distance from target organ, 32
  effect and, 30, 31–33
  localization of, 10, 33
  of morphine, 31–32
  of quinine, 29, 30, 31
  receptors at. *See* Drug-receptor interactions
  selectivity of, 35, 40, 41, 46
  specificity of, 35, 49
  of sulfa drugs, 33
Sites of loss of drugs, 105, 106
Skin
  absorption through, 74, 76, 89–91
  allergic manifestations of, 275
  drug application to
    for local effect, 91, 99
    poisoning from, 91
    toxic effects of caustics, 305
  structure and layers, 89–90
Small intestine
  absorption from 74, 80–84, 293
    area available for, 80, 81, 82, 83
    epithelium of, 80, 81, 82
    folds of Kerckring, 80, 81, 82
    pH in, 80
    villi of, 80, 81, 82
Sodium bicarbonate, 20, 33, 126–127, 434.
    See also Antacids
Sodium chloride
  as antidote for bromide poisoning, 334
  renal excretion of, 124
Sodium ion, in kidney, 115
  active transport (reabsorption), 125–133
    importance of, 125
    inhibition by
      benzothiadiazines, 440–441
      high-ceiling diuretics, 442–443
      mercurials, 439–440
  exchange with potassium ion, 128, 132
  excretion, 124
  glomerular filtration, 124
Solid dosage of drugs, 84–89. *See also* Sustained-release medications
  dissolution and disintegration of, 84–87
  enteric coatings for, 87–88
  inert constituents of, 85
  particle size, 85

water ingested with, 87
Somatic nervous system, 373–375
  autonomic nervous system vs., 374, 375
Species variations, 257–261
  in biologic half-lives, 259
  in biotransformation, 258–260
  destruction of uneconomic species and, 260–261
  drug responses and, 310–311
  in enzyme inducibility, 291
  evaluation of drugs and, 258–260, 401
Specificity of drugs
  in enzyme-substrate interactions, 140–142
  importance of, 197
  in mechanism and site of action, 35, 49
  side-effects and, 195–197
  species variations in, 302
  toxicity and, 307
Spinal cord
  cerebrospinal fluid, 109
  functional anatomy of, 344
Spironolactone, as diuretic, 442
Standard deviation, 188, 200
Standard safety margin, 193, 201
Stereoisomers, drug-receptor interactions and, 36, 43–44, 46
Steroids
  hepatotoxicity of, 307
  sources of, 393
Stimulants, 479–481. *See also specific drug, e.g.,* Amphetamine(s)
  character of dependence on, 351, 359–361, 367, 368, 480
  commonly abused, 359
  nature of action of, 359–360, 480
Stomach, 78–80
  absorption in, 74, 79, 80, 83
  anatomy of, 78, 290
  emptying rate, effects of, 79, 83, 290
  enteric coatings for drugs in, 87–88
  functions, 78, 79
  gastric fluid, 34, 45, 77
  pH of fluids in, 62, 79
Storage sites of drugs, 106
Streptomycin, 445. *See also* Antibacterials
  albumin binding of, 105
  as bactericidal agent, 404, 445
  resistance to, 270
  toxic effects of, 195, 308, 446
Strontium, half-life of, 223
Strychnine, absorption of, 63, 79
Subacute toxicity, 304. *See also* Toxicity, evaluation of
Subcutaneous (S.C.) administration, 76, 95–96. *See also* Blood flow, rate of
  absorption and, 95–97, 99
  advantages and disadvantages of, 96, 99

of depot preparations, 96, 99
of large fluid volumes, 96
time course of drug action and, 226, 227
Sublingual administration, 77-78, 99
Substrate(s), 140-142. See also Enzyme(s)
Succinylcholine biotransformation, abnormalities in, 251, 252
Sulfa drugs. See Sulfonamides
Sulfadiazine, particle size and absorption of, 85
Sulfanilamide
  biotransformation of, 148
  "elixir of sulfanilamide disaster," 401
  PABA and, 260
Sulfate conjugation, 145, 146, 148
Sulfathiazole biotransformation, toxic effect produced by, 148, 446
Sulfinpyrazone (Anturane), 443
Sulfobromophthalein in liver function tests, 139
Sulfonamides, 445. See also Antibacterials
  adverse interactions of, 289, 290
  bacterial resistance to, 270, 271
  biotransformation of, 148
    increased toxicity by, 148
  oral antidiabetics and diuretics developed from, 395
  toxic effects of, 446
Sulfur dioxide as air pollutant, 319, 320
Summation of drug effect, 284, 285, 286
Suramin, 106
Surface active agents as antiseptics, 447-448
Surface area of body in dosage determination, 242-243
Sushruta (Hindu physician), 3
Sustained-release medications
  absorption of, 88-89, 211, 228
  in glaucoma, 89
  for placement intravaginally, contraceptive agents, 89
  for subcutaneous administration, 96, 99
Sympathetic nervous system, 375, 377. See also Norepinephrine
  anatomy of, 375, 376, 377
  drugs affecting, 385-388
    pharmacologic significance of, 388
  functions of, 377-380
  neurotransmitter in, 380-381, 382-383
  parasympathetic nervous system vs., 375, 377-380
Synapse, 343
Synergism, 285, 286, 288-289

Tablets. See Solid dosage of drugs
Tachyphylaxis, 280, 281
Taste, variations in threshold of, 256, 257
Temporal lobe, cerebral, 347

Teratogens, 112, 308
  animal tests for, 399, 403
Termination of drug action, 117-168
  by biotransformation, 117, 139-165. See also Biotransformation
  by excretion, 117, 118-139, 165. See also Excretion
Tertiary amines, 60, 61
Testosterone pellets, absorption of, 211
Tetracaine, 458
Tetracycline, 445
  absorption of, 85
    antacids and, 290
  bacteriostatic activity of, 444, 445
  binding to tissue components, 105, 106
  toxicity of, 304, 308-309, 446
Tetrahydrocannabinols, psychologic effects of marihuana and, 363-366
Textbooks on pharmacology, 22, 25-26
Thalamus, 346
Thalidomide, teratogenicity of, 112, 308, 399
Theobromine, 438
Theophylline, 438
Therapeutic effect, lethal effect related to, 191-195, 200-201
Therapeutic ratio(s), 191-195
Thiamine, renal tubular secretion of, 128
Thiopental
  cumulative effects of, 234-236
  distribution rate and anesthesia onset, 225
  gastric absorption of, 79-80
  tissue redistribution of, 234-236
Thiosulfate for cyanide poisoning, 334
Threshold dose, 185
  elevation of, in poisoning therapy, 335-336
Thyroxine binding by cholestyramine, 290
  biotransformation of, 149
Time-response relations, 205-239
  absorption rate and, 209-211
  administration route and, 226-228
  blood drug levels and, 207-208
  cumulative toxicity and, 233-236
    in children and infants, 244-245
  duration of action in, 207. See also Duration of action
  elimination rate and, 211-224. See also Biotransformation; Elimination; Excretion
  latency in, 205-206
  multiple dosage and, 228-233. See also Multiple dose schedules
  peak effect in, 207, 227
  phases in, 203, 205-207
  single drug doses and, 224-228
Tissue components, drug binding to, 105, 106
Tissue redistribution, cumulative toxicity and, 234-236
Tolerance, 279-284, 350, 351

Tolerance–*Continued*
administration route and, 280–281
to alcohol, 283, 351, 354
to amphetamines, 280, 351, 360
to barbiturates, 280, 281, 283, 351, 354
cross-tolerance, 283
dose and, 354
to drugs affecting the central nervous system, 279, 280, 281
duration of action and, 280–281
to ephedrine, 280, 282
to glutethimide, 280
to LSD, 350, 351, 362, 364
to marihuana, 351, 364
mechanisms of, 279–284
drug disposition, 279–281
biotransformation and, 280, 282
enzyme induction and, 280, 282
pharmacodynamic, 279, 280, 281, 283
tachyphylaxis, 280, 281, 282
to morphine, 280, 281, 283, 356–357
to nitrites, 280, 281
nitroglycerin, 281
peak effect and, 280
to phenobarbital, 280
receptor reactivity and, 279, 281, 283
to sedative-hypnotics, 280, 351
to tranquilizers, 280, 351
Topical application, 91, 99
Toxic effect. *See* Toxicity
Toxicity, 301–337. *See also* Poisoning; Safety of drugs; *and specific drug*
age and, 245–247
air pollutants and, 319, 320
allergy vs., 277, 278, 279
of chemicals intended for use in humans, 307–309
of chemicals not intended for use in humans, 309–310
cumulative. *See* Cumulative toxicity
dose and, 18, 191–192, 200–201. *See also* Dose-effect (dose-response) curve
drug interactions leading to, 284
environmental, 318–319
evaluation of, 310–319. *See also* Lethal dose, median (LD50)
FDA guidelines, 398–400
interspecies variation and, 257–260
of gases, 305–306
of heparin, 197
incidence of, 307–309, 313, 319–326
industrial, 311–317
intensity of, as function of time, 326–328
nonselective, 306–307
pathologic changes in organs and, 307–308
potential for, 336
prevention of, 336–337
as relative concept, 301–303

selective, 260–261, 302
side-effects as criterion of, 194–195
specificity of drug and, 197
standards for
air pollutants, 319, 320
asbestos, 316
carcinogens, 316
polyvinyl chloride, 316
treatment of, 326–336. *See also* Antidote(s)
types of toxic effects, 303–310
local, 305–306
systemic, 306–310
withdrawal of enzyme-inducing drug and, 295
Toxicology, subdivisions of, 18–19. *See also* Poisoning; Toxicity
Trade (proprietary) drug names, 20, 21
Tranquilizers. *See specific drug, e.g.,* Meprobamate (Equanil, Miltown)
Transport mechanisms, 49–69
active transport, 66, 67–68. *See also* Active transport
in children and infants, 244
development of resistance and, 270, 271
distribution, 73
facilitated diffusion, 64–66. *See also* Facilitated diffusion
filtration, 68, 70
passive diffusion, 51–64, 69–70. *See also* Diffusion; Passive diffusion
pinocytosis, 67–68, 69
semipermeable membranes and, 49, 50, 51
in urine formation, 124–133
of weak electrolytes, 59–63, 70
Tranylcypromine, 478. *See also* Monoamine oxidase inhibitors
interactions of, 288, 384, 386, 387
Tromexan. *See* Ethyl biscoumacetate (Tromexan)
Tubules, renal. *See also* Urine formation
anatomy of, 119–122
reabsorption by, 124–134. *See also* Reabsorption, renal tubular
secretion by, 128, 134–135. *See also* Secretion, renal tubular
Tyramine
biotransformation of, 154
interactions with norepinephrine, 384, 385, 386, 387
monoamine oxidase inhibitors and, 262, 286
Tyrosine, as norepinephrine precursor, 382, 384

Undecylenic acid, 447
United States Adopted Name (USAN) Council for drugs, 20
United States Dispensatory and Physician's Pharmacology, The, 24

United States Environmental Protection
    Agency, 233
United States Pharmacopeia, The (U.S.P.),
    20, 22, 23, 398, 401, 470
Unlisted Drugs, 25
Urea, as diuretic, 438
  excretion of, 124, 126, 128
Ureter, 115, 120, 122
Uric acid, excretion of
  enhancement by probenecid, 395, 443
  interactions inhibiting, 292, 441, 443
  by tubular secretion, 128
Uricosuric agents, 443
Urine. *See also* Urine formation
  drug excretion in, 133–137. *See also* Ex-
      cretion, renal, of drug *and specific drug*
    concentration of drug in voided, 220–
      222
  pH of, 62, 133–134
    adjustment in therapy of poisoning, 134,
      332
  diuretics and, 292, 438–443
  tonicity of normal, 133
  water and solute loss in, 124
Urine formation. *See also* Excretion, renal, of
    drug; Reabsorption, renal tubular; Secre-
    tion, renal tubular; Sodium ion, in kidney
  ADH and, 130, 131, 132–133
  collecting duct in, 132–133
  concentration mechanisms in, 129–132
  distal convoluted tubules in, 132–133
  glomerular filtration in, 123–124, 133–
      134. *See also* Glomerulus, renal,
      filtration in
  hypertonic, 129-132
  hypotonic, 129, 132–133
  loop of Henle in, 129–132. *See also* Loop of
      Henle
  proximal tubule in, 125–129
  psychologic effects and, 263
  quantitative aspects of, 123–124
  transport mechanisms in, 124–135
  tubules in, 124–135
  volume of blood and, 123

Valmid. *See* Ethinamate (Valmid)
Van der Waals' forces
  drug-receptor interactions and, 40, 41, 42,
      43
  enzyme-substrate interactions and, 140
Vasoconstriction by drugs, 33, 93-94
Vasodilation by drugs, 33
Vasopressin. *See* Antidiuretic hormone
    (ADH)
Ventricles, brain, 109
Villi of small intestine, 80, 81, 82, 83
Vitamins
  active transport of, 67

genetic abnormalities and vitamin B_{12} ab-
    sorption, 253, 255–256
oxidation of vitamin A, 146, 154
renal tubular secretion of thiamine, 128
Volume of distribution, apparent, 102–105.
    See also Distribution of drugs
Vomiting
  induction
    by morphine, 462
    in poisoning, 329, 330–331
  inhibition by chlorpromazine, 476

Water
  diffusion through membranes,
      50-51, 52
  excretion
    ADH and, 126, 131, 132–133
    diuretics and, 438–443
    pulmonary, 93
    renal, 124, 125–126, 129–133
  filtration in kidney, 124
  hydrogen bonding of, 40, 54
  lipid/water partition coefficient, 56, 57
  reabsorption
    in large intestine, 84
    renal, 124, 125–126, 129–133
  transcapillary transport, 100–102
Water-soluble drugs
  active transport of, 67
  distribution to brain, 107–108, 110
  excretion routes of, 118
Weak electrolyte(s), 59-63, 69. *See also*
    Electrolyte(s)
Wepfer, John Jacob, 9
Withdrawal syndrome, 349–350, 351. *See
    also* Drug abuse and dependence *and
    specific drug*
  alcohol use and, 351, 354–355
  amphetamine use and, 351, 360-361
  barbiturate use and, 351, 354–355
  character of drug and, 349–351
  in newborn of drug-dependent mothers, 112
  opioid use and, 351, 357

Xanthine oxidase, 156
Xanthines, as diuretics, 438–439
Xenon, 45
X-ray irradiation, fetus and maternal, 112
Xylocaine. *See* Lidocaine (Xylocaine)

Zero-order kinetics, 144
  in absorption, 210, 237
    duration of action and, 228
  in biotransformation, 214–219
    of alcohol, 214–217
    of aspirin, 217–219
  in enzyme reactions, 144
  in excretion, 219